Clinical Handbook of
Child and Adolescent Psychiatry

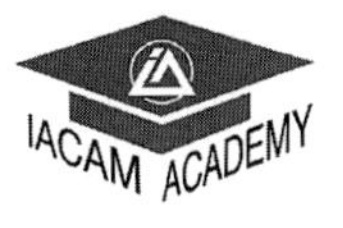

Clinical Handbook of Child and Adolescent Psychiatry

Editors

Savita Malhotra
MD PhD
Emeritus Professor of Psychiatry
Former Dean and Head
Department of Psychiatry
Postgraduate Institute of Medical Education and Research
Chandigarh, India

Nitin Gupta
MBBS MD
Consultant Psychiatrist and Therapist
Gupta Mind Healing and Counselling Centre
Chandigarh, India

Assistant Editor

Nidhi Chauhan
MD (Psychiatry) DM (Child and Adolescent Psychiatry)
Child and Adolescent Psychiatrist
Faculty of Psychiatry and Child and Adolescent Psychiatry
Department of Psychiatry
Postgraduate Institute of Medical Education and Research
Chandigarh, India

Foreword

Norbert Skokauskas

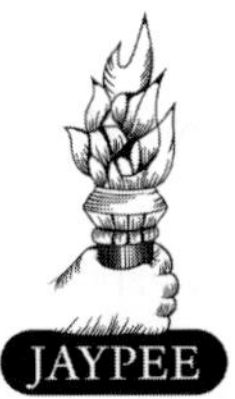

JAYPEE

JAYPEE BROTHERS MEDICAL PUBLISHERS
The Health Sciences Publisher
New Delhi | London

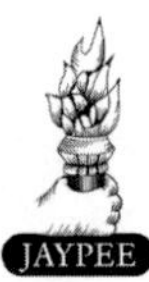

Jaypee Brothers Medical Publishers (P) Ltd

Headquarters
EMCA House, 23/23-B
Ansari Road, Daryaganj
New Delhi 110 002, India
Landline: +91-11-23272143, +91-11-23272703
+91-11-23282021, +91-11-23245672
e-mail: jaypee@jaypeebrothers.com

Corporate Office
4838/24, Ansari Road, Daryaganj
New Delhi 110 002, India
Phone: +91-11-43574357
Fax: +91-11-43574314
e-mail: jaypee@jaypeebrothers.com

Overseas Office
JP Medical Ltd.
83, Victoria Street, London
SW1H 0HW (UK)
Phone: +44-20 3170 8910
e-mail: info@jpmedpub.com

EU GPSR Authorised Representative
Logos Europe, 9 rue Nicolas Poussin
17000, La Rochelle, France
Phone: +33 (0) 6 67 93 73 78
e-mail: contact@logoseurope.eu

Website: www.jaypeebrothers.com
Website: www.jaypeedigital.com

Inquiries for bulk sales may be solicited at: jaypee@jaypeebrothers.com

Clinical Handbook of Child and Adolescent Psychiatry

First Edition: **2026**

ISBN: 978-93-7202-151-6

Printed at: Samrat Offset Pvt. Ltd.

Contributors

Aditya Agrawal MBBS MD (Psychiatry)
Consultant Psychiatrist
Department of Psychiatry
Agrawal Neuro-psychiatry Hospital
Palanpur, Gujarat, India

Akanksha Shukla MBBS MD (Psychiatry)
Senior Resident
Department of Psychiatry
All India Institutes of Medical Sciences
New Delhi, India

Akhila S Girimaji PhD
Speech Therapist and Audiologist
Department of Speech Pathology and Audiology
National Institute of Mental Health and Neurosciences
Bengaluru, Karnataka, India

Akhilesh Sharma MBBS MD (Psychiatry)
Department of Psychiatry
Postgraduate Institute of Medical Education and Research
Chandigarh, India

Anju Dhawan MBBS MD (Psychiatry)
Professor and Chief
Department of National Drug Dependence Treatment Center
All India Institutes of Medical Sciences
New Delhi, India

Bichitra Nanda Patra MD (Psychiatry)
Professor
Department of Psychiatrist
All India Institutes of Medical Sciences
New Delhi, India

BK Yamini PhD
Professor
Department of Speech Pathology and Audiology
National Institute of Mental Health and Neurosciences
Bengaluru, Karnataka, India

Chhitij Srivastava
MBBS MD DNB MRCPSYCH CCT (in Child and Adolescent Psychiatry)
Consultant Child and Adolescent Psychiatrist
Allahabad Child Development Centre
Prayagraj, Uttar Pradesh, India

Debasish Basu MD DNB
Consultant Psychiatrist
Department of Psychiatry
Fortis Medcentre
Chandigarh, India

Dhamodhara Pandian
MD (Psy) PDF (CAP) DM (CAP - ongoing)
Senior Resident
Department of Child and Adolescent Psychiatry
National Institute of Mental Health and Neurosciences
Bengaluru, Karnataka, India

Eesha Sharma
MBBS MD (Psychiatry) PhD (Environmental Determinants of Adolescent Temperament)
Associate Professor
Department of Child and Adolescent Psychiatry
National Institute of Mental Health and Neurosciences
Bengaluru, Karnataka, India

Gayatri Bhatia
MBBS MD (Psychiatry) DM (Addiction Psychiatry)
Consultant
Department of Psychiatry
Amaha Mental Health Centre
New Delhi, India

Harpreet Singh Dhillon
MD (Psychiatry) DM (Addiction Psychiatry)
Senior Resident
Department of Drug Deaddiction and Treatment Center
Postgraduate Institute of Medical Education and Research
Chandigarh, India

Harshini Manohar
MD (Psychiatry) PDF (CAP) DM (CAP)
Assistant Professor
Department of Child and Adolescent Psychiatry
National Institute of Mental Health and Neurosciences
Bengaluru, Karnataka, India

Henal Shah
MD MSc Health Professions Education (Maastricht)
Additional Professor
Department of Psychiatry
Topiwala National Medical College and
BYL Nair Charitable Hospital
Mumbai, Maharashtra, India

Himani Adarsh
MBBS MD (Psychiatry, PGIMER) DM (Child and Adolescent Psychiatry, PGIMER)
Consultant Psychiatrist
ClearMedi Bahra Multispeciality Hospital
Mohali, Punjab, India

Ira Domun MD (Psychiatry)
Ex-Senior Resident
Department of Psychiatry
Government Medical College and Hospital
Chandigarh, India

Janardhan Reddy YC MBBS DPM MD
Senior Professor of Psychiatry
Department of Psychiatry
National Institute of Mental Health and
Neurosciences
Bengaluru, Karnataka, India

Jasmin Garg MD (Psychiatry)
Department of Psychiatry
Government Medical College
Rajindra Hospital
Patiala, Punjab, India

Jai Ranjan Ram
MD MRC Psychiatry (UK) CCST in Child and Adolescent Psychiatry (UK)
Consultant
Department of Psychiatrist
Apollo Medical Hospital and
Mental Health Foundation
Kolkata, West Bengal, India

Jyoti Singh
MBBS MD DM (in Child and Adolescent Psychiatry)
Assistant Professor
Department of Psychiatry
ESIC Medical College and Hospital
Varanasi, Uttar Pradesh, India

Lakshmi Sravanti MD DM PGD (Music Therapy)
Assistant Professor
Department of Child and Adolescent Psychiatry
National Institute of Mental Health and
Neurosciences
Bengaluru, Karnataka, India

Manisha Bhattacharya
PhD MPhil in Clinical Psychology, MSc in Psychology
Consultant Clinical Psychology
Mental Health Foundation
Kolkata, West Bengal, India

Mansi Somaiya MD DNB (Psychiatry)
Consultant Psychiatrist
Department of Psychiatry
Mumbai, Maharashtra, India

Meghana Vijayanand MPhil PhD
Senior Clinical Psychologist
Center for Advanced Research and Excellence in
Autism and Developmental Disorders (CARE-ADD)
St John's Research Institute
St. John's National Academy of Health Sciences
Bengaluru, Karnataka, India

Mirza Sarwar Baig MBBS MD (Psychiatry)
DM Resident, Child and Adolescent Psychiatry
Department of Psychiatry
Postgraduate Institute of Medical Education
and Research
Chandigarh, India

N Prasanna Kumar
MD DM (Child and Adolescent Psychiatry)
Professor and Head
Department of Child and Adolescent Psychiatry
Government Hospital for Mental Care
Andhra Medical College
Visakhapatnam, Andhra Pradesh, India

Nidhi Chauhan
MBBS MD (Psychiatry) DM (Child and Adolescent Psychiatry)
Associate Professor
Department of Psychiatry
Postgraduate Institute of Medical Education and Research
Chandigarh, India

Nishant Goyal MD DPM
Professor of Psychiatry
In-charge Center for Child and Adolescent Psychiatry
fMRI Centre and Centre for Advanced Neuromodulation and Cognitive Neurosciences
Central Institute of Psychiatry
Ranchi, Jharkhand, India

Nishtha Chawla MBBS MD (Psychiatry)
Senior Resident (DM Psychosomatic Medicine)
Department of Psychiatry
All India Institutes of Medical Sciences
New Delhi, India

Nitin Gupta MBBS MD
Consultant Psychiatrist and Therapist
Gupta Mind Healing and Counselling Centre
Chandigarh, India

Prabhat Sitholey MD
Consultant Psychiatrist
Department of Psychiatry
King George's Medical University
Lucknow, Uttar Pradesh, India

Pragya Sharma PhD MPhil (Clinical Psychology)
Clinical Psychologist
Psyche in Motion
New Delhi, India

Pranshu Sharma MBBS MD (Psychiatry)
DM Resident, Child and Adolescent Psychiatry
Department of Psychiatry
Postgraduate Institute of Medical Education and Research
Chandigarh, India

Pratap Sharan MBBS MD (Psychiatry)
Professor and Head
Department of Psychiatry
All India Institute of Medical Sciences
New Delhi, India

Preeti Kandasamy MBBS DPM MD
Senior Professor of Psychiatry
Department of Psychiatry
National Institute of Mental Health and Neurosciences
Bengaluru, Karnataka, India

Prerna Sharma PhD MPhil (Clinical Psychology)
Associate Professor
Department of Clinical Psychology
Institute of Human Behavior and Allied Sciences
New Delhi, India

Priti Arun MD (Psychiatry)
Professor
Department of Psychiatry
Government Medical College and Hospital
Chandigarh, India

Rachna Bhargava PhD (Clinical Psychology)
Professor
National Drug Dependence Treatment Centre
All India Institute of Medical Sciences
New Delhi, India

Ragul Ganesh MD (Psychiatry)
Assistant Professor
Department of Psychiatry
Jawaharlal Institute of Postgraduate Medical Education and Research
Puducherry, India

Rajeev Jairam MBBS FRANZCP MD Cert Child Psych
Professor and Clinical Director
Department of Infant Child and Adolescent Mental Health Services
Sydney, New South Wales, Australia

Rajendra KM MBBS DPM MD DM
Additional Professor
Department of Child and Adolescent Psychiatry,
National Institute of Mental Health and Neurosciences
Bengaluru, Karnataka, India

Ram Pratap Beniwal MBBS MD
Professor, Centre of Excellence in Mental Health
Atal Bihari Vajpayee Institute of Medical Sciences
and Dr Ram Manohar Lohia Hospital
New Delhi, India

Rashmi Shukla MD DNB MRCPsych
Assistant Professor
Department of Psychiatrist
King George's Medical University
Lucknow, Uttar Pradesh, India

S Lokesh MPhil (Clinical Psychology)
PhD Scholar
Department of Clinical Psychology
National Institute of Mental Health and Neurosciences
Bengaluru, Karnataka, India

Sarthak Kukreja MBBS MD (Psychiatry)
Senior Resident
Department of Psychiatry
All India Institutes of Medical Sciences
New Delhi, India

Satish Chandra Girimaji MD (Psychiatry)
Former Senior Professor
Department of Child and Adolescent Psychiatry
National Institute of Mental Health and Neurosciences
Bengaluru, Karnataka, India

Satya Raj MD DPM DNB FRANZCP
Professor and Head
Department of Child and Adolescent Psychiatry Unit
Christian Medical College
Vellore, Tamil Nadu, India

Savita Malhotra MD PhD
Former Professor
Department of Psychiatry
Postgraduate Institute of Medical Education
and Research
Chandigarh, India

Savithri Suresh MPhil (Clinical Psychology)
PhD Scholar
Department of Clinical Psychology
National Institute of Mental Health and Neurosciences
Bengaluru, Karnataka, India

Shalini Naik MD (Psychiatry) PDF (Brain Stimulation)
Associate Professor
Department of Psychiatry
Postgraduate Institute of Medical Education
and Research
Chandigarh, India

Shekhar Seshadri MBBS DPM MD
Former Senior Professor
Department of Child and Adolescent Psychiatry
National Institute of Mental Health
and Neurosciences
Bengaluru, Karnataka, India

Shivanand Kattimani
MD (Psychiatry) DM (Child and adolescent Psychiatry)
Professor
Department of Psychiatry
Jawaharlal Institute of Postgraduate Medical
Education and Research
Puducherry, India

Shivangi Mehta MD (Psychiatry)
Assistant Professor
Department of Psychiatry
Government Medical College and Hospital
Chandigarh, India

Shivani Gusain MBBS MD
Senior Resident
Department of Psychiatry
Central Institute of Psychiatry
Ranchi, Jharkhand, India

Shivender Singh
MD DNB PDF (Child and Adolescent Psychiatry)
PGDMLE MRCPsych
Programme Co-ordinator (Psychiatry) National
Mental Health Survey 2 (NMHS-2)
Department of Psychiatry
National Institute of Mental Health and Neurosciences
Bengaluru, Karnataka, India

Shoba S Meera PhD
Associate Professor
Department of Speech Pathology and Audiology
National Institute of Mental Health and Neurosciences
Bengaluru, Karnataka, India

Shoba Srinath DPM MD (Psychiatry)
Consultant Child and Adolescent Psychiatrist
Retired Senior Professor
Department of Child and Adolescent Psychiatry
National Institute of Mental Health
and Neurosciences
Bengaluru, Karnataka, India

Shrinidhi Pratinidhi MBBS MD
Senior Resident
Department of Psychiatry
Central Institute of Psychiatry
Ranchi, Jharkhand, India

Smita Neelkanth Deshpande MD DPM
Professor (Research)
Department of Psychiatry
St John's Medical College Hospital
St. John's National Academy of Health Sciences
Bengaluru, Karnataka, India

Suresh Bada Math
MD DNB PGDMLE PGDHRL PhD in Law (NLSIU)
Professor of Psychiatry
Department of Psychiatry
National Institute of Mental Health
and Neurosciences
Bengaluru, Karnataka, India

Uma Hirisave MPhil PhD
Retired Senior Professor and Associate Dean
Department of Clinical Psychology
National Institute of Mental Health
and Neurosciences
Bengaluru, Karnataka, India

Ummul Fatima MPhil (Clinical Psychology)
Research Assistant
Department of Psychology
University of New Hampshire
Concord, New Hampshire, USA

Uttara Chari MPhil PhD
Associate Professor of Clinical Psychology
Department of Psychiatry
St. John's National Academy of Health Sciences
Bengaluru, Karnataka, India

Veena A Satyanarayana
MPhil PhD (Clinical Psychology)
Additional Professor
Department of Clinical Psychology
National Institute of Mental Health
and Neurosciences
Bengaluru, Karnataka, India

Velprashanth Venkatesan
MBBS MD (Psychiatry) DM (Child and Adolescent Psychiatry)
Assistant Professor
Department of Psychiatry
Sri Manakula Vinayagar Medical College and Hospital
Puducherry, India

Vijaya Raman MPhil PhD
Professor of Clinical Psychology
Department of Psychiatry
St John's Medical College and Hospital
Bengaluru, Karnataka, India

Vivek Agarwal MD
Professor and Head
Department of Psychiatry
King George's Medical University
Lucknow, Uttar Pradesh, India

Contributors

Foreword

Child and adolescent mental disorders are common and can be highly disabling. However, in many countries and regions, the number of trained child and adolescent psychiatrists remains far too small to meet the needs of the population. Because of this, it is essential to ensure that general psychiatrists and other mental health clinicians are equipped with the knowledge and skills to assess and manage these conditions in their everyday practice.

The need for such capacity-building is especially strong in India, where the population is very young and service demands are substantial. We also know that mental health conditions often begin early in life: Around 50% start before the age of 14 years and approximately 75% before the age of 25 years. Strengthening early identification and early intervention is therefore not only clinically important but also essential for long-term well-being.

In this context, the online *Certificate Course in Child and Adolescent Psychiatry for General Psychiatrists in India* has been a timely and impactful initiative. Now running for 5 years, it has supported clinicians across the country in developing practical, clinically grounded competencies in child and adolescent mental health care. I would like to sincerely congratulate Professor Savita Malhotra and her team for their leadership and committed work on this important program.

It is also very meaningful that the course is now complemented by the *Clinical Handbook of Child and Adolescent Psychiatry*, which provides a structured and comprehensive reference for participants. This Handbook spans the full range of developmental stages and clinical conditions. It offers guidance on assessment, formulation, therapeutic approaches, psychopharmacology, and care in special circumstances, including legal and ethical aspects. It brings together knowledge from many of India's leading experts and presents it in a way that is practical and accessible for everyday clinical use.

This resource will strengthen learning during the course, support retention of knowledge over time, and ultimately enhance the quality of care provided to children and adolescents, as well as the support given to their families.

Once again, I warmly congratulate the editors (Professor Savita Malhotra, Dr Nitin Gupta, and Dr Nidhi Chauhan) and their colleagues on this important achievement. Their work contributes significantly to the development of child and adolescent mental health services in India and will continue to benefit many young people in the years ahead.

Norbert Skokauskas MD PhD
Professor of Child and Adolescent Psychiatry
Norwegian University of Science and Technology
Secretary for Education and Scientific Publications
World Psychiatric Association

Preface

Mental healthcare services and systems of care for children and adolescents worldwide are deficient on account of a multitude of factors which include shortage of specialist manpower, lack of resources, and budgetary constraints. While prevalence of mental disorders among children and adolescents is no less than that in adults, the treatment gap is to the tune of 90%, more so in low- and middle-income countries (LAMIC). Low public awareness, poor literacy, high rates of social stigma, very high socioeconomic disparities, social discrimination, and lack of child-centric policies in LAMIC further compound the problem. Providing child and adolescent mental health (CAMH) services is recognized as a hugely challenging task globally in current times.

India, the most populous country in the world, is home to approximately 480 million children under 18 years and 560 million population under 25 years of age. There is a growing mental health crisis with a soaring number of conditions like depression, anxiety, suicidality, alcohol and substance-use disorders, road accidents, self-harm, etc., leading to high rates of disability and premature deaths. The number of qualified child and adolescent psychiatrists in India is very low, almost 1 per 5 million child population. Under these circumstances, the burden of care falls on either the general adult psychiatrists or the pediatricians who are often the first point of care for the children.

The Indian Association for Child and Adolescent Mental Health (IACAM) established an IACAM Academy in 2021 with the primary objective of capacity building by training general psychiatrists in child and adolescent psychiatry through an intensive 1-year online certificate course. This course has now been running continuously for 5 years and is a much sought after one, having provided training to nearly 500+ psychiatrists. The course faculty comprises the best academicians in the subject who are well recognized in India and the world not only for their teaching experience but also for their research acumen. Feedback has revealed that the participants of the IACAM Academy Course have demonstrated a significant change in their approach, competence, and skill in diagnosing and managing children and adolescents with mental disorders.

Keeping in view the demand for and success of the running of the IACAM Academy Course, and based on the extremely positive and encouraging feedback from the participants, it was felt that there was a need to bring together the richness of teachings in print form so that they are available in a utilitarian format for anyone with a (vested) interest in CAMH. Hence, this *book project* was envisioned following a series of discussions held within the IACAM Academy Core Group (www.iacamacademy.com/about/) and the IACAM Executive Committee (www.childindia.org/executive-council-members/) members.

This book is a compilation of chapters authored principally by the same faculty who have been teaching their respective topics which are covered in the IACAM Academy Course. However, while putting together the book chapters, it was soon realized by us that we needed to add a few more experts and a few more topics for completeness in order to prevent this book from looking as akin to a "half-baked dish". Hence, the same was done leading on to the development of a total of five sections and 34 chapters. We are indebted to all the authors not only from the IACAM Academy, but also those who have agreed to be part of this project due to their passion and expertise in child and adolescent psychiatry, for their continued support and commitment and contributing to this book.

The book has been conceptualized and divided into five broad sections, namely, Normal Development and Neurodevelopmental Conditions; Externalizing Disorders, Addictions, Mood, and Psychotic Disorders; Internalizing Disorders, Stress, and Trauma; Management and Aftercare; and Special Circumstances. The endeavor has been to prepare a comprehensive resource book, which can serve as a clinical guide for general psychiatrists, pediatricians, child psychologists, or other CAMH professionals, in their routine clinical practice. The content is focused more on interventions and treatment guidelines rather than around theoretical discussion. Child development and CAMH is majorly ethnocentric. Effort is made to include Indian experience and Indian solutions for Indian patients in a practical skill-oriented guidance made out in a simple format and language.

The brief matter written thereof should help in providing the reader a snapshot of the chapters solicited in order to gain some understanding about the scope, quality, and depth of the book: There are chapters on ethics, laws, disability assessment, and certification as applicable to children, and care of children living under special circumstances, with the objective to sensitize the readers about special precautions and considerations to be kept in mind. Chapters on pharmacotherapy elaborate the principles of use, indications, contraindications, dosages, special precautions, and side effects of drugs commonly prescribed and available in India. A series of chapters on various psychological interventions and psychotherapies recommended and useful for treating children and adolescents suffering from mental disorders have been included. Chapters on speech and language pathologies and related interventions as well as assessment and management of specific learning disabilities (SLDs) and intellectual disabilities provide an exhaustive account of common neurodevelopmental conditions for which interventions encompass complex psychosocial, family, and developmental remediation and rehabilitation services which are mostly unavailable to a large majority in the country. General psychiatrists can empower themselves or train their para-mental health professional staff in delivering these services. A chapter on infant and fetal mental health is included to highlight the importance of this period of life in influencing the course of developmental trajectory of brain and mental health, especially from the standpoint of launching primary preventive and promotive interventions early in life. There is a separate chapter on Internet/behavioral addictions, a newer mental health condition being encountered in recent years. Childhood trauma, sexual abuse, domestic violence, deliberate self-harm, and suicides are some of the other societal and mental health issues that psychiatrists are required to manage in emergencies or in medicolegal situations. These are highly sensitive issues which must be addressed very carefully.

Overall, we are of the opinion and belief that general psychiatrists as well as pediatricians and even child and adolescent psychiatrists will find this book an invaluable asset in their clinical practice. We also genuinely hope that it will empower psychiatrists (and other mental health professionals) and strengthen their commitment and competence to deal with childhood psychiatric disorders, additionally so in keeping with the comprehensive care approach to child and adolescent mental health as per the World Health Organization (WHO).

Savita Malhotra
Nitin Gupta
Nidhi Chauhan

Acknowledgments

We would like to take this opportunity to personally acknowledge all those who have been involved and supportive to this endeavor.

At the outset, we would like to personally thank each senior contributor who agreed to get involved in this project at a relatively short notice. Their involvement and commitment speak volumes not only to their dedication to this endeavor but more importantly the deep professional and personal relationship reflected and developed over time with the IACAM Academy. Further, this book becomes special in the very sense that each senior contributor *"is a well-known clinical and academic leader in the field of Child and Adolescent Psychiatry in India"*. We also place on record our thanks to each of the co-contributors for placing their confidence in *the book* and *us* by agreeing to be part of this exciting journey.

This project was envisioned as an outcome of myriad discussions held with the IACAM Academy Core Group (www.iacamacademy.com/about/) and the IACAM Executive Committee (www.childindia.org/executive-council-members/) members. It is difficult to thank and mention every colleague individually, but a Big Thank You to every member of both these core and key groups who not only were germane to this idea but also facilitated and encouraged it too all the way. A special mention is made of Dr Shekhar Seshadri (President, IACAM), Dr Devashish Konar (Immediate Past President, IACAM), Dr Henal Shah (Treasurer, IACAM and Course Consultant, IACAM Academy), and Dr Rachna Bhargava (Secretary General, IACAM) for supporting the activities of the IACAM Academy.

We are highly grateful to M/s Jaypee Brothers Medical Publishers (P) Ltd, New Delhi, India, for the professionalism displayed at every step of this project and for the exemplary involvement, commitment, and perfectionism in completing the work and ensuring delivery of a high-quality product in a time-bound manner.

Last but not least, our families have been a source of huge support for us; indeed, we are "indebted" to their "unsaid" sacrifices.

Contents

SECTION 1: Normal Development and Neurodevelopmental Conditions

SECTION 2: Externalizing Disorders, Addictions, Mood, and Psychotic Disorders

SECTION 1 Normal Development and Neurodevelopmental Conditions

Developmental Aspects-I: Neurodevelopment and Developmental Framework in Psychopathology

Savita Malhotra

INTRODUCTION

Psychopathology is the core science in psychiatry, defined as the scientific exploration of abnormal mental states, that concerns itself with the subjective experience of abnormal mental states. There are three main objectives of psychopathology, that are inter-related and interdependent: (1) Descriptive psychopathology; (2) clinical psychopathology; and (3) theoretical psychopathology. "Descriptive psychopathology" refers to distinction between "normal" and "abnormal" experiences and behaviors, and to describe the nature and development of these symptoms. Descriptive psychopathology, also called "phenomenology", is the systematic study of abnormal experience, cognition, and behavior. Psychiatric symptoms as experienced subjectively by patients are elicited, explored, and understood as to their meaning for the patient. "Clinical psychopathology" is based on the descriptive psychopathology, and refers to identification of symptoms and signs and their groupings in syndromic or diagnostic entities leading to nosological classificatory systems. In this process, efforts are made to name the psychiatric conditions, study the broad phenotypes for their course, outcome, and etiological underpinnings of clinical psychopathology; and develop guidelines for evidence-based treatments. However, mental disorders are neither distinct diagnostic entities nor do they exist per se. Mental disorders commonly share features which repeatedly bring into question the current nosological systems such as ICD and DSM. "Theoretical psychopathology", on the other hand, is the study of etiology and pathogenesis, which strongly links psychopathology to neuroscience. There is growing effort to delineate the neurological events that underly human experiential phenomenon or psychopathology. In this process, the language used by neuroscientists is located on one pole and that used by clinical psychiatrists is located on the other pole of human experience. This lack of common language and drift in two positions misses the point of continuum between neuroscience and psychopathology. There is need and call for integration of "mind" and "brain". In recent years, there is growing effort to produce adequate neurobiological and genetic targets of mental disorders that should inform studies of psychopathology and nosology.

It is clear that we learn more about pathology by studying normal functioning and learn about normal functioning by studying pathology. Psychopathology can be understood as disturbance, distortion, or degeneration of normal functioning. Great insights have been obtained by studying children and their growth trajectories in their naturalistic settings. There is an intimate link between the study of normal and abnormal ontogenesis. Normal development and abnormal development lie on a continuum. Therefore, it is absolutely crucial to know about the normal development of the brain and its vicissitudes.

DEVELOPMENT OF BRAIN AND MIND

Birth is the arbitrary starting point of human development, whereas development starts at conception. Development occurs as a function of two interacting forces and processes:

1. Evolutionary past that we share in common with our ancestors, providing a genetic blueprint that organizes the structure and functions of nervous system in a programmed manner, with its own developmental timetable. This is common to all individuals.
2. Environmental influences and experiences during the prenatal and postnatal phases of life that contribute to the development of individual differences in the structure and functions of the brain.

It is the contribution of the environment and lived experience before and after birth, that majorly shapes the uniqueness of personality, emotions, cognition, and behavior; and that represents the qualitative template of one's psyche. Each brain is uniquely customized, making each individual absolutely unique.

Although structural integrity of the basic brain structures like neurons and a well-functioning sensory apparatus occurs at a specific time period in the developmental process, and is an essential prerequisite, the experience and environmental stimulation contributes by generating and strengthening synaptic connections, thus adding both the bulk and the functional repertoire in the realm of cognition, emotions, and behavior.

It is evident that normal and pathological states are the part of the same neurodevelopmental continuum, which means that all the neuropsychopathology represents a deviance from the usual ontogenetic pathways. So, the study of abnormal development can enhance our understanding of normal development.

Environment organizes and modifies the capacities of the individual, wherein, individual is an active participant in one's own development. Individual exhibits, soon after birth, unique patterns of psychophysiological and behavioral reactions, arising out of brain's tendencies for excitation, inhibition, or neuroregulation. These innate patterns are construed as temperamental individuality, which impacts the environment and care giving. Infant's temperament evokes different behavioral or caregiving reactions by the mother which further influences the behavior of the child reciprocally.

Development of brain and mind in humans is a complex and intriguing process. The journey of the fetus/infant/child/adolescent from a single cell at conception to a reflex biological being at birth, and to a fully grown adult human being is fascinating. There are several (as given below) developmental theories that describe this complex process of mental development and explain normal from abnormal processes and mechanisms, simultaneously providing paradigms for intervention and treatments. These are discussed in detail in the subsequent chapters.

- Psychoanalytic Theory (Sigmund Freud, Anna Freud, Melanie Klein)
- Learning Theory (Ian Pavlov, Edward Thorndike, BF Skinner, J Watson)
- Temperament Theory (Stella Chess, Alexander Thomas)
- Attachment Theory (Rene Spitz, John Bowlby, Harry Harlow)
- Cognitive Developmental Theory (Jean Piaget, Lev Vagotsky, George Miller)

Progress in the fields of genetics and developmental neuroscience in the last 30 years have revolutionized our understanding of complex brain functions and its aberrations. There has been a growing shift from focus on manifestations to underlying neurobiological mechanisms. Synthesis of all earlier theories with neurobiology has given rise to a new discipline namely "Developmental Psychopathology" that integrates various disciplines such as embryology, developmental neuroscience, psychology, psychiatry, sociology, cultural anthropology, and epidemiology. It tries to ascertain how similar or different organizations of biological, cognitive, socioemotional processes contribute to expression of specific symptoms.

Structural neuroanatomy is taught in detail during initial years of medical school. However, functional neuroanatomy or the neuroanatomy of the functional systems of the brain is most crucial for our understanding of the brain mechanisms. Various functional systems in the brain are consciousness, attention, memory, language, sensory system, motor system, feeling states, emotions, association areas, cognition, and thinking. Behavior is sum of all these processes. These functional systems are subserved by one or many structural systems that are often interconnected, or even may be represented in the discreet or diffuse brain areas, whole of which is not understood as yet.

Development of the brain is complete by about 25 years of age. Brain is a highly dynamic organ that continues to change and has the potential to change throughout life. Learning and memory continues to grow with experience throughout life, reflecting the changes in synaptic organization. Different biological and social experiences possibly determine the changes according to gender, culture, and are responsible for individual differences in personality. So, the environment has a prolonged and major influence on brain development. Moreover, human neonate is not endowed with all the survival skills needed for life. These have to be acquired during the process of growing up supported by the environment through a prolonged process of education, training, and acculturation.

Brain Development

Brain development occurs in a programmed fashion with neurogenesis, synaptogenesis, neural migration, arborization, myelination, pruning, differentiation of neuronal functions, and so on.

MacLean (1985) gave a model of the brain called *"triune brain"* comprising a three-part system, phylogenetically linked to our evolutionary connection to reptiles and lower mammals.

Reptilian (primal) brain: At the central core, there is the reptilian brain, which is responsible for activation, arousal, homeostasis, and reproduction. These functions are subserved by basal ganglia and brain stem. This system is fully developed at birth. Phylogenetically, this is the oldest part of the brain.

Paleomammalian (primitive/emotional) brain: Middle layer is the paleomammalian brain or limbic system that wraps around the reptilian brain, and is responsible for learning, emotions, and memory. Anatomical structures involved are "limbic system, hippocampus, amygdala, and cingulate gyrus." This part of the brain develops early through early childhood experiences. Humans share this part with that in mammals.

Neomammalian (rational) brain: Outer layer is the neomammalian brain, required for conscious thought, self-awareness and higher cognition. It comprises cerebral cortex and corpus callosum. This is the youngest part of the brain, phylogenetically. This part of the brain is also much slower to develop than most other areas of the brain and continues to form into the third decade of life. This slowness of maturation of neocortex is also beneficial as it maximizes the influence of environment on human brain. **Figure 1** shows the broad representation of the proposed three layers of the brain.

All the three layers are linked together vertically and horizontally through complex neural networks, and may not function in synchrony. Although cerebellum is considered as a primitive brain structure, but it has networks with highly evolved neocortex.

Much of our emotional and interpersonal learning occurs during first few years of life when our primitive/emotional brain is in control, before the cortical system for conscious awareness and rational thought is available. Therefore, many important aspects of our lives are governed by reflexes, behaviors, and emotions that are learned outside of our conscious awareness, and thus, are not easily amenable to rational interpretation or conscious efforts at alteration.

There is successive differentiation between right and left-brain functions, as well as specialization of certain brain areas for specific skills such as language and spatial abilities. Learning one's own language requires categorizing sounds that make up language in first 12 months. Thereafter, babies lose the ability to distinguish between sounds to which they are not exposed.

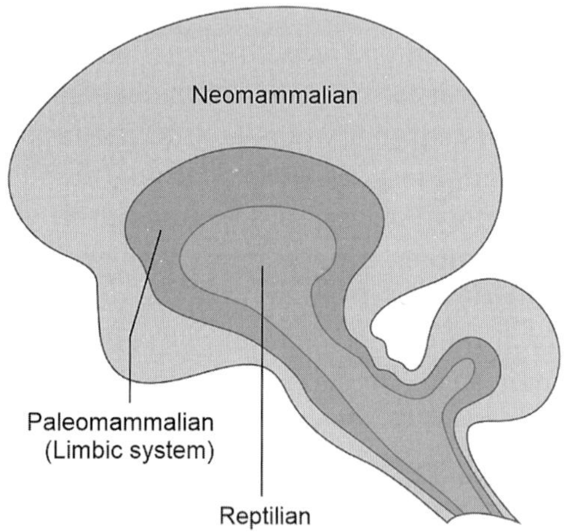

Fig. 1: Broad representation of the proposed three layers of the brain.[1]

Brain area specializations: **Figure 2** is a simplistic and pictorial representation of the various functions regulated by the frontal, occipital, parietal, and temporal lobes, respectively.[1]

Certain influences during early years of life make significant impact on the brain development. It is important to know and learn about these influences as these explain the development of various mental functions and eventually personality formation.

Sensitive Periods

Sensitive periods, also known as critical periods, are phases of exuberant neural growth and connectivity, where levels of metabolism are very high and learning is rapid. Sensitive periods are different for different neural systems. For example, sensitive period for language development is about 2 years of age. Right hemisphere develops rapidly in first 3 years, then asymmetry shifts to left hemisphere. During first year of life, close relationship with mother helps in development

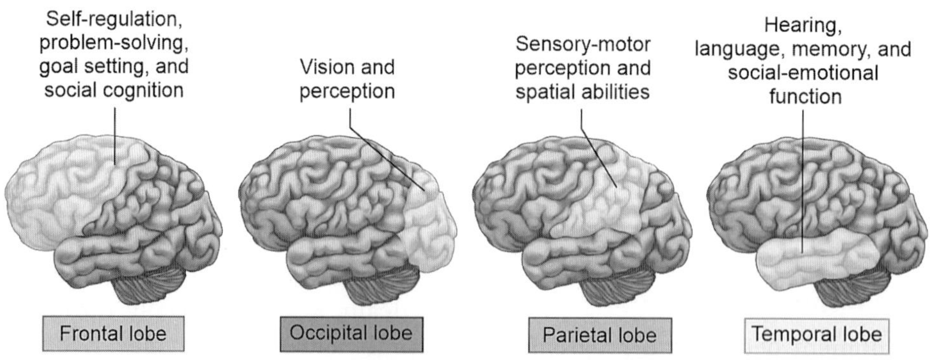

Fig. 2: The lobes of the brain and the function regulated by each.[1]

of neural networks that underly attachment and bonding, safety and danger, and core sense of self-identity. These serve the function of survival and self-preservation. Any disturbance during this phase can lead to severe impairments in identity formation, or interpersonal relationships in later life.

Neural Plasticity

Neurons grow and wire with one another in response to inner and outer stimuli, and in the process learn and memorize these networks as plastic changes. Repeated stimulations strengthen these interconnections through long-term potentiation (LTP) by which cell assemblies get organized into neural networks. Neural plasticity and LTP are crucial for consolidation of memory functions. Neuronal connections occur according to genetic programming, but their strength and effectiveness is altered by experience. Neurons that fire together wire together. Neural networks that are repeatedly stimulated get strengthened and those that are not stimulated die down. Following the principles of classical conditioning, simple forms of learning such as habituation, sensitization, and classical conditioning, is stored as plastic change in the structure and function of the brain as synaptic strength. Plastic changes are stored as memory and can persist for days.

There are two types of memory systems:

1. *Declarative/Explicit memory:* This is memory for facts and events. It is stored in medial temporal lobe.
2. *Procedural/Implicit memory:* This is memory for habits, habituation, sensitization, and conditioning. These are stored in amygdala, cerebellum, and basal ganglia.

Flowchart 1 describes the two types of memory systems in terms of their neural basis and functional characteristics.[1]

Social Cognition and Social Brain

Social cognition refers to the various psychological processes (both conscious and nonconscious)

Flowchart 1: Types, neural basis, and functional characteristics of memory systems.[1]

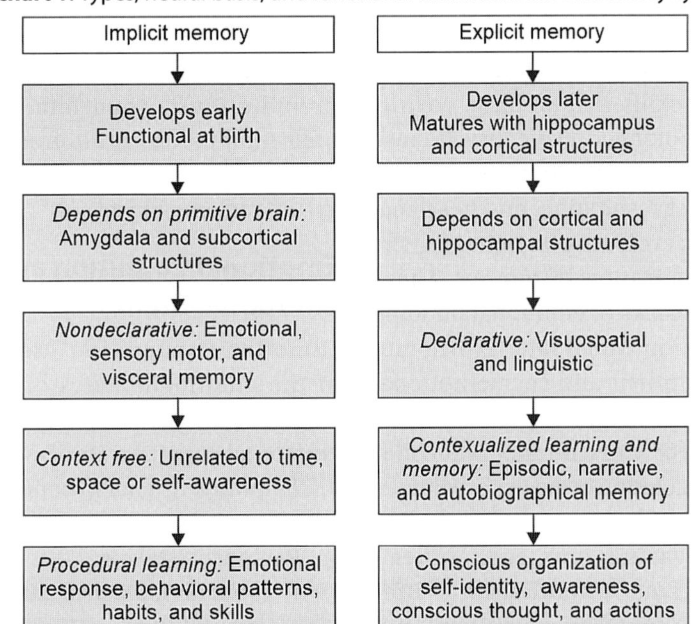

that underlie social behavior. Brain development takes place in interpersonal environment. Social cognition broadly includes the cognitive processes used to decode and encode the social world, and to understand and construct meaning about self and personal biography; and the social world, i.e., relationships, social norms, and morality.

Social cognition refers to:
- Perception of self
- Perception of others, and
- *Social knowledge:* Social knowledge can be of two types—
  1. Declarative knowledge (facts and concepts)
  2. Procedural knowledge (skills and strategies)
- Building of social brain is driven between 18 and 24 months by attunement between right hemisphere of the mother with the right hemisphere of the child; unconscious of the mother is transferred onto the unconscious of the child. Neonatal reflexes (controlled at birth by brainstem) serve the need for survival by enhancing physical and emotional connection of the newborn with the mother. These neonatal reflexes gradually get translated into more advanced skills like smiling, gazing, and imitating. Prolonged eye contact, close bodily contact with the mother, smell of the mother, feeling her respiration, and heartbeat contributes to developing schema in the infant for internalization of mother. These are the building blocks of emotional bonding and communication which later evolve into patterns of attachment and socioemotional interactions.
- Physical contact (between mother and child) sets the thermoregulation in the hypothalamus of the child.
- Mother–infant gazing into each other's eyes while nursing, establishes a life-long relationship between nutritional and emotional nurturance, linking their hearts and brains.
- Prolonged sharing of emotional gaze stimulates growth of networks of attachment in brain. As mother and child touch and separate and touch again, endorphin levels rise and fall leading to alternate feelings of well-being and distress.
- Mother–child interactions stimulate cascade of neurohumoral and neurochemical changes such as secretion of oxytocin, prolactin, endorphin, and dopamine. These biochemical changes stimulate structural maturation of orbitofrontal cortex.
- Internalization of mother occurs during childhood as a network of visceral, motor, sensory, and emotional memories. These memories get activated during the states of distress during adulthood. That is why whenever in distress, one tends to remember the mother.
- Thus, early experiences of bonding and attachment become imprinted within the circuits of social brain and continue in adulthood.

Figures 3 and 4 show the brain regions implicated in social cognition or social brain include temporoparietal junction, medial prefrontal cortex, orbitofrontal cortex, superior temporal sulcus, inferior frontal gyrus, fusiform gyrus, and amygdala.[3]

Emotional Cognition and Emotional Brain

"Emotional cognition" refers to awareness of the emotional states of self and of others. Brain mechanisms involved in development of emotional cognition are:
- *Empathy:* Crucial to bonding and altruism
- Theory of mind
- Perspective taking:
  - *First person perspective:* Awareness of own mental state

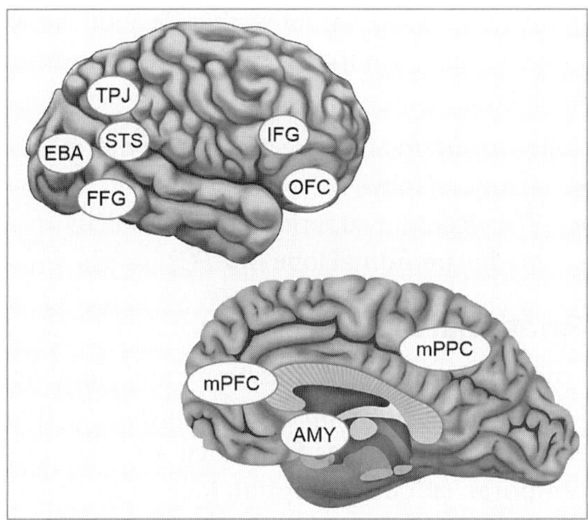

Fig. 3: Brain regions implicated in social cognition.[2] (AMY: amygdala; EBA: extrastriate body area; FFG: fusiform gyrus; IFG: inferior frontal gyrus; mPFC: medial prefrontal cortex; mPPC: medial parietal cortex; OFC: orbital frontal cortex; STS: superior temporal sulcus region; TPJ: temporoparietal junction)
Source: Pelphrey KA, Perlman SB. Charting brain mechanisms for the development of social cognition. Neuroimag Develop Clin Neurosci. 2009;73-90.

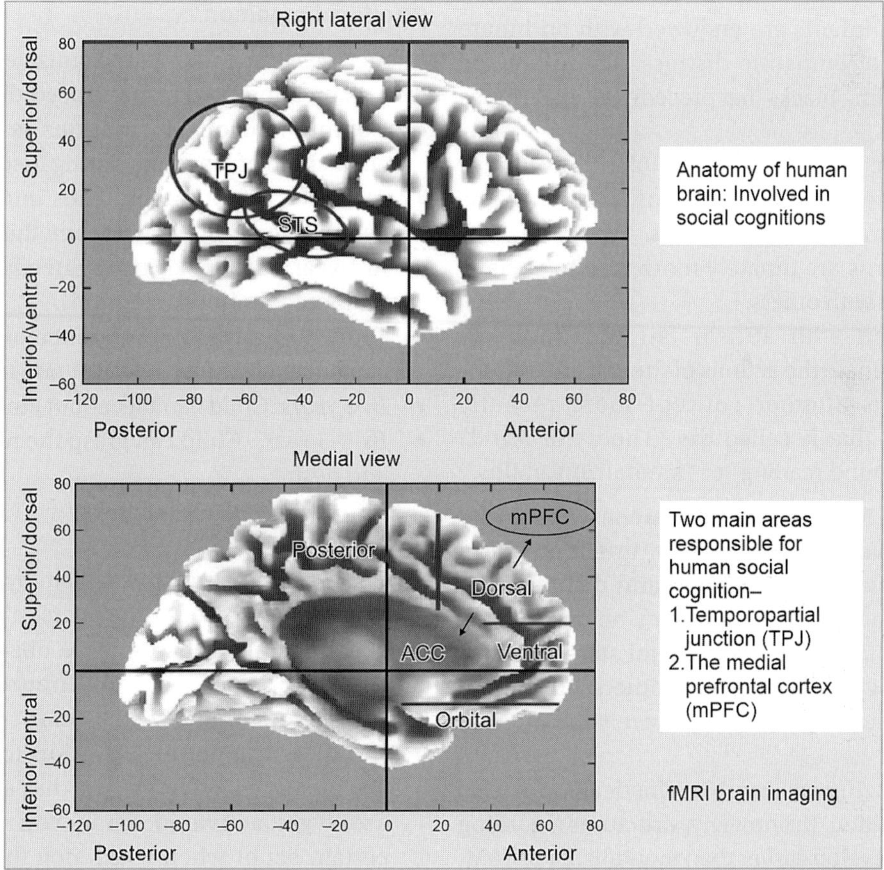

Fig. 4: Brain areas primarily involved in social cognition.[3] (fMRI: functional magnetic resonance imaging)
Source: Van Overwalle F. Social cognition and the brain: a meta-analysis. Hum Brain Mapp. 2009;30(3):829-58.

- *Third person perspective:* Awareness of others mental states

Empathy or emotional sharing between the infant and caretaker is immediately present from birth. This is an innate response and infants exhibit affective resonance manifesting as infant cry reaction to peer crying. Infants also experience emotional contagion through interaction with their caretakers. Von Economo's cells in anterior cingulate and anterior insula subserve the emotional contagion.

Newborn can perceive and discriminate between human emotions and also exhibit a variety of emotions in itself. By the first months of infanthood, infants recognize and mimic the distinct emotions of their mothers, a finding that shows that infants are endowed with an innate precursor of empathic distress. These are the initial building blocks that precede the experience of empathy.

- Discrete facial expressions of emotion have been identified in newborns, including joy, interest, disgust, and distress.
- Newborns are innately motivated to socially interact with others.
- Children with autism fail to effectively discriminate the actions of the self and other.

There is another concept more recently described, that is called the "Theory of Mind" (ToM) or "mind reading" or "mentalizing ability":

"Theory of Mind" refers to awareness that other people have thoughts, beliefs, intentions, and motivations that are different and distinct from our own and can explain other's behaviors. It is the ability to understand mental states such as intentions, goals, and beliefs of others. Attribution of mental states and ToM is severely impaired in autism.

Mentalizing is a more sophisticated form of social cognition. In ontogeny, structures regarding empathy develop earlier than mentalizing or ToM. So, empathy develops earlier than mentalizing. Mentalizing ability underlies frontal, prefrontal cortex, and temporal lobes that develop slowly, up to 25 years, compared to other regions during ontogeny.

Following brain areas are involved in the ToM:

- Temporal lobes
- *STS:* Posterior superior temporal sulcus
- Medial prefrontal lobe *(mPFC)*

Emotional Brain

Emotional brain comprises limbic and paralimbic structures, and develops early in phylogeny. Brain regions involving fusiform face area, superior temporal sulcus, occipital face area, mirror neuron system, as shown in **Figure 5**, comprise the emotional brain and subserve the functions of emotional cognition.

Infants have the ability to recognize emotions in facial expressions and respond accordingly.

- Comprehension of emotions is similar to acquisition of language during first year.
- At 1 year, infant understands intentionality, i.e., emotion is directed at something.
- At 1 year, baby looks in the direction in which mother looks (joint attention).
- Toddlers have social inference of emotions, can offer solace, can hurt or tease to provoke.
- *By 3 years:* Child can talk about emotions.
- *By 4–5 years:* Child can grasp the role of belief and desire.

Mirror Neuron System

- There exists neural mechanism by which one is able to represent other person's behavior, goals or intentions by mere observation of their actions. Various neuroimaging, functional magnetic resonance imaging (fMRI) and positron emission tomography (PET) studies have shown that same brain areas get activated when you perform a certain act or when you watch the same act being performed by someone else. So, there is similar common coding for production and

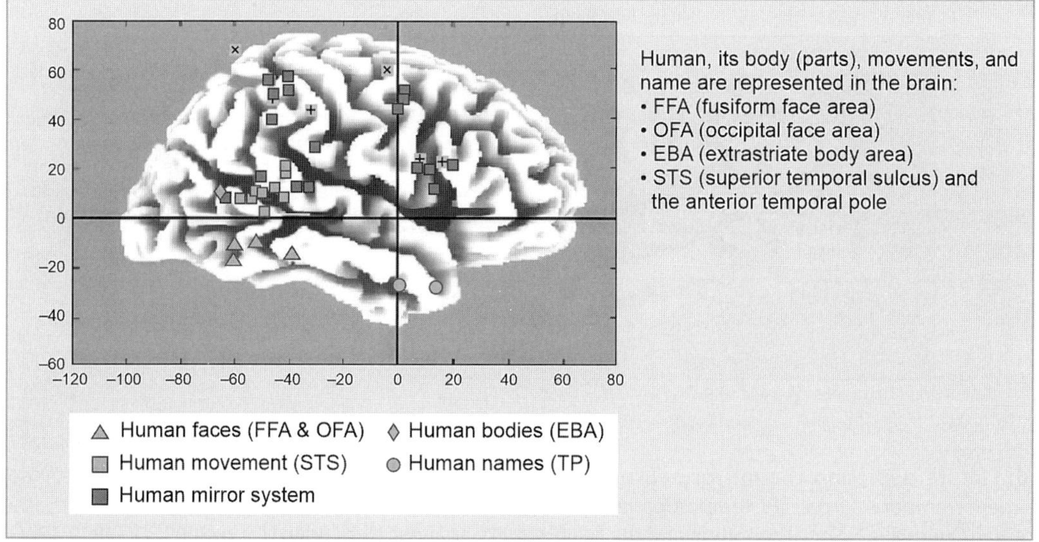

Fig. 5: Brain regions making the emotional brain.[3]

Source: Van Overwalle F. Social cognition and the brain: a meta-analysis. Hum Brain Mapp. 2009;30(3):829-58.

perception of the action. This is mediated through a set of neurons called "mirror neurons".

- Mirror system makes us understand other people's intentions by providing us with an automatic simulation of their actions, goals, and intentions.
- Mirror neurons represent neural basis for imitation and observational learning of gestures, phonetics, and actions.
- These neural mechanisms are also linked to emotional attachment, recognition of internal emotional states of others thereby serving to develop empathy and theory of mind.

Mirror neuron system comprises superior temporal sulcus, temporoparietal junction, inferior parietal lobe, and premotor cortex **(Fig. 6)**.

EXECUTIVE BRAIN: HIGHEST COGNITIVE AND EMOTIONAL PROCESSING

Executive brain refers to those parts of the brain that allow us to focus on a particular activity, filter out distractions, make decisions, and execute actions. Control of a large number of functions is routinely carried out unconsciously. This frees our conscious attention to turn toward other activities such as art, philosophy, religion, contemplation, self-awareness, imagination, etc., which are uniquely human. There are executive neural networks that process and combine inputs from sensory, motor, memory, emotional information to solve problems, and shape actions, plans, thoughts, and fantasies.

- Parietal cortex receives and combines sensory, motor, vestibular and internal bodily information, and sends projections to frontal lobe.
- Parietal lobe organizes body image and inner subjective experience.
- Temporal lobe integrates sensory information with socioemotional aspects and sends projections to frontal lobe.
- Frontal lobe networks integrate concepts of time, linking appraisal of past, present, and future memories.
- Frontal lobe is like CEO.

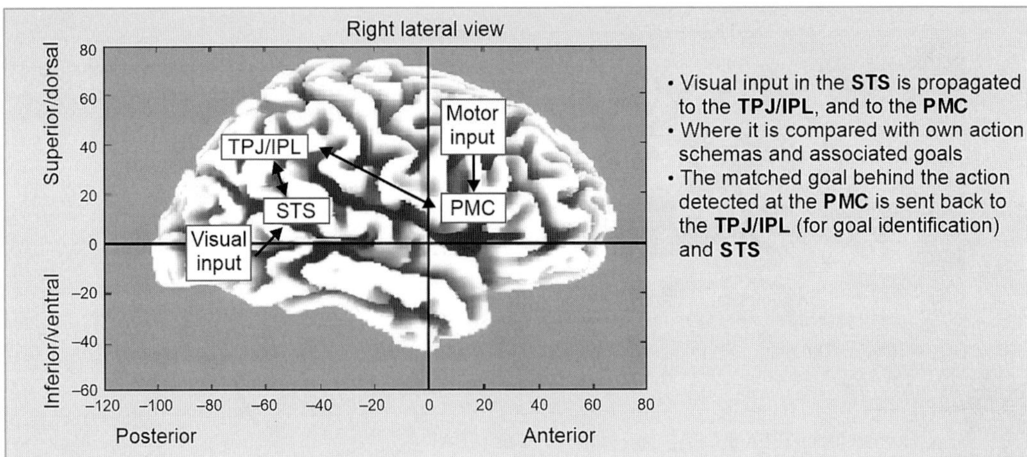

Fig. 6: Picture depicting the mirror neuron system.[3] (IPL: inferior parietal lobe; PMC: premotor cortex; STS: superiortemporal sulcus; TPJ: temporoparietal junction)
Source: Van Overwalle F. Social cognition and the brain: a meta-analysis. Hum Brain Mapp. 2009;30(3):829-58.

- Prefrontal cortex interprets intentions and beliefs of others.

Thus, frontal and prefrontal cortices are the prime seat for highest level of cognitive, emotional and behavioral executive functioning. Damage to prefrontal cortex leads to decrease capacity for empathy and emotional attachment, and psychopathy.

Moral Cognition

There are neural networks underlying normative morality. These are served by ventromedial prefrontal cortex and their connections particularly with the right hemisphere **(Fig. 7)**. Moral judgments are involuntary, rapid, and intuitive. Rational reasoning is post hoc.

Characteristics of normal brain development can be summarized as below.

- It is a self-organizing phenomenon. It constantly keeps adjusting to the environment and keeps changing.
- It is use-dependent. Brain functions that are used more are strengthened. You use it or lose.
- It is differentially specialized. Different parts of the brain subserve different functions.
- It involves self-constructive epigenetic process. Gene expression is altered by environmental factors leading to reciprocal interaction between gene and environment.
- It leads to divergent/convergent developmental paths. It is well-documented that various neurodevelopmental disorders such as autism spectrum disorders (ASD), attention-deficit/hyperactivity disorders (ADHD) and schizophrenia, share common genetic risk. Also, well-known environmental risk factors such as perinatal hypoxia, antenatal maternal and postnatal infections, and maternal smoking during pregnancy, are common to ASD, ADHD, and schizophrenia. There are shared phenotypic or endophenotypic traits cutting across diagnoses providing evidence for convergence of developmental pathways. There are variants in many genes that contribute to a specific disorder which means that risk genes converge on specific or multiple biological

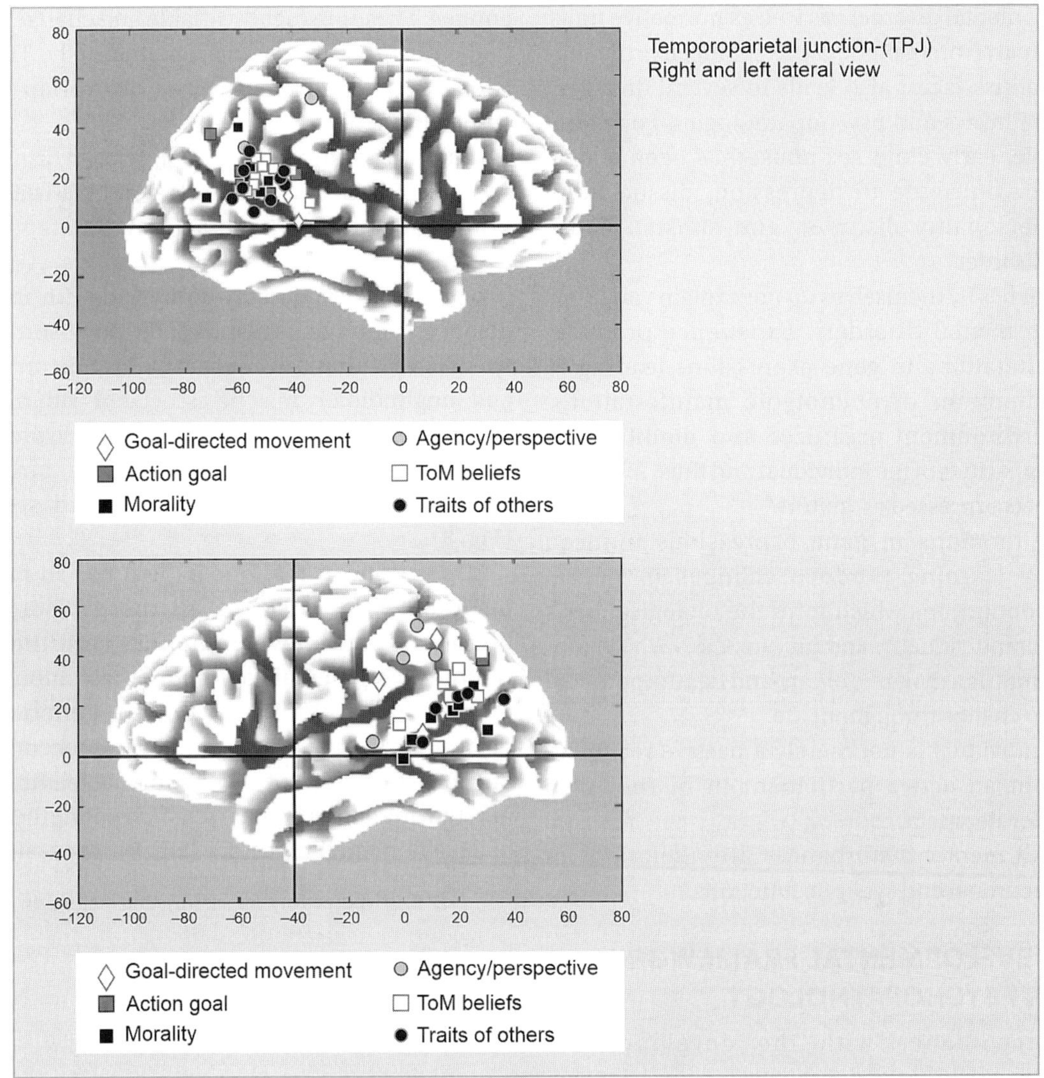

Fig. 7: Brain regions involved in moral cognition.
Source: Van Overwalle F. Social cognition and the brain: a meta-analysis. Hum Brain Mapp. 2009;30(3):829-58.

processes. There is another question as to what factors determine the development of one specific disorder rather than another. The risk genes may converge at the level of molecular pathways, neural circuits, or brain regions. There is also evidence for functional divergence between disorders despite their genetic overlap. This divergence could be due to relative contribution of rare versus common variants and on the timing of the expression of risk genes. There is an extensive overlap in common genetic variants in mental disorders where overlapping neurobiological mechanisms are implicated in development of mental disorders as well as normative traits. Apart from genetic factors, one environmental risk factor also leads to several divergent pathways and psychopathologies. For example, early child sex abuse has been shown to contribute to depression, dissociation, personality disorder, and substance use disorder.

- Genes by themselves do not explain variations in mental disorders. Experience produces alterations in gene expressions leading to alteration in phenotypic manifestations. Environment organizes and modifies the capacities of the individual and thus, "nurture" gets expressed as "nature".
- Alterations in gene expressions induced by learning produce changes in neural connections which form the biological basis for individuality and uniqueness.
- Brain is a dynamic organ, and has the potential to change throughout life.
- Individual is not merely a passive recipient, but an active participant in his/her own development.
- All mental disturbances are alterations of neuronal and synaptic functions.

DEVELOPMENTAL FRAMEWORK IN PSYCHOPATHOLOGY

In accordance with the developmental framework in psychopathology, it can be stated that normal and pathological states are part of the same neurodevelopmental continuum, and that neuropathology represents deviance from the usual ontogenetic pathways. There are bidirectional relationships between genetic, neural, behavioral, and environmental influences during development. Thus, various descriptive diagnostic categories can be seen to lie on a developmental continuum rather than as discreet conditions. Research has amply shown that most psychiatric disorders of childhood are not discreet entities. These are highly variable and changeable both cross-sectionally and longitudinally. There is also a considerable degree of overlap and co-occurrence.

Take the example of a well-described disorder such as ADHD. It is characterized by a triad of symptoms such as hyperactivity, inattention, and impulsivity. In clinical situations, ADHD is often cross-sectionally comorbid with many disorders such as autism spectrum disorders, specific learning disorders, conduct disorders; and longitudinally may be associated with many other disorders such as substance use disorders, bipolar affective disorders, depression, anxiety disorders, personality disorders, and so on **(Fig. 8)**.

Does it mean that one patient has so many disorders? No, basically all these disorders lie on a neurodevelopmental continuum. Neurodevelopmental continuum is a continuum of risk for brain insult (either genetic or environmental) of varying intensities, occurring at different stages of development, leading to different manifestations or outcomes along the line of developmental trajectory **(Fig. 9)**. Thus, all the

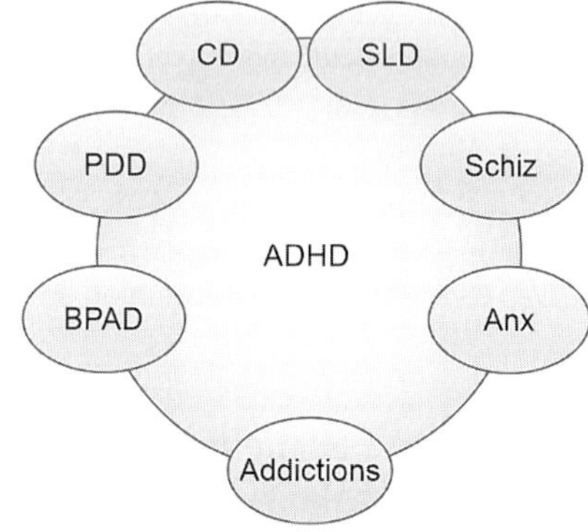

Fig. 8: Overlap and comorbidity of attention-deficit/hyperactivity disorder (ADHD) with other neurodevelopmental disorders and psychiatric conditions. (BPAD: bipolar disorder; PDD: pervasive developmental disorder; CD: conduct disorder; SLD: specific learning disorder; schiz: schizophrenia spectrum)

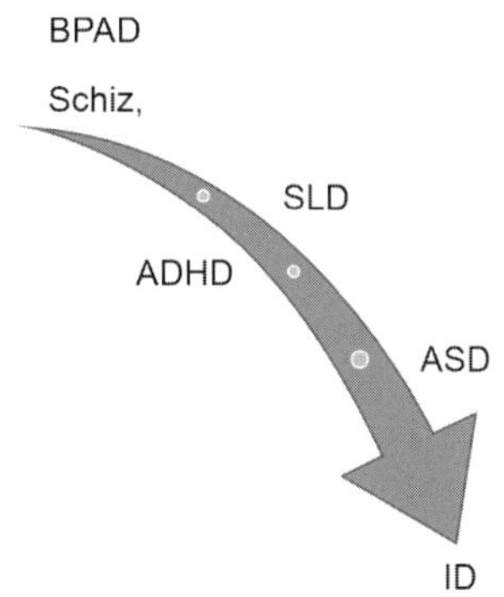

Fig. 9: Picture depicting neurodevelopmental continuum. (ADHD: attention-deficit/hyperactivity disorder; ASD: autism spectrum disorders; BPAD: bipolar disorder; ID: intellectual disability; Schz: schizophrenia spectrum disorder; SLD: specific learning disorders)

conditions on a neurodevelopmental continuum even though have different phenotypes but share common genetic and/or environmental risk or neurobiological underpinnings **(Fig. 9)**.

NEURODEVELOPMENTAL CONTINUUM

What happens in psychiatric disorders?

Brain comprises innumerable component parts which must be appropriately placed and function smoothly according to the genetic template supported by expectable/conducive environment. It is a task full of challenges and uncertainties. There are countless contingencies that can derail these complex developmental processes. This complexity of development and functioning of brain also makes it a fragile structure. There is a perpetual risk for lack of integration or dysregulation or disorganization of neural networks or neural functions at different stages of development.

Abnormalities occurring at the level of neural circuits and cellular and molecular functions in the form of:

- Disorganization
- Disintegration
- Dysregulation, and
- Hyperactivity/Hypoactivity

Lead to psychiatric disorders. This happens due to interplay of genetic, epigenetic, and environmental factors as discussed above.

Following neurobiological abnormalities can be described to contribute to causation of mental disorders:

1. *Aberrant neurodevelopment due to:*
    - Genetic defect
    - Brain insult such as trauma and infection particularly during sensitive periods
    - Physical environmental compromise such as exposure to toxins, infections, diet, and medications
    - Psychosocial environmental compromise such as experiencing stress, anxiety, mental trauma, deprivation, and abuse
2. Aberrant neurocircuitry
3. Neuronal loss
4. Neurohumoral abnormalities, i.e., release of stress hormones
5. Neurochemical abnormalities, i.e., neurotransmitter dysregulation

These neurobiological abnormalities can occur at any time during the course of development and they cut across diagnostic categories. These processes can be inter-related or even interdependent. For example, aberrant neurodevelopment due to any cause during fetal stage or infancy can lead to aberrant neurocircuitry as well as neurohumoral or neurochemical abnormalities impacting the brain functions in a manner that can lead to psychiatric disorder.

Underlying pathological processes include:

- Brain inflammation or systemic inflammation
- *Immune activation:* Occurs in all developmental stresses. Developmental stressors impact brain microglia. Microglia are primary immune cells of brain, they infiltrate brain during early embryo development, are involved in synaptic maturation and neural

circuit maintenance. These can drive the disease risk.

SUMMARY AND CONCLUSION

To summarize, human brain is a product of millions of years of evolutionary adaptations and modifications and continues to constantly evolve and change. Evolution is driven by physical survival of the species. Each individual brain reflects an adaptation to its unique environment, life history, and its unique individuality. Human neonate is totally dependent on environment for survival. This prolonged phase of dependency of newborn allows for growth of neocortex with all its complex functions. However, despite this massive neocortex, much of our lives remain under the influence of primitive emotional brain. Therefore, the knowledge of neurodevelopmental processes and mechanisms can significantly inform the clinical practice of child psychiatry.

In conclusion, it can be confidently said that brain is not a static structure, thus rendering considerable hope and opportunity to intervene at appropriate time to bring about amelioration or positive push to the developmental process. Even more so, understanding of the developmental pathways and trajectories is necessary for understanding psychiatric disorders. Psychiatric disorders, as we understand them today, are not discreet conditions. There is great deal of continuity and overlap which should be acknowledged and addressed in our clinical practice. One must explore the adverse disruptive influences in the course of development. This would help in understanding the genesis of problems, and in instituting the appropriate intervention approaches. One should always try to know the associated neurobiological conditions in each patient to inform the intervention strategies which must not be limited to mere symptom relief. Appropriate holistic approaches including preventive and promotive interventions must be targeted. This puts forth a very strong case for focusing on early years of life and for early intervention in practice of not just child and adolescent psychiatry but of the entire field of psychiatry.

REFERENCES

1. Martin A, Bloch MH, Volkmar FR. Lewis's Child and Adolescent Psychiatry: A Comprehensive Textbook. Gurugram: Wolters Kluwer; 2017.
2. Pelphrey KA, Perlman SB. Charting brain mechanisms for the development of social cognition. Neuroimag Develop Clin Neurosci. 2009;73-90.
3. Van Overwalle F. Social cognition and the brain: a meta-analysis. Hum Brain Mapp. 2009;30(3): 829-58.

SUGGESTED READING

1. Kandel ER. Psychiatry, Psychoanalysis, and the New Biology of Mind. VA, USA: American Psychiatric Publishing Inc; 2005.
2. Rey JM. (2015). IACAPAP e-Textbook of Child and Adolescent Mental Health. [online] Available from
    a. https://iacapap.org/iacapap-textbook-of-child-and-adolescent-mental-health [Last accessed November, 2025].
    b. https://www.google.com/url?sa=t&rct=j&q=&esrc=s&source=web&cd=&cad=rja&uact=8&ved=2ahUKEwij--3z-bnyAhWLILcAHZ2VDm8QFnoECAQQAQ&url=https%3A%2F%2Fiacapap.org%2Fj-m-reys-iacapap-e-textbook-of-child-and-adolescent-mental-health%2F&usg=AOvVaw0IUlcHUAPMM8VmJIVXjgon [Last accessed November, 2025].
3. Taylor E, Verhulst FC, Wong J, Yoshida K (Eds). Mental Health and Illness of Children and Adolescents. London: Springer; 2020.

Developmental Aspects-II: Developmental Theories Including Attachment Theory

Nidhi Chauhan, Velprashanth Venkatesan

INTRODUCTION

Have you ever wondered how an infant who was only able to lie on his/her back and make random noises, in a few months becomes a busy toddler making some sincere attempts at trying to put a block of Lego together purposefully and perhaps even make sense of it? Now looking back, we can either wonder or perhaps question if at all there is a process behind all this and whether there is anything random happening here. There are ways to understand this miraculous yet systematic process that unfolds in ways more complex than we can ever imagine. The field of science dedicated to understanding this is called *"Lifespan Development."*

LIFESPAN DEVELOPMENT

Lifespan development is the extensive field that examines patterns of growth, change, and in behavior that occurs across the lifespan. In its study of growth, change, and endurance of behavioral patterns, lifespan development takes up a scientific approach. Developmental theories make it possible to conceptualize large quantum of data regarding development, indicating which are the most salient and why.[1] Developmentalists assume that the process of development persists throughout every part of people's lives, beginning with the moment of conception and continuing until death. Developmental specialists assume that in some ways people continue to grow and change throughout the end of their lives, while in other respects the development once attained remains stable.[2]

Having said that, there are still certain issues that are challenging to understand. One of the primary issues is whether development proceeds in a *continuous or discontinuous* fashion. In continuous change, development is progressive and achievements are attained smoothly in gradually evolving process. Continuous change is quantitative; the basic underlying developmental processes that drive growth remain stable throughout the lifespan. In contrast, one can also view development as a discontinuous change, occurring in unique stages. Each stage brings about behavior that is understood to be qualitatively different from behavior at earlier stages. One of the enduring questions of development involves how much of people's behavior is due to their genetically determined *nature* and how much is due to *nurture,* the influences of the physical and social environment in which a child is raised.[3] This issue, which has deep philosophical and historical roots, has directed much work in lifespan development.

LIFESPAN DEVELOPMENT: THE VARIOUS SCHOOLS

Psychodynamic School

Proponents of the psychodynamic school, beginning from *Sigmund Freud* believe that much of behavior is pushed by inner forces, buried memories of events, and conflicts of which a person has no autonomy over. The inner forces, which may arise from one's childhood, continually influence behavior throughout the lifespan. Freud also believed that personality developed during childhood. He explained it via the *Psychosexual Stages of Development* **(Table 1)** which occur as children pass through discontinuous stages in which pleasure, or gratification, is focused on a particular organ and body part. He described that pleasure shifts *from the mouth (the oral stage) to the anus (the anal stage) and eventually to the genitals (the phallic stage and the genital stage).*[4] Psychoanalyst *Erik Erikson* provided another evolved psychodynamic view in his theory of psychosocial development, which emphasizes our social interaction with other people. In his *Psychosocial Stages of Development,* Erikson suggests that developmental stages occur all through our lives in eight distinct stages **(Table 2)**. The stages develop in a fixed pattern and are universal for all people irrespective for race and ethnicity. Erikson argued that each stage presents a crisis or conflict that the individual must resolve in order to develop a *virtue* that will allow his progress to the next stage. Although no crisis is ever fully resolved, making life increasingly complicated, the individual must find ways to deal with the crisis of each stage adequately to deal with demands made during the subsequent stage of development.[5]

TABLE 1: Freud's psychosexual stages of development.

Stage	*Oral phase*	*Anal phase*	*Phallic phase*	*Latent phase*	*Adolescent genital phase*
Age	Birth to 12–18 months	12–18 to 36 months	3–5 years	6–11 years	11 years plus
Features	Oral area primary site of gratification and tension • Nutritive sucking for nourishment • Non-nutritive sucking for soothing; oral gratification Mouth as site of exploration ("puts everything in the mouth") Biting as a tension release when upset or overstimulated • Child dependent and needy	The anal area is the primary site of gratification and tension • Conflict over control of bowels • Toilet training	Genitals as primary site of gratification and tension • Oedipus/ Electra complex (Attracted to opposite-sex parent; rivalry with same-sex parent) • Castration anxiety; fear of injury (Band-Aids needed for "boo-boos") • Sexual identity forming • Interest in genital exploration	Relative quiescence of libidinal drives • Sexual drives channeled into socially appropriate activities (e.g., school work and sports) • Further development of ego functions (judgment, frustration tolerance, etc.) • Formation of superego (conscience)	Final stage of psychosexual development • Recapitulate earlier phases • Separation and individuation from family • Identity formation • Biological capacity for orgasm and psychological capacity for true intimacy to develop

Source: Adapted from Tasman's Psychiatry, 4th edition, Chapter 7–A Psychiatric Perspective on Human Development.[33]

TABLE 2: Erik Erikson's psychosocial stages of development.

Stage/Age	*Crisis*	*Virtue*	*Features*
1. Birth to 12–18 months	*Trust* versus *mistrust*	Hope	• Trust depends on the reliability and quality of care provided. Optimism/hope from being able to trust that needs will be met. Basis of bonding/secure attachment. Promotes capacity for intimacy • Mistrust when basic needs are not met predictably, the infant feels helpless. Vulnerable to insecure attachment. Decreased capacity for intimacy • Frustration inherent in maturation—weaning, etc.
2. 12–18 to 36 months	*Autonomy* versus *shame*	Will	Autonomy—increased capacities and ability to "do it myself" such as motor, sphincter; language; etc. Increased self-esteem. Shame from lack of self-control. Self-doubt evolves from parental shaming (e.g., regarding toileting)
3. 3–5 years	*Initiative* versus *guilt*	Purpose	Initiative and enjoyment of activity and accomplishments. Self-esteem through being admired. New motor and language capacities. Expanding relationships/preschool. Guilt over aggressive urges. Feels the need to win at games. Role identification. Sibling rivalry is common
4. 6–11 years	*Industry* versus *inferiority*	Competence	• School success builds self-esteem. The child is busy creating, building, and accomplishing • The danger of a sense of inferiority and inadequacy if the child feels unable to compete for skills (e.g., academics, sports), and status among peers. Socially decisive age (building of social skills and competencies)
5. 11–18 years	*Identity* versus *role-confusion*	Fidelity	Group identity (peers) primary. Developing ego identity (sense of inner sameness). Preoccupation with appearance. Moodiness and affective reactivity. The danger of role confusion; and uncertainty about sexual and vocational identity
6. Early adulthood	*Intimacy* versus *isolation*	Love	Committed, interdependent, and intimate relationships are important. *Vocational identity:* Commitment, compensation, contentment, competence—feeling valued. Parenthood/ desire to nurture. Loneliness and poor self-esteem with disappointments in relationships and career
7. Middle aged adult	*Generativity* versus *stagnation*	Care	Selfless generativity with the capacity to care for and guide the next generation. Keeper of the meaning—imparting wisdom versus rigid competitiveness. Stagnation—insecurity in self; inability selflessly to nurture children or share what has been learned
8. Old age	*Integrity* versus *despair*	Wisdom	The feeling of dignity and satisfaction in life well lived. Imparting of wisdom. Despair—preoccupation with regrets and bitterness about life's disappointments

Source: Adapted from Tasman's Psychiatry, 4th edition, Chapter 7–A Psychiatric Perspective on Human Development.[33]

Humanistic School

This school was revolutionary as it rejected the notion that an individual's behavior is largely determined by unconscious drives; the humanistic perspective contends that people have a natural capacity to make decisions about their lives and to control their behavior. According to this approach, everyone has the capacity and needs to reach more advanced levels of maturity, and people will always seek to reach their full potential.[6] The humanistic perspective emphasizes *free will*, the ability of humans to make choices and come to decisions about their lives and thereby defeat the shackles of instincts and inevitability of fate. The key proponents of this theory include *Carl Rogers* and later *Abraham Maslow* who gave his *Hierarchy of Needs.*[7] Despite making strides in sociopolitical movements, the humanistic perspective is yet to make a mark in terms of explaining the factors determining the development from birth.

Behavioral School

Behavioral school suggests that ways to understand and determine development are only via descriptive and observable behavior in response to external stimuli in the environment. The key proponent of this movement includes *Ivan Pavlov (Classical Conditioning), JB Watson and BF Skinner (Operant Conditioning).* If we know the stimuli, we can predict the behavior. In this respect, the behavioral perspective imparts the view that nurture is more important to development than nature.[8] Behavioral theorists reject the idea that people universally go through a series of stages. Instead, people are explained to be influenced by the environmental stimuli in which they happen to be a passive recipient. Developmental patterns, then, are individualized, reflecting a particular set of environmental stimuli, and behavior is the result of continuing exposure to these unique factors in the environment. The most influential of the behavioral theories is the *Social Learning Theory* by *Albert Bandura* where behavior is learned primarily through observation and not merely through stimuli-responses leading to trial and error, as it is with operant conditioning. He emphatically demonstrated via *Bobo Doll Experiment* that children do not need to experience the consequences of a behavior themselves to learn it. Social learning theory holds that when we see the behavior of a model being rewarded, we are attuned to imitate that behavior.[9]

Cognitive School

The cognitive perspective explains how people mentally represent and symbolize about the world. They seek to learn how cognitive abilities change as people develop, such as how the intellectual abilities are constructed as different faculties, and how different cognitive abilities are inter-related to one another. Cognitive development inherently induces development in various domains such as thought, emotions, judgement, and overall social development as well. The pioneering effort in the cognitive perspective came from *Jean Piaget's Theory of Cognitive Development.* He suggested that not only does the amount of perceived information increase in each stage **(Table 3)**, but the qualitative properties of this knowledge and its interpretations change as well. Piaget suggested that human cognition is organized into *schemes*, that is, structured mental patterns that represent behaviors and actions. In infants, such schemes represent concrete behavior—a scheme for rooting, for grasping, and for each separate behavior.[10] In older children, the schemes become more sophisticated and abstract, such as the set of skills involved in riding a cycle or playing a game in one's mobile phone. Piaget suggested that the growth in children's conceptualization of the world can be explained

TABLE 3: Piaget's cognitive stages of development.

Stage	*Age*	*Description*
Sensorimotor stage	Birth to 1st month	*Substage 1—simple reflex:* During this period, the various reflexes that determine the infant's interactions with the world are at the center of its cognitive life
	1–4 months	*Substage 2—primary circular reactions:* At this age, infants begin to coordinate what were separate actions into single, integrated activities
	4–8 months	*Substage 3—secondary circular reactions:* During this period, infants take major strides in shifting their cognitive horizons beyond themselves and begin to act on the outside world
	8–12 months	*Substage 4—coordination of secondary circular reactions:* In this stage, infants begin to use more calculated approaches to producing events, coordinating several schemes to generate a single act. They achieve object performance during this stage
	12–18 months	*Substage 5—tertiary circular reactions:* At this age, infants develop what Piaget regards as the deliberate variation of actions that bring desirable consequences. Rather than just repeating enjoyable activities, infants appear to carry out miniature experiments to observe the consequences
	18 months to 2 years	*Substage 6—beginning of symbolic thought:* The major achievement of substage 6 is the capacity for mental representation or symbolic thought. Piaget argued that at this stage the infants begin to imagine that objects might be present at places even when they cannot see it
Preoperational stage	3–6 years	Language acquisition with symbolic reasoning *Egocentrism*: Sees the world exclusively from own perspective. *Transductive thinking*—causality is inferred from temporal or spatial proximity. Magical thinking (prelogical). Animism
Concrete operational stage	6–11 years	Emergence of logical, cause-and-effect thinking *Reversibility* of events and ideas. Switch from egocentric to social speech. Ability to see another's point of view. *Conservation* of volume and quantity. Rigid interpretation of rules
Formal operations stage	From 12 years	*Hypothetical/deductive abstract reasoning*. Elaboration of information processing. *Metacognitive capacity*—able to think about thinking. Ability to grasp the concept of probabilities. Ability to consider options and weigh relative risk and relative benefit

Source: Adapted from Tasman's Psychiatry, 4th edition, Chapter 7–A Psychiatric Perspective on Human Development.[33]

by the two basic principles of *Assimilation and Accommodation*. Assimilation is the process in which people understand an experience in terms of their present schemes of cognitive development and way of thinking. Assimilation occurs when people use their current schemes about the world to perceive and understand a new experience. In contrast, accommodation refers to change in existing schemes to encounter with new stimuli or events. Assimilation and accommodation work in tandem to bring about cognitive development.[11]

Another branch of psychology that is cognitively based is the field of "Moral Psychology" and the pioneer of this field was a person inspired by Piaget. He was *Lawrence Kohlberg* who, in 1958, began the study of the development of moral judgment far beyond the ages studied earlier by Piaget, who also claimed that logic and morality develop through constructive stages which he called as *heteronormative morality*.[12] Expanding on Piaget's work, Kohlberg determined that the process of moral development was mainly concerned with justice and that it continued throughout the individual's life, a notion that led to a discourse on the philosophical implications of such research. The six stages of moral development occur in phases of preconventional, conventional, and postconventional morality[13] **(Table 4)**. The major criticism of cognitive theories is that they suggest discontinuous development which has in recent times led to the *Information Processing Theory*. Information processing approaches grew out of developments in the electronic processing of information, particularly as carried out by computers. They assume that even complex behavior such as learning, remembering, categorizing, and thinking can be broken down into a series of individual, specific steps or mental faculties. Just like computers, children are assumed by information processing approaches to have limited capacity for processing information. As they develop, however, they employ increasingly sophisticated strategies that allow them to process information more efficiently.[1]

Evolutionary School

The evolutionary concept seeks to describe behavior that is the result of our genetic inheritance from our ancestors and is built on the ground-breaking work of *Charles Darwin* who argued that behaviors can get inherited based on utility in survival through the process of *Natural Selection*[14] and such that it occurs over long epochs of time working its way through long bloodlines of genetic pool. The evolutionary perspective also inspires the science of *ethology*, which examines how our biological makeup influences our behavior that are observed in animals as soon as they are born without any prior exposure to environment outside the womb. A primary proponent of ethology was *Konrad Lorenz (1903–1989)*, who discovered that newborn geese are genetically preprogramed to become attached to the first moving object they see after birth.

TABLE 4: Kohlberg's stages of moral development.

Moral stage	*Age*	*Description*
Premoral period	Birth till 1 year	Inborn emotions of anger, fear, sadness, and joy emerge as premoral primary emotions
Emergence of moral emotions	1–2 years	Embarrassment, shame, and guilt. Emergence of normative standards. Distress at disappointing parents
Level 1: Preconventional morality	2–5 years	*Right and wrong are determined by rewards and punishments:* • *Stage 1:* Punishment/obedience. What leads to punishment is wrong • *Stage 2:* Rewards. Whatever is right is rewarded
Level 2: Conventional morality	6–11 years	*Seek approval; avoid blame:* • *Stage 3:* Good intentions = good behavior • *Stage 4:* Obedience to authority and "doing one's duty"
Level 3: Postconventional morality	12–18 years	*Abstract notions of justice; rights of others override obedience to rules:* • *Stage 5:* Difference between moral and legal rights—rules should sometimes be broken • *Stage 6:* Individual principles of conscience. Takes into account likely views of others affected by moral decisions

Source: Adapted from Tasman's Psychiatry, 4th edition, Chapter 7–A Psychiatric Perspective on Human Development.[33]

His work, which demonstrated the importance of biological determinants in influencing behavior patterns, ultimately compelled developmentalists to consider how human behavior might reflect inborn genetic patterns[15,16] and even lead to current concepts of *Behavioral Phenotypes.* The evolutionary approach has indeed been a source of impetus for major genetic research in twin studies and genomic studies to understand behavioral patterns in inheritance.

Sociocultural School

Last but not least among the theoretical perspectives is the impact of one's sociocultural and environmental factors that directly shape behavior through "Nurture." Thus, several theories address development through the rubric of cultural-contextual factors. The most influential among them all is the *Attachment Theory by John Bowlby* who held that the child's bond (attachment) to the nurturer (attachment figure) is primary and inborn. All humans and nonhuman primates require close interpersonal contact to survive. Bowlby's attachment theory was equally influenced by *Ethological* experiments of Lorenz and also experiments of *Harry Harlow in rhesus monkeys,* thus having biological roots that explain attachment being an entity that is inborn. But as much as the origin being innate, Bowlby explained that the fate of one's attachment is fully dependent on the experiences a newborn received from its caretaker. He along with further works by *Mary Ainsworth and Mary Main* describes stages and types of attachment from birth till preschool age **(Table 5)** and beyond that. These eventually shape the formation of *Secure Attachment.* Bowlby (1973) conceived of individual differences in attachment as rooted in inner representations of the self, important others (e.g., attachment of figures, usually the parents), and relationships. From birth, the interactions of an infant with his/her primary caregivers will make way for personality development and will shape the nature and quality of subsequent close relationships, including expectations of social acceptance and attitudes regarding rejection. A secure base is formed when an attachment figure (usually a parent) provides stability and safety to the infant in moments of distress consistently and in a sensitive manner. This allows the infant to feel that it is safe to venture into the unknown surroundings.[2,3,17] The disruption of this process may lead to *Insecure Attachment Patterns* **(Table 6)**.

Other theories describe the larger context of culture in development, the two of which are *Urie Bronfenbrenner's Bioecological Model of Development*[1] and *Lev Vygotsky's Socio-cultural Theory of Development.* We will see the latter in detail. Vygotsky, who lived a brief life from 1896 to 1934, gave the notion that children's understanding of the world is acquired through

TABLE 5: Bowlby's stages of attachment.

Stage	*Age*	*Description*
Preattachment	0–2 months	Infants cannot discriminate. No established symbiosis with mother
Attachment in the making	2–6 months	The infant directs particular signals to the primary caregiver. Begins to identify the attachment figure. But, no separation protest
Clear cut attachment	6 months to 3–4 years	Discriminate signals to primary attachment figure with separation protest. Formation of secondary attachment figures with stranger's anxiety
Goal corrected partnership	3–4 years onward	Multiple attachments formed. Able to understand caregiver's availability and thus reduce separation anxiety with clear signs of a secure base

Source: Adapted from Tasman's Psychiatry, 4th edition, Chapter 7–A Psychiatric Perspective on Human Development.[33]

TABLE 6: Types of attachment.

Secure attachment	*Anxious attachment*
• Children with a secure attachment use their mother as a safe base to explore their environment • They are moderately distressed when their mother leaves the room (separation anxiety) and seek contact with their mother when she returns • They also show moderate stranger anxiety; they show some distress when approached by a stranger	• Children with this type of attachment are clingy to their mother in a new situation and are not willing to explore—suggesting that they do not have trust in her • They are extremely distressed when separated from their mother. When the mother returns, they are pleased to see her and go to her for comfort, but they cannot be comforted and may show signs of anger toward her. This type of attachment style occurs because the mother is inconsistent
Avoidant attachment	***Disorganized attachment***
• Children with this attachment do not use the mother as a safe base; they are not distressed on separation from their caregiver and are not joyful when the mother returns. They show little stranger's anxiety • This type of attachment occurs because the mother ignores the emotional needs of the infant	• They display attachment behaviors typical of avoidant children, becoming socially withdrawn and untrusting of others • If the child and caregiver were to be separated for any amount of time, on the reunion, the child would act conflicted. They may initially run toward their caregiver but then seem to change their mind and either run away or act out • In the eyes of a child with a fearful avoidant attachment, their caregivers are untrustworthy

Source: Adapted from Tasman's Psychiatry, 4th Edition, Chapter 7–A Psychiatric Perspective on Human Development.[33]

their problem-solving interactions with adults and other children. In his description, children play and cooperate with others, they learn what is important in their society and, at the same time, advance cognitively in their understanding of the world. Consequently, to understand the course of development, we must consider what is meaningful to the immediate members of one's culture. More than most other theories, sociocultural theory emphasizes that development is a reciprocal transaction between the people in a child's environment and the child.[18] Vygotsky believed that people and settings (*Scaffolding*) influence the child, who, in turn, influences the setting and so on. This pattern continues in an endless loop, with children being both recipients of external influences and sources of influence (*Zone of Proximal Development*) both interacting in a dynamic equilibrium. For example, a child raised with his joint family in collectivistic societies will have own rules of self-esteem development compared to child who grows up in a nuclear family with individualistic morale.[19] The relatives, too, are affected by that situation and that child, depending on how close and frequent their contact is with the child.[20] Thus, the system allows for mutual development through interactions.

Cognitive Neuroscience School

The current school of developmentalists are keen on building a bridge between the various cognitive abilities hypothesized from a faculty psychology point of view and then to connect these functions to a well-defined neural activity in a localized brain area/circuit. With advancements in functional neuroimaging by use of fMRI, EEG, functional near infrared spectroscopy and many such advancements, a live person while performing a mental task, his cognitive functions can be mapped spatially and temporally to a brain activity.[21] A key challenge is to further understand molecular genetic changes that occur through one's experience that, in turn, encompass these neural changes. This field has, henceforth, contributed toward the concept of *Critical Periods*—a time limited epoch in development when specific experiences must occur to drive normal development and *Sensitive Periods*—a time limited epoch in development when experiences have maximal effect on learning. These concepts have evolved into a more complex division in learning called the *Experience-expectant learning* (common processes across species that emerge from universal experience like language) and *Experience-dependent learning* (unique processes in individuals that emerge from specific sociocultural experiences like visuospatial orientation in hunting tribes).[22]

DEVELOPMENT ACROSS AGES

Having considered the various theoretical aspects of "Lifespan Development" we can try to look at the domains of development across four areas namely *Physical, Cognitive, Emotional, and Social* where we shall see how the above theories can apply at various levels and further see them from chronological perspective divided into four epochs namely: *(1) Infancy, (2) Preschool age, (3) Middle school age, and (4) Adolescence.*

Lifespan Development: Infancy

Physical Development: Infancy

The development of gross and fine-motor skills proceeds along a predictable pattern in normal children, with substantial individual and cultural variations determined by the reinforcements, social learning, and the cultural exposure for same. The infant's physical growth encompasses certain guiding principles which we will see as follows. *The cephalocaudal principle* states that growth follows a direction and order that begins with the head and upper regions of head and then proceeds down toward feet and to the rest of the body. The cephalocaudal growth principle means that we attain our visual abilities (located in the head) well before we master the capacity to walk (closer to the end of the body). *The proximodistal principle* states that development proceeds from the center of the body toward the extremities in the periphery. The proximodistal principle means that the trunk develops before the arms and legs. Furthermore, the development of the ability to utilize parts of the body also follows the proximodistal principle. For instance, sitting without support is then followed by development of pincer grasp. *The Principle of Hierarchical Integration* states that simple skills typically develop distinctly and independently but that these simple skills are constructed into more elaborate ones. Thus, the relatively complex skill of grasping something in the hand cannot be mastered until the developing infant learns how to control—and integrate—execute the movements of the individual fingers. Finally, *The Principle of the Independence of Systems* suggests that different body systems grow at different rates. For instance, the patterns of growth for brain cortical maturity and sexual maturation are quite different.[2] Developmentalist *Esther Thelen* has created an innovative theory to explain how motor skills develop and are coordinated. *Dynamic systems theory* describes how motor behaviors are assembled.[23] By "assembled," Thelen means the integration of a variety of skills that develop in a child, ranging from the development of an infant's musculature, its sensory abilities and motor system, as well as its motivation to carry out motor activities with support from the environment. According to dynamic systems theory, motor development in a particular sphere, such as "grasping" is not just dependent on the brain initiating a "grasping program" that permits the muscles to grab things. Instead, grasping requires the coordination of muscles, perception, cognition, and motivation. The theory emphasizes how children's abundant exploratory activities, which produce new challenges as they interact with their environment, lead them to advancements in motor skills.[24]

Cognitive Development: Infancy

During the sensorimotor period (refer to **Table 3**) (birth to about 2 years) with its six substages, infants progress from the use of simple reflexes, through the development of repeated and coordinated actions that gradually increase in complexity, to the ability to generate meaningful outcomes from their actions. By the end of the sixth substage of the sensorimotor period, infants are beginning to engage in symbolic thought.[7,10] Infants, in this period, begin prelinguistic use of words. Prelinguistic communication involves the use of nascent vocalizations, babbling, deictic gestures, facial expressions, imitation, and other nonlinguistic means to express thoughts and states. Prelinguistic communication prepares the infant for speech. Infants typically produce their first words between the ages of 10 and 14 months. At around 18 months, children typically begin to connect words together into primitive sentences that express single thoughts. Beginning of speech is characterized by using holophrases (child saying "milk" to demand milk), telegraphic speech (incomplete sentences like "Varun want ball"), etc. The development of language is also influenced by both genetic and contextual factors in this age. The learning theory approach to language acquisition assumes that adults and children use basic behavioral processes—such as conditioning, reinforcement, and shaping/prompting—in language learning with the famous model of *Verbal Operants by Skinner* which comprise *Manding, Tacting, Echoing, and Inraverbals* used in training of children with "Autism." A different approach proposed by *Noam Chomsky* holds that humans are genetically endowed with a *language-acquisition device*, which permits them to detect and use the principles of universal grammar that underlie all languages in order to fill in the innate gaps within one's language device to proceed with an accepted word usage.[25]

Emotional Development: Infancy

Beginning of the basic emotions of contentment, distress, and interest, which may be reliably observed in the first 2 months of life, begin after the transition at 2–3 months. By the time infants have reached 6 months of age, they exhibit a detailed evolution of a primary expression of contentment into a more elaborate joy and contentment; similarly of interest into surprise and interest, and of distress into sadness, disgust, and anger.[26] Because of the relational context of emotion expression in early infancy, emotional regulation now is both a within-the-infant and a relational property such that they are largely reactive with respect to the regulation of emotional expression.[3]

Social Development: Infancy

Through *social referencing*, infants from the age of 8 or 9 months use the expressions of others to clarify ambiguous situations and learn appropriate reactions to them as they have inherently provided with capacity to watch other's reaction to a situation to adopt one's own. Early in life, infants develop the capability of nonverbal decoding: determining the emotional states of others based on their facial and vocal expressions if the environment is also sufficiently stimulating.[27] Infants also begin to develop a *Theory of Mind* in a basic form that enables imitation skills: thus, initiating a knowledge and beliefs about how they and others may think. Mothers' interactions with their babies are particularly important for social development. Mothers who respond effectively to their babies' social overtures appear to contribute to the babies' ability to become securely attached and this *secure base,* in turn, ensures the child show *stranger's anxiety and separation anxiety* and later the capacity to form differential attachments and object relations.[28] Through a process of reciprocal socialization, infants and caregivers interact and affect one another's behavior, which strengthens their mutual relationship. From an early age, infants engage in rudimentary forms of social interaction with other children, and their level of sociability rises as they age.[29]

Lifespan Development: Preschool

Physical Development: Preschool

In addition to gaining height and weight, the bodies of preschool children go through changes in form and structure. Children grow slenderer, and their bones and muscles strengthen. Children in the preschool years are generally quite healthy.[30] This rapid burst of energy gives rise to the *Terrible twos* where every child suddenly becomes a version of *Flash* the superhero from the DC comics. The greatest health threats are accidents and environmental factors because of the immature brain's failure to regulate the unbridled physical energy of a toddler. Brain growth is particularly rapid during the preschool years, with the number of interconnections among cells and the amount of myelin around neurons increasing greatly. The halves of the brain begin to specialize in somewhat different tasks—a process called *lateralization.*[31] Both gross and fine motor skills advance rapidly during the preschool years thus emergence of drawing, writing, bicycle riding all begin to smoothly emerge if opportunities are provided. Gender differences begin to emerge in the genitalia, fine motor skills are honed, and handedness begins to assert itself.[32]

Cognitive Development: Preschool

During the stage that Piaget has described as *Preoperational,* children are not yet able to engage in organized, formal, and logical thinking. *Conservation* is the knowledge that quantity is unrelated to the arrangement and physical appearance of objects. Because they are unable to conserve, preschoolers cannot fathom the fact that changes in one dimension (such as a change in appearance) do not necessarily mean that other dimensions (such as quantity) change. For example, children who do not yet understand the principle of conservation feel quite comfortable asserting that the quantity of liquid changes as it is poured between glasses of different sizes. They simply are unlikely to realize that the transformation in appearance does not imply a transformation in quantity. Another hallmark of the preoperational period is egocentric thinking. *Egocentric thought* is thinking that does not consider the viewpoints of others. Preschoolers although can imitate others and assume the perspective of others, they still do not understand that others have different perspectives from their own. Egocentric thought takes two forms: the lack of awareness that others see things from a different physical perspective and the failure to realize that others may hold thoughts, feelings, and points of view that differ from theirs. Egocentric thinking is what is behind children's lack of concern over their overt gestures, nonverbal behavior and some ridiculous comments made inappropriately leading to several moments of fun and the impact it has on others. However, their development of symbolic function permits quicker and more effective thinking as they are freed from the limitations of sensorimotor learning. According to Piaget, children in the preoperational stage engage in intuitive thought for the first time, actively applying rudimentary reasoning skills to the acquisition of world knowledge. Yet, preschoolers are unable to consider all available information about a stimulus. Instead, they focus on superficial, obvious elements that are within their sight (e.g., if a child's father arrives and it rains soon after, the child ponders if at all his father has brought the rain). These external elements come to dominate preschoolers thinking, leading to inaccuracy in thought. To Piaget, the root of this belief is centration, a key element, and limitation, of the thinking of children in the preoperational period. *Centration* is the process of concentrating on one limited aspect of a stimulus and ignoring other aspects.[2,11] Children during this phase rapidly progress from two-word utterances to longer, more sophisticated expressions that reflect their growing vocabularies and emerging grasp of grammar. The development of linguistic abilities is affected by socioeconomic status. The result can be lowered linguistic—and, ultimately, academic—performance by vulnerable children in poverty. Lev Vygotsky's theory proposed that the nature and progress of children's cognitive development are dependent on the children's social and cultural context and there is evidence accumulating to emphasize this fact across the world.[19]

Emotional Development: Preschool

Preschoolers are quite good at several component skills of emotional competence. They begin to express a range of diverse emotions as they learn the rules of emotional expression and gain the ways necessary for appropriate and effective expression and regulation of emotion through daily interactions with their parents, including how parents react to their emotional displays.[33] Explicit awareness of emotion regulation strategies likely emerges between ages 3 and 5 years.[34] Affective perspective taking, particularly the identification of emotions in others that differ from one's feelings in those situations, also allows the child to begin to take another's cognitive perspective. This capacity of "theory of mind[35] further evolves in order to bring a more elaborate understanding in more than one perspective without centration." This allows them to conceive of a situation from another's point of view, in addition to their own. They are beginning to be able to delay impulsive responses in rule-governed ways. Children independently attempt to regulate their display of emotion without adult support and 3- and 4-year-old who have developed an understanding of appropriate, effective strategies are well poised to deploy these strategies to manage the frustrations of a school classroom.[36]

Social Development: Preschool

According to Erik Erikson,[5] preschool-age children initially are in the autonomy-versus-shame-and-doubt stage (18 months to 3 years) in which they develop independence and mastery over their physical and social worlds or feel shame, self-doubt, and unhappiness. Later, in the initiative-versus guilt stage (ages 3 to 6 years), preschool-age children face conflicts between the desire to act independently and the guilt that comes from the unintended consequences of their actions. Preschoolers' self-concepts are formed partly from their own understanding and evaluation of their characters, partly from their parents' behavior toward them, and partly from cultural influences. The social role of one's gender identity roughly emerges from 3 to 4 years of age. The strong gender expectations held by preschoolers are explained in different ways by different theorists. One of the earliest theories on development of *Gender Identity evolving in to Gender Constancy* was proposed by Kohlberg.[37] Some point to genetic factors as evidence for a biological explanation of gender expectations. Freud's psychoanalytic theories use a framework based on the subconscious. Social learning theorists focus on environmental influences, including parents, teachers, peers, and the media, while cognitive theorists propose that children form gender schemas, cognitive frameworks that organize information that the children gather about gender.[1,2] As per *Mildred Parten's* social aspects of play **(Table 7)**, older preschoolers

TABLE 7: Parten's social aspects of play.

Type of play	*Description*
Parallel play	Children use same kind of toys in an imitable manner at the same time but do not interact with each other. Typical during the early preschool years and toddlerhood
Onlooker play	Children just observe others at play but not initiate a participation. They may look quietly, and they may make comments of encouragement or advice. Common among preschoolers and can be helpful when a child is inclined to join a play group
Associative play	Two or more children in sync will be sharing or borrowing toys or materials, although they do not cooperate for a same goal. They will enjoy each other's company and play in their own way
Cooperative play	Children genuinely play with one another, taking turns, making exchanges, following a common theme/goal by playing games, or by competing with one another

Source: Adapted from 'Development Across the Lifespan—Robert S Feldman', 8th edition, Chapter 8 – Social and Personality development in the Preschool Age.[1]

engage in more constructive play than functional play. They also engage in more associative and cooperative play than younger preschoolers, who do more parallel and onlooker playing.[38,39] Aggression, which involves intentional harm to another person, begins to emerge in the preschool years. As children age and improve their language and social skills, acts of aggression typically decline in frequency and intensity. Albert Bandura[9] and his colleagues illustrated the power of models in a classic study of preschool-age children to demonstrate *Social Learning.* One group of children watched a film of an adult playing aggressively and violently with a *Bobo doll* (a large and inflated plastic clown designed as a punching bag for children that always returns to an upright position after being pushed down). In comparison, children in another group watched a film of an adult playing sedately with a set of "Tinker toys." Later, the preschool-age children were allowed to play with several toys, which included both the "Bobo doll" and the "Tinker toys." But first, the children were led to feel frustrated by being refused the opportunity to play with a favorite toy. As predicted by social learning theory, the preschool-age children modeled the behavior of the adults. Those who had seen the aggressive model playing with the Bobo doll were remarkably more aggressive than those who had watched the calm, nonaggressive model of playing with the "Tinker toys."[40] Piaget and Kohlberg believed that the moral conduct of preschool-age children is characterized by a belief in external, unchangeable rules of conduct and sure-immediate punishment for all misdeeds which, in turn, is largely influenced by parenting and culture as well. This, in turn, leads to many preschoolers believing in *Immanent Justice Reasoning*, the framework where prior deeds will determine a justification of punishment.[13]

Lifespan Development: School Going Age

Physical Development: School Going Age

During middle childhood, children develop many types of skills that earlier they could not perform well. For instance, most school-age children can readily learn to dance, roller skate, swim, and skip rope. Further, there is now an increased coordination of fine motor skills as well. Typing at a computer keyboard. Playing an instrument. Writing in cursive handwriting with pen and pencil. Drawing detailed pictures and doodles. These are just some of the accomplishments that depend on improvements in fine motor coordination that occur during early and middle childhood. Children of 6- and 7-year-old can tie their shoes and fasten buttons; by the age of 8 years, they can use each hand independently; and by 11- and 12-year-old, they can manipulate objects with almost as much capability as expected from an adult. One reason for advances in fine motor skills is that the amount of myelination in the brain that increases significantly between the ages of 6 and 8 years.[41] In part, growth is genetically determined, but societal factors such as economic status, dietary habits, nutrition, and disease also contribute significantly. Cultural expectations appear to underlie most gross motor skill differences between boys and girls.

Cognitive Development: School-going Age

According to Piaget,[11] school-age children enter the "Concrete Operational" period and for the first time become capable of applying logical thought processes to concrete problems. The stage is marked by the achievement of conservation, reduced egocentrism, and centration. Children at the level of concrete operations can consider two aspects of a problem simultaneously and have multiple facets of a situational perception. In their social interactions, they consider not only what they are saying but also the needs of the listener. When they perform conservation experiments, they consider not only the most obvious change but also a compensating change. The coordination of two perspectives forms the basis of both their social and scientific thinking.[7] According to information processing approaches, children's intellectual development in the school years can be attributed to substantial increases in memory capacity and the sophistication of the "programs" children can handle.[2] The language development of children in the school years is also considerably sophisticated, with improvements in vocabulary, syntax, and pragmatics. Children learn to control their behavior through linguistic strategies, and they learn more effectively by seeking clarification when they need it. Bilingualism often seen in India can be beneficial in the school years. Children who are taught all subjects in the first language, with simultaneous instruction in English, also appear to experience few deficits and attain several linguistic and cognitive advantages.[42]

Emotional Development: School-going Age

By middle childhood, children begin to imbibe a set of expectations for themselves and can generate complex emotions such as pride and shame independent of adult prompting. Middle childhood is a period of rapid growth in emotional self-regulation. The capacity to self-regulate is made possible by greater representational and cognitive abilities allowing school-age children to anticipate the consequence of their choices.[33] As their involvement in sports, music, and other activities increases, they may worry about their performance in athletic games or recitals. This increased expectation from other's perception may, in turn, leads to increased presentation of anxiety issues in children of this age. Psychodynamic concepts talk about modulation of emotion by new cognitive structures during latency was thought to occur because of a signal of anxiety triggered by perceived dangers concerning bodily injury. At times, the revival of behavioral separation anxiety through any object loss can present with behavioral reactions/conversions that may present in form of regression. Later school avoidance and school reluctance, which are forms of separation anxiety, or dissociative episodes after any distress become the major features of manifest anxiety seen in the clinic.[43]

Social Development: School-going Age

In addition to language skills, conversational skills continue to develop during middle childhood. Children become more competent in their use of pragmatics, the rules governing the use of language to communicate in each social setting. According to Erikson, children in the middle childhood years are in the industry-versus-inferiority stage, focusing on achieving competence and responding to a wide range of personal challenges.[5] Children in these years are developing self-esteem; those with chronically low self-esteem can become trapped in a cycle of failure in which low self-esteem feeds on itself by producing low expectations and poor performance. According to Kohlberg (refer to **Table 4**), people pass from preconventional morality (motivated by rewards and punishments), through conventional morality (motivated by social reference), to postconventional morality (motivated by a sense of universal moral principles).[7] Children's friendships also display progress through status hierarchies, and their understanding of friendship passes through stages, from an initial focus on mutual liking and time spent together, through to the consideration of personality features and the benefits that friendship provides, to finally an appreciation of intimacy and loyalty.[44]

Lifespan Development: Adolescence

Physical Development: Adolescence

The adolescent years are characterized by a physical growth spurt, which for girls begins around age of 10 years, and for boys, around the age of 12 years. Puberty begins in girls at around age of 11 years and in boys at around age of 13 years. The physical changes of puberty often have psychological impacts, such as an accentuation in self-esteem and self-awareness, along with conflicts and uncertainty about sexuality. Premature pubertal changes have different effects on boys and girls. For boys, being bigger and more developed can lead to increased athleticism, greater popularity, and a more positive self-concept. For girls, this can lead to increased popularity and an enhanced social life but also insecurity over their bodies, which all of a sudden look different from everyone else's. In the short term, late maturation can be a physical and social setback that affects boys' self-image. Girls who develop pubertal changes with a delay may suffer neglect by their peers, but ultimately, they appear to suffer no major issues and may even benefit.[1,2] Excessive concern about obesity can cause some adolescents, especially girls, to develop an eating disorder, such as anorexia nervosa or bulimia which are classically known for their body image disturbances.

Cognitive Development: Adolescence

Changes in the brain give rise to rapid cognitive growth of adolescence, especially changes in the prefrontal cortex. These changes permit sophisticated thought, evaluation, and judgment, enabling the complex intellectual achievements of adolescence. Adolescence coincides with Piaget's formal operations period of development when people begin to engage in abstract thought and scientific reasoning.[7,11] By bringing formal principles of logic to be applied on problems they face, adolescents can consider them in the abstract rather than only in concrete terms. They can experiment their understanding by systematically carrying out hypothetical experiments on problems and situations and observing what their experimental "interventions" bring about. Adolescents' emerging cognitive abilities may also promote a form of *adolescent egocentrism*, a self-absorption related to their developing sense of themselves as independent identities. This can make it hard for adolescents to accept criticism and tolerate authority figures. Adolescents may play to an *imaginary audience* of critical observers, and they may develop *personal fables,*[7] the view that what happens to them is unique, exceptional, and not relatable to others. According to information processing approaches, cognitive development during adolescence is gradual and quantitative, encompassing improvements in memory capacity, mental faculties, metacognition, and other aspects of cognition. Adolescents also grow in metacognition, which permits them to monitor their thought processes and accurately make sense of their cognitive capacities.

Emotional Development: Adolescence

Adolescence creates a rapid rise in openness to experience, resulting in significant increase in higher rejection sensitivity, negative emotionality, greater sensitivity to peer-related social interactions, greater reward-seeking and greater commitment to long-term and socially rewarding goals.[33] While these changes create a need to develop the skills necessary for greater independence from the family and the establishment of developmentally important peer and romantic relationships, they are also hypothesized to create greater risk for emotional and behavioral dysregulation. As adolescents begin to assert their autonomy and broaden their horizon, they are at increasing vulnerability for emotional breakdowns, even from "drama" with friends, relationships, and expectations of teachers and coaches, and mostly with parents. Thus, it is not rare to see parents of teenagers often being clueless as to how their emotional outburst be managed. In addition, adolescents' increased autonomy means that they are also likely to be more responsible for regulating their affective responses.[45] Lastly, adolescents' greater emotionality could also be contributed by cognitive developments that render them more vulnerable to self-consciousness and apprehension as well as more ability to empathize with and, hence, take on the emotional experiences of others.[46]

Social Development: Adolescence

Adolescents' capacity to reason abstractly, emboldened by their use of formal operations, leads to a change in their daily behavior. Whereas earlier they may have unquestioningly accepted rules and explanations set out for them, their increased abstract reasoning abilities may lead them to question their parents and other authority figures far more rebelliously.[7] Developments in abstract thinking also led to greater idealism, which may make adolescents impatient with imperfections in institutions, such as schools and the government. According to Erik Erikson,[5] adolescents are in the identity versus-identity-confusion stage, seeking to discover their individuality and identity. They may become confused and exhibit irrational reactions, and they may rely for help and information more on friends and peers than on adults. Adolescents' quest for autonomy often brings confusion and tension to their relationships with their parents, but the actual "generation gap" between parents' and teenagers' attitudes is usually not very significant. Peers are vital during adolescence because they provide social comparison and reference groups against which to judge social success. Relationships among adolescents are characterized by the need for affiliation. During adolescence, boys and girls begin to spend time together in groups. In general, segregation between people of different races and ethnicities increases in middle and late adolescence, even in schools with a diverse student body. Degrees of popularity during adolescence include popular and controversial teenagers (the notorious and popularity) and also neglected and rejected adolescents (the less popular). Peer pressure is not a small phenomenon. Adolescents conform to their peers in areas in which they feel their peers are experts and to adults in areas of adult expertise. As adolescents grow in confidence, their conformity to both peers and adults decrease. During adolescence, dating and finding partners in romance, leads to intimacy, entertainment, and prestige. Achieving psychological intimacy, which is difficult at first, becomes easier as adolescents mature, gain confidence, and take commitments to relationships and fidelity seriously.[2,46] For most adolescents, masturbation is often the first step into sexuality. The age of first intercourse, which is now in the teens, has declined as the double standard has faded and the norm of permissiveness with affection has gained ground.[47]

SUMMARY AND CONCLUSION

To summarize, development in all domains occur depending upon the age and stage of the child/adolescent and the same is depicted in **Table 8**.

In conclusion, an individual's development is a lifelong and dynamic process that unfolds across multiple interconnected domains—physical, cognitive, emotional, social, and moral. Growth in one area often influences and strengthens progress in others, highlighting the importance of a holistic approach to nurturing potential. Physical development provides the foundation for exploration and independence, while cognitive growth enhances thinking, problem-solving, and decision-making skills. Emotional and social development shape relationships, self-awareness, empathy, and the ability to navigate

TABLE 8: Summary of lifespan development (based upon the authors understanding of the topic).

Developmental stage	*Physical development*	*Cognitive development*	*Emotional development*	*Sociocultural development*
Infancy (Birth till 3 years)	Cephalocaudal, proximodistal development. Hierarchical integration. Simple skills are integrated into more complex systems. Exploratory activity of children helps them to interact with environment and help motor skill advancements	Constructivist theory by Piaget talks about sensorimotor cognitive stages, evolve through six substages culminating in the development of symbolic thought. Prelinguistic communications occur. Nativists like Chomsky mentions the existence of "Language-Acquisition Device" that prepares language emergence	Basic emotions of contentment, distress and interest can be observed by 2 months. Further differentiation of above emotions into joy, surprise, sadness, disgust, and anger evolves from 6 months	Social referencing begins with emergence of "Theory of Mind." Attachment patterns are initiated, and formation of secure base occurs by 2–3 years. The psychosocial stage of "Trust versus Mistrust" occurs with a development of virtue of hope. Then, the crisis of "Autonomy versus Shame" begins with development of will
Preschool (3–6 years)	Rapid brain growth occurs in this period with lateralization and specialization, thus further learning of skilled fine motor activities like writing, drawing, climbing, etc.	Preoperational stage begins with ability to engage in early logical thinking. But, reasoning is transductive, while thinking is egocentric with centration and lack of conservation.	Diverse emotions emerge with cultural context governing the rules of expression. Explicit awareness of emotion regulation emerges from 3 years	Children face the conflict between desire to act independently and the guilt that come from unintended consequences. More elaborate cooperative

Contd...

Contd...

Developmental stage	*Physical development*	*Cognitive development*	*Emotional development*	*Sociocultural development*
		Environment influences language development with beginning of "private speech" as per Vygotsky		play emerges with active social learning, within the zone of proximal development
School going (7–12 years)	Increased strength and highly coordinated motor skills that culminate in several accomplishments in performance of arts and play behaviors. Sophistication of executive functions begin with improved inhibition, control and speed of coordination attributed to rapid myelination from 6 years. Cultural expectations may create variations in skill development	Concrete operational stage of Piaget begins with emergence of conservation, increased use of scientific inductive reasoning. Substantial improvement in language and vocabulary with rapid learning of languages. Shift from preconventional to conventional morality occurs leading to more adherence to rules and response to rewards/punishments	Complex emotions of pride and shame emerge. Capacity to self-regulate between with emotional self-perception and perception in others emerge, leading to anticipation of consequences of one's actions. More understanding of other's emotions occurs leading to expectations and fears of judgment. More propensity to have multiple anxiety provoking situations	More competent use of pragmatic communication with social stimulation. The psychosocial conflict of "Industry versus Inferiority" with emerging virtue of competence. Self-esteem develops with their competence which can influence friendship and status hierarchies. Early understanding of loyalty and intimacy emerges
Adolescence (12 years and above)	Growth spurt with puberty occurs marking significant changes in physique with gender variations. Greater need for nutrition influenced by social status occurs. Sexual maturity occurs with overwhelming changes in states of arousal and regulation of autonomic systems	Cortical changes emerge with capacity for formal operational stage. Adolescents have increased hypothetico-deductive reasoning, leading to more need for experimentation. Challenges of adolescent egocentrism, imaginary audience, and personal fables. Metacognitive abilities emerge with initiation of self-awareness and introspective abilities	Nascent prefrontal cortex coupled with increased need for experimentation, leads to constant reward seeking engagement and greater vulnerability for emotional and behavioral dysregulation. More ability to empathize with others can create intense emotional group affect with peers	Psychosocial crisis of "Identity versus role-confusion" emerges which can continue for several years till one's fidelity is found. Increased need for peer validation and loyalty paves way for need of psychological intimacy. Quest for autonomy brings conflicts with authority figures. Understanding of morality may evolve into postconventional morality and lesser regard for rules within one's cultural context

complex social environments. Moral development guides values, ethics, and responsible behavior.

In addition, neurosciences approach at present are actively assessing the quantitative changes in brain cortical maturity and connectivity, that can be accounted from "Gene-environment" influences, which may help to identify and delineate various systems. These systems can integrate in various hierarchy to create behaviors that are explained within the context of sociocultural meanings and motivations. The more metaphysical explanations from psychodynamic and humanistic "free-will" would thus add to these contexts to create a rich understanding of actions that drive one's lifespan development. But, in the end, it is wise to always remember the "Blind men and the elephant" analogy while bringing together various theories of development and thus to not fall into the trap of trying to grasp a complex process using a single perspective and continue to assimilate while we concurrently accommodate new knowledge holistically.

REFERENCES

1. Feldman R. (2011). Life span development. [online] Available from http://docmerit.s3.amazonaws.com/uploads/document/40796/1707297268non.pdf [Last accessed November, 2025].
2. Berk LE. Development through the Lifespan. London: Sage Publications; 2022.
3. Humphreys KL, Zeanah CH, Scheeringa MS. Infant Development: The First 3 Years of Life. In: Tasman A, Kay J, Lieberman JA, First MB, Riba MB (Eds). Psychiatry, 1st edition. United States: Wiley; 2015. pp. 134-58.
4. Elkatawneh H. (2013). Freud's Psycho-Sexual Stages of Development. [online] Available from http://dx.doi.org/10.2139/ssrn.2364215. [Last accessed November, 2025].
5. Orenstein GA, Lewis L. Eriksons stages of psychosocial development. In: StatPearls [Internet]. Treasure Island (FL): StatPearls Publishing; 2022.
6. DeRobertis EM, Bland AM. Lifespan human development and "the humanistic perspective": A contribution toward inclusion. Human Psychol. 2020;48(1):3-27.
7. Crain W. Theories of Development: Concepts and Applications, 7th edition. United Kingdom: Routledge; 2024.
8. Schneider SM, Morris EK. A History of the Term Radical Behaviorism: From Watson to Skinner | Perspectives on Behavior Science. Behav Analyst. 1987;10:27-39.
9. Bandura A. Social foundations of thought and action. Englewood Cliffs, NJ. 1986;1986(23-28):2.
10. Piaget J. Piaget's Theory. Handbook of Child Psychology. New York: Wiley. 1983. pp. 41-102.
11. Loewen S. Exceptional intellectual performance: a neo-Piagetian perspective. High Ability Studies. 2006;17(2):159-81.
12. McNamee S. Moral Behaviour, Moral Development and Motivation. J Moral Edu. 1977;7(1): 27-31.
13. Kohlberg L, Hersh RH. Moral development: A review of the theory. Theory Pract. 1977;16(2):53-9.
14. Charlesworth WR, Costall A, Ghiselin MT. Darwin and Developmental Psychology: 100 Years Later. Hum Develop. 2009;29(1):1-35.
15. Richard KJ, Sjölander S. Obituary: Konrad Zacharias Lorenz, 7 November 1903 – 27 February 1989. Biogr Mems Fell R Soc. 1992;38:209-28.
16. Tzschentke B, Plagemann A. Imprinting and critical periods in early development. World's Poultry Sci J. 2006;62(4):626-37.
17. Dykas MJ, Cassidy J. Attachment and the processing of social information across the life span: Theory and evidence. Psychol Bull. 2011;137(1):19-46.
18. Verenikina I. Vygotsky's Socio-Cultural Theory and the Zone of Proximal Development. Facul Social Sci Papers (Arch). 2003:4-14.
19. Daneshfar S, Moharami M. Dynamic Assessment in Vygotsky's Sociocultural Theory: Origins and Main Concepts. JLTR. 2018;9(3):600.
20. Wexler BE. Brain and Culture: Neurobiology, Ideology, and Social Change. Cambridge, Massachusetts: MIT Press; 2008.
21. Jessell TM, Sanes JR. Development: The decade of the developing brain. Curr Opin Neurobiol. 2000;10(5):599-611.
22. Munakata Y, Casey BJ, Diamond A. Developmental cognitive neuroscience: progress and potential. Trends Cogn Sci. 2004;8(3):122-8.

23. Thelen E. Dynamic Systems Theory and the Complexity of Change. Psychoanalytic Dialogues. 2005;15(2):255-83.
24. Corbetta D, Snapp-Childs W. Seeing and touching: the role of sensory-motor experience on the development of infant reaching. Infant Behav Develop. 2009;32(1):44-58.
25. Bolhuis JJ, Tattersall I, Chomsky N, Berwick RC. How Could Language Have Evolved? PLoS Biol. 2014;12(8):e1001934.
26. Lewis MD. Cognition-Emotion Feedback and the Self-Organization of Developmental Paths. Hum Develop. 2010;38(2):71-102.
27. Schmitow C, Stenberg G. Social referencing in 10-month-old infants. Eur J Develop Psychol. 2013;10(5):533-45.
28. Evans T, Whittingham K, Boyd R. What helps the mother of a preterm infant become securely attached, responsive and well-adjusted? Infant Behav Develop. 2012;35(1):1-11.
29. Meltzoff AN, Waismeyer A, Gopnik A. Learning about causes from people: observational causal learning in 24-month-old infants. Develop Psychol. 2012;48(5):1215.
30. Largo RH, Fischer JE, Rousson V. Neuromotor development from kindergarten age to adolescence: developmental course and variability. Swiss Med Weekly. 2003;133(13-14):193.
31. Scharoun SM, Bryden PJ. Hand preference, performance abilities, and hand selection in children. Front Psychol. 2014;5:82.
32. Dundas EM, Plaut DC, Behrmann M. The joint development of hemispheric lateralization for words and faces. J Exper Psychol General. 2013;142(2):348.
33. Tasman A, Kay J, Lieberman JA, First MB, Riba M. Psychiatry, 2 Volume Set. New Jersey: John Wiley & Sons; 2015.
34. Denham SA, Kalb S, Way E, Warren-Khot H, Rhoades BL, Bassett HH. Social and emotional information processing in preschoolers: indicator of early school success? Early Child Dev Care. 2013;183(5):667-88.
35. Wellman HM, Cross D, Watson J. Meta-Analysis of Theory-of-Mind Development: The Truth about False Belief. Child Dev. 2001;72(3):655-84.
36. Blair C, Diamond A. Biological processes in prevention and intervention: The promotion of self-regulation as a means of preventing school failure. Develop Psychopathol. 2008;20(3):899-911.
37. Ruble DN, Taylor LJ, Cyphers L, Greulich FK, Lurye LE, Shrout PE. The role of gender constancy in early gender development. Child Develop. 2007;78(4):1121-36.
38. Parten MB. Social participation among pre-school children. J Abnorm Soc Psychol. 1932;27(3):243.
39. Dyer S, Moneta GB. Frequency of parallel, associative, and cooperative play in British children of different socioeconomic status. Soc Behav Personal Int J. 2006;34(5):587-92.
40. Bandura A, Grusec JE, Menlove FL. Vicarious extinction of avoidance behavior. J Personal Soc Psychol. 1967;5(1):16.
41. Cratty BJ. (1979). Perceptual and motor development in infants and children. [online] Available from https://eric.ed.gov/?id=ED164540 [Last accessed 16 November, 2025].
42. Hoff E. Interpreting the early language trajectories of children from low-SES and language minority homes: implications for closing achievement gaps. Develop Psychol. 2013;49(1):4.
43. Shapiro T, Perry R. Latency Revisited: The Age 7 Plus or Minus 1. Psychoanal Study Child. 1976;31(1):79-105.
44. Damon W, Hart D. (1991). Self-Understanding in Childhood and Adolescence. CUP Archive; 1991. [online] Available from https://books.google.com/books?hl=en&lr=&id=jO4zAAAAIAAJ&oi=fnd&pg=PR7&dq=Damon,+W.,+%26+Hart,+D.+(1988).+Self-understanding+in+childhood+and+adolescence.+New+York:+ Cambridge+University+Press.&ots=UBEyZPVdU_&sig=Rf_oZjLeVy_FOUxNPIwS_m8tBvI [Last accessed 16 November, 2025].
45. Steinberg L. Cognitive and affective development in adolescence. Trends Cogn Sci. 2005;9(2):69-74.
46. Nelson EE, Leibenluft E, McClure EB, Pine DS. The social re-orientation of adolescence: a neuroscience perspective on the process and its relation to psychopathology. Psychol Med. 2005;35(2):163-74.
47. Centers for Disease Control and Prevention (CDC). Trends in HIV-and STD-related risk behaviors among high school students–United States, 1991-2007. MMWR Morb Mortal Wkly Rep. 2008;57(30):817-22.

Assessment and Formulation: History Taking, Clinical Assessment, and Case Formulation, Interacting with the Child and Family

Eesha Sharma, Shekhar Seshadri

INTRODUCTION

A thorough clinical assessment is one of the major pillars of child psychiatry. No diagnostic laboratory test or psychometric test gives as much information about the child and family as spending time with them, using clinical skills in a developmentally appropriate and comprehensive manner covering all aspects of history and mental status examination (MSE). The quality of clinical assessment also sets the stage for long-term therapeutic relationships between the clinician and the child, as well as the clinician and the family. For budding child psychiatrists, it is important to hone skills in establishing rapport with the child, developmentally appropriate interviewing skills, eliciting information on developmental, personal, past, family, and presenting history, and case formulation.

This chapter will first delve into the conceptual underpinnings of clinical assessment in child psychiatry. These would be concepts that determine why child psychiatrists do what they do. This will be followed by areas of clinical assessment for both history and mental status examination. The utility of structured assessment tools will be discussed towards the end of the chapter. Readers are encouraged to look at the references at the end of the chapter for further reading. Throughout the chapter, the term "child" is used whenever the text is relevant for ages 0–11 years, i.e., young children and preadolescents; the term "adolescents" is used for ages 12–17 years.

OBJECTIVES OF CLINICAL ASSESSMENT

Objectives of clinical assessment can vary depending upon the context of a child's clinical presentation. Consider the following presentations—a 15-year-old boy presenting around the time of school examinations to get disability certification for a specific learning disorder; a 6-year-old presenting with speech delay; a 17-year-old presenting with long-standing irritability, self-harm behavior, and sleep disturbance. The emphasis on developmental history, psychometric assessments, and building a therapeutic alliance is likely to differ across these presentations. When approaching them the clinician needs to make an active decision about what the specific objectives of clinical assessment in each case will be. Broadly speaking, four key objectives can be listed that apply in varying degrees to almost all presentations in child psychiatry. These include case formulation, therapeutic alliance, identification of multidisciplinary roles, and understanding the nature and impact of previous interventions.[1] Case formulation, therapeutic alliance and eliciting information about previous interventions will be dealt with in greater depth in the upcoming sections. Here, we look at the role of multidisciplinary teams in child psychiatry. Multidisciplinary teams are vital in child psychiatry. Without the able contribution of, say, a clinical psychologist and a psychiatric social worker, a child psychiatrist may find it difficult to comprehensively assess developmental or learning issues, or to factor in myriad psychosocial and systemic factors and interventions relevant for a given child, respectively.

DIFFERENCE BETWEEN ASSESSMENTS IN ADULT AND CHILD PSYCHIATRY

Children are Generally not "Self-referred"

Generally, children and adolescents are not self-referred. Parents or caregivers note certain behavioral changes or concerns that make them seek a consultation. Unlike adult psychiatry consultations, the "problem" is not defined by the "patient". This one fact has a major role to play in the first consultation, as well as the long-term therapeutic alliance. It is the onus of the child psychiatrist to bear this in mind, build a mutually agreeable context with the child or adolescent, and then turn the consultation and treatment into a largely child-centric process. An honest, open, and unhurried approach usually aids the child or adolescent to gradually warm up to the situation. It is alright for the child psychiatrist to spend a few consultations in getting to know the child and building the common context. Even though parents may feel anxious and impatient, they need to be educated about the key role that the child's positive involvement will play in the process.

With some adolescent consultations, it is possible that they themselves identify, say, academic or internalizing difficulties, and, interestingly, in some of these situations, the parents may not agree with the need for a consultation. Here, the child psychiatrist must be the adolescent's advocate and work with the parents' knowledge, attitude and practices. So, unlike adult psychiatry, child psychiatry practice needs specific skills to enable collaborative participation of the child or adolescent and family members in the evaluation and treatment process. Nonparticipation of either party would impact long-term positive outcomes.

Externalizing Problems are a More Common Reason for Referral

Parents or caregivers initiate referrals based on what behaviors they observe in the child or adolescent. Visible behavioral changes are most often characteristic of externalizing presentations that can be seen in a spectrum of childhood psychiatric disorders, including neurodevelopmental, mood, anxiety, and even psychotic disorders. It is important that externalizing presentations do not curtail the evaluation for internalizing problems in children and adolescents. If one considers how very young children express distress, it is apparent that, e.g, crying which can often be accompanied by disruption and mild aggression, can result from all sorts of distress that the child may be experiencing. This behavior pattern can be seen when children fight over toys, or when they are scared to leave their parents and go to school, or when a stranger approaches them, and so on. Psychological distress in young children is typically expressed externally and serves the essential purpose of keeping the parents involved in the child's life and garner their support for coregulation that ultimately paves the way for the development of socioemotional regulation. As children grow older, their expressions of distress in externalizing or internalizing patterns may follow variable trajectories. For the child psychiatrist, it is important to keep a developmental lens while evaluating for the range of diagnostic possibilities.

Neurodevelopmental Disorders are the Most Common Underlying Reasons for Referral

Depressive and anxiety disorders are the most common mental health problems in adults.

Among children, and even adolescents, neurodevelopmental disorders, either as the primary concerns for presentation or as the key underlying vulnerabilities, are common. Whatever behavioral concerns the parents report, it is important to gather a detailed developmental history, and evaluate the possibility of the behavior resulting from cognitive, language, and social or emotional developmental deficits. In young children, developmental deficits may be apparent as a gross delay in observable milestones. Among adolescents, developmental deficits may be more apparent from a "life skills" perspective. While they may not have a history of milestone delay, an assessment of their current functioning and behavioral repertoire may indicate difficulties with problem-solving, emotional regulation, coping with stress, time management, social skills, etc.

CASE VIGNETTE 1

To illustrate neurodevelopmental underpinnings in adolescents, let us consider the difficulties that Ajay, a 16-year-old boy, presented with. His mother had brought him with concerns of excessive mobile use, a declining interest in academic tasks and irritability in the last 1 year. The mother said that Ajay would spend the better part of his day on the phone and got irritated anytime she objected to his excessive use. When mother asked about his declining academics, he would say he "will do it" but then in the past several months he did not seem to be putting in any consistent effort, rather he would keep procrastinating. During evaluation, Ajay's childhood developmental history did not reveal any gross delays. However, from around the age of 6–7 years, he was known to be a "shy" child, generally reserved and having some difficulties in adapting to increasing grade levels at school. Teachers would point out that he would not participate in extracurricular activities, however, they were supportive and would allow him to engage in tasks that he was comfortable with. Academic issues became increasingly prominent since class 7 or 8. His marks started to decline but he would attend school regularly and follow through on all classwork and homework. He managed to write his class 10 board examinations. The mother had to take leave from her place of work, and sit with him for months, helping him learn subjects "by rote". Now Ajay was in class 11. He was finding it difficult not only to cope up with the amount of study material in the science stream that he was pursuing, but also to conceptually understand the study materials. Mother would keep asking him to spend more time studying "to catch up", but Ajay was becoming increasingly withdrawn from studying. Ajay was also noted to have difficulties with his peers. Mother said that he never had any fights, but his peers generally treated him "like a young boy" explaining him things and guiding him. She felt that he was fortunate to have such friends. She also noted that it was difficult for him to make decisions about managing his time, about undertaking small responsibilities for household chores, and had little clarity about what career path he wanted to take. During the clinical evaluation, while Ajay was cooperative and spoke relevantly, it was noted that his responses were brief and concrete. As the evaluation progressed, it became apparent that Ajay's cognitive and socioemotional skills were not adequately developed to face all the challenges that were coming his way. As a result, there was significant avoidance as far as academics were concerned, and given his limited extracurricular interests, "having nothing much to do" he resorted to using the mobile phone for games and general browsing social media and YouTube. While he was aware of his difficulties, he was unable to think of any solutions. He denied feeling depressed and did not have signs and symptoms to indicate any mental health disorder.

Clearly, Ajay was struggling developmentally, but the parental concerns were about the changes in his behavior. Rather than a behavioral modification, limit setting approach, Ajay would benefit more from a developmental intervention focusing on cognitive, socioemotional and academic skills. Perhaps he would also need guidance on academic choices and future planning.

Need for Information from Multiple Sources

Traditional psychiatric teaching emphasizes the importance of an ideographic phenomenological approach that places an individual's self-reported experience at the center of the diagnosis making process. For children and adolescents, this may not always be ideal. While a child-centric focus is critical in planning and conducting interventions, in order to comprehensively understand the presentation, information from multiple sources must be sought. This could include both parents, grandparents, schoolteachers, and any significant others who know the child well and have observed the concerning behaviors. This is important since children may not be adequately developed in verbally processing and reporting their mental states and experiences. There is a need to record the child's description of the problem, alongside gathering what other people's observations and interpretations of the child's behaviors are in order to then put all these information together and make clinical interpretations. While it may be a time-taking process, it is important that the child psychiatrist openly discusses the importance and relevance of these endeavors with the family and proceed.

Therapeutic Alliance with both Child and Caregivers

Children's mental health problems have significant contributions from both individual and environmental factors. Treatment almost always includes working with the child and family separately. Therefore, treatment goals and therapeutic alliance must be specifically built with both the child and the family. The child psychiatrist needs to retain objectivity and be able to join with both the child and the family, even in the presence of noncorroborative information, or parent-child relational difficulties.

Review and Revision of Treatment Goals and Case Formulation

Development can have a significant impact on symptom manifestations, on the child's skills, on their ability to talk about and understand their difficulties, and on participation in treatment. Over time, environmental factors may also undergo significant changes such that a revision in case formulation is mandated with a reidentification of predisposing, precipitating, perpetuating, and protective factors. A child who had come with significant hyperactivity and difficulties settling down in school at the age of 7 years, may now, at 15 years, have a very different presentation, largely determined by bullying experiences that are mediated by the child's social skill deficits and impulsivity.

Homotypic and heterotypic continuities determined by developmental psychopathology can be observed over age and require the child psychiatrist to be open to reconceptualization and formulation informed by the changing factors.

Emphasis on a Strength-based Approach

Earlier a point was made about the commonality of neurodevelopmental factors in child psychiatric presentations. Whereas neurodevelopmental disorders are defined by the presence of developmental delays and functional deficits, it is important to take a strength-based approach. For example, in a child with a specific learning disorder, the focus is not on how the child cannot learn, but rather on what learning modalities work for the child. The latter needs to be identified and enabled in the child's learning environment. Similarly, in adolescents presenting with mood disorders and parent-child attachment problems, the evidence-informed attachment-based family therapy lays emphasis on strengthening intact aspects of the parent-child relationship that can be honed to support the adolescent in their recovery from the mood disorder.

A strength-based approach not only capitalizes on the capabilities that can be therapeutically utilized, but it also aids in the preservation and nurturing of positive familial relationships. Families can respond quite variably to the occurrence of mental health issues in children and adolescents. They may even go through a grief-like reaction with prominent denial and anger that impact relationships, treatment seeking, and follow-up. In such situations, orienting toward strengths and abilities can be helpful in maintaining hope and therapeutic alliance.

CONCEPTUAL UNDERPINNINGS

Child Friendly Space

Attending formal spaces like a doctor's clinic can be quite intimidating, especially for young children. They may not have any prior experience of such a space, and may not know either what to expect from the space or what they are expected to do. For a genuine interaction with the child where his strengths and difficulties will be observable, the child must feel comfortable. Therefore, the concept of a child-friendly space. A child-friendly space is characterized by a sense of familiarity, easy access to and provisions for children of all ages and abilities, and capable of holding children's interest. When children enter the space, they must "see" and "hear" things that look and sound familiar and that hold their interest. Often parents engage children with cartoons, or story books, or books with animal and object pictures, etc. The clinic space could be populated with similar content to give children a sense of familiarity and make them feel interested and engaged. These would complement the clinician's age-appropriate engagement skills.

Sitting and waiting is not becoming of children. They like to move around and explore. A child-friendly space must have enough room for the same such that their natural activity and exploratory behaviors can be supported and also become important observations for the clinical assessment. In addition, amenities for care and feeding of babies and children of different abilities must be provided.

Therapeutic Alliance

Therapeutic alliance is bidirectional. It comprises a reciprocal positive relationship between the clinician and the patient, along with an agreement on the goals of treatment and the tasks to be undertaken in order to achieve those goals **(Fig. 1)**.[2] Therapeutic alliance may take some time to establish, as a common understanding forms about the child's or adolescent's difficulties. Over the course of treatment, the alliance may experience multiple ruptures and repairs that help it grow and move toward the goals. It is like an attachment relationship wherein disappointments, and setbacks in the context of the relationship, with a rediscovery of the positive bond each time strengthens the relationship.

The child psychiatrist needs to be conscientious of the multitude of factors that contribute to a therapeutic alliance. To begin with, introductions in the very first meeting must convey the who, why, and what of the consultations clearly to the child. **Table 1** lists areas that the child psychiatrist needs to cover

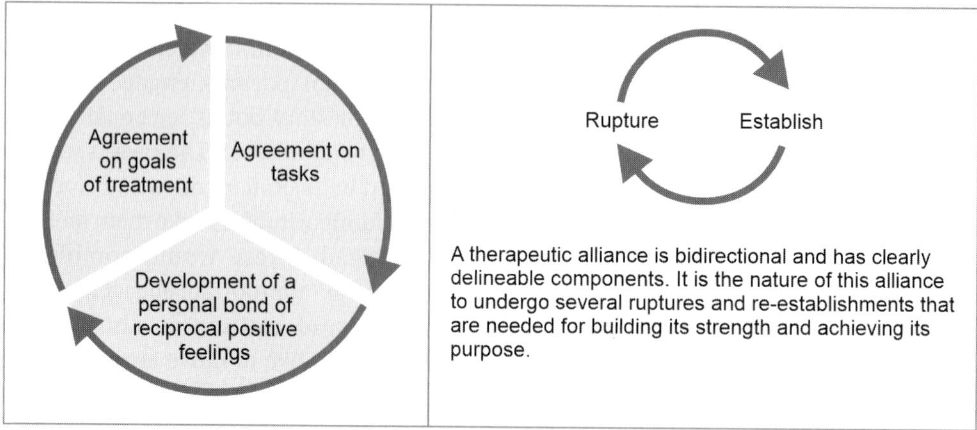

Fig. 1: Components of a therapeutic alliance.

TABLE 1: Introductions—the first step in therapeutic alliance.

What the child psychiatrist must talk about themselves?	*What the child psychiatrist must explore about the child?*
• Who are you? • Who are you to this child? • Why do you want to speak to him/her? • What do you want to speak about? • What will you do with what the child tells you? • Will you believe the child? • Will you tell someone else? • Will you "solve" the problem?	• What is the child's name? • How old is the child? • Where is the child's home? • Who all live there? • What does the child do? – Go to school/study at home (online) – Any other place the child visits • How does the child feel about school? • What are the child's hobbies? – Favorite pastime? • What does the child's personhood comprise? – Identities – Aspirations – Thoughts – Emotions – Recent changes

TABLE 2: Dos and don'ts while interacting with a child.

Dos	*Don'ts*
• Address child by name • Simple—one thought per sentence • Honesty, curiosity, and patience • Meta-thinking (values and reactions) • Nonverbal communication • Have something fun to do	• Negatively worded statements • Why? questions • Adult language concepts • Suggestive statements • Leading questions

when initially talking to the child. It is important to note that the first goal of the consultation is not to quickly find solutions. The child psychiatrist needs to address the parent's anxiety and needs for quick solutions, while working toward building a sustainable relationship with the child.

What transpires between the child psychiatrist and the child, in terms of both language and activity, is important in determining the ease with which a therapeutic alliance builds. Some "dos" and "don'ts" are listed in **Table 2**. The interaction is likely to be influenced by myriad factors. Some of these (including the chronological age, developmental age, emotional state, emotional skills, and any disability) determine the developmentally appropriate skills and techniques that the clinician needs to employ. Some others (child's motivation and perception of the purpose of consultation, child's current physical and emotional needs, and familiarity with the spaces and methods) determine the pace of the interaction. In addition, the clinician needs to be familiar with background cultural factors and the presence of others in order to make clinical interpretations and decisions.

Case Formulation

Case formulation is central to understanding a child's difficulties and determines the therapeutic plans and timelines. To simply describe it, a case formulation is the process by which the clinician assimilates the available information from history and examination, to identify salient features that interact, and the mechanisms through which they interact, in order to "explain" the child's presenting concerns.[3,4] Understandably, in formulating the clinician must take into account all the developmental, personal, and familial factors that could directly or indirectly play a role in the manifestation of the behavioral and emotional difficulties that the child has come with. Essentially, the case formulation arises from a biopsychosocial and cultural framework and seeks to answer three questions:

1. *"What is wrong?"*
2. *"How did it get this way?"*
3. *"What can be done about it?"*

It is generally not possible to understand everything about a child and family in a few detailed evaluations. The case formulation can evolve over time. It could be dynamic and even revised as new insights are gained about the child and his/her life circumstances. The process of building a case formulation is illustrated below with the help of a case of a 10-year-old boy with developmental issues and mental illness.

CASE VIGNETTE 2: HOW TO BUILD A CASE FORMULATION

Vijay is a 10-year-old boy. He was born preterm. While he has not had any major medical or neurological issues, there has been developmental delay across all domains, more pronounced in the social and communication domains. Vijay's father has alcohol dependence syndrome, with impaired personal, social, and occupational functioning; he is largely uninvolved as far as parenting roles and responsibilities are concerned. Vijay mother is the breadwinner for the family and is significantly stressed with her parenting role. She has found it hard to find appropriate help for Vijay. In the last 8–9 months, on top of the developmental difficulties that Vijay had, mother reports that he had become quite irritable, had difficulty sleeping, was demanding "to go out" multiple times a day, and she found it harder to engage him in any one-to-one activities that had been possible earlier for almost 15–30 minutes at a time.

Current and Ongoing Concerns

The first step in building a case formulation is to delineate presenting from ongoing concerns **(Fig. 2)**. There may have been developmental or minor behavioral issues that the parents noticed the child to have since a young age. The parents would have been utilizing personal, familial, social, or systemic resources to respond to them. The current presentation may be for reasons very different from the ongoing developmental concerns. The presenting concerns are what needs to be conceptualized and formulated. They are the treatment-seeking needs and need to be addressed on priority.

Vijay has had developmental difficulties, but those are not the reasons for which the mother brought him for consultation. Her reasons for seeking help are the changes in Vijay's behavior that began 8–9 months ago.

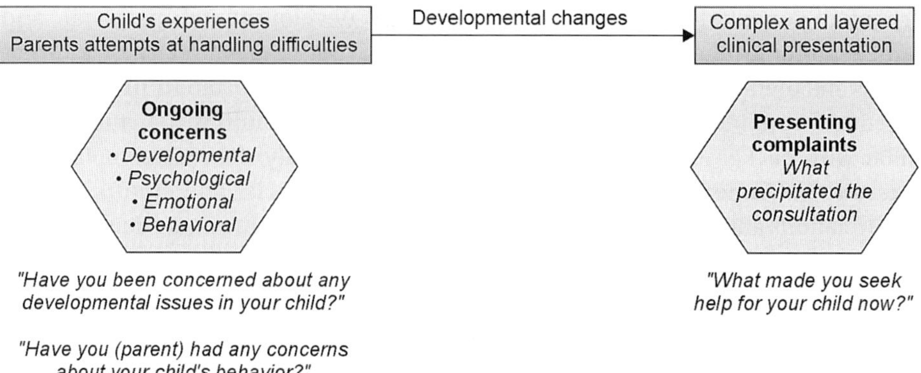

Fig. 2: Delineating presenting concerns from ongoing concerns.

Often, in children with developmental disorders, *diagnostic overshadowing* can result in all concerns being attributed to the developmental disorder. This leads to missed comorbidities and undertreatment, contributing to high morbidity and burden of care. To avoid this, the clinician must always enquire for the presenting problems, and characterize their onset, look for quantitative and qualitative behavioral changes, and look for changes in appetitive behaviors such as sleep, food intake, and sexual behaviors that are more likely indicative of a comorbid disorder, atop the ongoing developmental concerns. To start formulating an approach to assist with a child's difficulties, we must ask the question:

"What factors in the child's history have either contributed to or are moderating the presenting concerns, and through what mechanisms do they seem to be doing that?"

Symptom Dimensions in Child Psychiatry

It is not uncommon for clinical presentations in child psychiatry to be either polymorphic or changing over time. Changing picture over time is illustrated by neurodevelopmental disorders that typically follow a pattern of decreasing symptom severity with age, childhood onset depression may switch to bipolar disorder in follow-up, and obsessive compulsive and related disorders often show prominent symptom migration. An example of a polymorphic presentation is irritability, and sleeplessness, along with repetitive behaviors, all of which keep fluctuating over weeks to months; and on a background of developmental deficits. Long-term outcomes in such presentations may be unpredictable, nevertheless close follow-up is a necessity for treatment, developmental support, and monitoring. Common symptom dimensions observed in child psychiatric presentations and their behavioral manifestations are detailed in **Table 3**.

It is important that the child psychiatrist does not rush into final diagnoses if such polymorphic and multidimensional symptoms are evident. While this may pose dilemmas in decisions around medication and psychotherapeutic interventions, it may be prudent to take a dimensional approach to interventions while monitoring over long term for various possible differential diagnoses.

In Vijay's case, the presenting concerns—irritability, sleep disturbance, distractibility, and demanding behaviors are perhaps suggestive of a mood disorder. However, given the global developmental delay, differential diagnoses could be considered, as neurodevelopmental comorbidities, anxiety, disruptive behavior disorders, obsessive-compulsive spectrum, and even

TABLE 3: Common symptom dimensions and their behavioral manifestations in children.

	Developmental disorders	*Mood/anxiety symptoms*	*Disruptive behavior disorders*	*Learning disabilities*
Young children	• Cannot sit/walk even in the 2nd year of life • Cannot speak like children his/her age • Does not make eye contact • Does not respond to name call • Does not play with children his/her age • Keeps daydreaming • Does not complete any activity he/she starts • Is usually restless and fidgety • Does not sit in the seat in class, wants to repeatedly go out to the toilet or elsewhere	• Very cranky, irritable when sent to school • Becomes quiet, tried to hide in front of outsiders • Refusal to eat or go to sleep	• Does not obey commands • Answers back to elders • Teases, troubles other children • Is demanding • Frequently starts fighting and is aggressive • Frequent complaints from school about classroom behavior	• Cannot identify alphabets correctly • Confuses alphabets • Avoids writing
Older children/ adolescents	• Cannot make friends • Lags behind in studies • Gets bullied by other children • Poor academic performance	• Is very shy • Feels scared to talk to teachers and outsiders • Does not answer in class • Irritability • Self-harm behaviors • Stays aloof	• Is very argumentative • Lies and steals • Troubles and bullies other children in class • Hurts animals • Is demanding and very often becomes aggressive when demands are not met • Drug use	• Makes a lot of silly mistakes • Spelling mistakes • Learns everything orally but cannot write • Is very slow with calculations simple for his/ her age

psychotic disorders could share these symptoms. So, if one were to look at his symptoms dimensionally, mood, sleep, executive functioning, and behavioral disinhibition can be noted. In planning dimensional interventions—medications and nonpharmacological interventions that support mood regulation, sleep, and behavioral engagement with gentle limit setting could be planned.

Inner Voice

Behavior typically does not arise in a vacuum. There are identifiable biological, psychological, or social triggers for behavior. Without elucidating the triggers and addressing them, behavior modification approaches are likely to be ineffective. The clinician has to trace back the journey of a behavior **(Fig. 3)** to its emotional concomitants, the thoughts underlying the behavior, and further back to the experience that triggered that thought and the context in which the experience occurred. The thoughts underlying the behavior are the "inner voice" that arise from experiences that children have and that are evoked in situations where the behavior

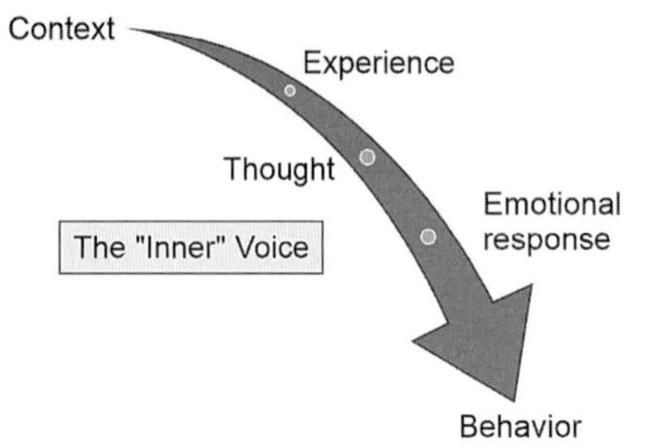

The questions that the clinician needs to ask and to understand the "inner voice" are:
"When do these behaviors occur?"
"Are there specific scenarios when these behaviors do not occur?"
"What is the parent's assessment of the child's emotional state when this behavior occurs?"
"What makes the behavior come down?"
"When was the first time these behaviors were seen?"
"What had been happening in the child's life at that time?"

Fig. 3: Concept of "inner voice".

of interest is evident.[5,6] Resolution of problematic behaviors requires modification of the child's inner voice.

In Vijay's case too, it would be pertinent to examine the situations in which the problematic irritability and demanding behaviors arise. The "inner voice" can be elicited in children as young as toddlers, so even children with mild-moderate developmental delays need to be engaged so as to elicit their emotions, experiences, and contexts that would give us insights on their possible inner voices.

Biopsychosocial Factors

Psychiatry training dwells upon the role of biological, psychological, and social factors in the occurrence of psychiatric disorders. In the case of children, these factors span not just the immediate space that the child inhabits, but multi-layered ecologies around the child that directly or indirectly impact the child, the child's caregivers, or the spaces that the child occupies. Bronfenbrenner's socioecological framework is pertinent in this regard. **Figure 4** lists some examples of areas to be explored in deciphering the biopsychosocial and cultural factors relevant in a particular case.

In Vijay's case, what if we get to know that the symptoms started when the mother switched jobs around 9 months ago. Her new job required her to travel out of station, stay away from the child for longer hours, sometimes even overnight. Vijay had earlier never stayed away from her for such long periods of time. In the mother's absence, Vijay's father or his maternal grandmother were responsible for him. The father was largely uninvolved and with his alcohol use disorder was himself quite dysfunctional. Even though the grandmother was physically present she found it hard to soothe him or engage him in any tasks, so she would give up after a few minutes.

Clearly, not just Vijay's biological and developmental vulnerabilities, but also the nature of caregiving, familial and extrafamilial support systems, joblessness and the need for the mother to take up a tedious and challenging job, etc. all are contributing toward his symptoms. The case formulation needs to take into account all these aspects as all of them would be critical intervention targets.

Case Formulation for the Illustrated Case of a 10-year-old Boy with Developmental and Mental Health Concerns

Vijay has biological predispositions to mental illness. A family history of mental illness, in the form of alcohol use disorder in his father, poses genetic risk. With a preterm birth, his brain was already at a maturational disadvantage that would have been further escalated with vulnerability to nutritional, and other early childhood health risks. The genetic vulnerability and all these factors nonconducive to brain growth and development would have contributed to the

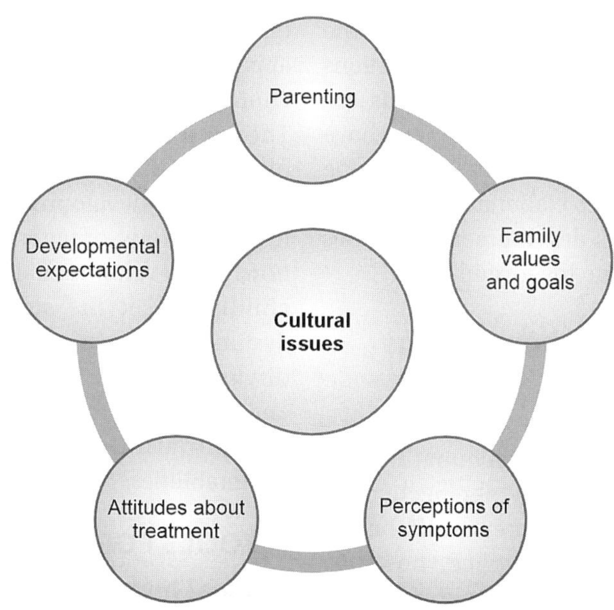

Biological factors	Psychological factors	Social factors
• Family history • Genetics • Physical development • Constitution • Intelligence • Temperament • Medical comorbidities	• Emotional development • Personality structure • Self-esteem • Insight • Defenses • Patterns of behavior • Patterns of cognition • Responses to stressors • Coping strategies	• Family constellation • Peer relationships • School • Neighborhood • Socioeconomic issues • Culture(s) • Religion(s)

Fig. 4: Biopsychosocial and cultural factors to be considered in case formulation.

reported global developmental delay. Parental mental illness and the compromised familial and extrafamilial financial and social support systems would have compromised early developmental intervention and a nurturing environment. Multiple changes about 9 months ago resulted in further impediments in caregiving. The child's irritability, sleep disturbance, demandingness, and difficulty in sustaining attention could be a manifestation of the emotional disturbance in response to these changes. They could also be serving as a means of keeping the mother closer to him for longer, as mother would take leaves when he was "more unwell". In terms of interventions, medication could support with restoring sleep and decreasing the intensity of the child's emotional disturbance. Active liaison is needed with the mother's current place of work to enable her presence during the acute phase of the child's treatment. In the intermediate term, it would be critical to look at possible occupational options for the mother, and to also assess the scope of training and garnering support from other family members. Child's father would need a detailed evaluation and initiation of treatment for his mental health challenges. The child needs long-term follow-up to assess treatment response, symptom course, developmental support, and psychosocial interventions with the family.

So, the clinician needs to put together the myriad factors in mechanistic conceptualizations that "explain" the child's presenting concerns and what can be done about them. While the above is an illustrative formulation, there is still scope for the reader to delve into elaborate enquiry and inclusion of, e.g., Vijay's developmental abilities and family dynamics, into the formulation.

A Developmental Psychopathology Perspective

Several authors have written about the significance of "developmental psychopathology". It has become one of the key perspectives to understand the origins of mental ill health and the sustenance of resilience, not only among children and adolescents, but across all ages. The developmental psychopathology perspective states that *"psychopathology is an outcome of development and once it emerges, it affects future development".*[7,8] This implies that psychopathology, in a way, is development gone awry, and the developmental deficits and deviations that result affect further developmental course in an individual. Given the evident deficits and deviations that accompany the apparent psychopathology, further development could have a rather constrained potential. The perspective takes into account the myriad bi- and multidirectional factors that interact with innate developmental potentials to result in the various outcomes. **Figure 5** illustrates how the developmental vulnerabilities in early childhood set the stage for difficulties and dysfunction in school, and how these deficits and disruptions then interact with environmental and familial contingencies to result in further psychopathologies and developmental vulnerabilities.

TOOLS FOR ASSESSMENT

Clinical Interview

Clinical assessment with a delineation of all aspects of the child, and family history is the most effective and comprehensive tool available to the clinician. Specific information needs elicitation in each area, as depicted in **Table 4**. Even for aspects such as developmental milestones and temperament, specific questions can be used, as depicted in **Tables 5 and 6**. All the information

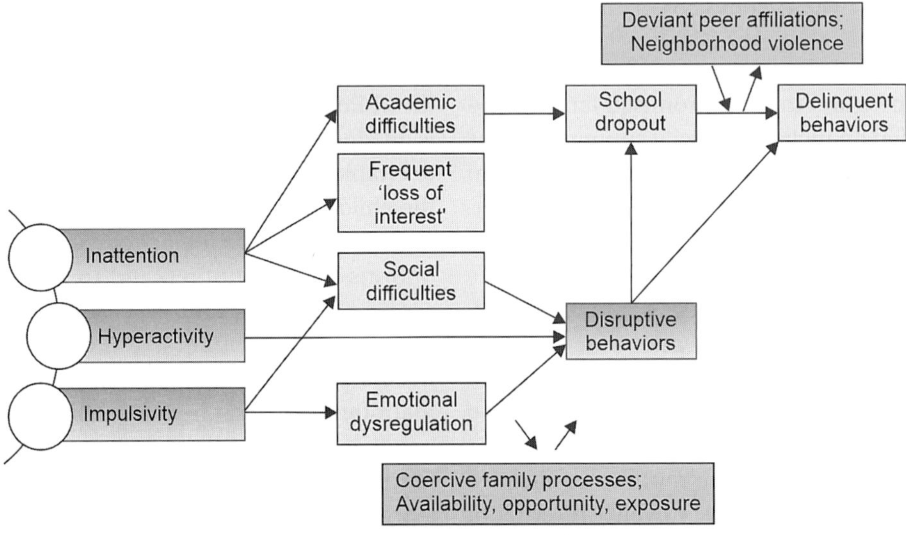

Fig. 5: Illustration of developmental psychopathology.

TABLE 4: History taking in child psychiatric clinical assessment.

Component	*Details can include*
Sources of information	Patient and caregivers, collateral information from school/significant others, medical records
Chief complaints	What brought the patient in now?
History of present illness	Symptoms, course, severity, triggering events, and pertinent negatives
Past psychiatric history	Previous evaluations, therapies, hospitalizations, medications, and treatments; history of aggression or harm toward self or others; substance use history
Past medical history	Illnesses, hospitalizations, surgeries, and medications, including folk and alternative remedies, etc.
Family psychiatric and medical history	Pertinent positives and negatives in the family's psychiatric and medical history, especially substance use, suicide, cardiac history (e.g., sudden deaths)
Social history	Family constellation, peer relations, interactions with the law and social services, key events such as migration, birth of siblings, and loss in the family
Education history	Schools, grades, report cards, special or regular education, changes in schools, and suspensions
Developmental history	Mother's pregnancy and labor, delivery, milestones during infancy; stages of motor, cognitive, social, and behavioral development
Psychological testing	IQ, tests of adaptive functioning, speech, and language evaluations
Mental status examination	
Assessment	Diagnoses and hypotheses of causality
Plan	Treatment goals and options, other persons or agencies to contact

TABLE 5: Clinical assessment of development.

Developmental domain	*Example questions*
Motor	• When did the child start walking? • What sports/activities does the child do? Which ones have gone well? Which ones not so well?
Cognitive	• Did the child show interest in things you pointed to? Did the child point out things to you? • At what age did the child begin play school/nursery? Were there any difficulties? • How does the child do in reading? In arithmetic? With writing? • Has the child had any difficulties in any specific subject? • Has the child ever failed in school? • Has the child ever been suspended from school, or has ever refused to go to school?
Social	• How does the child relate to you? • How did the child respond to your directions? • When did the child start to show interest in other children? How did that go? • What kind of friends does the child have now? How does the child get along with them?

Contd...

Contd...

Developmental domain	*Example questions*
Emotional	• Does the child recognize when he/she is feeling sad, anxious, angry? • How does the child soothe himself/herself when in a bad mood or anxious? • What is the child's most common mood state? • How does the child respond to unexpected changes? Disappointments? Frustrations?
Moral	• Does the child recognize right from wrong? • How does the child react when confronted with mistakes or doing something wrong? • Has the child deliberately hurt other people? Animals? Property? • Does the child consider consequences of his/her decisions on others? • Does the child show remorse after hurting others? • Is the child too perfectionistic or morally rigid?

TABLE 6: Clinical assessment of temperament.

Developmental domain	*Example questions*
Activity levels	• How active/energetic is the child generally? • Are there periods when the child can sit still or is there constant movement? Fidgetiness? • What kind of games does the child prefer? Calm and quiet? Or, noisy and energetic?
Rhythmicity	• Does the child eat/sleep regularly? • Are the sleeping and feeding patterns predictable?
Distractibility	• Is the child able to concentrate on the activity he/she is doing? • Is the child easily distracted by, say, someone coming into the room or some noise outside?
Approach/withdrawal	• How does the child respond to new situations? People? Places? Things? • Does the child show interest in new situations? People? Places? Things?
Adaptability	• Does the child adjust to changes in his/her environment? • Does the child become upset if something in his/her environment changes?
Attention span and persistence	• Does the child complete the activities he/she starts? • Does the child get easily frustrated if he/she faces some difficulties in a task?
Intensity of reaction	• Does the child show intense reactions, when he/she likes something? Is happy about something? Or, is upset by something? Or, is the child calm and not very emotional in his/her reactions to pleasant/unpleasant situations?
Responsiveness threshold	• Is the child sensitive to sounds, tastes, smells, touch? • Does the child react to even minor changes in his/her surroundings? • Are even minor changes in his/her surroundings bothersome?
Mood	• How is the child's mood most of the time? • Is he/she generally cheerful, pleasant, friendly? Or, generally cranky and prone to crying?

need not necessarily be elicited in one session. In fact, the child and family are themselves able to determine the pace and extent of evaluation under each area, given their comfort and rapport at the time of a specific session. A clinician's collaborative stance greatly assists this process.

Performing mental status examination (MSE) in children may often be challenging given children's limitations in language and verbal processing of their experiences. However, it is important that the clinician understand that developmental abilities limit assessment in only some aspects of the MSE, such as thought possession and content. Most other aspects—general appearance and behavior, mood, speech, perceptual abnormalities—and even developmental capabilities can be quite fruitfully observed in a nondirective play setting. **Box 1** lists some salient features that can be observed even when children do not engage in a lot of verbal exchange with the clinician.

Structured Tools for Assessment

There are several tools available, a lot of them at significant costs, for various types of assessments. Broadly, these could be (1) parent or self-report questionnaires [mini-international neuropsychiatric interview, depression rating scales, attention-deficit/hyperactivity disorder (ADHD) rating scales, etc.], (2) observational measures (e.g., autism diagnostic observation schedules, parent-child dyadic interaction, etc.), and (3) performance measures (intelligence tests). Published tools have undergone testing with clinical population, several of them have age norms, and other psychometric properties data. Overall, they are valid and reliable measures of whatever they intend to measure. However, they are not a replacement for a thorough clinical assessment. The formulation processes described above are best undertaken through clinical and collaborative dialogues over multiple sessions. Structured assessment tools have specific utility for monitoring symptom severity over course of treatment, and in research.

BOX 1: Observational features during clinical assessment of young children.

- Physical appearance
- Gait and posture
- Behavioral organization
- Psychomotor activity
- Involuntary movements
- Repetitious activity
- Disturbances of attention
- Exploratory behavior
- Playfulness
- Relatedness
- Eye contact
- Behavioral evidence of emotion
- Speech
- Disturbances of speech melody

SUMMARY AND CONCLUSION

To summarize, clinical assessment, interview, and formulation in child psychiatry are critical in diagnosing and planning interventions. The clinician needs to be well-versed with the developmental and multifactorial underpinnings of psychopathology in children, to suitably apply clinical skills in the context of a presentation.

In conclusion, while there are several structured tools available for developmental and psychopathological evaluations, none of them supersede a thorough clinical assessment. The clinician needs to hone skills in eliciting historical data and mental status examinations of young children that may not entirely be language dependent. Clinical assessment is the first step in and, perhaps, a strong predictor of long-term therapeutic alliance that determines positive clinical outcomes. Readers are encouraged to refer the reference list at the end of the chapter for further nuanced understanding.

REFERENCES

1. Srinath S, Jacob P, Sharma E, Gautam A. Clinical practice guidelines for assessment of children and adolescents. Indian J Psychiatry. 2019; 61(Suppl S2):158-75.

2. Ardito RB, Rabellino D. Therapeutic alliance and outcome of psychotherapy: historical excursus, measurements, and prospects for research. Front Psychol. 2011;2:270.
3. Henderson SW, Andrés Martin. Case formulation and integration of information in child and adolescent mental health. In: Rey JM (Ed). IACAPAP e-Textbook of Child and Adolescent Mental Health. Geneva: International Association for Child and Adolescent Psychiatry and Allied Professions; 2014.
4. Winters NC, Hanson G, Stoyanova V. The case formulation in child and adolescent psychiatry. Child Adolesc Psychiatr Clin N Am. 2007;16(1): 111-32, ix.
5. Firestone RW. Combating Destructive Thought Processes: Voice Therapy and Separation Theory. India: Sage Publications, Inc.; 1997.
6. Wieland S. Hearing the Internal Trauma: Working with Children and Adolescents Who Have Been Sexually Abused. housand Oaks, CA: Sage Publications; 1997.
7. Cicchetti D, Rogosch FA. Equifinality and multifinality in developmental psychopathology. Dev Psychopathol. 1996;8:597-600.
8. Cicchetti D, Cannon TD. Neurodevelopmental processes in the ontogenesis and epigenesis of psychopathology. Dev Psychopathol. 1999;11(3): 375-93.

CHAPTER 4

Fetal and Infant Mental Health

Satya Raj

INTRODUCTION

India is the most populated country in the world, with nearly a fifth of the world's population. The infants and toddlers up to the age of 0–4 years account for 9.32% of the population (UN World Population Prospects).

The Infant Mortality Rate (IMR) in India is estimated to be 27 per 1,000 live births, as per the 2021 estimates.[1] This steady decline in the IMR can be attributed to the better access to healthcare facilities, improved antenatal, perinatal and neonatal care, strengthened immunization and breastfeeding practices. With the physical health of infants showing better outcomes, recently there has been an increasing focus on the mental health of infants. Emphasis has been on positive mental health, i.e., the holistic development of healthy infants and toddlers and promoting secure attachment in the infant and toddler with the primary caregiver. The well-being of the infant starts early, soon after conception, and fetal well-being is very closely interrelated with maternal well-being, both physically and mentally.

MATERNAL MENTAL HEALTH AND ITS IMPACT ON THE DEVELOPING FETUS

Maternal mental health during both the antenatal and postnatal period is shown to have a profound impact on the fetal, infant, and child mental health outcomes. The emotional well-being of mothers during the antenatal period is associated with neurodevelopmental outcomes in the child. Anxiety or depression in mothers during the antenatal period can affect the temperament of the child.[2-5]

Maternal mood during the antenatal period is associated with variation in the brain structure and corticolimbic connectivity of the offspring.[6] Depressive symptoms in the mother during the antenatal period are associated with cortical thinning, primarily in the right frontal lobes in children. Maternal well-being has an impact on fetal physiology as well.[7] Few studies have shown that maternal adversity and stress activates the glucocorticoids (stress mediators), and this in turn affects fetal development; however, it needs to be studied further, to show the exact link between maternal mental health and specific fetal and infant outcomes. Perceived stress in the mother is a heritable trait, and it can affect the stress reactivity of the offspring.[8]

Prenatal adversity may increase the sensitivity of the offspring to postnatal environmental influences. The term "metaplasticity" therefore refers to the degree to which the developing organism is susceptible to future environmental influences.[9] Therefore, in this chapter, we shall discuss the importance of fetal well-being and infant mental health.

FETAL WELL-BEING

The DOHaD hypothesis, "developmental origins of health and disease" affirms that the quality of fetal development is related to chronic illness over the life span of the individual. Maternal well-being during the antenatal period and fetal wellness can significantly alter the mental health trajectories of the individual. Therefore, when there is a disruption in the same, it can lead to adverse mental health outcomes. There are multiple studies[10,11] to show that fetal growth, measured by birth weight, is associated with specific psychopathology in children. For example, when the birth weight is <2.5 kg, there is an increased risk of the child developing ADHD.[12,13]

Aizer et al.,[14] in their study, showed that birth weight was also associated with intelligence and academic performance. Therefore, though there are epidemiological studies that reveal associations between fetal growth and mental health outcomes, there is very little evidence for specific disorders.[15]

INFANT MENTAL HEALTH

The early years in the development of the child are very important. We discussed the importance of maternal well-being and its impact on fetal health. Similarly, the first 5 years of life are also very important. The term "infant mental health" was coined by Selma Fraiberg.

Definition of Infant Mental Health

Fraiberg et al. defined infant mental health as the "social, emotional, and cognitive well-being of a baby within the context of a caregiving relationship".[16] "Infant" refers to children <3 years of age. "Mental" includes social, emotional, and cognitive well-being. "Health" implies wellness. It therefore focuses on the positive mental health, secure attachment, and holistic development of the infant, in the context of a caregiving relationship.

Zero to Three National Center for Infants, Toddlers, and Families, 2012, defines infant mental health as "the healthy social and emotional development of a child from birth to 3 years; promotion of healthy social and emotional development, prevention of mental health problems, and treatment of the mental health problems of very young children in the context of their families."[17]

Prevalence of Infant Mental Health Problems

Prevalence rates of infant mental health problems are difficult to assess, due to lack of awareness and difficulty in diagnosing the same.[18] Epidemiological studies reveal the prevalence of mental health disorders in the 1–5-year age group to be 16–18%.[19]

Skovgaard et al., in the Copenhagen Child Cohort 2000 study opined that the most common diagnoses in the age group up to 1.5 years were disturbances of emotion, behavior, eating, and regulatory disorder, and parent-child relationship disturbances were noted in about 8%.

Wichstrøm et al., in a study, reported that the prevalence of any psychiatric disorder in preschoolers was 12.5%, and the most common disorders noted in this age group were attention-deficit/hyperactivity disorder (ADHD) (1.9%), oppositional defiant disorder (1.8%), anxiety disorders (1.5%), and depressive disorders (2.0%).[20]

In a study done in India, Vengadavaradan et al.[21] reported that bonding disorders was 24% among healthy postpartum mothers and 45.2% in mothers with psychiatric disorders. Another study done in India among 237 mother-infant dyads, reported that 41% of mothers with mental illness had a bonding disorder.[22]

COMMON PROBLEMS IN INFANTS AND TODDLERS

The common problems in infants and toddlers are feeding problems, sleep problems, and regulatory difficulties. Behavioral problems,

ADHD, depression, and anxiety are common in preschoolers.

Attachment-related difficulties and problems in the relationship with the primary caregiver are also common reasons for referral to an infant mental health specialist.

Diagnostic Classification for Infants and Toddlers

The infants' emotional and developmental needs and the clinical presentations are very varied and therefore require developmentally sensitive descriptors; hence, a focused, specific diagnostic system like the DC zero to five (DC:0–5), tailored to address the same is essential.[23]

It has been highlighted earlier that "infant mental health" is explicitly relational in its focus, and therefore, a diagnostic classification system for early childhood disorders should focus not only on the child's psychopathology but also on the relationship between the child and the caregiver, and the relational framework must also be included.[24] DC:0–5 provides a multiaxial diagnosis which helps not only in a holistic understanding of the child's needs but also gives a framework for multidisciplinary input. The DC:0–5 multiaxial diagnosis includes:

- *Axis I:* Clinical diagnosis
- *Axis II:* Relationship classification
- *Axis III:* Medical and developmental disorders and conditions
- *Axis IV:* Psychosocial stressor
- *Axis V:* Emotional and social functioning

The DC: 0–5 has a few additions, like an Axis I "Relationship Specific Disorder of Early Childhood." An axial characterization is continued from the DC:0–3R, but two major changes are introduced. First, the DC:0–5 proposes to simplify ratings of relationship adaptation/maladaptation and to expand what is rated so that, in addition to characterizing the child's relationship with his or her primary caregiver, there also is a characterization of the network of family relationships in which the child develops.

CORE CONCEPTS IN INFANT MENTAL HEALTH

The child's development should be viewed within the context of the system of relationships that form their environment.[25] There are multiple complex "layers" of the environment, each influencing a child's healthy development. Infant mental health systems should therefore address the adverse influences on the early relationship between the primary caregiver and child.

The primary focus of work in infant mental health is the "mother-infant dyad". Dyadic reciprocal exchanges between the mother and the infant form the foundations for the development. Infants and young children typically negotiate a series of dyadic relationships, creating unique and intimate patterns of interaction with important people in their lives.

Multiple models exist in infant mental health, namely the (1) Serve return model, (2) Neurosequential model, (3) Mutual regulation model, (4) Dyadic states of consciousness, (5) Brazelton's touch points, (6) Neurorelational model, and (7) Attachment models.[26]

The serve and return model can be explained as the "mother-infant reciprocity"[27] and "two-way interchanges"; this "serve and return" between a child and an important adult in his or her life is considered essential for neural wiring, and it is the most essential experience needed for shaping the architecture of the developing brain. The core neural networks organize as a reflection of early experience, and therefore, any disruption in this like in the case of early developmental trauma and neglect will have a disproportionate influence on brain organization and later brain functioning.

Each model highlights a specific feature of the dyad and therefore gives us a framework to deal with the infant's mental health problems holistically.

ASSESSMENTS IN INFANT MENTAL HEALTH

Depending on the reason for referral, the assessments must be planned. Comprehensive assessment of the infant or toddler, the parents, and the family within the framework of the sociocultural context is essential. A detailed history of the infant, the parents, and the family background must be collected. A comprehensive assessment must be done, keeping in mind the biopsychosocial framework.

The development of the child is always the result of continuous dynamic interactions between the child and the environment, and the experience provided by the family.[28] The assessment aims to understand the problems of the infant and the family, their strengths and vulnerabilities, and to frame interventions to maximize the parenting capacity and the developmental potential of their child. Risk assessment is also vital to identify any potential risk of harm to the infant and developmental risk. Recent stressors and supports must also be assessed.

The unique feature of an infant assessment is that the infant or young child has "no words to tell their side of the story"; therefore, observation of their behavior, their responses, and the interaction with the primary caregiver is crucial in helping the clinician understand the child's current difficulties.

Infant mental status examination is needed to get a holistic understanding of the infant or toddler.[29] The appearance of the infant, level of nourishment, and any dysmorphic features must be noted. The apparent reaction to the situation, the initial reaction to the setting and strangers, and later adaptation must be assessed. State regulation, sensory regulation, activity level, attention span, and frustration tolerance must be assessed. Motor functioning and speech and language must be assessed. Thought, mood and affect, modes of emotional expression, range, and responsiveness need to be assessed. Cognition, play behavior, and relatedness to caregivers and attachment behaviors, are crucial areas that need careful assessment.

There are many structured and semistructured assessments available for infants, the modified Crowell procedure can be used to assess the parent-infant dyadic interaction.[30]

Other tools that can be used to assess the infant or toddler are as follows:
- Child Behavior Checklist (CBCL) for 1.5–5 years
- Strengths and Difficulties Questionnaire (SDQ)
- The Ages and Stages Questionnaire (ASQ-3)
- The Ages and Stages Questionnaire: Social Emotional (ASQ:SE)
- Preschool Age Psychiatric Assessment (PAPA)

The commonly used developmental assessments include:
- The Neonatal Behavioral Assessment Scale (NBAS)
- The Bayley Scales of Infant Development (BSID)
- Gesell's developmental schedule
- The Wechsler Preschool and Primary Scale of Intelligence (WPPSI)
- The Vineland Adaptive Behavior Scales

Parenting assessment may also be required at times, depending on the nature of the problem. Assessment of parenting capacity, parental stress, and parent reflective capacity can be done. The parenting stress index, parent development interview, and parent reflective functioning questionnaire are a few of the assessments that can be used.

Following the completion of the assessment process, a diagnostic formulation needs to be done, and this is explained to the family, and an intervention plan is made. The 4P (*P*redisposing, *P*recipitating, *P*erpetuating, and *P*rotective factors) model is useful in understanding the different aspects of the problem at hand and the strengths of the family. This aids in planning an effective intervention tailored to the specific needs of the infant and the family.

INTERVENTIONS IN INFANT MENTAL HEALTH

The basic principles of the therapeutic strategies in infant mental health are that they work with the mother-infant dyad, and focus on improving attachment, working on infant regulation, improving the reflective capacity of the primary caregiver, and help in enhancing the sense of safety and security in the infant.

Caregiving must be well-attuned, gentle, and responsive. There are many parenting programs, like Triple P: Positive Parenting Program, Incredible Years, Parent-Child Interaction Therapy, and Promoting First Relationships. Infant-Parent Psychotherapy; Child-Parent Psychotherapy; Mindful Parenting; Watch, Wait, and Wonder are a few of the evidence-based interventions, working on the reflective capacity of the parent.

Parent-child interaction Therapy, Video Intervention Therapy, Floor-time, Filial Play Therapy, Theraplay, and Circle of Security are therapeutic models that are more directive and offer behavioral training, and parental skill building.

Structure of therapy: The therapy has three components, the therapeutic gateway, the pathway, and the Zone of reflection and plane of transformation.[26] The therapist can start working with explicit behaviors and then move to the internal feelings and thoughts, or we can move from feelings to actions as well. For example, if the therapist observes that the parent is hitting the child, then the reflection can start from there, through the "explicit gateway" and move to the feelings and emotions. The parents are asked to reflect on their feelings or behavior, and the therapist facilitates this process and aids in the transformation.

Infant mental health practice must include aspects of primary, secondary, and tertiary prevention. Primary prevention consists of health promotion, and this must begin in the perinatal period.[31] The main aim is to develop maternal reflective capacities and enhance the mother's capacity to keep the baby in mind. Mother-infant dyads are screened for the emergence of infant-parent challenges and early intervention is provided, depending on the need. Psychoeducation regarding sensitive parenting and best mother-infant dyadic practices are provided to all mother-infant dyads, and focused targeted interventions are provided as required.

SUMMARY AND CONCLUSION

Infant mental health is an area that is rapidly gaining importance in India, and other Asian countries. Tomlinson has highlighted in his article the paucity of research in the field of infant mental health in the developing world. More than 90% of infants live in low- and middle-income countries, but research and data on infant mental health in these countries is very little.[32]

India is home to the largest number of children and considering the WHO theme of "survive and thrive", it is very important for us to now help our children thrive in this country. We need to recognize the importance of infant mental health and initiate services for the same. This can be done in a very systematic and organized way by integrating the infant mental health service into the existing postnatal care follow-up visits and immunization clinics. This early screening will aid early intervention and hence better outcomes.

In addition to this, we must also focus on comprehensive care for the mother-infant dyad at the community level and this can be done only if there are more resources in the form of increased personnel trained in infant mental health. This will also mean that we need to look at it from a top-down approach wherein there are clear infant mental health policies developed by the government and increased utilization of the existing community mental health resources for health promotion activities in the mother-infant dyad. There also must be significant input into creating awareness about the importance of infant mental health services among the public and mainly among our medical fraternity, obstetricians, and pediatricians who happen to be the first port of call for the mother and baby.

There needs to be research into this area looking into the prevalence of infant mental health problems in our population, where the presentation, sociocultural factors, and challenges may be very different from the West.

REFERENCES

1. National Family Health Survey (NFHS-5), 2019–21, India Fact Sheet, Ministry of Health & Family Welfare, Government of India.
2. Glover V. Maternal depression, anxiety, and stress during pregnancy and child outcome: what needs to be done. Best Pract Res Clin Obstet Gynaecol. 2014;28:25-35.
3. O'Donnell KJ, Glover V, Barker ED, O'Connor TG. The persisting effect of maternal mood in pregnancy on childhood psychopathology. Dev Psychopathol. 2014;26:393-403.
4. Huizink AC, de Medina PG, Mulder EJ, Visser GH, Buitelaar JK. Psychological measures of prenatal stress as predictors of infant temperament. J Am Acad Child Adolesc Psychiatry. 2002;41:1078-85.
5. Werner EA, Myers MM, Fifer WP, Cheng B, Fang Y, Allen R, et al. Prenatal predictors of infant temperament. Dev Psychobiol. 2007;49:474-84.
6. Qiu A, Anh TT, Li Y, Chen H, Rifkin-Graboi A, Broekman BF, et al. Prenatal maternal depression alters amygdala functional connectivity in 6-month-old infants. Transl Psychiatry. 2015;5:e508.
7. Monk C, Myers MM, Sloan RP, Ellman LM, Fifer WP. Effects of women's stress elicited physiological activity and chronic anxiety on fetal heart rate. J Dev Behav Pediatr. 2003;24:32-8.
8. Wüst S, Federenko I, Hellhammer DH, Kirschbaum C. Genetic factors, perceived chronic stress, and the free cortisol response to awakening. Psychoneuroendocrinology. 2000;25:707-20.
9. Pluess M, Belsky J. Prenatal programming of postnatal plasticity? Dev Psychopathol. 2011;23:29-38.
10. Schlotz W, Phillips DI. Fetal origins of mental health: evidence and mechanisms. Brain Behav Immun. 2009;23:905-16.
11. Räikkönen K, Pesonen AK, Roseboom TJ, Eriksson JG. Early determinants of mental health. Best Pract Res Clin Endocrinol Metab. 2012;26:599-611.
12. Breslau N, Chilcoat HD. Psychiatric sequelae of low birth weight at 11 years of age. Biol Psychiatry. 2000;47:1005-11.
13. Banerjee TD, Middleton F, Faraone SV. Environmental risk factors for attention-deficit hyperactivity disorder. Acta Paediatr. 2007;96:1269-74.
14. Aizer A, Currie J. The intergenerational transmission of inequality: maternal disadvantage and health at birth. Science. 2014;344:856-61.
15. O'Donnell KJ, Meaney MJ. Fetal Origins of Mental Health: The Developmental Origins of Health and Disease Hypothesis. Am J Psychiatry. 2017;174(4):319-28.
16. Fraiberg S. Clinical Studies in Infant Mental Health. The First Year of Life. New York: Basic Books Inc.; 1980. p. 279.
17. Zero to three National Center for Infants, Toddlers and Families: Early childhood mental Health, 2012.
18. Klitzing K von, Doehnert M, Kroll M, Grube M. Mental disorders in early childhood. Dtsch Arztebl Int. 2015;112:375-86.
19. Skovgaard AM, Houmann T, Christiansen E, Landorph S, Jørgensen T, et al. CCC 2000 Study Team. The prevalence of mental health problems in children 1(1/2) years of age - the Copenhagen Child Cohort 2000. J Child Psychol Psychiatry. 2007;48(1):62-70. Erratum in: J Child Psychol Psychiatry. 2008;49(2):219.
20. Wichstrøm L, Berg-Nielsen TS, Angold A, Egger HL, Solheim E, Sveen TH. Prevalence of psychiatric disorders in preschoolers. J Child Psychol Psychiatry. 2012;53:695-705.

21. Vengadavaradan A, Bharadwaj B, Sathyanarayanan G, Durairaj J. Frequency and correlates of mother-infant bonding disorders among postpartum women in India. Asian J Psychiatry. 2019;44:72-9.
22. Chandra PS, Desai G, Reddy D, Thippeswamy H, Saraf G. The establishment of a mother-baby inpatient psychiatry unit in India: Adaptation of a Western model to meet local cultural and resource needs. Indian J Psychiatry. 2015;57(3):290-4.
23. Egger HL, Emde RN. Developmentally sensitive diagnostic criteria for mental health disorders in early childhood: the diagnostic and statistical manual of mental disorders-IV, the research diagnostic criteria-preschool age, and the diagnostic classification of mental health and developmental disorders of infancy and early childhood-revised. Am Psychol. 2011;66(2):95-106.
24. Zeanah CH, Lieberman A. Defining relational pathology in early childhood: the diagnostic classification of mental health and developmental disorders of infancy and early childhood DC:0-5 Approach. Infant Ment Health J. 2016;37(5): 509-20.
25. Bronfenbrenner U. The Ecology of Human Development: Experiments by Nature and Design. ambridge, Massachusetts: Harvard University Press; 1979.
26. Brandt K (2014). Core concepts in infant-family and early childhood mental health. In Brandt K, Perry BD, Seligman S, Tronick E (Eds.) Infant and early childhood mental health: Core concepts and clinical practice (pp. 1–20). American Psychiatric Publishing, Inc.
27. Brazelton TB, Tronick E, Adamson L, Als H, Wise S. Early mother-infant reciprocity. Ciba Found Symp. 1975;(33):137-54.
28. Sameroff AJ, Fiese BH. Models of development and developmental risk. In: Zeanah CH Jr. (Ed). Handbook of Infant Mental Health, 2nd edition. New York: The Guilford Press; 2000. pp. 3-19.
29. Thomas JM, Benham AL, Gean M, Luby J, Minde K, Turner S, et al. Practice parameters for the psychiatric assessment of infants and toddlers (0-36 months). American Academy of Child and Adolescent Psychiatry. J Am Acad Child Adolesc Psychiatry. 1997;36(10 Suppl):21S-36S.
30. Crowell JA, Feldman SS. Mothers' internal models of relationships and children's behavioral and developmental status: a study of mother-child interaction. Child Dev. 1988;59(5):1273-85.
31. Zeanah CH, Handbook of infant mental health, Fourth edition.
32. Tomlinson M, Morgan B. Infant Mental Health Research in Africa: a call for action for research in the next 10 years. Glob Ment Health (Camb). 2015;2:e7.

Intellectual Disability: Concept, Definition, Assessment, Diagnosis, Formulation of Management Plan, and Management

Satish Chandra Girimaji

INTRODUCTION

Concept, Definition, and Description

The hallmark of intellectual disability (ID) is impaired global cognitive development leading to diminished intellectual capacity. Intellectual capacity plays a crucial role in our lives and diminished intellectual functions obviously puts lifelong limitations on functioning. It is one of the most common neurodevelopmental disorders (NDDs), with prevalence around 2%.[1]

Though the term ID is widely used currently, ICD-11 and DSM-5 have their own labels for the condition—disorders of intellectual development (DID) in ICD-11 and intellectual developmental disorder (IDD) in DSM-5. These terms replace old terminologies often with pejorative connotation such as mental retardation.

There are three ways of conceptualizing ID:

1. *Statistical or psychometric model:* ID as an extreme variation in the lower end of Gaussian or bell-shaped normal distribution of intelligence, considered to be <2 standard deviations below the mean. But in reality, this distribution is skewed to the left with a hump in the lowest ranges, implying that there are more people in lower ranges of intelligence.
2. *Biomedical model:* This "disorder perspective" considers ID as a NDD, a disorder secondary to an impairment in the maturation and development of brain. Anything that significantly interferes with the smooth, orderly, orchestrated process of brain maturation and development is likely to cause impairments in development of intelligence and thereby lead to ID.
3. *Sociocultural model:* This is a "disability perspective" that considers people with lesser intelligence having deficits in adaptive behaviors and thereby face disadvantages in their societies. In other words, they have higher support needs to carry on with their lives in the society in which they live. Adaptive behaviors are considered to have three components—(1) *conceptual,* (2) *practical,* and (3) *social domains.*

Modern classificatory systems consider all these three aspects in defining ID.

- DSM-5 defines ID or IDD as a disorder with onset during developmental period that includes intellectual *and* adaptive functioning deficits in conceptual, practical, and social domains. It further characterizes deficits in intellectual functioning as deficits in *reasoning, problem solving, planning, abstract thinking, judgment, academic learning, and learning from experience.* Intelligence can be ascertained clinically or through individualized, standardized IQ tests. Likewise, adaptive function deficits are conceptualized as failure to meet the developmental and sociocultural standards for personal independence and social responsibility.[2]

- ICD-11 defines DID as "group of etiologically diverse conditions originating during the developmental period characterized by significantly below average intellectual functioning and adaptive behavior that are approximately two or more standard deviations below the mean (approximately less than the 2.3rd percentile), based on appropriately normed, individually administered standardized tests. *Where appropriately normed and standardized tests are not available, diagnosis of DID requires greater reliance on clinical judgment based on appropriate assessment of comparable behavioral indicators.*" Detailed behavioral descriptions (behavioral indicators) are provided for both intellectual and adaptive functioning.[3]

Both systems make it amply clear in their hierarchical structure that ID belongs to parent category of NDDs.

CLASSIFICATION BY SEVERITY

Both systems provide four severity levels of mild, moderate, severe, and profound ID. Current trend is to downplay the importance of IQ bands in classifying ID based on severity and rely more on *behavioral indicators* or age-wise detailed behavioral descriptions for different severity levels. In India, these behavioral indicators assume a great importance for clinicians in their practice, because of the lack of availability of standardized tests across different ages and severity levels.

- In a major departure from earlier approaches, DSM-5 has done away with IQ altogether for ascertainment of severity of ID and has employed level of *adaptive skills* (that indicate the level of support required) as the criterion for determining severity levels. Adaptive skills comprise of conceptual, social, and practical domains.
- ICD-11 persists with IQ bands, but provides for exercising clinical judgment when standardized tests are not available **(Table 1)**. Behavioral indicators for both intellectual and adaptive functioning are provided to assist the clinician in such a situation.
- Both systems recognize difficulties in diagnosing ID in very young children and have a separate category for them—global developmental delay (GDD) for children under 5 years in DSM-5 and provisional DID for children under 4 years in ICD-11.

Clinician needs to have a working knowledge of the modern classificatory approach and how it comes into play in clinical practice. **Table 1** summarizes ICD-11 approach from this perspective along with descriptions, which can also serve as a rough guide to prognosis by severity.

Etiologic Factors

Anything that interferes with orderly, orchestrated development of the brain can lead to impaired cognitive development thereby leading to ID. It is worth noting here that growth, maturation, and development of the brain is under tight genetic control; but it is also influenced by environmental factors. Thus, a host of genetic and environmental factors operating during pre-, peri- and postnatal periods of development can give rise to ID.[4] Elucidating etiologic factors becomes relevant at many points in management. **Table 2** summarizes these etiologies.

A known cause is more likely to be found in more severe forms ID than in milder forms. Overall, etiology is untraceable in about one-third of cases.

A number of syndromes are recognizable based on physical phenotype, and the clinician needs to be aware of them. These are described in **Table 3**.

TABLE 1: Classification of ID (DID) in ICD-11.

Severity	*Criterion*	*Alternative*	*Brief description*
Mild	IQ and adaptive functions 2–3 SD below mean	Clinical judgment based on behavioral indicators	Can acquire basic self-care, domestic, and practical activities, relatively independent living employment as adults with some support; Difficulties in complex language concepts/academic skills
Moderate	IQ and adaptive functions are 3–4 SDs below mean	Same as above	Can acquire basic language and academic skills, basic self-care, domestic, and practical skills; require consistent support for independent living/employment as adults
Severe	IQ and adaptive functions are four or more SDs below mean	Same as above	Very limited language and academic skills; Can acquire basic self-care with intensive training; Need daily support and supervision
Profound	IQ and adaptive functions 4 or more SDs below mean based on BI	Same as above	Mostly nonverbal communication; can acquire some basic self-care with supervision; Sensory, motor impairments +; Need continuous support/supervision
Provisional	GDD present, but age <4 years or in age >4 years when assessment is not possible		
Unspecified	Residual category		

(DID: disorders of intellectual development; BI: behavioural indicators; GDD: global developmental delay)

TABLE 2: Overview of etiologies of ID.

Category	*Subgroup*	*Type*	*Examples*
Prenatal	Genetic	Chromosomal	Down syndrome, trisomy 18, and Turner syndrome
		Microdeletion	Prader–Willi syndrome and Angelman syndrome
		Single gene disorders	• *Autosomal dominant:* Tuberous sclerosis • *Autosomal recessive:* Primary microcephaly and classical phenylketonuria • *X-linked:* Hunter syndrome, Rett syndrome, and Fragile X syndrome
		CNV	17q21.31 microdeletion and 1q21.1 microdeletion
	Environmental	Deficiencies	Iodine deficiency and folate deficiency
		Teratogens	Medications (valproate, phenytoin, and warfarin), heavy metals (mercury), and abortifacients
		Infections	TORCH infections, HIV, and syphilis
		Substances	Alcohol (fetal alcohol spectrum disorder)
		Others	Severe malnutrition and Rh isoimmunization
	Multifactorial		Neural tube defects and congenital hydrocephalus
Perinatal		Third trimester	Eclampsia, diabetes, and placental dysfunction
		Labor	Prematurity, very low birth weight, hypoxic-ischemic encephalopathy, and birth trauma
		Neonatal	Septicemia and severe prolonged jaundice
Postnatal			Meningoencephalitis and traumatic brain injury

(CNV: copy number variation; HIV: human immunodeficiency virus; TORCH: toxoplasmosis, rubella, cytomegalovirus, and herpes simplex virus)

TABLE 3: Recognizable syndromes in IDD.

Syndrome	*Key features*
Down syndrome	Typical facies, short stature, up-slanting eyes, clinodactyly, simian crease, and cup-shape ears
Fragile X syndrome	Elongated, triangular face, protruding/prominent ears, and macro-orchidism in postpubertal boys
Rett syndrome	Normal development till 1 year of age in a girl child followed by plateauing and regression, loss of hand functions, and mid-line hand stereotypies
Cornelia de Lange syndrome	Synophrys, bushy eyebrows, long eyelashes, microcephaly, flat philtrum, and hirsutism
Prader–Willi syndrome	Obesity, hypogonadism, small hands and feet, and skin picking
Tuberous sclerosis	Sebaceous adenomas, ash-leaf spots, shagreen patches, and seizures
Congenital hypothyroidism	Lethargy, growth failure, coarse and dry skin, constipation, protuberant abdomen, and bradycardia
Mucopolysaccharidoses	Coarse facial features, macrocephaly, coarse skin, and regression
Homocystinuria	Marfanoid features and behavioral changes
Phenylketonuria	Light colored iris and hair, abnormal smell of urine, microcephaly, and seizures
Primary microcephaly	Severe congenital microcephaly with only mild to moderate ID
Rubinstein–Taybi syndrome	Prominent beak-shaped nose, broad thumb and hallux

(ID: intellectual disability; IDD: intellectual developmental disorder)

Comorbidities

A variety of other disorders frequently co-occur with ID:

- *Other NDDs*, such as speech and language disorders, autism spectrum disorder, and attention-deficit/hyperactivity disorder (ADHD) commonly co-occur with ID. Both ICD-11 and DSM-5 permit the diagnosis-specific learning disorders along with ID, based on significant discrepancy between general intellectual functioning and academic skills.
- *Medical disorders (excluding those causing ID):* These include cerebral palsy, seizure disorder, and sensory impairments. Other conditions such as cardiac anomalies, endocrine disorders, skeletal anomalies, and nutritional disorders also can occur.
- *Psychiatric disorders and problem behaviors:* These are an important aspect of clinical presentation and need careful attention for evaluation and management.
  - Overall, comorbid psychiatric disorders are at least three times more common in ID.[5]
  - Full range of psychiatric disorders are known to occur with ID, viz., internalizing, externalizing, stress-related conditions, severe mental illness, and sleeping and feeding disorders. It is worth emphasizing that modern classificatory systems allow for diagnosis of full range of psychiatric disorders at all levels of severity of ID.
  - Nonsyndromic problem behaviors, that do not conform to the pattern of a psychiatric disorder, such as self-injurious behaviors, aggression, impulsivity, and socially/sexually inappropriate behaviors are also common.

- Many genetic disorders are accompanied by specific pattern of behaviors, the so-called *behavioral phenotypes*. For instance, Prader–Willi syndrome is associated with obesity, compulsive behaviors, skin picking, and mood changes.
- Psychiatric disorders and problem behaviors are a major source of stress and distress for children and families, and lead to many negative consequences such as social exclusion. Hence, prompt recognition and management of these conditions is essential. The same diagnostic criteria that apply to neurotypical children, with some modifications, are employed. These modifications are necessitated by the fact that clinical picture may be influenced by the presence and severity of ID and limited verbal capacity.
- They tend to be underdiagnosed, because of *diagnostic overshadowing*—a clinician error of misattribution of symptoms of comorbid disorder to ID itself.
- Another factor resulting in underdiagnosis or misdiagnosis is "psychosocial or diagnostic masking", i.e., manifestations of the disorders are modified or masked by the presence of ID, especially in more severe forms.

Clinical Presentation

Children with ID often present to psychiatrists with complaints of:

- Delayed milestones of development, especially language delay, lagging behind in mental development compared to other children of same age
- Slow in learning everything
- Poor intelligence, poor memory, easily forgets, slow in grasping, and remembering
- Poor scholastic performance from the beginning
- Not able to take care of self

In addition, children also are brought for consultation for the following reasons:

- Parents already know about the condition and want guidance and advice regarding further management, such as education, training, and vocation
- For management of comorbid problems behaviors and mental health problems, especially recent-onset behavior changes
- For letters to schools and authorities, and for IQ/disability assessment and certification

Clinical evaluation has to take into consideration the needs of the particular child and family and proceed accordingly.

CLINICAL EVALUATION

This starts from the moment the child and family come in, and is geared toward answering the following questions:

- What precipitated the consultation?
- Is there significant developmental delay? Is it global (affecting all areas of development, viz., motor, cognitive, social, and language) or restricted (for instance only motor or speech), how severe?
- What could be the cause/s? What about recurrence risk?
- Are there associated medical problems?
- Are there associated behavioral or psychiatric problems? If so, what are the contributing factors?
- How much do parents know about the condition? What are their expectations? What are the difficulties/stressors faced by them? How about coping?

Collection of relevant clinical history and psychiatric examination is a dynamic process and calls for skillful collection of historical information, interview/observation and synthesizing it to develop a formulation, comprehensive diagnosis and also management plan. Clinician needs to be flexible and structure the consultation to suit the given context. Information from multiple sources—parents, other caregivers, previous consultation notes, school report, and from the child herself or himself whenever possible enhances the quality and reliability of the information.

History

It is preferable to let the parents "tell their story", and take leads from it for further exploration, rather than forcing a structure. Gaps in information can be filled as one goes along. Note-keeping helps in documentation and for clarifying the information. Open-ended questions ("wh" questions such as what, who, when, where, how) fetch valuable information and can be followed by more directed queries. **Box 1** provides a standard format to record the history.

BOX 1: Format for history-taking in intellectual disability (ID).

- *Complaints* with duration, onset, and evolution of current problems
- *Family history:* Three generation genetic diagram; family history of ID, epilepsy, other developmental problems, early deaths, etc.; Current living arrangement; Health and harmony in family; Family stress, coping, and adaptation
- *Personal history:* Pre-, peri-, and postnatal details, developmental milestones, developmental course or trajectory (onset of delay, dates of acquisition of key milestones, delay in all areas or not, severity of delay, schooling history, and puberty/menstrual history)
- *Medical history:* Seizures, feeding problems, recurrent infections, etc.
- *Psychiatric history:* Details of onset, evolution, and current status of behavioral and other psychopathological disturbances
- *Treatment history:* Past efforts by the family in seeking help, nature, and response to past treatment, and current medication if any
- *Current developmental attainments:* In motor, cognitive, language and social areas; Adaptive skills; Parents' estimation of mental age of the child

Psychiatric Examination

This needs to be modified to suit the context and includes both interviewing and observation. It is always a good idea to start the consultation by interacting with the child, verbally and/or nonverbally, irrespective of the age, as it helps in getting an initial impression that can be developed as the evaluation proceeds. Making the child comfortable first, using simple language, making sure that child had understood the question, giving ample time to respond, and taking the help of parents whenever necessary enhance the quality of information obtained from verbal interview.

The purpose of psychiatric examination is manifold, viz.,

- To ascertain presence and severity of ID
- To supplement the historical information about comorbidities such as other NDDs [for instance ADHD and autism spectrum disorder (ASD)] and psychiatric disorders (for e.g., social anxiety)
- To get to know the "child behind ID", and "family behind the child". This will help in developing a sound therapeutic relationship and individualizing the management.

A quick evaluation of current intellectual and adaptive skills is an essential part of clinical evaluation and helps the clinicians to get an idea of presence and severity of ID, as well as areas of good functioning and skills.

- An overall impression of current intellectual functioning can be obtained clinically by taking into account different competencies that include verbal/nonverbal comprehension and expression, speed of thinking, reasoning/problem-solving abilities, depth of understanding of events and situations, fund of knowledge, and academic skills.
- Current adaptive functioning can be assessed by exploring the attainment of practical (self-care and domestic skills), social (shopping,

TABLE 4: Clinical interview/mental status examination (MSE).

Aspect	*Details/examples*
Setting for interview	Child-friendly ambience and arrangement; Keep toys, books, pictures, paper, and pencil; Space to move around; Safe from danger
Building rapport with child	Make kid and parents comfortable; Be ready to get up from seat to interact and engage; find something child has learnt and comment
Initiate collaborative work with parents	Allow them to speak and listen; Value their opinions, impressions, and efforts; Appreciate parents for the right things they have done.
Observations (ask parents to comment on observed behaviors—how much it reflects what they see at home)	• *Basics:* Vision, hearing, locomotion, and physical health • *Response to interview situation:* Excited, fearful and tense, and shy • *Alertness:* Over-aroused, withdrawn • *Sociability:* Approachability, social responsiveness, and eye contact • *Motor activity:* Fidgetiness, restlessness, hyperactivity, lethargy • *Impulse control:* Climbing, interfering, temper tantrum, and aggression • *Attention and concentration:* Persistence with tasks and distractibility • *Communication:* Receptive/expressive, verbal/nonverbal • Intellectual abilities • *Mood:* Inhibited, excessively cheerful, crying, and irritable • *Others:* Play behaviors, stereotypies, and self-injury
Verbal interviewing	Simple, structured, and brief; use clear and concrete questions; Avoid leading questions; Take parents' help when necessary
Parent-child interactions	Quality of engagement with child, communication patterns, degree and quality of control over the child behavior
Parent-parent interaction	Participation in interview, quality of communication, consulting each other, and consensus-building

mobility, money management, relationships, gullibility, and naivety), and conceptual (time, space, distance, directions, etc.) skills.

Table 4 describes a format for examining and recording various aspects of psychiatric examination.

Physical Examination

- This is an essential part and parcel of the evaluation, and helps in elucidating etiologic factors, and associated physical comorbidities.
- It needs to be carried out after the child is comfortable and relaxed. **Table 5** describes a format for physical examination.
- Minimum points to note are height, weight, head circumference, vision, hearing, locomotor skills, and major and minor congenital anomalies. Presence of four or more minor congenital anomalies is suggestive of genetic cause. Syndromes are identified by a set of key features, and not on the basis of a single finding.

CLINICAL DIAGNOSIS

In most cases, diagnosis of ID can be made clinically by establishing significant deficits in intellectual and adaptive functioning based on history and examination. Specific pointers to diagnosis are GDD, a developmental trajectory highly suggestive of suboptimal development compared to same-age peers, parents' estimation of mental age, and current intellectual/adaptive

TABLE 5: Physical examination in a child with intellectual disability (ID).

Body part	*Examples of anomalies/findings*
Height and weight	Short/tall stature, increased arm span, gigantism, obesity, and emaciation
Facial gestalt	Typical face (Down, coarse, and progeroid), triangular, and mid-facial hypoplasia
Skull	Micro-/macrocephaly, brachycephaly, trigonocephaly, and plagiocephaly
Eyes/vision	Deeply set/prominent, microphthalmia, upslanting/downslanting, hypertelorism, epicanthal folds, light-colored iris, strabismus, ptosis, bushy eyebrows, synophrys, corneal clouding, and visual impairment
Ears	Low-set, large, malformed, protruding, cup-shaped, and hearing impairment
Nose	Short/beak-shaped, depressed nasal bridge, and flaring/hypoplastic nostrils
Palate	High arched, shallow, clefting, and bifid uvula
Skin	Dry and coarse, café-au-lait spots, abnormal pigmentation, and ichthyosis
Hair	Hirsutism, light-colored, and low anterior/posterior hairline
Neck	Short, webbed, and torticollis
Other facial	Short/long philtrum, micrognathia, and sloping forehead
Hands/fingers	Simian crease, clinodactyly, arachno/syn/polydactyly, and broad thumb
Chest	Pectus excavatum, pectus carinatum, nipple anomalies, and gynecomastia
Abdomen	Protuberant, umbilical hernia, hepatosplenomegaly, and inguinal hernia
External genitalia	Hypogenitalism, macro-orchidism, and ambiguous genitalia
Feet	Pes planus, pes cavus, hallux valgus/varus, and broad hallux
Skeletal	Increased carrying angle, kyphosis, scoliosis, and spina bifida
Neurological	Hypo-/hypertonia, spasticity, involuntary movements, and gait problems

deficits noted during mental status examination (MSE) as detailed above.

- Diagnostic difficulties are sometimes encountered in very mild forms of ID, to set it apart from borderline intelligence and specific learning disability (SLD). In such situations, standardized psychological testing for intellectual/adaptive functions is required. Vineland scales, Binet-Kamat test, Wechsler Scales and Bhatia Battery are commonly used. A synthesis of information from all three sources—history, examination, and report of psychological testing—is called for to ascertain the diagnosis in such cases. Unnecessary and erroneous labeling of child must be avoided.
- *IQ score of <70 is suggestive, but not conclusive* of presence of ID, and as mentioned, should be interpreted along with historical information and MSE.
- The diagnosis of GDD is meant only for very young children, and should not be used as a substitute for ID.
- Special attention must be given to look for *comorbid psychiatric problems*. Symptoms such as hyperactivity, impulsivity, tantrums, withdrawal, disinterest in usual activities, sleep and appetite disturbances, and "meltdowns" are often reported by parents and should alert the clinician to the possibility of comorbid disorder. *A recent-onset behavior change is highly indicative of a comorbid problem.* Thorough clinical evaluation—history eliciting duration, onset, and course, contexts where symptoms occur, baseline behaviors

and temperament, stressors and life events, parent-child relationships and parenting practices, qualitative and quantitative behavioral and mood changes, disturbed daily routines and biological functions, along with a good cross-sectional MSE, especially paying attention to nonverbal behavioral patterns will help the clinician to narrow down and establish the diagnosis. Clinician must make sure that behavioral symptoms are inappropriate for developmental age of the child to be considered significant. In this context, the concept of "behavioral equivalents"—behavioral patterns that are suggestive of underlying psychopathology—would help the clinician arrive at the diagnosis. Few examples of behavioral equivalents are given below:

- *Depression:* Recent-onset crying, clinging, irritability, downcast face, self-injury, and loss of appetite.
- *Hypomania:* Recent-onset increased energy, increased socialization, overtalkativeness, demanding, impatience, excessive laughing, and roaming away from home.
- *Stress and trauma-related problems:* Recent-onset fearfulness/frightened look on face, clinging, getting scared of and avoiding certain situations and activities, and sleep disturbances.

It is essential to make a comprehensive diagnosis to guide the management accordingly, with following elements:

- Severity of ID
- Possible etiology/etiologic factors
- Comorbid medical conditions such as epilepsy and sensory impairments
- Comorbid psychiatric disorders/problem behaviors
- Family/psychosocial factors, such as issues in parenting, stress and coping, and health and harmony in families

(Note that this is very different from Rutter's multiaxial diagnosis, which is no longer recommended.)

Differential Diagnosis

Several NDDs can be misdiagnosed as ID and vice versa. Situation is further complicated by the fact they frequently co-occur with each other. *A developmental diagnostic exercise eliciting developmental trajectory and current level of development in motor, cognitive, social and language areas, and other associated features brings in diagnostic clarity.*

- Developmental language disorder is considered when delayed language development (receptive and/or expressive) is unexplained by or disproportionate to the current cognitive/intellectual functioning. For example, a 7-year-old child with the intellectual level of 6 years, whose language development is around 3 years, has developmental language disorder and not ID. On the other hand, a 7-year-old child with intellectual level of around 4 years and language level of 2 years has *both* ID and developmental language disorder.
- SLD is characterized by *circumscribed cognitive impairment* affecting academic skills, in the background of otherwise typical intellectual functioning. Diagnostic errors happen when academic skills are equated with or taken as a substitute for global intellectual functioning.
- There is a recent tendency to overdiagnose ASD and many children with ID with no autistic features are being mistakenly labeled as having ASD. Clinician has to guard himself/herself from making such diagnostic errors, as it may have grave consequences for the child and parents. This often happens when a child with ID also has language delay and cannot communicate verbally or has isolated symptoms such as poor eye contact and

stereotypies. A careful evaluation of child's capacity for nonverbal interaction and communication will settle the issue and avoid diagnostic pitfall.

- ASD is primarily a disorder of social development with impairments in social interactions and communication, and may be accompanied by ID. Careful evaluation of child's memory, learning, problem-solving ability, and fund of information in nonsocial areas will help the clinician to decide whether there is comorbid ID.
- Other conditions sometimes mistaken for ID are visual/hearing impairments, cerebral palsy, and severe emotional withdrawal.
- Neuroprogressive disorders with childhood onset such as lysosomal storage disorders have deteriorating course, unlike the overwhelming majority of children with ID who improve with age. In addition to the underlying medical condition, a diagnosis of ID can be made if the criteria are satisfied.

Figure 1 depicts different current developmental scenarios and corresponding appropriate diagnoses.

Physical Investigations

These have to be planned based on clinical presentation and after due consideration of yield of information over and above clinical evaluation, and in consultation with parents.[5-7] *Routine brain imaging such as MRI is not recommended, as they do not add any meaningful information in most cases to a good clinical evaluation.* Common contexts that require physical investigations are noted in **Table 6**.

Standardized Psychological Assessment for Intellectual/Educational Functions

This is useful for many reasons:

- For diagnosis and differential diagnosis in children who are "slow learners", a group of children where it may not be possible clinically with certainty to differentiate between borderline intelligence, mild ID, and SLD.
- To get an accurate idea of child's assets and liabilities, strengths and vulnerabilities, to help in planning education/training

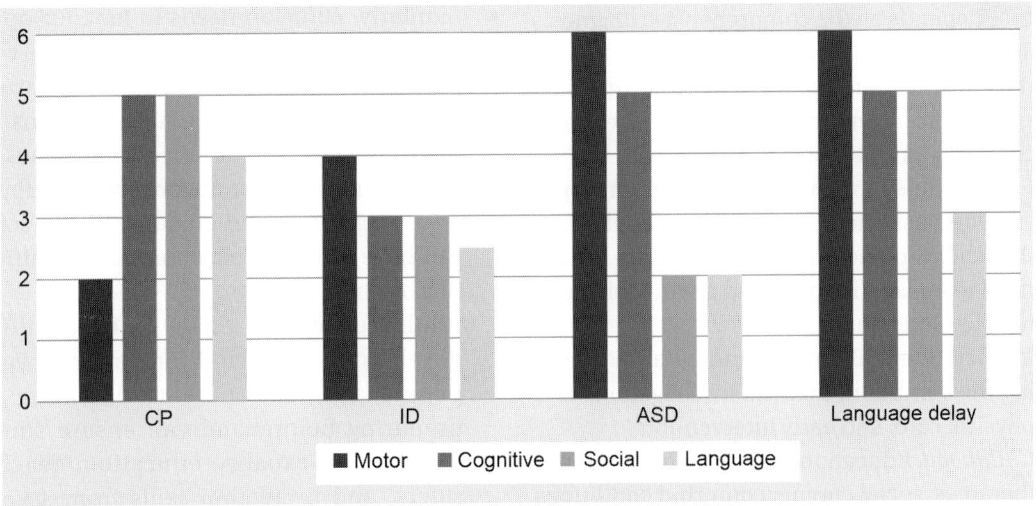

Fig. 1: Developmental diagnosis based on current developmental profiles in four children aged 6 years.

TABLE 6: Clinical situations that necessitate physical investigations.

Situation	*Comment/explanation*	*Examples*
For genetic counseling	Recurrence risk for next child, mother in early pregnancy, clinical picture suggestive of genetic cause, and strong family history of similar illness	Whole exome/targeted sequencing, chromosomal micro-array, and noninvasive prenatal genetic testing
Possibility of a treatable cause	Many inherited metabolic disorders are treatable in early stage. Examples are phenylketonuria (PKU), galactosemia, hypothyroidism, organic acidemias, and Hurler syndrome	Tandem mass spectroscopy, amino acid profiles, enzyme studies, and genetic studies
Better management	Tuberous sclerosis complex, epileptic encephalopathies, and sensory impairments	MRI, EEG, and hearing/visual evaluation
Parents' request	Parents are keen to know the cause even though the cause may be untreatable	MRI, exome sequencing, and metabolic testing

- For disability assessment and certification, which is based on IQ score.

Assessment also becomes a basis to track the child's progress over time. Available tests in India and their utility is discussed in detail in a recent publication.[7]

FORMULATION OF MANAGEMENT PLAN

- Formulation of management plan and prioritization of steps of management in a given case depends on the comprehensive diagnosis and other key variables such as child's age, reason and context for consultation, past consultations and treatments, and stress and coping in families.
- From a life-span perspective, different stages are often associated with unique challenges that children and parents have to face. These need to be kept in mind and adequately dealt with by clinicians.
- *Infancy:* Survival, understanding and accepting the condition, medical investigations and physical care, and early intervention
- *Childhood:* Education and schooling, training/therapies, social coping, comorbid conditions such as ADHD and problem behaviors, peer relations, schooling experiences, and parental expectations
- *Adolescence:* Sexuality, puberty and menstruation, vocational training, psychiatric and behavioral disturbances, independence, and transition to adulthood
- Home-based and parent-mediated interventions should always be part of management. Clinician needs to utilize every opportunity to educate, empower, and train parents.
- Similarly, clinician needs to look for opportunities to provide necessary support and guidance to families to negotiate through many difficult and stressful situations that they often face. For instance, a courteous and nice-sounding letter advocating for support, encouragement, and guidance to the school can have favorable effect on school's attitude toward the child.
- Adolescence may prove to be a difficult developmental period for both the young people and their parents. Planning and preparing beforehand can ensure smooth transition. Sexuality education, teaching safety, and protection skills from a young age, detection and management of new

onset comorbid problems, meaningful and productive daily routines, social skills training, opportunities for social participation, and recreational/sports activities are some of the key interventions that help them to enjoy their adolescence and transition well to adulthood.

Usual steps in the management in a given case are as follows:

- Educate and counsel parents about the condition
- Educate the child wherever possible
- Check for presence of treatable underlying cause and make necessary referrals[8]
- Teach parents home-based intervention/training skills
- Identify and manage comorbid behavioral and psychiatric problems
- Identify and manage comorbid medical problems
- Check about the need for genetic counseling and refer
- Help parents to access social welfare benefits
- Refer for requisite therapies and interventions
- Emphasize the need for safety and self-protection skills and facilitate
- Emphasize the need for formal education in inclusions schools, special schools, open schooling [National Institute of Open Schooling (NIOS)], and facilitate the same
- In adolescents help transition from schooling to vocational training
- Address any other concerns of parents such as future planning and guardianship[9]

MANAGEMENT

From a clinical perspective, given the developmental nature of ID, the aims of management are twofold:

- Ensure optimum health, development, well-being of individuals
- Ensure good family adaptation (family empowerment)

To this, *a third aim*, viz., to create a socially conducive and facilitative environment could be of interest to psychiatrists who are specially interested in this field. Management is guided by certain *key principles and philosophies*, that are laid down in **Table 7**.

- Clinician attitudes, approaches, and perceived quality of clinical encounter make enormous difference to the well-being of children and families. Basic approach should be one of *having a good knowledge base* and *building*

TABLE 7: Key philosophies and principles that guide management.

Philosophy/principle	*Explanation*
Rights-based approach	People with intellectual disability (ID) enjoy the same rights as others. Society as a whole and Government is committed to provide affordable and accessible services and supports to them and their families
Inclusion	Participation within family and social participation; inclusion in education, workforce, leisure activities, recreation, sports, public spaces; antistigma measures
Family empowerment	Enables families to manage an often-stressful situation effectively and thrive; highly relevant in India because family-based care is the rule and institutionalization is an exception
Early detection and intervention	Ensures best possible development and well-being and prevents secondary complications
Parent mediated, home-based interventions	Transfer of intervention skills to parents; a collaborative approach in which parents are partners in care and learn to carry out interventions at home

hope and optimism. Thus, management calls for both *scientific and humanistic approach*.

- Ideally, management has to be multidisciplinary; but in reality, it is often not possible because of lack of availability and access. Hence, it is always a good idea for the clinician to have some basic knowledge and expertise beyond his routine clinical skills in aspects such as early intervention techniques, speech and language therapy, and developmental behavioral interventions. Some basic messages about such interventions can be very useful for parents.
- Ready-at-hand set of leaflets, guidelines and tips for parents, and authentic web resources comes in handy and is much appreciated by parents.
- Clinician needs to guard himself/herself from errors that can vitiate the management. These are listed in **Box 2**.

There are several dimensions and components of management; they are summarized in **Table 8**, and some of these aspects are described below.

Parent Psychoeducation and Counseling

This is a crucial and initial step in management and serves as a foundation for further interventions. Psychoeducation builds on what parents already know about the problem and covers nature of comprehensive diagnosis, prognosis, clarification of misconceptions, treatment

BOX 2: Common errors to avoid in clinical work.

- Negative, pessimistic attitude and therapeutic nihilism ("nothing can be done"/"it is too late")
- Underestimation of future attainments and erroneously painting a gloomy picture
- Not treating the individuals with respect and dignity
- Implicitly or explicitly blaming parents
- Lack of adequate knowledge base
- Cursory and incomplete evaluation
- Missing or misdiagnosing comorbid psychiatric and medical conditions
- Not providing treatment options
- Giving false reassurances ("he will be normal when he grows up")
- Recommending unproven treatments and unnecessary, often expensive medications

TABLE 8: Dimensions of management.

Dimension	*Examples of components*
Parent psychoeducation and counseling	Diagnosis, prognosis, clarifying misconceptions and faulty perceptions/expectations, supporting parents, building hope and confidence, explaining treatment options, addressing health and harmony issues in family, optimizing parenting practices, teaching stress management and better coping/adaptation, and teaching techniques of home-based intervention
Child education and counseling	Exploring lived experiences, explaining limitations in simple terms and highlighting assets, conveying that "not your fault, it is a problem", teaching coping, and motivating for working on problems
Medical interventions	Genetic counseling, management of treatable causes, and medical comorbidities
Psychiatric/behavioral interventions	Identifying and managing comorbid psychiatric disorders/problem behaviors
Developmental interventions	Early intervention, speech and language therapy, individualized training program, education/schooling, and vocational training
Others	Assisting in certification/accessing social security benefits, liaising with other professionals and schools, addressing developmental stage-specific issues, e.g., adolescence

options, and addresses any other queries that parents have. One frequent task for the clinician is shifting parents' explanatory model for the condition from a "medical model" (a disease of brain that can be cured by medicines, injections, operations, etc.), to a "developmental model" (a condition that has occurred due to damage to some parts of the developing brain, which gets better by stimulation, education, and training). Use of figures, graphs, and examples are useful to conveying the message effectively.

Counseling also involves supporting parents when the diagnosis comes as disturbing news, leading to many reactions such as shock, denial, self-blame, disillusionment and a sense of loss. A sensitive, compassionate handling of the situation, allowing for ventilation, a supportive, empathic stance, reassurance that child will continue to improve (instilling a realistic hope), will help parents feel better and prepare them to face the situation with confidence. **Table 9** describes a few approaches on how to build hope and optimism.

The stages, process, and content of parent counseling are described in detail elsewhere.[10] Identifying and appreciating the positive efforts, addressing maladaptive parenting patterns such as overinvolvement and overprotection, skills transfer for home-based training and strengthening parents' coping and adaptation are the other major steps in counseling. **Box 3** lists a few key messages to be conveyed to parents during counseling.

Child Education and Counseling

This is a neglected area, because of the faulty assumption that children with ID do not have the necessary capacity for it. It should always be attempted wherever possible. Older children with milder forms of ID can immensely benefit from education and counseling. Interviewing and educating techniques need to be adapted to suit the given child. Child education needs to focus both on their limitations such as some difficulties in learning as well as their strengths. Attempt must be made to get an idea of their

TABLE 9: Building hope, optimism, and confidence in parents in clinical practice.

Technique	*Comment/explanation*
Respect and dignity for children and families	This is an absolute ethical requirement; it puts them at ease and sets the tone for further work
Positive engagement—helpful concern, interact positively, and build rapport	During consultation, parents tend to view the child "through the eyes" of the clinician; when clinician shows interest, and takes pleasure in interacting with child, parents also feel happy and hopeful
Focus on current attainments	Shift the focus from what the child cannot do *to what the child has already learnt;* asking parents how the child learnt it, and appreciating parents for it. This emphasis on "success experiences" of parents having been able to teach something, opens up the topic of child's potentialities and capabilities and how parents can teach the child
Appropriate way of addressing the question "Will she/he be normal?" through a balanced positive framing	Give a range of outcomes, rather than painting a uniformly negative picture. For example, "he will be independent like a normal person in such and such aspects and will require only a little support in such and such areas, and perhaps a lot of support in some areas."; also emphasize that child will definitely keep improving over time, especially with good education/training inputs and opportunities for learning

BOX 3: Some key messages to parents during counseling.

- Child will continue to develop, though at a slower pace
- Child may be slow in learning, but still can be taught with patience, persistence, repetition, encouragement/praise, and the correct approach.
- Look at abilities rather than deficits (what the child is able to do and what can be taught, rather than what he or she is not able to do)
- Have realistic expectations; do not criticize the child for his/her shortcomings
- Learn the techniques of training and practice them
- There is no need to feel ashamed or embarrassed about the child's condition
- Do not blame yourself or other family members for the child's condition
- Do not overprotect the child; encourage the child to become independent
- Do not waste money unnecessarily on dubious/ unproven treatments
- Find out about services that are available and utilize them
- Connect with other parents and join parent associations/networks
- Keep your normal life intact, and work together as a family to solve problems
- Arrange daily routines such that everybody gets some time off from the child
- Keep your social life intact; do not socially isolate yourself from relatives/friends

"lived experiences" and any stressful experiences such as stigmatization, bullying, and harassment, which need to be addressed in management. They also can be encouraged and motivated to work on realistic goals and taught relevant coping skills.

Early Intervention and Stimulation

All young children with delays of whatever degree need to receive home-based parent-mediated early intervention and stimulation. Most parents are motivated and are very keen to learn and practice what they can do to help this child, and it is the clinician's job to guide, educate and teach them early intervention skills. This is in addition to center-based intervention such as physiotherapy, occupational therapy, and speech and language therapy, wherever these therapies are available. A few relevant approaches are described below with examples:

- Engage with child through all five senses in as many different ways as possible, note their response, reinforce and repeat.
- Watch the child's gestures, facial expressions, and body language to understand what she is communicating and respond appropriately.
- Notice and respond to child's noises and utterances (parallel vocalization)
- Use gestures, facial expressions, and body language (like "actors in a drama") while interacting
- Give a "running commentary" of ongoing activities
- Engage in mutually enjoyable play (mother-infant games)—(gentle swinging, peek-a-boo, rocking in the lap with a song, and tickling game)
- Improve hand functions (grasp, release, transfer, pick, pour, build, push, pull, throw, and catch)
- Teach simple social skills—come, go, take, give, show, bring, pick up, point to something (light and body parts), follow your direction of pointing, etc. Use modeling and hand-on-hand technique if needed
- Take the child out and show familiar sights and sounds such as animals, birds, vehicles, etc.
- Encourage the child to do simple communicative gestures—hi-fi, namaste, ta-ta, and bye-bye
- Teach the child how to perform simple actions—clap-clap, how crow/dog/auto makes sounds, how bird flies, how you eat/ sleep/drink water, how Mom combs her hair/ applies powder
- Point to people, objects, pictures, and names and encourage her to repeat it. Notice, praise and appreciate even the slightest attempt. Similarly, teach the child to name actions.

- Always wait for a few seconds for the child to respond, do not bombard the child
- Recite nursery rhymes, sing lullabies so that the child learns to anticipate familiar sounds and rhymes. Get her to mimic related actions.
- *Reduce screen time to <15 minutes per day.* Avoid screen to feed.
- Play interactive/turn-taking games with child—run and catch, ball and bat, kicking ball back and forth, catch and throw, and hide and seek
- Encourage imaginative activities—pretend play, driving play, doll play, and cooking and serving play
- Teach concepts—big/small, long/short, sweet/sour, soft/hard, hot/cold, up/down, right/left, and now/later. Use sorting, classifying, arranging, building, recognizing, and naming to teach concepts.
- Teach self-care from early age—eating, drinking, handwashing, dressing, toileting, and brushing teeth.

Skills Training

Even children with very severe forms of ID can acquire new skills by using the appropriate techniques, and such skills training is a key step in intervention starting from early years. Self-care, domestic, social, and other practical skills are the usual areas to focus on. Providing opportunities and encouraging learning ensures that children's capacities are optimally utilized. Behavioral techniques are widely employed for this purpose. Clinicians need to be aware of these techniques and make their best efforts to transfer these skills to parents. **Table 10** describes these behavioral techniques for building new skills.

TABLE 10: Behavioral approaches to build new skills.

Technique	*Brief definition*	*Example/comment*
Goal specification	Specific description of behavior to be learnt, based on current level and needs	Drinks from a glass and eats pieces of roti by self
Task analysis	Breaking activity into sequential steps	Number of steps depends on child's learning capacity
Rewarding	Pleasant event following a given desired behavior; should be immediate, consistent, appropriate, and contingent	*Praise:* "Good job", an appreciative clap, "Shabbash!" *Material:* A small bit of cookie
Modeling	Showing how, or demonstrating, so that the child imitates and learns	Works well in children who have learnt to imitate
Shaping (successive approximation)	Teaching the simplified version of the total task and gradually increasing complexity; useful when a skill cannot be broken down into discrete steps	To teach pincer grasp, start with bigger objects such as a small ball and move on to smaller and smaller objects
Back-chaining	Breaking down the task into several small steps and teaching the last step first and then going backward; Very effective; Applicable to most activities of daily living (ADLs)	*Drink by self:* Parent fills glass with a little water, gives to child to drink; next to pick up glass from table, and so on
Forward chaining	Teaching the first step first; teach first step of the task first	Brushing teeth (easiest step comes first)
Prompting	Verbal/physical assistance, hand-on-hand, and gradually fading of assistance	Works well when child cannot imitate or is clumsy

Management of Comorbid Psychiatric and Behavior Problems

These are common reasons for consultation and are a major source of parental stress. *As noted earlier, full range of psychiatric disorders can co-occur with ID, and are as amenable for treatment as in typical children.* Recent-onset behavior change is often a clue to onset of comorbid problem. A judicious combination of pharmacological and behavioral/psychosocial interventions works best.

Pharmacological interventions: Indications and choice of medication is similar to their use in typical children, with some special precautions:[5,11]

- Parents have to be taken into confidence and medication started with their consent.
- The principle of "start low and go slow" is particularly applicable. Indiscriminate use of higher doses or multiple medications makes the child vulnerable for physical and behavioral side effects.
- Special care in choice of medication is necessary in the preexisting medical conditions such as epilepsy, cerebral palsy, neurological problems, and cardiac problems. For instance, clonidine up to 5 μg/kg/day is useful in comorbid ADHD with or without epilepsy.
- Drug interactions, especially with antiepileptics, need careful consideration.
- Careful monitoring of response to medication and titration of the dose is necessary to ensure best possible response.
- Similarly, careful monitoring for adverse effects is necessary as these children are more prone for neurological and other adverse effects.
- By and large, psychotropic medications work as well in ID as in other children, with a few exceptions.

Medication can be considered in moderate to severe nonsyndromic disruptive behaviors such as irritability, aggression, and self-injury. Risperidone in doses up to 1 mg/day (0.04 mg/kg/day) or aripiprazole up to 2 mg/day is usually effective.

Behavioral and psychosocial interventions: These are used either solely or in combination with medication depending on the needs of the given case.

- A good number of problem behaviors are "learnt behaviors", and respond well to behavioral interventions following a thorough functional analysis, which is a more refined form of antecedent-behavior-consequence (ABC) analysis.
- Most parents are eager to learn and practice these techniques (behavioral parent training or parent management training) and clinician needs to keep this as an important agenda in the management. Demonstrating or modeling is a powerful method to teach parents.[10]
- Common behavioral techniques that are useful to manage problem behaviors are laid down in **Table 11**.
- Other psychosocial interventions for problem behaviors include undue stress reduction, environmental support, teaching coping skills, improving parent-child relationships and parenting practices, and addressing health and harmony issues in families. An in-depth understanding of factors contributing to problem behaviors will help the clinician to choose appropriate techniques.
- Very frequently, problem behaviors are embedded in faulty interaction patterns between parents/other significant adults and the child. Understanding and breaking these patterns and putting in place healthy patterns often leads to substantial reduction in the problem behaviors.
- Many mothers are stressed out, even showing signs of burnout. In such situation, arranging for a consultation becomes necessary.

TABLE 11: Behavior techniques to reduce problem behaviors.

Technique	*Brief description*
Disregarding	Ignoring the behavior (as if it is not occurring at all) but continuing the attention to child
Ignoring	Ignoring both the child and behavior
Redirecting	Catching the child just as an odd behavior is beginning and guiding toward appropriate behavior
Limit-setting	Clearly communicating what is acceptable and unacceptable behaviors to child and enforcing limits
Blocking	Preventing the behavior from being completed (example aggression)
Gradual guidance	Waiting for the child to stop resisting physically and then guiding toward completion
Time-out (from positive reinforcement)	Removal of attention/reinforcement contingent upon occurrence of a specified/ undesirable behavior
Differential reinforcement of other behavior	Noticing and rewarding when child shows desirable behavior or when undesirable behavior is absent (catching the child being good and praising)
Overcorrection	Child has to not only restore but do something more to set right whatever damage or disturbance that has occurred as a result of undesirable behavior
Response cost	Withholding a privilege that child enjoys contingent upon the occurrence of undesirable behavior

- Many children with problem behaviors have deficient skills that contribute to problem behaviors. Teaching these skills, for example communication training, can reduce problem behaviors (**Table 10** on building new skills).

Some representative case examples of comorbid psychiatric disorders are given below:

- A 15-year-old thinly built boy with moderate ID attending a special school presented with 6-month history of episodes of being very restless, talkative, sleepless, and interfering with others' activities and occasional aggression lasting for about 10 days once in a month. Parents sought consultation as this became very troublesome, when he was in "restless period". On psychiatric examination, he was noted to be cheerful, restless, inattentive, trying to pick things from the table and getting irritable with parents when they tried to restrain him.
- A provisional diagnosis of bipolar affective disorder with brief-lasting manic episodes was made. He responded well to olanzapine 5 mg/day.
- Aruna (not her name) is a 16-year-old girl with moderate ID secondary to a rare genetic disorder. Till 2 years, she was attending a special school regularly and learnt basic literacy skills and was friendly with teachers and classmates. At home, she managed almost all self-care activities by herself and could even fetch milk from a nearby shop. She presented 2-year history of gradually becoming withdrawn, lost interest in going to school, laughing and cry to herself for no reason, and muttering irrelevant things and deteriorating self-care. On examination, she was noted to be withdrawn, noncommunicative, continuously mumbling, as if talking to someone. She would answer a couple of questions meaningfully, but after that would lapse into irrelevant talk. A provisional diagnosis of schizophrenia in the background

of moderate ID was made, and she was given aripiprazole starting with 2.5 mg initially and was titrated up to 10 mg/day. Parents were also counseled about retraining/rehabilitation and activity therapy. A remarkable improvement was noted by 8 weeks: psychotic symptoms subsided, there was better interaction with family and self-care markedly improved. Dose was reduced to 7.5 mg/day as she developed extra-pyramidal symptoms and trihexyphenidyl 2 mg/day was added. She was maintaining improvement at the end 6 months of follow-up.

- Geetha (not her name), a 9-year-old girl with severe ID and difficult-to-treat epilepsy on multiple antiepileptic drugs was referred for problem behaviors. Parents reported severe behavioral dysregulation with restlessness, shouting, screaming, irritability, throwing things around, decreased sleep, and severe impulsive aggression such as pinching, and biting. A provisional diagnosis of ADHD with ODD symptoms (because of over-protectiveness and permissive parenting, often seen in such children) was made and she was started on clonidine 0.025 mg at bed time and built up to 0.125 mg/day. Parents were also counseled about activity scheduling, limit-setting, differential reinforcement, and skills training. Significant improvement was noted in her problem behaviors and skill levels by 3 months.

SUMMARY AND CONCLUSION

To summarize, ID is a common NDD with significant impairments in intellectual and adaptive functioning, that often leads to lifelong impairments. It can result from any significant genetic and/or environmental adverse influence on brain maturation and development during pre-, peri-, or postnatal periods. Its severity can vary from being very mild to very severe. Other NDDs, medical conditions, and psychiatric/behavioral problems frequently co-occur with ID. A thorough clinical evaluation consisting of history, physical examination, and psychiatric examination needs to be conducted to arrive at a comprehensive diagnosis that comprises severity, etiologic factors, comorbid disorders, and significant family and psychosocial factors. Clinician has the task of educating and counseling children and parents, building hope and optimism, alleviate family stress and enhance coping, transfer skills for home-based management, manage comorbid mental health/behavioral problems, and attend to medical issues such as genetic counseling. Another essential management task is developing detailed plan for individualized developmental intervention/education/training. Effective management ensures optimum development and well-being of children as well as optimal coping and adaptation of the families.

In conclusion, ID is a common NDD, often leading to lifelong disability as it significantly impairs intellectual and adaptive development. It is frequently accompanied by other neuro-developmental, physical, psychiatric, and behavioral comorbidities. A thorough clinical evaluation from multiple sources and a comprehensive diagnosis pave the way for an effective management. Clinician has the task of instilling hope and optimism and empowering children and families, which help them to adapt and thrive and this calls for a blend of both scientific and humanistic approach.

Conflict of interest: The author declares that there is no conflict of interest.

Financial disclosure: There is no relevant financial disclosure of funds linked with the chapter.

REFERENCES

1. Russell PSS, Nagaraj S, Vengadavaradan A, Russell S, Mammen PM, Shankar SR, et al. Prevalence of intellectual disability in India:

A meta-analysis. World J Clin Pediatr. 2022;11(2): 206-14.
2. American Psychiatric Association, DSM-5 Task Force. (2013). Diagnostic and statistical manual of mental disorders: DSM-5™ (5th ed.). [online] Available from https://psychiatryonline.org/doi/book/10.1176/appi.books.9780890425596 [Last accessed 20th November, 2025].
3. World Health Organization. International Classification of Diseases 11th Revision. [online] Available from https://icd.who.int/en [Last accessed 20th November, 2025].
4. Girimaji SC, Basheer S, Biswas A, Gangadharan SK. Intellectual Disability—Concepts, Aetiology, and Genetics. In: Bhaumik S, Alexander R (Eds). Oxford Textbook of the Psychiatry of Intellectual Disability. Oxford: Oxford University Press; 2020. pp. 23-34.
5. Siegel M, McGuire K, Veenstra-VanderWeele J, Stratigos K, King B; American Academy of Child and Adolescent Psychiatry (AACAP) Committee on Quality Issues (CQI); et al. Practice Parameter for the Assessment and Treatment of Psychiatric Disorders in Children and Adolescents With Intellectual Disability (Intellectual Developmental Disorder). J Am Acad Child Adolesc Psychiatry. 2020;59(4):468-96.
6. Girimaji SC. Clinical Practice Guidelines for the Diagnosis and Management of Children With Mental Retardation. Indian J Psychiatry. 2008;43-67.
7. Kishore Mt, Udipi G, Seshadri S. Clinical practice guidelines for assessment and management of intellectual disability. Indian J Psychiatry. 2019;61(8):194.
8. Arun P, Mahajan S. Addressing the Visible and Invisible Gaps and Challenges in the Diagnosis and Management of Intellectual Disability. J Indian Assoc Child Adolesc Ment Health. 2023; 19(1):75-80.
9. Sivakumar T, Thirthalli J. Future Care Planning for Persons with Intellectual Developmental Disorder in Resource-Poor Settings. J Psychosoc Rehabil Ment Health. 2022;9(3):235-8.
10. Girimaji SC. Counsellors Manual for Family Intervention in Mental Retardation. New Delhi: Indian Council of Medical Research; 1996.
11. Santosh PJ, Baird G. Psychopharmacotherapy in children and adults with intellectual disability. Lancet. 1999;354(9174):233-42.

Developmental Speech and Language Disorders: Concept, Definition, Assessment, Diagnosis, Formulation of Management Plan, and Management

Shoba S Meera, Akhila S Girimaji, BK Yamini

INTRODUCTION

Developmental speech and language disorders encompass a range of conditions where children have difficulties with speech and/or language development, i.e., difficulty acquiring and using language or speech skills at the expected developmental stage. These disorders typically manifest during early childhood and can significantly affect a child's ability to communicate effectively, thus impacting their social, academic, and emotional well-being. These disorders can occur in isolation or alongside other developmental conditions, the latter being more common. As with most neurodevelopmental disorders (NDDs), early identification and intervention are crucial for managing developmental speech and language disorders to improve overall communication skills and quality of life. The prevalence of developmental speech and language disorders in India varies widely based on different studies and methodologies. One study suggests that around 7–11% of children may be affected by speech and language disorders.[1] While speech and language disorders share several common features, they have distinct identifying characteristics. In this chapter, they will be discussed as developmental speech disorders and developmental language disorders.

DEVELOPMENTAL SPEECH DISORDERS

Developmental speech disorders refer to a group of conditions that affect a child's ability to produce speech sounds correctly or speak fluently, impacting their ability to communicate effectively. While developmental speech sound disorders (SSDs) encompass a range of difficulties related to producing sounds correctly and clearly, developmental speech fluency disorders involve disruptions in the flow of speech, such as repetitions, prolongations, or blocks of sounds, syllables, or words.

There are two main types of SSDs: (1) Phonetic (articulation disorders) and (2) phonemic (phonological disorders). Articulation disorder (phonetic) involves difficulty in physically producing specific speech sounds, i.e., the issue lies in the motor aspects of speech production. Some of the most common errors in the phonetic type of SSD include errors of substitution, i.e., replacing one sound with another [e.g., /θun/ (thun) for /sun/]; omission, i.e., leaving out sounds [e.g., /gi:n/(geen) for /gri:n/(green)]; distortion, i.e., altering the sound so that it sounds incorrect [e.g., /ʃku:l/(s*ch*ool) – ch is weak or sounds distorted, for /sku:l/ (school)]; and addition, i.e., adding extra sounds into words [e.g., /sʌneIk/(sanake) for /sneik/(snake)]. Phonological disorder (phonemic) type involves difficulty in understanding the sound system and rules of language. It is about how the brain organizes sounds into meaningful patterns. Some common types of phonological-type SSD include fronting: substituting sounds produced at the back of the mouth with sounds produced at the front [e.g., /ti/(tey) for /ki/ (key)]; stopping, substituting a stop sound (like "t" or "d") for a fricative (like "s" or "f") [e.g., /pΛn/(pan) for / fΛn/(fan)]; final consonant deletion: omitting the last consonant of a word [e.g., /kΛ/(cu) for /kΛp/ (cup); cluster reduction: omitting one or more consonants in a cluster [e.g., /pu:n/(poon) for / spu:n/(spoon)], etc. All children may have these difficulties when they start to first learn to speak. However, if the difficulties persist past the age at which mastery must happen, they need attention and intervention.[2,3] In addition to children with/ without co-occurring NDDs who may have SSDs, children with cerebral palsy (dysarthria), apraxia of speech, cleft lip and palate, and hearing impairment among other disorders may have SSDs and need targeted treatment.

Developmental speech fluency disorders are interruptions in the flow of speaking. The characteristic types of dysfluencies in stuttering include repetitions of sounds, syllables, and monosyllabic words; prolongations of speech sounds; and blocks. The onset of stuttering typically occurs in childhood, with the average age being around 33 months.[4] Children with stuttering may develop secondary behaviors, which are observed only during dysfluent speech. These behaviors include motor actions such as eye blinking, flaring of nostrils, head movement, whole-body movement, and distorting the mouth. They may also include physiological responses, avoidance, and expectancy.[5] Additionally, these children may develop social anxiety, a sense of loss of control, and negative thoughts or feelings about themselves or communication in general.[4] The dysfluencies in stuttering may be influenced by the situation and the languages spoken (native/first language—L1, second language—L2, and so on). Developmental stuttering in children must be differentiated from neurogenic stuttering, psychogenic stuttering, and cluttering.

DEVELOPMENTAL LANGUAGE DISORDERS

Developmental language disorders involve difficulties with understanding and/or producing language. This can affect a child's ability to understand others, express thoughts, and use language in socially appropriate ways. Language is a complex system used for communication, and it comprises several interrelated components that enable individuals to convey and comprehend meaning effectively. These components include phonology, morphology, syntax, semantics, and pragmatics. Understanding these components is essential for diagnosing and treating language disorders, as difficulties in any one of these areas can significantly impact overall communication.

As per International Classification of Diseases (ICD)-11,[6] persistent deficits in the acquisition, understanding, production, or use of language in at least one of the following specific components of language warrant a diagnosis of developmental language disorder: (1) The ability to decompose words into constituent sounds and mentally manipulate those sounds (i.e., phonological awareness); (2) the ability to use language rules, e.g., regarding word endings and how words are combined to form sentences (i.e., syntax, morphology, or grammar); (3) the ability to learn, understand, and use language to convey the meaning of words and sentences (i.e., semantics); (4) the ability to tell a story or have a conversation (i.e., narrative or conversational discourse); and (5) the ability to understand and use language in social contexts, e.g., making inferences, understanding verbal humor, and resolving ambiguous meaning (i.e., pragmatics). While language disorder is the term used in Diagnostic and Statistical Manual of Mental Disorders, 5th Edition (DSM-5),[7] developmental language disorder is used in ICD-11.[6] Irrespective of the terminology used, both classification systems place language disorders under the broad category of NDDs. Other terms used in clinical spaces and often used interchangeably include language impairment, spoken language disorder, receptive expressive language disorder, etc.

Language disorders may present as (1) receptive and expressive language difficulties, i.e., difficulty in understanding or processing language and expressing themselves; (2) expressive language difficulties only, i.e., expressing thoughts or ideas using spoken or written language; and (3) difficulty with pragmatic language only, a diagnosis often considered as diagnosis by exclusion and must not be made in the presence of disorders such as autism where social communication deficits are a core symptom.[8] In disorders of pragmatic language (also referred to as a social communication disorder), difficulties are in the understanding and use of language in social contexts, e.g., speaking in turns, making inferences, making friends, negotiating. Here receptive and expressive language skills are relatively unimpaired, but pragmatic language abilities are markedly below the expected level for the individual's age and interfere with communication.

Developmental language disorders may occur in isolation (primary), formerly called specific language impairment [LI], or co-occur with other NDDs (secondary) like autism spectrum disorder (ASD), attention-deficit/hyperactivity disorder (ADHD), and intellectual disability (ID). This diagnostic overlap is not limited to cross-sectional findings but also occurs over time in that receiving one neurodevelopmental diagnosis predicts receiving other related diagnoses later over the life course.[9] As with most NDDs, some of the common etiology and risk factors include genetic influences, neurological factors, environmental factors (like language exposure/stimulation), etc.

Language Difficulties in Other Neurodevelopmental Disorders

Some of the most common language difficulties and presentation in children with NDDs like ASD, ADHD, ID include the following:

- Delay in speech and language development, and the delay can range from mild to severe, with some children being nonverbal or minimally verbal, i.e., having very limited speech[10]
- Significant communication problems in 50% of preschool children with ADHD[11]
- Limited vocabulary; that is, children with NDDs may have a smaller vocabulary compared to their typically developing peers,[12] and deficits in semantic reception and expression may be evident too[13]
- Challenges in understanding spoken or written language. For instance, they may struggle with following multistep directions or grasping the meaning of more complex language[14]
- Difficulties in grammar and syntax like trouble constructing grammatically correct sentences, often using shorter and simpler sentence structures. Further, they may omit necessary grammatical elements, such as articles, pronouns, or verb endings.[15] Deficits in tense markers; sentence types; homonym, synonym, and antonym judgment may be evident too.[16]
- Phonological processing issues including difficulty in distinguishing between similar sounds, which can affect their speech clarity and literacy skills[17]
- Narrative difficulties, that is, difficulties in constructing coherent narratives (telling stories or describing events). Children with NDDs may struggle with organizing their thoughts, maintaining a logical sequence, and including essential details

- Pragmatic language, which refers to the social use of language, is often impaired in children with NDDs, especially those with ASD. They may have trouble with topic maintenance, turn-taking in conversation, understanding social cues, or using appropriate language in social situations.[18,19]

Assessment

Assessment of developmental speech and language disorders requires a nuanced understanding of speech-language developmental milestones **(Box 1)** and various ways in which speech and language can be impaired. Play-based

BOX 1: Key speech-language developmental milestones.

Prelinguistic stage (0–12 months):
- Cooing and babbling
  - Vocal play and cooing sounds
  - Canonical babbling (e.g., "bababa" or "dadada")
- Gesture use
- Joint attention
- Imitation
- Early understanding of turn-taking in communication
- Blows raspberries
- Tries to imitate the sounds made

First words (12–18 months):
- Single words (around 12 months)
  - Emergence of first meaningful words (usually names of familiar people or objects)
  - Typically, around 50 words by 18 months
- Holophrastic stage
  - Use of single words to express complete ideas or requests (e.g., "milk" to mean "I want milk")
  - Emphasis on nouns and verbs
- Uses long string of sounds, syllables, and real words with speech-like inflection

Vocabulary explosion and two-word sentences (18–24 months):
- Vocabulary growth
  - Rapid increase in the number of words known and used
  - Typical vocabulary of 200–300 words by the age of 2 years
- Combining words
  - Start of two-word combinations (e.g., "big car")
- Uses consonants at the beginning of the words
- Speech may not be clear and will have substitution or omission errors

Early sentences and grammar (2–3 years):
- Three-word sentences
  - Use of simple sentences with subject–object–verb structure [e.g., SOV: Indian languages "/ΛmΛ ka:r kodu/ ("Maa, Give me car"); /mΛ khana ðo/ ("Ma, give me food"]
  - Incorporation of adjectives, pronouns, and prepositions
- Grammar and syntax development
  - Use of plurals, past tense, and other grammatical markers
  - Increasing complexity in sentence structure
- Correctly produces most vowels in words
- Has correct production of /p,b,m,h,w,d and n/ in words
- Speech is intelligible to familiar listeners but may not be to unfamiliar listeners

Contd...

Contd...

Narrative and conversational skills (3–5 years):
- Storytelling and descriptive language
  - Ability to tell simple stories and describe events.
  - Use of conjunctions (e.g., "and," "but," "because") to connect ideas
- Question asking and answering
  - Frequent use of questions (e.g., "Why?" "How?")
  - Improved ability to answer questions and follow conversations
- Pragmatics and social language
  - Understanding and using polite forms of address
  - Ability to take turns and maintain a topic in conversation
- By 5 years, the child produces most consonant sounds correctly, though a few errors are developmentally appropriate (ex: wabbit for rabbit)
- Should be able to blend word parts like cup + cake
- Identifies rhyming words

School-age language development (5+ years):
- Advanced vocabulary and complex sentences
  - Continued growth in vocabulary, including more abstract and academic words
  - Use of more complex and varied sentence structures
- Reading and writing integration
  - Development of literacy skills
  - Understanding of written language supporting oral language skills
- Metalinguistic awareness
  - Ability to think about and manipulate language (e.g., understanding jokes, puns, and wordplay)
- Social and academic language use
  - Adaptation of language use to different contexts (e.g., formal vs. informal settings)
  - Mastery of language required for academic success
- Child's speech is understandable in conversation
- Child would have acquired all the speech sounds correctly

assessments form an important part of assessing children.

Some of the earliest signs of language delay before the child's first birthday include the following: Child has not yet started to:

- Make sounds back and forth with you
- Babble with changes in tone, e.g., dadadadadadadada
- Use gestures like waving "bye bye" or shaking head for "no"
- Try to imitate/copy sounds that you make
- Respond to her/his name
- Recognize the names of some people (family members and objects)
- Communicate in some way when s/he needs help with something

As with most conditions, mapping and understanding the pathway to care are crucial. Equally important is to understand care pathways to NDDs, including developmental speech language disorders. This includes the coming together of a multidisciplinary team. Specifically in developmental speech language disorders, key decisions are made by the Speech-Language Pathologist (SLP) in consultation with the team of professionals and with the parents/caregivers of children.

Key steps included in detailed evaluation of speech and language disorders are as follows:

- *History and screening:* Quick checks to identify children who may need a full evaluation. This involves brief interactions or standardized screening tests to spot potential issues.

- *Standardized testing:* Use of norm-referenced tests to compare a child's performance to that of peers. Examples include the Assessment for Language Development.[20]
- *Observational assessment:* Evaluating the child in natural settings (e.g., during play, conversation). This approach provides insights into how speech and language issues manifest in everyday activities.
- *Speech-language sampling:* Collecting and analyzing samples of the child's spoken language
- *Hearing tests:* Audiological evaluations are crucial since hearing issues can impact language development
- Oral–vocal mechanism examination including speech cranial nerves examination
- Speech subsystem analysis such as assessing the phonatory system, articulatory system, and so on
- Swallowing assessment
- Instrumental and perceptual analysis of speech

Diagnosis

Diagnosis of developmental speech and language disorders involves integrating information from detailed developmental and medical history, assessments that are based on parent report, and direct observation of the child. Some of the key steps in the diagnosis include the following:

- *Differential diagnosis:* Distinguishing between different types of speech and language disorders
- Next is identifying if the disorder is primary (not due to another condition) or secondary to other issues (e.g., hearing loss, neurological conditions).
- *Severity classification:* Assessing how severe the disorder is and its impact on daily functioning. Categories often include mild, moderate, severe, or profound.
- *Identifying comorbidities:* Recognizing other co-occurring conditions, such as IDD, ASD, ADHD, or learning disabilities. This is crucial in intervention planning
- *Functional impact:* Evaluating how the disorder affects the child's ability to communicate, learn, and interact socially. This too helps in planning interventions that are tailored to the child's needs.

Prognosis

Prognosis varies widely depending on the type and severity of the disorder, comorbidities, the age at which intervention begins, and the intensity of the support provided. Early diagnosis and intervention are crucial for improving outcomes.

Management

A management plan is a package of intervention strategies proposed depending on the diagnosis arrived at by the clinician. The overall purpose of a management plan is to improve the speech and/or language in the child, thus enhancing communication. Ultimately, the goal of speech and language interventions is effective communication—whether verbal or nonverbal—because communication is key.

Key objectives of intervention as described by Owens et al.[21] include the following:

- Making intervention sessions fun for the child
- Helping children not only learn skills in the session but also generalize learnings to their real-world environments, such as home, school, and work
- The child should not have to think about what has been learned; in large part, it should be automatic.
- The child must be able to self-monitor. Although modifications should be automatic, they will still require monitoring. The child should be able to listen to and observe himself or herself and make corrections as needed, without the interventionist being present.

- Intervention should be sensitive to the personal and cultural characteristics of the child and the child's family.

Speech and language intervention for children include a variety of practices. Interventions can be carried out in various settings such as home, hospitals/clinics, early years setting (preschool/nursery), school, early intervention centers, etc. The method of delivery of intervention can be direct (clinician-child) and parent mediated (parent-child). In direct intervention, the focus is between the clinician and the child individually or in a group setting based on the developmental age and the diagnosis.[22] The intervention can be parent mediated, or caregiver mediated, where the focus is on delivering the intervention through the caregiver who then works with their child (e.g., LiL' STEPS, UPPA).[23,24] Rightfully so, these interventions are gaining momentum in India, since families of ASD children face significant barriers to care in terms of dearth of trained resources, lack of government or state funding, social stigma, etc. Another barrier to services is geographic location and travel to intervention services. Recent interventions have been able to address this aspect too by demonstrating that it is feasible and acceptable to provide caregiver-mediated interventions online.[23]

INTERVENTION FOR DEVELOPMENTAL SPEECH DISORDERS

As discussed in the earlier section developmental speech disorders are classified into (1) phonetic (articulation disorders) and (2) phonemic (phonological disorders); hence, the intervention approaches are also dichotomized accordingly. However, it is important to understand that the normal speech sound production involves both the production of the sound at a motor level and its use in accordance with the rules of language. Thus, the two skills are intertwined. Both the approaches follow the establishment phase, generalization phase, and maintenance phase. Phonetic/articulation approaches target the correct production of the target sound and are the sounds that are often selected when the errors are assumed to be motor based. It focuses on the placement and movement of articulators of the target sound in combination with auditory stimulation (e.g., ear training, focused auditory input).[25] Few of the very well-established articulation approaches are imitation, phonetic placement, successive approximation, etc. Phonemic/phonological-based approaches target group of sounds with similar error patterns than individual sounds. The effort is to help the child internalize the phonological rules of the language and generalize these rules. The focus of the phonological-based approaches is to (1) establish sound and feature contrasts and (2) replace error patterns with appropriate phonological patterns.[25] Few of the well-established phonological approaches are minimal pair contrast therapy, metaphon therapy, etc. Explaining the phonetic/phonemic approaches is beyond the scope of this chapter; however, few guidelines have been provided in **Box 2**. SSDs in severe form might also require use of augmentative and alternative communication (AAC). The details of AAC are provided later in this chapter. AAC may be recommended for those children with severe apraxia of speech and limited improvement with speech output.

Interventions to improve fluency for children with stuttering include indirect approaches, direct approaches, hybrid method, and use of analogies. Indirect approaches focus on counselling families on modifying their speech and the child's environment (reducing the rate of speech, using indirect prompts, etc.). Direct approaches focus on using fluency-shaping strategies like airflow management, slow rate of speech using prolongation, etc. This approach also focuses on changing the child's speech, attitudes, and beliefs

BOX 2: Some of the most important techniques for SSDs that families can start with.

- Modeling correct sounds
- Create a communicative environment by enjoying conversations and showing interest in what they say regardless of speech difficulties
- Use of multimodal (visual, tactile, and auditory) to help them learn articulation
- Using a gesture to represent a sound (e.g., "hissing sound of a snake" for /s/')
- Play sound games such as rhyming words or activities that enhance auditory discrimination
- Incorporating sound practice into play. For example, "I spy" using target sounds
- Use a combination of play + drill to enhance the involvement of children in sessions
- Reading books and emphasizing the target sounds as you come across them
- Acknowledge and celebrate your child's efforts
- Short and regular sessions at home than longer sessions
- Be patient and positive

BOX 3: Some of the most important techniques for developmental fluency disorders that families can start with.

- Reducing the communication rate of both the family member and the child
- Rephrasing to model fluent speech
- Asking the child to control the breathing to improve speech—use of analogies
- To insert natural pauses when talking
- Use of shorter clearer sentence
- Giving the child time to complete the sentences
- Reduce conversational demands on the child
- Decrease questions
- Listen carefully to what the child is saying
- Do not interrupt
- Acknowledge and encourage when speech is difficult
- Involve peers in the communication
- Use of play-based activities to enhance participation from the child
- Playing fun speech games such as "charades", where a child describes a picture using pauses

to manage stuttering or facilitate fluency.[26] Hybrid approach includes a combination of fluency shaping, stuttering modification, and cognitive behavioral objectives to reduce the stuttering dysfluencies.[27] The use of analogies such as "garden hose", "blown up ballon", and "lily pad" are excellent ways to help the child visualize and understand their sound system, thus helping in reduction of stuttering behavior. Along with these techniques, there are several instrument-based approaches available—delayed auditory feedback, auditory masking, metronome timed speech, Dr. fluency, etc. The secondary behaviors such as body movements, facial grimaces, and distracting sounds also need to be addressed during the intervention sessions. **Box 3** provides certain techniques for healthcare professionals to begin with.

Intervention for Developmental Language Disorders

The goal of intervention is maximally effective use of language (verbal or nonverbal) to accomplish communication goals in everyday situations. Effective language intervention involves a great deal of thought and a wide variety of decision making. Intervention for children with language disorders is influenced by the nature and severity of the disorder, the age of the child, and environmental considerations as well as personal, linguistic, and cultural background of the child. A current gap in intervention for developmental language disorders as with other behavioral interventions is evidence-based practices suited for our socioeconomic, cultural, and linguistic environment. While there are some interventions that have been evaluated/are being evaluated that include language and social communication as key target areas,[23,24,28,29] there is a lot of work that needs to be done in this space. Providing specific intervention techniques and describing intervention plans based on the age and severity of the language disorder or the comorbid conditions are beyond the scope of this chapter. However, we have provided general principles for intervention and the most important speech-language techniques healthcare professionals can get families started **(Box 4)** with while they navigate the process of finding a speech-language pathologist and settle into intervention programs.

Intervention for language disorders should be guided through several principles that may help the child holistically rather than one deficit area.[30] These principles are as follows:

- The goal of intervention should be greater facility of language use in conversation, narration, exposition, and other textual genres in hearing, speaking, reading, and writing.
- Deficit areas are rarely, if ever, the only areas of language that should be targeted in an intervention program.
- Select goals that stimulate the child's language acquisition or development rather than goals based on deficit areas.
- Select goals based on the child's readiness and need for that particular target.
- Manipulate the context to create more opportunities for the language target to appear.
- Exploit different modalities to develop appropriate context for intervention targets.
- Manipulate clinical discourse so that targeted areas are more noticeable and important in various contexts.
- Contrast a child's language performance with mature adult usage by recasting a child's utterance.
- Provide good models of easily comprehended well-formed phrases and sentences.
- Use various modalities (verbal and nonverbal) to elicit and modify a child's language.

BOX 4: Some of the most important speech-language techniques that families can start with.

- Encourage all forms of communication (a good foundation in nonverbal communication will help the child with verbal modes)
- Use of gestures and signs
- Use visual supports (pictures, gestures, signs)
- Use simplified and clear instructions with emphasis on keywords
- Use of repetition and consistent routines
- Imitate the child's vocalizations or words and encourage them to imitate you
- Label and comment on things around the child
- Describe and comment on daily activities
- Use parallel talk (talk about the activity and describe what the child is doing)
- Use songs and rhymes to interact and build language and imitation skills
- Introduce and expand vocabulary
- Provide choices
- Expansion and extension (repeat what the child says and add new words or information)
- Recasting (correct the child's grammar in a nonintrusive way, e.g., if the child says, "I goed to the park," you respond with, "Oh, you went to the park?)
- Turn-taking conversations (encourage turn-taking in conversations by pausing and giving the child time to respond—remember a response can be nonverbal too. Encourage all forms of communication!)
- Encourage pretend play and role-playing
- Encourage peer interactions and group play
- Model correct speech without pressure to imitate
- Create opportunities for successful communication
- Break tasks into manageable steps
- Celebrate small progress and provide positive reinforcement

Augmentative and alternative communication in developmental speech and language disorders: Augmentative and alternative communication includes all forms of communication that are used to express thoughts, needs, wants, and ideas. Augmentative means to supplement or facilitate the existing verbal communication and alternative means a type of communication that can be used instead of verbal speech. Augmentative communication must start at the beginning of the intervention or early years of the child's life for those who are at risk of speech and language delay, those who are minimally verbal, and those whose speech is difficult to understand. Alternate forms of communication can also be introduced early in life instead of waiting and seeing whether the child will develop verbal communication.

AAC tools can support various communication needs—from simple requesting or complementing information to expressing complex ideas. AAC is used not only by those with communication challenges, but also by neurotypical group to achieve or get a message across. AAC is used mainly to facilitate communication and is used across the lifespan. There are various types of AAC—unaided (no tech) and aided (high tech and low tech). Unaided AAC includes gestures, facial expressions, finger spelling, gestures, vocalizations, and verbalizations. Aided AAC requires some form of tool, either electronic (high tech—communication apps, text to speech, speech-generating devices) or nonelectronic (low tech—communication boards, objects, pictures, visual schedules, etc.). An individual may use one AAC device or a combination of devices. To select a device for an individual, a thorough assessment has to be carried out including detailed case history, sensory and motor history, detailed speech and language assessment, social communication, cognitive assessment, etc. Based on the assessment, the type of device suitable for the individual is chosen. An evaluation by a speech-language pathologist prior to initiating AAC is highly recommended since all AACs do not fit all children. Few strategies that the communication partner/family can inculcate for persons using AAC are given in **Box 5**.

Awareness of speech and language disorders has come a long way, but some persistent myths still cloud understanding of speech-language development and intervention. In **Table 1**, we have highlighted a few of these misconceptions. With increased education and better access to resources, we are hopeful that these myths can

BOX 5: Strategies families can inculcate during conversing with AAC partner.

- Pay attention to what the speaker is communicating
- Choose a quiet environment with minimal background noise initially
- Face the person you are talking with
- Start with concrete subject/or the current situation
- Please wait for the reply of the AAC user
- Keep the remarks simple and short
- Do not finish the sentences off for the AAC user
- Introduce one topic at a time
- Using augmented input to facilitate communication
- Increasing wait time for conversational turn-taking

(AAC: augmentative and alternative communication)

TABLE 1: Myths and facts surrounding speech and language intervention.

Myth	*What is correct?*
Children will outgrow speech and language disorders without intervention	Not all children outgrow speech and language delays without intervention. Early intervention is important and often needed
Intervention should start only after diagnosis of a severe disorder	Speech and language intervention can start as soon as possible, be it a minimal problem or severe problem
Parents should wait and see before seeking help	No. Parents should not wait and see before seeking intervention. Research shows early intervention is the best for speech and language development considering brain plasticity and critical window for learning
Once a child starts speaking, intervention is no longer needed	The intervention has to continue until the child acquires age-appropriate communication, language, and speech skills
Speech intervention can fix all speech problems quickly	It definitely helps to enhance, develop, and build the communication, language, and speech skills but is not a quick fix for all the speech problems

Contd...

Contd...

Myth	*What is correct?*
Speech intervention only focuses on pronunciation	No. The main focus of any speech-language intervention is to enhance the communication (both verbal and nonverbal) and language skills. Speech intervention does focus on production of speech sounds. However, it does not entail only the pronunciation
Therapy is not effective for nonverbal children	Intervention is effective irrespective of the mode of communication. In fact, it helps in communication skills with the introduction of AAC, language skills, and social interaction abilities
Speech intervention is a one-size-fits-all approach	Speech and language intervention is tailor made for each child based on the child's development, language age, his abilities, and also child's strengths and weaknesses
AAC will prevent a child from learning to speak	No. In fact research suggests that AAC helps with a child's language and speech development
AAC is only for people who are completely nonverbal	No. AAC is beneficial for anyone with difficulty communicating whether due to developmental, cognitive, physical, or sociobehavioral condition. It works as a facilitator to verbal speech
Once a person starts using AAC, they will never speak	Using AAC does not prevent a person or child from learning to speak
AAC should only be introduced after speech intervention fails	No. AAC can be introduced as early as 1 year so that it facilitates the language development of the child
Children with language disorders should only learn one language	There is no difference in language development in bilingual children with and without language disorders. So, there is no need for children with language disorders to learn only one language, provided there is enough training in both the languages
Bilingual children with language disorders get confused by two languages	Learning two languages does not confuse the child. It has many advantages—enhanced communication, social interaction, etc.
It is better to wait until a child masters one language before introducing another	Children can learn two languages simultaneously. Children are quite adept at learning and sorting rules of two/multiple languages from an early age
Parents should speak only the dominant language at home	Parents can speak the dominant language along with the regional language or other languages the parents and the child are most comfortable with. This does not at any point hinder the child's language development

be busted—paving the way for better support for children and their families.

SUMMARY AND CONCLUSION

In summary, this chapter highlights key definitions of developmental speech and language disorders and their assessment and management with a focus on clinical aspects. It is imperative and crucial for a speech-language pathologist to be part of a multidisciplinary team that works with children with NDDs and their families.

REFERENCES

1. Arora NK, Nair MKC, Gulati S, Deshmukh V, Mohapatra A, Mishra D, et al. Neurodevelopmental disorders in children aged 2-9 years:

Population-based burden estimates across five regions in India. PLoS Med. 2018;15(7):e1002615.

2. Bowen C. Children's Speech Sound Disorders, 2nd edition. New York: Wiley-Blackwell.
3. Shriberg LD, Kwiatkowski J. Developmental phonological disorders. I: A clinical profile. J Speech Hear Res. 1994;37(5):1100-26.
4. ASHA. (n.d.). Stuttering, cluttering, and fluency. [online] Available from https://www.asha.org/practice-portal/clinical-topics/fluency-disorders/ [Last accessed November, 2025].
5. Shipley KG, McAfee JG. Assessment in Speech-Language Pathology: A Resource Manual. Plural Publishing, Inc.; 2021.
6. World Health Organization. (2022). ICD-11:International Classification of Diseases (11th revision). [online] Available from https://www.who.int/news/item/11-02-2022-icd-11-2022-release [Last accessed November, 2025].
7. American Psychiatric Association. (2013). Diagnostic and Statistical Manual of Mental Disorders, Fifth Edition (DSM-5).
8. Adams C. Practitioner review: The assessment of language pragmatics. J Child Psychol Psychiatry. 2002;43(8):973-87.
9. Manohar H, Meera SS, Nair DB, Srinath S. Language disorders in children: Complementary role of child psychiatrists and speech-language pathologists. J All India Inst Speech Hear. 2022;41(1):3-16.
10. Paul R, Norbury C. Language disorders from infancy through adolescence: Listening, speaking, reading, writing, and communicating. In: Language Disorders from Infancy through Adolescence: Listening, Speaking, Reading, Writing, and Communicating, 4th edition. Philadelphia: Elsevier; 2012.
11. Girimaji AS, Meera SS, Keshavaprasad YB, Jacob P, Philip M, Rajgopal H. Use of Children's Communication Checklist-2 to identify Communication Problems in Kannada Speaking Preschool Children with Attention Deficit Hyperactivity Disorder: A Preliminary Study. Indian J Psychol Med. 2023;45(5):539-41.
12. Rice ML, Hoffman L. Predicting Vocabulary Growth in Children With and Without Specific Language Impairment: A Longitudinal Study From 2.6 to 21 Years of Age. J Speech Lang Hear Res. 2015;58(2):345.
13. Sebastian S, Oviya MP, Thejesh R, Chengappa SK. Semantic and Syntactic Deficits in Malayalam-Speaking children with Learning Disability. Lang India. 2024;24(2):42-55.
14. Bishop DVM. Developmental cognitive genetics: How psychology can inform genetics and vice versa. Q J Exp Psychol. 2006;59(7):1153.
15. Leonard LB. Children with Specific Language Impairment. Cambridge, MA: MIT Press; 2014.
16. Tiwari S, Karanth P, Rajashekar B. Specific language impairment in a morphologically complex agglutinative Indian language—Kannada. J Commun Disord. 2017;66:22-39.
17. Snowling MJ, Hulme C. Interventions for children's language and literacy difficulties. Int J Lang Commun Disorders. 2012;47(1):27-34.
18. Shah RZ. Pragmatic language skill deficits among children with autism spectrum disorder. Int J Indian Psychol. 2022;10(2). https://doi.org/10.25215/1002.034.
19. Tager-Flusberg H, Paul R, Lord C. Language and communication in autism. In: Handbook of Autism and Pervasive Developmental Disorders. New York: Wiley; 2005.
20. Lakkanna S, Venkatesh K, Bhat J. Assessment of Language Development: A Manipal Manual, 1st edition. Manipal: Manipal University Press; 2021.
21. Owens Jr RE, Farinella KA, Metz DE. Introduction to Communication Disorders. A Lifespan Evidence-Based Perspective, 5th edition. England: Pearson Education Limited; 2000.
22. Law J, Dennis JA, Charlton JJV. Speech and language therapy interventions for children with primary speech and/or language disorders. Cochrane Database Syst Rev. 2017(1):CD012490..
23. Meera SS, Srikar M, Raju R, Swaminathan D, Johnson RE, Watson LR. Feasibility and acceptability of a caregiver-mediated early support program, delivered online, for infants at elevated familial likelihood for autism: A feasibility randomized controlled trial. Autism Res. 2024;17(9):1853-66.
24. Sengupta K, Mahadik S, Kapoor G. Glocalizing project ImPACT: Feasibility, acceptability and preliminary outcomes of a parent-mediated social communication intervention for autism adapted

to the Indian context. Res Autism Spectrum Disorders. 2020;76:101585.

25. Bernthal J, Bankson NW. Articulation and Phonological Disorder: Speech Sound Disorders in Children, 8th edition. Pearson.
26. Yaruss JS, Quesal RW. Overall Assessment of the Speaker's Experience of Stuttering (OASES): documenting multiple outcomes in stuttering treatment. J Fluency Disorders. 2006;31(2):90-115.
27. Baumeister H, Caspar F, Herziger F. Treatment outcome study of the stuttering therapy summer camp 2000 for children and adolescents. Psychother Psychosom Med Psychol. 2003; 53(11):455-63.
28. Karanth P, Shaista S, Srikanth N. Efficacy of communication DEALL—an indigenous early intervention program for children with autism spectrum disorders. Indian J Pediatr. 2010;77(9):957-62.
29. Rahman A, Divan G, Hamdani SU, Vajaratkar V, Taylor C, Leadbitter K, et al. Effectiveness of the parent-mediated intervention for children with autism spectrum disorder in south Asia in India and Pakistan (PASS): a randomised controlled trial. Lancet Psychiatry. 2016;3(2):128-36.
30. Fey ME, Long SH, Finestack LH. Ten principles of grammar facilitation for children with specific language impairments. Am J Speech-Lang Pathol. 2003;12(1):3-15.

Specific Learning Disorders (Reading, Writing, Arithmetic, and Mixed) and Motor Coordination Disorders

Henal Shah, Mansi Somaiya

INTRODUCTION

Poor academic performance is one of the most common reasons for referring children to health services. Specific learning disorders (SLDs) are one of the important causes of this presentation. SLD encompasses a range of neurodevelopmental conditions characterized by persistent difficulties in acquiring and using specific academic skills significantly below age-level expectations. These difficulties are not primarily attributable to intellectual disabilities, sensory deficits, or inadequate educational opportunities. SLDs include disorders related to reading (dyslexia), writing (dysgraphia), arithmetic (dyscalculia), and mixed disorders involving deficits across multiple domains.

Motor coordination disorders (MCDs) refer to conditions characterized by difficulties in motor coordination that significantly interfere with academic achievement or daily activities. Developmental coordination disorder (DCD) is one such disorder that affects motor skills acquisition, including coordination, balance, and fine or gross motor movements. It is one of the disorders mentioned under neurodevelopment disorders.

How common are these disorders?

Specific learning disorder, a prevalent neurodevelopmental condition, impacts approximately 3–10% of children, making it among the most widespread disorders of its kind. In India, 8% of children up to 19 years have SLD.[1] Dyslexia affects around 6.20% of children and adolescents, with dysgraphia impacting a similar percentage at 6.30%. Meanwhile, dyscalculia's prevalence is lower, estimated at 4.90%.[2] The male-to-female ratio for learning disorders is 2.3:1.[3] Another notable fact is that comorbidities occur very often, along with SLD and DCD.

Developmental coordination disorder affects 5–10% of children in school, making it one of the most common disorders in this age group. The main issue observed in children with DCD is the presence of motor difficulties that hinder both the learning and execution of motor-related tasks.[4]

DEFINITION

Specific Learning Disorder

In the 1960s, Samuel Kirk (2014)[5] introduced learning disability (LD), who described dyslexia as a "learning disability" and LD as "unexpected difficulty in mastering academic skills." Kirk suggested that LD affects language and academics across ages due to emotional, behavioral, or cerebral factors. Individuals with LD often show a notable gap between their presumed and actual intellectual capacity, regardless of neurological dysfunction, with causes unrelated to mental, educational, cultural, emotional, or sensory factors.

Over the years, there have been changes in the understanding and diagnosis of these disorders. As our knowledge of SLD progresses, so do the diagnostic criteria. Fundamentally, SLD is recognized as a disability rooted in the central nervous system, primarily affecting academic skills. According to the Individuals with Disabilities Education Act, SLD disrupts fundamental psychological processes related to language comprehension or usage, manifesting in difficulties with listening, thinking, speaking, reading, spelling, or mathematical calculations. This encompasses conditions such as dyslexia, brain injury, and developmental aphasia but excludes challenges stemming from visual, auditory, or motor impairments, intellectual disability, emotional disturbance, or socioeconomic factors.[6]

Developmental Coordination Disorder

Developmental coordination disorder manifests as motor skills below the expected level for the individual's age, often characterized by clumsiness and delays in early motor milestones such as walking and crawling. These difficulties can affect both gross and fine motor movements, hindering academic progress and daily activities. Importantly, DCD is not caused by other medical conditions such as cerebral palsy or intellectual disability, although it may coexist with them. In cases where intellectual disability is present, the motor challenges exceed what would be anticipated based solely on intelligence quotient (IQ). In Diagnostic and Statistical Manual of Mental Disorder (DSM)-5, DCD is classified as a motor disorder within the broader category of neurodevelopmental disorders (NDDs), with the requirement that symptom onset occurs during the developmental period. The DSM-5 criteria underscore that the condition of "learning and executing coordinated motor skills below the expected level for age" is only applicable when the child has had "opportunities for skill learning." It is important to realize that the development of motor skills depends on the child, environment, and task factors **(Fig. 1)**. If the environment has not supported the learning of motor skills, there would be deficits, but not necessarily DCD.[7]

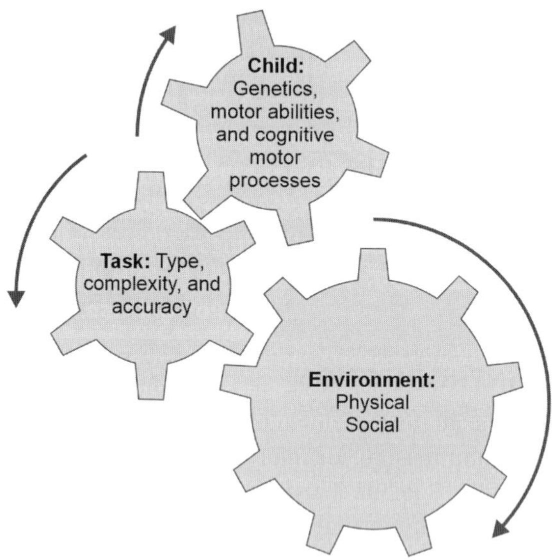

Fig. 1: Development of motor skills.

CHARACTERISTICS

Dyslexia has the following features **(Figs. 2 and 3)**:

- Difficulty in understanding the sounds of letters, poor phonological awareness, and poor decoding
- Reading slowly and word by word, monotonously
- Following text with fingers, losing place in the text
- Not heeding punctuation in the sentence—monotonous reading
- A child may be able to break up the word but cannot blend it to make a word.
- Mispronouncing common words—laying stress on wrong syllables
- Substituting with similar-looking words that may or may not fit into the text
- Reversing letters in a word (b for d, p for q) or putting them in the wrong order ("on" for "no", "saw" for "was", "who" for "how", "dog" for "God").

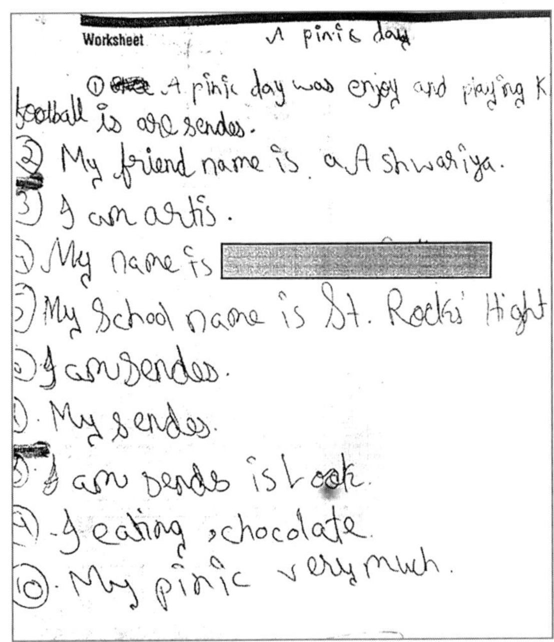

Fig. 2: A written sample showing grammatical errors, omissions of letters and words, substitution, and spelling errors.

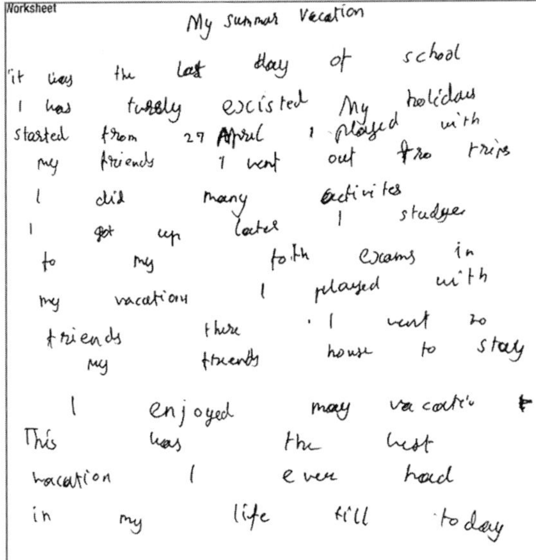

Fig. 3: A written sample showing spelling errors, missing punctuation, additions, incorrect capitalization, and poor handwriting.

- Omissions such as "Practise" instead of "Practising"
- Additions such as "Defeated" instead of "Defeat"
- Poor reading comprehension

Dysgraphia

Typical writing errors/difficulties are as follows:
- Difficulty in putting thoughts into writing
- Written sentences are jumbled, although spoken sentences may be correct.
- Difficulty in forming letters
- Muscle control may be poor; writing may be very small or large and may be impossible to read.
- Has handwriting problems, incomplete written work
- Writes very hard, often digging holes in the paper
- Has spelling problems, can be a poor speller because of poor phonics or poor visual memory or both
- A child with good phonic skills might spell words according to their sound. Such as Monkey as Munky, Bridge as Brig and Enough as Enuf
- Has trouble in blending sounds of double consonants, e.g., Gl in Glass and Bl in Blast
- Mirror writes words—i.e., reversals [writing "b" for "d", "p" for "q".]
- Inverts letters, writing "n" for "u", "m" for "w", "d" for "q", "p" for "b", "f" for "t"
- Bizarre spelling—totally unrelated to the original word, just using some of the alphabet.

Dyscalculia presents as:
- Poor number sense
- May have difficulties in small, big, and understanding number line
- Reads 13 for 31
- Tables are difficult.
- Time, day, and month may be confusing.
- Money concepts difficult

- Counts on fingers
- Abstract thinking is poor (mental sums)
- Some students reverse the direction of calculations and work from left to right.
- Symbol confusion occurs.
- Word problems may be difficult.

Developmental coordination disorder:

- A walk, which is unsteady
- Difficulty descending stairs
- Dropping objects
- Bumping into others
- Tripping often
- Difficulty tying shoes, putting on clothes, buttoning and other self-care activities
- Difficulty in performing activities such as writing, coloring, and using scissors.[6]

It is important to note that a child may have a single or a combination of the above. Further, the severity and comorbidities vary, making each child's presentation unique.

What is not specific learning disorder?

Academic difficulties arise due to many causes. Before diagnosing SLD, the assessment should exclude the following factors as primary contributors to academic problems:

- Intellectual difficulties such as borderline intellectual functioning and intellectual disability
- Other NDDs, such as attention-deficit/hyperactivity disorder (ADHD) and autism spectrum disorder (ASD)
- Psychiatric conditions that affect academics such as mood disorders, anxiety disorders, separation anxiety, and psychosis
- Perceptual difficulties such as hearing impairments and visual impairments
- Poor exposure to language and academics due to discrepancy between language spoken at home and language used in schooling, first-generation learners lacking sufficient social support, or inadequate educational resources
- Chronic school absences due to medical conditions
- Neurological conditions that impair writing, such as myopathy or writer's cramp.

ETIOLOGY

Specific Learning Disorder

No single cause is implicated in the emergence of SLD. Various causes have been implicated.

Box 1 illustrates the etiology of SLD.[8]

Various theories have been implicated in the emergence of SLD.

The connection between academic difficulties in SLD and other cognitive skills has long been acknowledged. A substantial body of research on cognitive models of SLD lays out following key concepts:[9]

- SLDs are componential, meaning that their academic challenges stem from specific weaknesses in certain cognitive processes rather than a general intellectual disability.

BOX 1: Etiology of specific learning disorder (SLD).

Prenatal factors:
- Chromosomal abnormalities, genetic factors
- Congenital infections—rubella, HIV, cytomegalovirus (CMV)
- Teratogens
- Malnutrition in mother
- Radiation
- Exposure to alcohol

Perinatal factors:
- Asphyxia
- Hypoxia at birth
- Mechanical birth trauma
- Hypoglycemia
- PREMATURITY

Postnatal factors:
- Trauma
- Hypoxic ischemic encephalopathy
- Infections (meningitis and encephalitis)
- Environmental—lower social class, poverty, poor housing, and unstable family environment

- These cognitive components linked to SLD, much like academic skills, exist along a continuum in the general population. Understanding typical development can shed light on the genesis of SLD.
- Each academic and cognitive component is likely to have a distinct footprint in the brain and genetic makeup. These signatures may overlap due to correlation, but they are not interchangeable.
- This overlap helps explain the high rates of comorbidity among different SLD.
- Deficiencies in these cognitive and academic processes often persist throughout life, particularly without intervention.

Phonological deficit theory: Reading and writing difficulties in spellings stem from impairment in the ability to identify or manipulate the components' sounds in speech, otherwise called phonological awareness. A failure in phonological awareness leads to poor association of written representations of speech elements. Children with dyslexia are known to have difficulty in basic phonological tasks such as manipulating speech sounds.[10]

Abnormal sensory processing: The deficit is a result of auditory processing affecting the processing of sounds or disturbing sounds being kept in the memory long enough to be processed. Hence, individuals with dyslexia were noticed to have number of auditory tasks such as frequency discrimination and temporal order judgement.[10]

Magnocellular theory: Impaired visual processing in the magnocellular visual pathway. The pathway is involved in directing visual attention and visual research skills. There are deficits in synchronization of visual information during the reading process.[10,11]

Neurobiological theory: Differences in neuronal connectivity, neurotransmitter function, and neural plasticity may contribute to difficulties in learning and academic performance.[10] When it comes to reading, decoding, or recognizing words at sight, three regions spanning the four lobes of the brain play a significant role: The left inferior frontal gyrus located in the frontal lobe, the left temporoparietal cortex, and the left occipitotemporal region. Differences in brain activation patterns between typically developing children and those with reading disorders, such as specific word reading disability (SWRD) and differences in brain structure, suggest challenges in forming the neural systems necessary for reading. These structural differences affect the development of cognitive processes such as phonological, orthographic, and semantic representations crucial for reading. While some argue that these differences are due to reading instruction, evidence suggests they can be observed even before formal reading instruction begins. Without proper instruction during critical periods of development, readers may develop inefficient neural systems. However, successful interventions can often normalize these neural processes. Children with dyslexia demonstrate less growth in brain activity within the temporoparietal and occipitotemporal regions when engaged in reading and rhyming activities compared to their counterparts.[12]

Similarly, mathematical difficulties, such as specific math disability (SMD), are associated with distinct functional brain networks involved in various mathematical processes. In children without any math difficulties, certain brain regions play crucial roles in processing quantitative information. Firstly, the intraparietal sulcus, posterior parietal cortex, and areas in the pre-frontal cortex are significant for representing and dealing with quantitative data. Secondly, regions in the medial temporal lobe and hippocampus are vital for recalling math facts. Thirdly, other important areas include visual regions that are responsible for judging visual forms and processing symbols. Lastly, prefrontal regions are engaged in higher-level functions such as error monitoring, maintaining, and manipulating information. As children become more proficient in math, they rely less on the parietal network and more on the frontal network for these processes. Disruptions in these networks or their interactions can lead to SMD, but successful interventions can normalize these neural networks.[9]

Genetic: Both reading and math difficulties have strong genetic components, with certain genes implicated in their development.

Environmental factors: They play a significant role in influencing literacy and numeracy rates, socioeconomic status, schooling practices, family literacy environments, and peer influences. The interplay between genetic predispositions and environmental factors can exacerbate reading difficulties, but there is evidence that neural plasticity allows for improvements even in challenging circumstances.

Developmental Coordination Disorder

Children and adults with DCD exhibit a widespread pattern of impairment across various measures.[13] These include:

- Difficulties in controlling gaze during reaching or walking
- Integrating cognitive tasks with motor activities and their associated brain functions
- Learning motor skills that rely heavily on practice intensity and type
- Predicting and controlling movements internally
- Exhibiting more inconsistent movement patterns and adopting a cautious approach to movement, especially when navigating obstacles. This cautiousness probably compensates for underlying motor control deficits, affecting tasks like reaching and walking.

A common thread among these deficits is a breakdown in visual-motor integration. This impacts tasks involving eye-hand coordination and navigating complex terrain. Additionally, challenges with cognitive control and its incorporation into motor planning are evident.

COMORBIDITIES

Learning difficulty may be accompanied by various comorbidities. Owing to the difficulties faced with learning, the child may face various difficulties in school, at home, and in social settings. The comorbidities are listed in **Table 1**. Different presentations are possible: sometimes children may present with behavioral and emotional conditions masking the learning difficulty, which gets uncovered with evaluation or may present as learning difficulty along with emotional or behavioral conditions.[3] The clinician must keep an eye on these conditions. The various presentations and their impact are discussed in **Table 2**.

TABLE 1: Prevalence of comorbidity in specific learning disorder (SLD).

Comorbid disorders	*Prevalence*
Behavioral and emotional disorders	30%
Attention-deficit hyper-activity/disorder (ADHD) • Inattention difficulties • ADHD and dyslexia	Variable; 10–60% 20–40%
Conduct disorder	6%
Depressive disorder	33%
Anxiety disorders	20–30% 28%
Autism spectrum disorders and dyslexia	6%
Language disorders	*Varies:* Around 30–40% of patients with SLD have a reading disorder. Patients with dyslexia with a specific language disorder vary from 55 to 77%

TABLE 2: Comorbidity in specific learning disorder (SLD) and its impact.[3]

Comorbid disorders	*How comorbidity affects SLD presentation*	*How testing is impacted in presence of a comorbidity*	*How remediation is affected in presence of a comorbidity*
Attention-deficit/ hyperactivity disorder	• Behavioral issues • Poor attention span	• Drop in IQ scores • Gives up easily in the tests • Hurry to finish tests • Spacing and letter formation is affected • Omissions are more in spellings • Organization of ideation is affected • Dysgraphia—handwriting is affected, alignment is affected • Visuospatial errors are often seen	• Longer time to drive in a concept • Memory issues • Forgets the learnt matter quickly • Frequent breaks • Process slows down • Repetitions are more because of inattention • Behavior—impulsive and can lead to avoidance • Counseling the parents must be included in the IEP • Behavior management/ modification is also to be included • Gives up easily • Fine motor skills and handwriting skills may also require inputs
Conduct disorder	• Hyperactivity • Disruptive in class • Frequent anger outbursts • Poor academic performance	• Disinterested and irritable • Rapport building is difficult • *Mazes:* Poor planning and impulsivity • *Similarities subtest:* Mostly give superficial answers followed by "that's all I know", "That's it, and nothing else", "nothing is same" • Out rightly denied answering on the same • *Arithmetic:* Inattention • Disinterest, lack of motivation or casual attitude to testing • Impulsivity • Manipulating and faking bad in testing	• Projecting negative feelings toward the examiner as he is perceived as an authority figure • Defiance or not complying with the instruction • Irritability and hostility when probed • Answering back, arguing, or asking impertinent questions • Giving up easily • Process of remediation slows down • Behavior management
Depressive disorder	• Disinterest in studies • Poor academic performance • Prefers to be her/himself • Poor interest • Slow in responding • Soft speech	• Hesitant to respond • Gives up very easily • Answers very softly • Downward gaze • Delayed reaction time • Random marking	• Hesitant to respond • Give up very easily • Answer very softly • Downward gaze • Delayed reaction time • Random marking

Contd...

Contd...

Comorbid disorders	*How comorbidity affects SLD presentation*	*How testing is impacted in presence of a comorbidity*	*How remediation is affected in presence of a comorbidity*
	• May have a poor eye contact • Low self-esteem	• Overall time fatigue • Forgetfulness • No clarifications • Hesitance to clarify • Low motivation • Shallow processing • Organization skills are affected • Not elaborate sentences • Sadness in content • Thought productivity in essays—poverty of content in essays	• Overall time fatigue • Forgetfulness • No clarifications • Hesitance to clarify • Low motivation • Shallow processing • Slow process
Anxiety disorders	• Anxiety impacts performance • Disrupts attention/ information processing • Avoidance to write	• Gives up very easily • Delayed reaction time • Answers hastily or may have hesitations • Random marking • Overall time fatigue • Forgetfulness • No clarifications • Hesitance to clarify • Shallow processing • Organization skills are affected • Not elaborate sentences • In a hurry to finish	• Gives up very easily • Delayed reaction time • Answers hastily or may have hesitations • Forgetfulness • Hesitance to clarify • Organization skills are affected
Autism spectrum disorders and dyslexia	• Minimal eye contact • Rigidity of thought • Difficulty in comprehension and completing papers in exams • Difficulty to do complex tasks • Many children with autism have excellent basic reading skills. Some even have what we call "hyperlexia." However, understanding is poor • Visual and auditory processing difficulties, often associated with ASD	• Poor concept of time lapse • Wanting perfection • Answers to only what is asked • Rigidity of thought • Mechanical • Concrete thoughts • Poor abstraction • Factual information • Short sentences • Vocabulary is simple • Minimal spelling errors • Poor receptive language • Math reasoning is affected	• Social skills training should be included as well • Avoidance for math is often seen • Rigidity in behavior • Refusal to therapy • Behavioral modification may also be required • Prepare for schedule changes in settings • Slows down the process • Wanting perfection • Stuck with redundant details

Contd...

Contd...

Comorbid disorders	*How comorbidity affects SLD presentation*	*How testing is impacted in presence of a comorbidity*	*How remediation is affected in presence of a comorbidity*
	• "Islets of ability" – strengths in particular areas, such as design, logic, and creative skills		
Language disorders	• Reading difficulties often associated with nonspecific language impairment—nonverbal and language deficits • Expressive language disorder-hard to put thoughts and feelings together, limited vocabulary, leave out key words, mix up tenses • Mixed receptive—expressive language disorder—difficulty in understanding and expression, difficulty understanding verbal directions/longer sentences, trouble understanding basic vocabulary, have reading comprehension difficulties • Auditory processing disorder—trouble recording different sounds in words, frequent asking for repetition of words/sentences, drop word endings and certain syllables, at risk for reading disabilities • Social communication disorders—difficulty in making appropriate conversations, interrupt often/speak too little, at risk of reading comprehension issues	• Reading comprehension difficulties • Omissions may be present	Work on language deficits is important and needs to be implemented with remediation

Comorbidity with Specific Learning Disorder

Table 2 shows the comorbidity in specific learning disorder and its impact.

Comorbidity with Specific Learning Disorder and the Impact

Table 3 shows the various tests used for assessment of specific learning disorder.

TABLE 3: Various tests used for assessment of specific learning disorder (SLD).

Name of test	*Domains tested*	*Who can assess*	*Advantages*	*Disadvantages*	*How to access*	*Adapted/ validated in Indian population (yes/no)*
NIMHANS Index for SLD—Level I (5–7 years) and Level II (8–12 years) (Used in conjunction with MISIC)	• *Level I:* Assessment of preacademic skills; attention, visual and auditory discrimination, visual and auditory memory, speech, and language, visuo-motor and language, writing and number skills • *Level II:* Assess areas of attention, reading, spelling, perceptuo-motor, visuo-motor integration, memory, and arithmetic skills	Clinical psychologists and special educators	• Used to confirm SLD diagnosis and certification • Used to monitor progress after remediation • Wide range of pertinent areas covered • Easily available and administered • Good for early identification of learning issues • Mostly paper pencil tests	• Limited age range as it can only be used ages between 5 and 12 years • Available in English, Kannada, and Hindi	Purchase from NIMHANS, Bengaluru	Yes
Wide range achievement test (WRAT)-4	• Reading composite = Word reading + Reading comprehension • Spelling • Math computation	Psychologist, special educator, and teacher	• Screening and diagnosis of difficulties in academic areas • Takes 15–30 minutes • Parallel forms allowing for retesting • Age and grade-based norms	• No applied math assessment • No broad writing skills assessed	Available on purchase/ even online purchase	No
Test of written language (TOWL-4)	• Vocabulary • Spelling • Style (punctuation and grammar) • Logical sentences	Anyone with formal training in assessment and English proficiency	• Helps in identifying students with writing difficulties	• Time-consuming scoring • Subjectivity in scoring procedures in some domains	Available on purchase/ even online purchase	No

Contd...

Contd...

Name of test	*Domains tested*	*Who can assess*	*Advantages*	*Disadvantages*	*How to access*	*Adapted/ validated in Indian population (yes/no)*
	• Sentence combining • Contextual conventions • Contextual language • Story construction		• Strong conceptual model of writing • Good reliability	Between 7 and 8 poor discriminations		
Wechsler Individual Achievement Test (WIAT) III	• Listening comprehension • Oral expression • Word reading • Pseudo word decoding • Reading comprehension • Oral reading fluency • Spelling • Sentence composition • Essay composition • Math problem solving • Numerical operations • Math fluency	Psychologist, special educator, and teacher	• Good overview of students' strengths and weaknesses • Good ceiling and basal of subtests	• English fluency needed • No college adult norms	Available on purchase/ even online purchase	NO
Woodcock-Johnson III tests of achievements (WJ-III)	• Reading • Writing • Mathematics • Academic fluency • Academic skills • Oral comprehension • General academic knowledge	Psychologist and educator	• Range of academic capacities correlated with Cattell–Horn–Carroll theory: Wide range of areas covered. Can be used between the age of 2–90 years and grade	• English proficiency required • Subjectivity in some scoring • Training needs to be thorough to be able to administer	Available on purchase/even online purchase	Not standardized on the Indian population; hence, not culture friendly

Contd...

Contd...

Name of test	*Domains tested*	*Who can assess*	*Advantages*	*Disadvantages*	*How to access*	*Adapted/ validated in Indian population (yes/no)*
			• Kindergarten to grade 18 • Intraindividual comparison of scores • Used for diagnosis of SLD • Computerized scoring			
Kaufman Test of Educational Achievement (K-TEA)	• Phonological processing • Math concepts and applications • Letter and word recognition • Nonsense word decoding • Writing fluency • Silent reading fluency • Math fluency • Reading comprehension • Written expression • Associational fluency • Spelling • Object naming facility • Reading vocabulary • Letter naming facility	Psychologist, special educator, and teacher	• Sound error analysis guidelines that are normed • Looks at all areas of IDEA • Alternate forms good for re-evaluations • Offers recommendations for writing IEPs • New norms for ages 4:0 through 25:11 and for grades pre-K through 12	• Extensive training needed to learn the test • American idiomatic vocabulary, hence difficult to those with limited proficiency of nonfamiliarity with American English	Available on purchase/even online purchase	No, has been normed and validated on a representative sample of the United States

Contd...

Contd...

Name of test	*Domains tested*	*Who can assess*	*Advantages*	*Disadvantages*	*How to access*	*Adapted/ validated in Indian population (yes/no)*
	• Listening comprehension • Word recognition fluency • Oral expression • Decoding fluency					
Peabody Individual Achievement Test-Revised (PIAT-R)	• General knowledge • Math • Reading recognition • Reading comprehension • Spelling	Special educator, psychologist, and teacher	• Easy to administer and score • Useful for decision making for interventions • Good for screening	• Limited questions hence not reliable measure for domains • Norms are national norms, hence regional differences not recognized	Available on purchase/even online purchase	No
Aston Index Battery	• Visual and auditory discrimination • Motor coordination • Written language • Reading and spelling • General ability and attainment	Teacher, psychologist, special educator, and speech pathologist	Good tool for screening and diagnosis of language difficulties	• Ceiling effects on some subtests • Time consuming for classroom administration • No math testing • Ages 5–14 only	Available on purchase/even online purchase	No

Comorbidity with Developmental Coordination Disorder[14]

- Specific language impairment (up to 70%)
- *ADHD (50%):* Some researchers suggest that DCD and ADHD share symptoms, as children with ADHD often exhibit motor challenges. At the same time, executive dysfunctions and slow processing speed, characteristics of ADHD, are also common in children with DCD. Therefore, distinguishing between the difficulties specific to each disorder is uncertain. However, ADHD and DCD are still regarded as distinct disorders due to their unique core deficits.[15]
- Specific learning disabilities (17.8–27.5%)
- Anxiety (16.7–33.8%)
- Depression (9.1–11.8%)
- ASD (4.1–8.2%)

DIAGNOSIS

For identification of SLD, the following two approaches have been used.[16]

1. *Cognitive dissonance model:* These frameworks assess cognition and identify disparities through different methods. They try to tap into the unexpectedness of academic difficulties. They are faulted for the "waiting to fail approach," and that dissonance may not occur with higher IQ. They include:
   a. Ability-achievement discrepancy (AAD)
   b. Evaluating processing strengths and weaknesses (PSW)
2. *Instructional framework:* This approach incorporates response to intervention (RTI). This more preventive approach suggests that intervention be provided when a child has difficulties. This may be progressively from group to individual help. If the problem persists, academic testing is indicated. Here, the need for cognitive assessment is not mandatory unless intellectual disability is suspected.

The DSM IV initially proposed diagnosing SLD through an aptitude-achievement gap assessment, akin to the International Classification of Diseases 10. However, this approach has been revised in DSM-5, shifting focus to persistent struggles in acquiring essential academic skills during schooling, with difficulties persisting even after the intervention, the RTI method.

Diagnosis necessitates a comprehensive evaluation using standardized academic achievement tests and data from various sources. SLD diagnosis relies on the unexpected nature of educational difficulties, excluding explanations such as intellectual disability, motor disorders, or environmental factors. Confirmation requires evidence of academic underperformance compared to age norms, typically 1.5 standard deviations below the mean on appropriate tests.

DSM-5 uses the term "specific learning disorder" (SLD).[17]

Specific learning disorder is characterized by persistent difficulties in learning and applying academic skills, including:

- Slow, inaccurate, or effortful reading
- Difficulty comprehending written material
- Spelling challenges
- Problems with written expression
- Difficulties with number sense, arithmetic facts, and mathematical reasoning

These difficulties must persist for at least 6 months despite interventions targeting them. The affected skills must be substantially below the expected level for the individual's age (at least 1.5 standard deviations below the population mean). SLD significantly interferes with academic or work performance and daily activities. Diagnosis requires the use of standardized achievement tests and comprehensive clinical assessment.

Specific learning disorder typically manifests during school years but may only become apparent once academic demands exceed individual capacities. Diagnosis relies on historical information, school reports, and psychoeducational evaluations.

Impairments within specific academic domains include:

- *Reading:* Word reading accuracy, reading rate/fluency, and reading comprehension
- *Written expression:* Spelling accuracy, grammar, punctuation, and clarity of expression
- *Mathematics:* Number sense, arithmetic facts memorization, calculation accuracy/fluidity, and mathematical reasoning.

Severity levels range from mild to severe:

- *Mild:* Some difficulties in one or two academic areas are manageable with accommodations or support services, especially during school years.
- *Moderate:* There are marked difficulties in one or more academic skills, requiring intensive teaching and support at school and home.
- *Severe:* Severe difficulties across multiple academic areas, unlikely to become proficient despite intensive teaching and support services

The DSM-5 approach to learning disorders is broad, considering them a spectrum rather than distinct categories. Studies on twins and families show that reading, math, and writing difficulties share genetic and environmental factors. This leads to an approach combining different types of learning disorders instead of separating them, simplifying the diagnostic process. For instance, test scores may vary across subjects, sometimes just falling short of clinical thresholds.

The new criteria no longer include the IQ-achievement gap, and intellectual assessments are only necessary when intellectual disability is suspected. Emphasis is placed on early access to interventions rather than extensive diagnostic evaluations. This involves educating parents and consulting with them and teachers.

Additionally, the DSM-5 now considers the effects of interventions and the persistence of symptoms, though implementing these changes may present practical challenges. The severity of SLD is determined by the extent of support needed, ranging from mild to severe, although precise quantification remains elusive.

On the other hand, ICD 11 calls the condition a "developmental learning disorder." This encompasses difficulties in reading, writing, mathematics, and other learning areas. The criterion remains centered around the gap between achievement, chronological age, and intellectual functioning level.

Developmental Coordination Disorder

Confusion over its terminology persisted until 1994, when the term DCD was universally accepted, leading to a global agreement on defining, assessing, and treating it. Since then, there has been significant advancement in understanding the performance issues associated with DCD.[18] In the earlier edition of the DSM (DSM-IV-TR), DCD was categorized among "learning disorders." However, in DSM-5, it is redefined as a motor disorder within the broader scope of "neurodevelopmental disorders." Additionally, DSM-5 introduces a new criterion that specifies the onset of symptoms during the developmental period.[4] Despite its high prevalence among school-aged children, DCD often goes undiagnosed. Unlike conditions such as cerebral palsy, the symptoms of DCD may not be readily apparent, making it easy for them to be overlooked in terms of their impact on daily functioning compared to more obvious pediatric movement-related conditions. Even in affluent nations, healthcare professionals may lack sufficient awareness of DCD. Consequently, obtaining a diagnosis and accessing therapy poses significant challenges for children with DCD and their families.

What helps in early identification?

It is essential to monitor for this condition and intervene early when difficulties are observed. It is imperative not to wait for the child to outgrow them. If risk factors, as seen in **Box 2**, are present, one has to be vigilant.

Various screening instruments are available. Dr Nandini Singh and her team at NBRC, with support from the Department of Science and Technology, Government of India, recently developed the Dyslexia Assessment for Languages of India (DALI). It is a comprehensive screening and assessment tool for dyslexia among children in grades 1–5. DALI consists of two screening tools: one for ages 5–7 (grades 1–2) and another for ages 8–10 (grades 3–5). It includes testing in both English and the child's mother tongue, aiding in distinguishing between dyslexia and language difficulties. DALI has undergone standardization and validation across four languages (Hindi, Marathi, Kannada, and English) in schools across five centers, involving 4,840 children from grades 1–5. Efforts are underway to expand the assessment to grade X and to include mathematics. The evaluation will also cover Bengali, Urdu, and Tamil languages.[3]

The GOI has published an instrument for teachers **(Fig. 4)** to complete when children are in grade 3 or 8, whichever is earlier.[19]

The screening must be followed up by referring the indicated children to the necessary centers for diagnostic confirmation.

Risk factors for DCD:

- Male sex
- Preterm birth (<32 weeks)
- Low birth weight (<1,500 g)
- Small-for-gestational age
- Walking independently at 15 months or later
- Attention difficulties
- Social communication issues
- Difficulties in nonword repetition, spelling, and reading

BOX 2: Risk factors in specific learning disorder (SLD).

- *Perinatal conditions:*
  - Low Apgar scores
  - Low birth weight and/or preterm birth
  - Hospitalization for >24 hours in a neonatal intensive care unit
  - Difficulty with suckling, sucking, and swallowing
  - Chronic otitis media that may result in intermittent hearing loss
- *Genetic or environmental conditions:*
  - Family history of SLD
  - Family history of speech/language delays
  - Exposure to environmental toxins or other harmful substances
  - Limited language exposure in home, childcare, and other settings
- *Developmental milestones:*
  - *Delay in cognitive skills:*
    - Not demonstrating object permanence
    - Limited understanding of means–ends relationships (e.g., using a stool to reach a cookie jar)
    - Lack of symbolic play behavior
  - *Delay in comprehension and/or expression of spoken language:*
    - Limited receptive vocabulary
    - Reduced expressive vocabulary ("late talkers")
    - Difficulty understanding simple (e.g., one-step) directions
    - Monotone or other unusual prosodic features of speech
    - Reduced intelligibility
    - Infrequent or inappropriate spontaneous communication (vocal, verbal, or nonverbal)
    - Immature syntax
  - *Delay in emergent literacy skills:*
    - Slow speed for naming objects and colors
    - Limited phonological awareness (e.g., rhyming and syllable blending)
    - Minimal interest in print
    - Limited print awareness (e.g., book handling and recognizing environmental print)
  - *Delay in perceptual-motor skills:*
    - Problems in gross or fine motor coordination (e.g., hopping, dressing, cutting, and stringing beads)
    - Difficulty coloring, copying, and drawing

Form A

Screening for learning disability

Name of student: ....

Date of birth: ....

Class: ....

Name of school: ....

How long has the teacher been familiar with the student: ....

Dear teacher

Have you observed in your day-to-day teaching that the student has some of the following difficulties?

Answer with "X" in appropriate column.

S. no.	*Statement*	*Never*	*Sometimes**	*Frequently***
1	*Makes mistakes in reading like:* • Omits words • Substitutes words • Adds words • Skips lines • Reads sentences repeatedly			
2	Can answer questions orally but has difficulty in writing answers or oral work is better than written work			
3	Writes or reads figures or letters in wrong way, for example, 15 for 51, 6 for 9, b for d			
4	Difficulty in differentiating letter sounds for vowels and blends, example "E" for "I"; "ch" for "sh"			
5	Difficulty in rhyming words and repeating them			
6	Reads in past tense, while the text is written in present tense or vice-versa; example replaces "is" with "was"			
7	Changes the sequence of alphabets while reading; example says "neerg" instead of "green"			
8	Replaces long words with compact one; example "musim" for "museum"			
9	Difficulty in taking notes or copying them from blackboard and books			
10	Confusion with mathematics symbols (+, –, ×, ÷) while solving word problems and mathematics computation			
11	Difficulty in spellings			
12	Difficulties with spatial orientation and direction; example confusion between left and right, east and west, up and down, etc.			
13	Misplaces upper- and lower-case letters, example BeTTer, n for N, i for I			
14	Writes in mirror images; example "ram"—"mar"			

*Sometimes: Up to 6–7 times in 2–3 months

**Frequently: More than 7 times in 2–3 months

Fig. 4: Screening form for teachers.[19]

Questions for screening for DCD: Movement Assessment Battery for Children (MABC) checklist and DCD-Q are parent-reported questionnaires that have been used to screen. The following questions would be useful to ask to elicit possibility of DCD[4]:

- Was your child born prematurely? If so, how many weeks early?
- What was your child's birth weight?
- At what age did your child begin walking independently?
- Would you, or anyone else, describe your child as "clumsy"?
- Are daily tasks such as dressing (including buttoning shirts and tying shoelaces), brushing teeth, and using utensils while eating difficult for your child?
- At what age did your child learn to ride a bike without training wheels?
- Does your child struggle with fine motor activities such as handwriting (cursive), printing, or cutting with scissors? Do they switch hand dominance?
- Does your child face challenges with gross motor activities such as throwing or kicking a ball, participating in team sports at school or in the community, or succeeding in physical education classes?
- Has anyone else in your family received a diagnosis of DCD, ADHD, or specific learning disabilities?

How do I assess?

Assessment of children with SLD involves a thorough clinical evaluation, followed by standardized psychometric testing of the child's cognitive abilities and academic skills.

During the clinical evaluation, children with SLD may be brought in by their parents or referred by schools. Unfortunately, these children are often unfairly labeled as "lazy" or "stupid" and may face disciplinary actions both at home and at school due to comorbid behavioral symptoms. Their clinical presentation varies, with some primarily expressing concerns about poor academic performance, while others exhibit secondary symptoms such as school refusal, oppositional behavior, and low self-esteem. Academic difficulties commonly observed include slow writing, incomplete classwork and homework, poor handwriting, difficulty completing tasks within deadlines, spelling errors, slow reading, and challenges in mathematics.

Before psychological testing, the psychiatrist gathers a detailed history from parents and children and conducts a thorough examination. The clinical evaluation should be structured to cover the components listed in the provided **Box 3**.[3]

TESTING

This is a highly debated issue, with the newer DSM suggesting that intelligence assessment is

BOX 3: History taking in SLD.

History taking in specific learning disorder (SLD):

- Presenting complaints and their progression
- History of any behavioral or emotional problems
- *Schooling history:* School attendance, classroom behavior, any change of school, any change of curriculum, the type of academic difficulties, whether any intervention or accommodations in school for the same, impact of the interventions, etc.
- Family history of any neurodevelopmental disorders or psychiatric illness or neurological disorders
- Family life and relationships
- Medical history
- History of any evaluation and intervention
- Family's awareness and perception of the child's problems
- Behavioral observation and mental status examination of the child
- Informal assessment of reading, writing, spelling, and arithmetic skills
- Physical examination of the child, especially neurological and sensory system examination
- Screening for common comorbid disorders including ADHD, ODD, depression, and anxiety disorders
- Report from class teacher

optional except in specific cases. In the Indian setting, the discrepancy model is often used due to the lack of resources for early intervention.

Standardized IQ tests can assess a child's intelligence level. Options include the Binet–Kamat test, Malin's Intelligence Scale for Indian Children (MISIC), Wechsler's Intelligence Scale for Children, and the Cognitive Battery of the Woodcock-Johnson test. Following the assessment of IQ, tests evaluating academic abilities must be administered. Various tests, outlined in **Table 3**, are valuable for this purpose. They include the National Institute for Mental Health and Neurosciences (NIMHANS) Index for SLD, wide range achievement test, test of written language, Wechsler Individual Achievement test, Woodcock-Johnson tests of Achievement, Kaufman Test of Educational Achievement, and Peabody Individual Achievement Test-Revised, among others.

To diagnose DCD, the following four diagnostic criteria are required to be met:

1. Impairment in the ability to acquire and execute motor skills at an age-appropriate level
2. Significant interference with activities of daily living, academic performance, leisure, and play
3. Onset is early in the developmental period.
4. The movement difficulties are not better explained by intellectual disability, visual impairment, or other neurological conditions affecting movement

To assess the age-inappropriate motor skills in children with DCD as defined by criterion A, researchers and clinicians commonly use the Movement Assessment Battery for Children, 2nd edition (MABC-2) and the Bruininkse Oseretsky Test for Motor Proficiency, 2nd edition (BOT-2). These assessments are well established in both research and clinical settings for evaluating motor performance levels due to their strong psychometric properties.[4]

The diagnostic process for children suspected of having DCD involves using various assessment tools such as the MABC-checklist, DCD-Q, and DCD-Daily to evaluate motor skill difficulties and their impact on daily activities. While the MABC-checklist and DCD-Q are parent-reported questionnaires, the DCD-daily includes both a questionnaire and standardized tasks. Early signs of motor difficulties are identified during history taking, and a multidisciplinary approach is taken if other medical conditions are suspected. Standardized tests confirm diagnosis, but task performance analysis is essential for understanding specific challenges and planning treatment.

DISORDER TO DISABILITY

Specific learning disorder is one of the 21 disorders listed in the Rights of Persons with Disabilities, RWPD.[19]

To qualify as a disability and avail of a unique disability identification card (UDID) card and specified help, getting certified as having SLD using the discrepancy model is necessary. The gazette specifies that for diagnosis, IQ should be more than 85. The suggested tests for academic achievement are the NIMHANS battery or grade level assessment device (GLAD). Regarding academic achievement, three standards below age on the NIMHANS battery or below 40% on GLAD are the suggested cut-off for diagnosis. The discrepancy would indicate the presence of SLD, and in the absence of a reliable quantification method, the occurrence implies a benchmark disability. Initially, the certification was to be done by a disability board consisting of government doctors. A recent change in the gazette allows the chair of the board to include private practitioners if no government physician is available. The certification will be done for children aged 8 years and above only. The child may require repeat certification during the academic year of class X and the academic year of class XII. The certificate

Flowchart 1: Assessment of specific learning disorder (SLD).

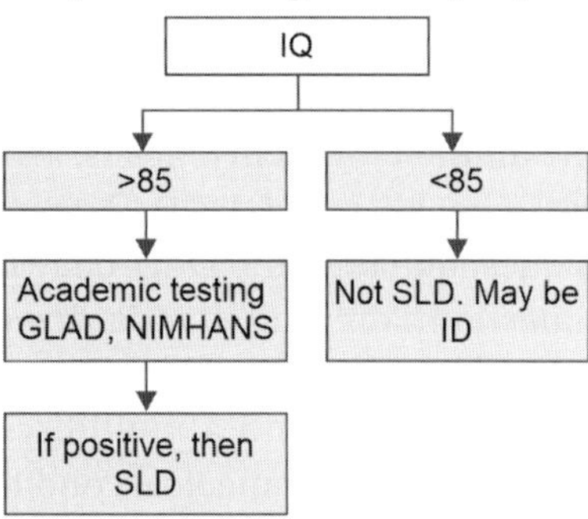

issued at 18 years or more will be valid lifelong. The process is highlighted in **Flowchart 1**.

How to get a Unique Disability Identification Card?

The "Unique ID for Persons with Disabilities" initiative aims to establish a comprehensive National Database for PwDs and provide each individual with a unique disability identity card. This undertaking seeks to enhance transparency, efficiency, and accessibility in delivering government assistance to people with disabilities while ensuring consistency across all levels of implementation, from local villages to the national level. Additionally, it will facilitate the monitoring of both the physical and financial progress of beneficiaries throughout the implementation hierarchy, spanning from grassroot levels up to the national scale. The card helps persons with benchmark difficulties (>40%) who then become entitled to avail certain provisions as laid by law. These vary from educational help to reservations in educational institutions and places of work.[1]

The following are the steps to obtain a card. (https://www.swavlambancard.gov.in/cms/online-application-guide)

- *Step 1:* Individuals with disabilities will click on the registration link to sign up on the UDID web portal.
- *Step 2:* Using their credentials, they log in to the system and select "Apply online for Disability Certificate." They then read the instructions and complete the online application form.
- *Step 3:* They upload a color passport photo and other necessary documents such as income proof, identity proof, and SC/ST/OBC proof, as required.
- *Step 4:* The individual submits the data to the CMO office/medical authority.
- *Step 5:* The CMO office/medical authority verifies the submitted data.
- *Step 6:* The CMO office/medical authority assigns relevant specialist(s) to assess the individual's disability.
- *Step 7:* The specialist doctor evaluates the disability of the individual and provides an opinion on the disability.
- *Step 8:* The medical board reviews the case and assigns a disability percentage. The CMO office then prepares the disability certificate and generates the UDID along with the disability certificate.
- *Step 9:* The UDID datasheet is sent for UDID card printing, and the card is dispatched to the individual with disabilities.

Currently, the government gazette mentions dyspraxia under SLD; no method of quantification or assessment is specified for benchmark disability.

MANAGEMENT AND INTERVENTION

Children and adolescents who present with learning difficulties usually present to a pediatrician or a psychiatrist. Many times, the school sensitively picks up and screens for learning difficulties and refers them to a psychiatrist. A multidisciplinary setup in ideal circumstances shall include a psychiatrist, pediatrician, psychologist, special educator, and occupational therapist. A holistic and comprehensive management enables holistic evaluation and management **(Box 4)**. Whether one is in a tertiary or periphery setup or a stand-alone psychiatrist, some handy techniques can be discussed.[3]

BOX 4: Management in specific learning disorder (SLD).[3]

- *Accommodations:* Facilitate the student to access the educational material. Grippers, special papers providing tactile feedback, spell checkers, audio books, and technological devices. Technological devices include voice recognition devices, touchpad devices, and calculators. Allowance of breaks. Extra time can be availed.
- *Modification:* Tasks given to the child are actually changed. Change a delivery, content or instructional level of subject matter or tests are implemented.
  - Oral assignments
  - Writing in short
  - Focus on content and spelling
  - Not having to read aloud
  - Extra time
  - Learning lower-level math
  - Dropping a language
- *Remedial education:* Process to help the child acquire age-appropriate skills in all his foundation areas for attaining knowledge at his pace and potential.

Overall, the focus on intervention would include:

- Determining SLD and its type. Also, include the impact of SLD and appropriately liaison with the various disciplines. For example, ruling out a medical disorder, psychotherapeutic support, and a pharmacological approach in case of emotional and behavioral conditions.
- Determining the associated comorbidity and treating the same
- Intervention in core deficits which include remedial education

Remedial Education[3]

The process involves an understanding of the child's current level. It starts with making an individualized education plan, keeping in mind the strengths and weaknesses. It can be made for 3 months, 6 months, or for a year. On the basis of SMART (Specific, Measurable, Achievable, Realistic, and Timely), goals can be set. IEP goals are made for all areas—reading, writing, and mathematics. It uses multisensory stimulation techniques such as visual, auditory, kinesthetic, and tactile stimuli (VAKT).

In the early years, the focus is on learning language skills, basic skills of reading, writing, and mathematics. In secondary years, the focus shifts to basic skills; children learn concepts, critical thinking, and problem solving. Modifications and accommodations to help the child cope.

Remediation techniques include the following:

Reading: In problems of decoding, phonological awareness must be increased. This means the ability and understanding to manipulate the sound structure of words. Focus on phonemes, which are the smallest unit of speech, such as K in Kit and b in Bat. This would involve the ability to hear and manipulate individual phonemes.

Isolation—training is in recognizing the individual sounds in words, e.g., say the first sound in the letter hat.

Phoneme identity—ability to distinguish the same sound in differing words, e.g., same sounds in pan and pond.

Phoneme substitution—replace one phoneme for another to create a new word (cat-mat, bad-bat)

Oral segmenting—break the word in different sounds (ban b/a/n)

Oral blending—join the sounds to form words (c/a/n)

Writing: Eye hand coordination and ability to segment phonemes are important. Basic motor functioning—hand exercises—such as working with clay, beading, and finger tapping. Improve spelling, phonic instructions, and teaching of letter writing used. Numbered arrow cues, hiding letters and visualizing writing letters, utilizing numbered cues to write letters, and finally checking letters compared to the sample. Master automatically the ability to retrieve letters, educational games, and activities can also be used to make them learn. With this as the base, planning, organizing, reviewing, and editing skills, practice using concept maps and different aids and strategies.

Mathematics: Strategies that can be used to practice number syntax are linking numbers to related digits such as 1,2,3,4. Drill and practice help in remembering number facts. Verbalization of arithmetic concepts, procedures, and operations are helpful in explicit instruction.

Motor coordination disorder: The aim is to reduce the impact of the disorder on well-being and daily functioning. Neurorehabilitation or motor-based interventions such as physical therapy and occupational therapy are used **(Box 5)**. Evidence for almost all therapies is being established.

Sensory integration: The approach involves appropriate sensory stimulation to promote motor adaptation and higher cortical learning. Sensory integration involves the organization of sensation from one's own body and environment but makes it possible to use the body effectively within the environment.

Process-oriented treatment: Laszlo and Bairstow proposed this approach. Kinesthesia is integral to the acquisition and performance of skilled motor behavior.

Perceptual motor training enhances sensory motor experience by giving children such tasks **(Box 6)**. It is used for mild motor problems.[20]

BOX 5: Bottom-up approaches to intervention.[20]

Goal: Remediation of underlying deficits:
- Sensory integration
- Process-oriented treatment
- Perceptual motor training
- Combination

BOX 6: Top-down approaches to intervention.[20]

Goal: Problem-solving approach to motor skill acquisition:
- Task-specific intervention
- Cognitive approaches

Task-specific intervention: Direct teaching of the task to be learned. Performance is the result of learning, and learning is optimal when the task is specified. Task accomplishment is achieved in steps by breaking it down into smaller units, teaching each unit separately and linking the units for the entire task performance. Generalization of the task is important.

Cognitive approaches: Problem-solving approach to guide skill acquisition. The five interrelated steps guide motor skills acquisition.

Boufard and Wall: Problem-solving approach to guide skill acquisition:
- *Problem identification:* Identify the nature of problem to be solved.
- *Problem representation:* Appropriate, accurate, and depiction of the motor problem
- *Plan construction:* Solve the movement problem and explore alternatives. Complex evaluation and revision of plan until a new suitable plan emerges
- *Plan execution:* Execution of plan
- Evaluation of progress

Cognitive orientation to daily occupational performance:
- Child centered
- Verbal self-instructional program
- Increasing functional performance through strategy use

Most therapists use a combination of approaches. Generalization and skills transfer, as well as larger studies, are needed.[20] **Flowchart 2** shows the flow of interventions in SLD.

Provisions to a Child with Specific Learning Disorder[21]

A child with SLD is given various provisions. As an example, in the state of Maharashtra across different boards and curricula, a child is given various provisions as mentioned in **Table 4**.

Flowchart 2: Interventions for specific learning disorders (based on the content of the chapter).

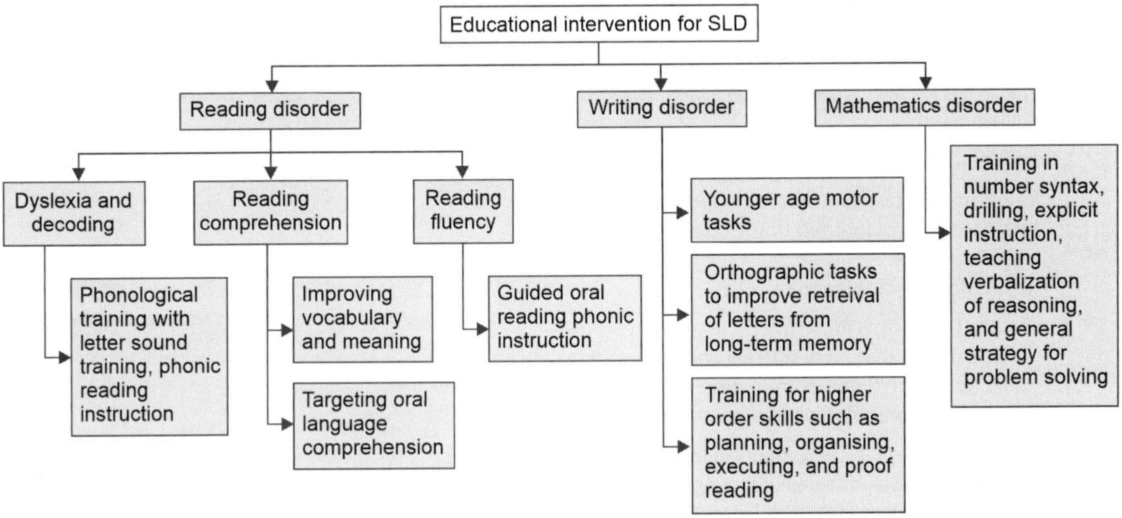

TABLE 4: Provisions in specific learning disorder (SLD).

	Provisions	*10th Std*			*12th Std*	*Degree colleges**
		SSC	*ICSE*	*CBSE*		
1	Nearest examination center of student's choice	√	√	√	√	√
2	Total 20 grace marks in either 1 subject or maximum of 3 subjects will be given	√	√	√	√	√
3	Answer books have to be sent in separate covers	√	√	√	√	√
4	Students will get 25% additional time to write exams	√	√	√	√#	√
5	Teachers who supervise are requested to read out the question paper as and when the student needs help (dyslexia)	√	√	√	√	√
6	Students can opt to get a writer/amanuensis at the time of examination (dysgraphia)	√	√	√	√	√
7	Student will be condoned from spelling mistakes/errors (dyslexia/dysgraphia)	√	√	√	√	√
8	Student will be exempted from directional mistakes in maps, drawing figures, maps, charts, diagrams, graphs, etc., and marks will be based on rest of the paper (dyslexia/dysgraphia)	√	√	√	√	√
9	Allowed to use the calculator (dyscalculia)	×	√	√	–	–
10	Student can opt to take/do Std. VII arithmetic with one work experience subject (dyscalculia)	√	×	×	–	–

Contd...

Contd...

	Provisions	10th Std			12th Std	Degree colleges*
		SSC	ICSE	CBSE		
11	Students can opt to drop mathematics and can take any other subject (dyscalculia)	×	√	√	–	–
12	Students can opt for dropping science and can take physiology, hygiene, and home science instead of regular science (dyslexia/dysgraphia/dyscalculia)	√	√	√	–	–
13	If the student opts for regular science instead of practical examination in science and technology (part I and part II) oral examination will be allowed (dyslexia/dysgraphia/dyscalculia)	√	√	√	–	–
14	Permitted to opt avoid appearing for practical but should submit certificates of having completed the concerned course of studies from related authorities in subjects such as practical work—experience, social service, technical subjects, etc. (dyslexia/dysgraphia)	×	×	×	√	–
15	Student can opt to drop 1 language and do 1 work experience subject instead (dyslexia/dysgraphia)	√	√	√	√	√

*Govt aided/professional and nonprofessional colleges in nonagricultural universities/engineering/polytechnics and teachers training colleges.

#Students will get an extra half hour (30 minutes) time for each examination paper.

School Liaison[3]

Along with the focus on identification, evaluation, and intervention, a psychiatrist makes an attempt to reach out to the school in the following ways for various purposes:

- Identification of academic issues and other comorbid issues
- Advocate for the child
- Educate the teachers about SLD and create awareness.
- Facilitate screening of SLD in school.
- Encourage the school to help the child and provide the academic modifications and arrangements that are rightfully deserved. Empower the school system.
- Teacher training to identify, refer, and use classroom strategies.
- Provide opportunities to develop motor learning and create awareness of DCD in the school setting.

SUMMARY AND CONCLUSION

To summarize, professionals should acknowledge that specific methods to identify and treat SLDs have scientific backing. It is crucial to assess promptly to prevent delays in aiding assistance. These evaluations should consider any additional comorbid and environmental conditions a child might have. Practitioners utilizing this assessment data can ensure that intervention programs are grounded in evidence and tailored to the individual. It is important to be aware of DCD and look for it and refer for interventions.

In conclusion, SLDs encompass a range of neurodevelopmental disorders characterized by persistent difficulties in acquiring and using specific academic skills significantly below age-level expectations. It typically manifests during school years with impairment in areas such as reading, writing, and mathematics. A clinician must keep an eye on different conditions that contribute to learning difficulties. Learning difficulties are not primarily attributable to intellectual disabilities, sensory deficits, or inadequate enrichment. MCDs are also characterized by difficulties in motor coordination, cause impairment in daily activities, and interfere with academic achievement. The multifactorial model integrates various etiological factors, including genetic, neurobiological, neuropsychological, obstetric factors, and environmental influences are implicated in development of SLD. Assessment of children with SLD involves a thorough clinical evaluation, followed by standardized psychometric testing of the child's cognitive abilities and academic skills. Intervention involves accommodations, modification, remedial education, and provision of academic benefits.

REFERENCES

1. Scaria LM, Bhaskaran D, George B. Prevalence of Specific Learning Disorders (SLD) among children in India: A systematic review and meta-analysis. Indian J Psychol Med. 2023;45(3):213-9.
2. Joseph JK, Devu BK. Prevalence and pattern of learning disability in India: A systematic review and meta-analysis. Indian J Psychiatr Nurs. 2022;19(2):152-62.
3. Shah HR, Sagar JK, Somaiya MP, Nagpal JK. Clinical practice guidelines on assessment and management of specific learning disorders. Indian journal of psychiatry. 2019;61(Suppl 2):211-25.
4. Harris SR, Mickelson EC, Zwicker JG. Diagnosis and management of developmental coordination disorder. CMAJ. 2015;187(9):659-65.
5. Kirk SA. Republication of "Learning Disabilities: A Historical Note". Interv School Clin. 2014;50(2): 125-8.
6. https://sites.ed.gov/idea/statute-chapter-33/subchapter-i/1401/30#:~:text=The%20term%20%E2%80%9Cspecific%20learning%20disability,spell%2C%20or%20do%20mathematical%20calculations
7. Smits-Engelsman B, Verbecque E. Pediatric care for children with developmental coordination disorder, can we do better? Biomed J. 2022;45(2): 250-64.
8. Bhate S, Wilkinson S. Aetiology of learning disability. Psychiatry. 2006;5(9):298-301.
9. Grigorenko EL, Compton DL, Fuchs LS, Wagner RK, Willcutt EG, Fletcher JM. Understanding, educating, and supporting children with specific learning disabilities: 50 years of science and practice. Am Psychol. 2020;75(1):37-51.
10. Mugesh T, Arthi J, Dutt S. Specific Learning Disabilities: Revisiting the theories, research and rehabilitation in the current perspective. Int J Creative Res Thoughts. 2023;11:e474-484.
11. Frank Y. Specific Learning Disabilities. Oxford University Press; 2014.
12. Kearns DM, Hancock R, Hoeft F, Pugh KR, Frost SJ. The Neurobiology of Dyslexia. Teaching Exceptional Children. 2019;51(3):175-88.
13. Subara-Zukic E, Cole MH, McGuckian TB, Steenbergen B, Green D, Smits-Engelsman BC, et al. Behavioral and neuroimaging research on developmental coordination disorder (DCD): A combined systematic review and meta-analysis of recent findings. Front Psychol. 2022;13:809455.
14. Lino F, Chieffo DPR. Developmental Coordination Disorder and most prevalent comorbidities: A narrative review. Children. 2022;9(7):1095.
15. Lachambre C, Proteau-Lemieux M, Lepage J-F, Bussières E-L, Lippé S. Attentional and executive functions in children and adolescents with developmental coordination disorder and the influence of comorbid disorders: A systematic review of the literature. PLoS ONE. 2021;16(6):e0252043.
16. Shah H, Dhillon S, Shelke S. Cognitive assessment of a Child with Specific Learning Disorder: IQ tests & Beyond. In: Subramanyam A, Sagar J (Eds). Specific Learning Disorder(s) An Indian

perspective. New Delhi: Jaypee Brothers Medical Publishers (P) Ltd.; 2024. pp 108-22.
17. American Psychiatric Association. Diagnostic and Statistical Manual of Mental Disorders, 5th edition. Arlington, VA American Psychiatric Association Publishing; 2013.
18. Jane JY, Burnett AF, Sit CH. Motor skill interventions in children with developmental coordination disorder: a systematic review and meta-analysis. Arch Phys Med Rehab. 2018;99(10):2076-99.
19. Guidelines for the purpose of assessing the extent of following specified disabilities http://www.ccdisabilities.nic.in/actsguideline/new-guidelines-purpose-assessing-extent-specified-disability-person-included-under the RPwDAct2016.
20. Mandich AD, Polatajko HJ, Macnab JJ, Miller LT. Treatment of children with Developmental Coordination Disorder: what is the evidence? Phys Occup Ther Pediatr. 2001;20(2-3):51-68.
21. Shah HR, Trivedi SC. Specific learning disability in Maharashtra: Current scenario and road ahead. Ann Indian Psychiatr. 2017;1:11.

Autism Spectrum Disorders: Concept, Definition, Assessment, Diagnosis, Formulation of Management Plan, and Management

Jai Ranjan Ram, Manisha Bhattacharya

INTRODUCTION

"Autism" as a term was initially introduced to describe a behavioral symptom of self-withdrawal in patients with schizophrenia. In 1943, psychiatrist Dr Leo Kanner and pediatrician Dr Hans Asperger adopted the term autism in the 1940s to introduce a syndrome in children with behavioral differences in social interaction and communication, and restrictive and repetitive interests.

In the following 80 years, the growth in understanding the various aspects of this enigmatic condition has been exponential. The current chapter offers a very selective review of clinically relevant aspects of the autism spectrum disorder (ASD), which is relevant for clinicians who are well versed with the basic theoretical knowledge about the condition.

The content of this chapter presupposes basic knowledge about ASD and highlights some specific clinical aspects, which the authors feel is often missed or not discussed. Additionally, some parts of the text are highlighted to make it easy for readers to remember the key learning points. The text is also interspersed with "practice points". This portion highlights how the theoretical knowledge about the condition translates into daily clinical practice.

THE ENIGMA OF RISING PREVALENCE

One of the fundamental questions about ASD is whether the prevalence is "truly" increasing.[1]

In countries where regular epidemiological data is available, the prevalence has steadily increased. In the USA, the percentage of children with ASD has steadily increased since the 1970s, when it was <0.4%. It is currently estimated to be between 1% and 2%. This reflects an increase of 150% to 400% in 50 years. The available data on the prevalence of autism in Indian studies varies depending on the methodology, population sampled, and geographic focus. Estimates vary widely—from 0.09 to over 1%.

The answer to the question whether it is increased prevalence against improved detection is complex. The consensus opinion is that it is most likely due to improved detection. However, here are some indicators that it may be due to true increase in prevalence. Some studies suggest that environmental factors, such as air pollution and maternal stress, may play a role in increasing autism diagnoses, although more research is needed to clarify these relationships.

Better detection and awareness are huge drivers. The evidence tilts toward detection as the main engine. A 2020 global review in The Lancet concluded most of the rise stems from awareness, diagnostic shifts, and service access.[2,3]

Diagnostic criteria have expanded—DSM-IV's rigid categories gave way to DSM-5's spectrum approach in 2013, capturing milder cases like Asperger's that once slipped through. Screening tools (e.g., M-CHAT) and professional training have spread, especially in high-income countries.

Awareness has exploded. Popular TV shows now have characters who have autism, prompting more parents to seek diagnosis. Studies adjusting for these factors, such as a 2015 US analysis, attribute over 50% of the rise to reclassification and better case finding.[4] Historical under-diagnosis is clear: A UK study found adults in their 60s with undiagnosed autism at rates same as diagnosis being made in children during the same time period. This suggests that many cases were missed before.[5]

But a true increase is not off the table. Environmental factors—air pollution, pesticide exposure, and maternal inflammation—keep popping up in research. A 2022 Harvard study linked prenatal PM2.5 exposure to a 1.5-fold autism risk.[6] Advanced parental age, rising globally, correlates with higher odds too. Genetic studies hint at de novo mutations, though their frequency has not clearly increased.[7]

Key Learning Points

- *Increased prevalence of ASD:* The number of individuals with ASD has risen, regardless of the cause, leading to a significantly larger patient population for psychiatrists to treat.
- *Shift in demographics:* There are now more adults with ASD than children, requiring long-term psychiatric care and support.
- *Training gaps:* Traditional psychiatric training often lacks focus on skills for working with adults and families affected by ASD, as it was historically viewed as a childhood condition.
- *Need for updated skills:* Current and future psychiatrists must refine their management and understanding of ASD to address this growing need effectively.
- *Broader perspectives:* Skills should align with demographic changes and incorporate human rights considerations in ASD care. The phrase "nothing about us, without us" holds true when we are planning care for everyone affected with ASD. Voices of the people with the condition has to be incorporated.

What is ASD?

It is a common, highly heritable, and heterogeneous neurodevelopmental disorder that has common cognitive and clinical features. It commonly co-occurs with other conditions.

Why can diagnosis be complex?

For clinicians, diagnosing ASD in a young child with prototypical presentation may not pose any challenge. The more overt the presentation is, the earlier is the possibility of a correct diagnosis. In our clinical experience, once the age range of 6–8 years is crossed and ASD is not detected, the diagnosis becomes more complex. Extending this logic, the diagnosis is even more complex in young adults or adults, if they have been missed. The diagnostic difficulty in diagnosing ASD arises from several facts

- The significant variability in presentation. The dictum, if you have seen 1 person with autism, you have seen 1 person with autism. Each person with autism has variable set of difficulties and presentation, which evolves with age.
- The milder end of the spectrum may have less of "abnormal' behavior than absence of "normal" behavior.
- The symptoms of comorbidities frequently mask the detection of core ASD features. Additionally, multiple comorbidities can co-occur in persons with ASD.
- Girls with ASD have less prominent prototypical symptoms and hence slip through the net.
- In undiagnosed adults, the features of ASD may take a backseat because the severe symptoms of comorbidity [mood disorder or psychosis or obsessive-compulsive disorder (OCD)] need urgent redressal. After the initial presenting symptoms start improving with treatment, the core symptoms of ASD, emerges. However, if the clinician is not mindful of the subtle or overt signs and symptoms of ASD, the condition may remain undiagnosed.

- ASD symptoms (e.g., deficit in social interaction) may not fully manifest until social demands exceed capacity, i.e., in late childhood or adolescence or even as adults (postmarriage).

Key Learning Points

- *Variability and evolution:* ASD presentation varies widely between individuals and changes with age, making it harder to spot, especially if missed by ages 6–8 when symptoms may become subtler or more complex.
- *Subtle signs and masking:* Milder cases may show an absence of "normal" behavior rather than obvious "abnormal" behavior, and comorbidities (e.g., mood disorders, OCD) or gender differences (e.g., girls with less typical symptoms) can hide core ASD features.
- *Late detection challenges:* In undiagnosed adults or older children, ASD symptoms may only emerge when social demands exceed capacity (e.g., adolescence or adulthood), and a lack of early developmental history complicates identification after severe comorbidities are treated.

ASSESSMENT FOR AUTISM SPECTRUM DISORDER

For any clinician, the queries that need to be answered are:

- Does the person have autism?
- What is the cognitive and developmental level of the person with autism?
- What are the medical comorbidities?
- What are the psychiatric comorbidities?

To diagnose autism, a clinical interview based on diagnostic criterion for ASD in DSM-5 suffices. The questionnaires which augment assessment can be subdivided into screening tools and diagnostic tools.

For screening, the most common tool used is MCHAT, which most clinicians are familiar with. A 20-item tool in Bengali for use by Anganwadi workers have also been developed by a group of clinicians in West Bengal, and it has been field tested for sensitivity, specificity and has been used to screen >2 lakh children in the state.

For diagnosing autism, Indian Scale for Assessment of Autism (ISAA), Childhood Autism Rating Scale Version 2 (CARS 2) are the most commonly used scales. Autism Diagnostic Observation Schedule (ADOS) and Autism Diagnostic Interview-Revised (ADI-R) are infrequently used in India because of cost and training implications. ISAA is the scale which is most widely used in government settings.

For developmental assessment, the most common tool which is used in India is Vineland Adaptive Behaviour Scales (VABS). It is also useful to track the changes in adaptive behavior following intervention.

For IQ assessments, the tools which are commonly used are:

- Binet-Kamat Test of Intelligence (BKT)
- Malin's Intelligence Scale for Indian Children (MISIC),
- Wechsler Intelligence Scale for Children—Fourth Edition, India (WISC-IV India)
- Raven's Progressive Matrices (RPM)
- Seguin Form Board Test (SFBT)

As a practitioner, deciding which tool to use involves clinical judgment. There are multiple, interlinked factors which need to be taken into consideration. The key factors are described here.

Purpose of the Assessment

Screening versus diagnosis: If the goal is to flag potential issues (e.g., autism or intellectual delay), a screening tool like the M-CHAT-R (for autism) or Raven's Progressive Matrices (for IQ) might suffice. For a definitive diagnosis or detailed cognitive profile, diagnostic tools such as the ISAA (autism) or WISC-IV India (IQ) are preferred.

Intervention planning: Tools such as the VABS (adaptive behavior) or MISIC (IQ with subtest breakdown) provide detailed insights into strengths and weaknesses of the assessee, aiding in more individually tailored support plans.

Monitoring progress: VABS might be chosen to track changes over time.

Age and Developmental Level

Tools are age specific. WISC-IV India suits school-aged children (6–16 years). A 2-year-old would not be assessed with the MISIC, which starts at age 6.

Developmental stage matters too. A nonverbal child might need the Raven's CPM or SFB rather than a verbally heavy tool such as the BKT.

Tools, such as the MISIC or BKT, adapted for Indian languages, might be chosen over imported tools if language alignment is critical. If language is not a barrier, the WISC-IV India could work.

Practical Constraints

Time: Quick tools such as the Seguin Form Board (10–15 minutes) suit busy settings, while the ADI-R (2–3 hours) demands more commitment which is feasible in research and some private settings.

Training: Some tools (e.g., ADOS-2 and WISC-IV) require certified administrators, limiting their use to specialized settings. Simpler tools such as the CARS-2 need less expertise.

Resources: In rural India or underfunded clinics, low-cost options such as the BKT might be prioritized over pricier tools such as the WISC-IV India.

Child's behavior and engagement: A restless or uncooperative child might do better with short, engaging tasks (e.g., Raven's CPM).

Therefore, it is clear that choosing which tool/s to use for a particular individual requires clinical judgement. Additionally, many young people and adults now come with a self-diagnosis of ASD. Therefore, clinicians now have to be adept at evaluation of ASD across the life span. The basic principles of assessment remain the same. The propensity of more people coming with self-diagnosis is bound to increase over years to come. Evaluating the individual's concern with sensitivity and respectfully is mandatory in these circumstances, even if the clinician is skeptical about the process.

Key Learning Points

- *Core Questions:* Clinicians must determine:
  - Does the person have autism?
  - What is their cognitive/developmental level?
  - What medical and psychiatric comorbidities exist?
- *Diagnosing autism:* A clinical interview using DSM-5 criteria is usually enough; tools such as ISAA and CARS-2 are widely used in India, while ADOS and ADI-R are less common due to cost/training.
- *Screening tools:* MCHAT is the most popular screening tool; a 20-item Bengali tool by West Bengal clinicians has screened over 2 lakh kids effectively.
- *Developmental assessment:* VABS is the go-to tool in India for assessing and tracking adaptive behavior changes postintervention.
- *IQ tools:* Common options include BKT, MISIC, WISC-IV India, RPM, and SFBT.
- *Choosing tools:* Depends on:
  - Purpose (screening, diagnosis, intervention, or monitoring)
  - Age/developmental stage
  - Practical constraints (time, training, and cost)
  - Child's behavior
- *Key factors:* Screening uses quick tools (e.g., MCHAT-R); diagnosis needs detailed ones (e.g., ISAA); VABS helps plan interventions; age-specific tools like WISC-IV fit school kids (6–16).
- *Practical tips:* Short tools (e.g., Seguin Form Board) suit busy clinics or restless kids; language-adapted tools (e.g., MISIC) work better in diverse settings.
- *Self-diagnosis trend:* More people, especially youth/adults, present with self-diagnosed autism; clinicians must evaluate respectfully across all ages using the same principles.
- *Clinical judgment:* Selecting the right tool requires balancing purpose, practicality, and patient needs—there's no one-size-fits-all approach!

Medical Assessments

First and foremost, routine EEG and brain scan or genetic tests are not required. These need to be done only if they are clinically indicated.[8]

Core Medical Assessments

The aim is to assess the status of physical health, identify co-occurring medical conditions, and rule out mimics without unnecessary medical tests.

Medical assessments need to be tailored, keeping in mind the age and the source of referral. By source of the referral, the authors mean that in many new referrals, a basic medical evaluation may have already been done (i.e., referrals from pediatricians or other physicians).

The template given below is meant for young children, who have not been medically evaluated earlier and have come with suspected ASD or developmental delay. For every such scenario, it is important to not miss any genetic syndrome, epilepsy, cerebral palsy, hearing, or vision impairment.

Physical Examination

What: A general head-to-toe check, including:

- Head circumference (to detect macrocephaly, linked to autism in some cases).
- Neurological examination (e.g., muscle tone, reflexes, and coordination)
- Dysmorphic features (e.g., facial asymmetry and large ears) suggest genetic syndromes.
- Hearing and vision screening. Brain auditory evoked potential (BAER) if possible.

Neurological Screening

What: Assess for:

- Seizures (history of staring spells and jerking movements)
- Gross motor abnormalities (e.g., unsteady gait and tremors)

Nutritional Assessment

Measure weight and height. It is important to track changes if the person is started on psychotropic medicines.

Check for signs of malnutrition (e.g., pallor, thin hair, and stunting). Malnutrition is prevalent in rural India and can exacerbate developmental challenges or mimic delays.

Some routine blood tests such as hemoglobin (for anemia).

Thyroid function (TSH, if symptoms such as lethargy or poor growth are present) can be done.

These tests might indicate treatable conditions such as anemia or hypothyroidism which can affect behavior and development; lead poisoning can mimic autism.

Key Learning Points

- *No routine tests:* EEG, brain scans, or genetic tests are not needed unless clinically indicated—avoid unnecessary procedures.
- *Core goals:* Assess physical health, identify co-occurring conditions (e.g., epilepsy), and rule out mimics of autism or delay without overtesting.
- *Tailored approach:* Customize assessments based on age and referral source (e.g., new cases vs. kids already seen by pediatricians).
- *Target group:* Focus is on young children with suspected ASD or delay who have not had prior medical evaluation.
- *Physical examination:* Head-to-toe check—measure head circumference (for macrocephaly), neurological examination (tone and reflexes), and look for dysmorphic features (e.g., facial asymmetry), hinting at genetic syndromes.
- *Sensory screening:* Test hearing (BAER if possible) and vision to catch impairments that could affect development.
- *Neurological signs:* Screen for seizures (e.g., staring spells) and motor issues (e.g., unsteady gait)—do not miss epilepsy or cerebral palsy.
- *Nutritional check:* Measure height/weight (track if on psychotropics), look for malnutrition signs (pallor and stunting), common in rural India and can mimic delays.

- *Basic blood tests:* Hemoglobin (for anemia) and TSH (thyroid, if lethargy/growth issues) to spot treatable conditions such as anemia or hypothyroidism that impact behavior.
- *Key conditions:* Rule out genetic syndromes, epilepsy, cerebral palsy, and lead poisoning—treatable mimics matter!

The assessment for psychiatric comorbidities will be discussed in later part of the chapter, where comorbidities are discussed.

It is vitally important that during assessments, the individual's views, hopes, and expectations are explored. Medical practitioners are notorious to presume incompetence of young people or people with disabilities. For each individual, even if they are nonverbal or deeming to have severe retardation, definite attempts to make them feel welcomed are essential.

It is our experience that many young people and adults feel their voice was not heard during an assessment process and more credence was paid to their carer's version, who may only be concerned about the disruptive behavior or their ward not following societal norms.

An attempt must be made to speak with young people and adults in private. It is especially important to keep in mind the fact that many of them are more prone to various forms of abuse, including sexual abuse. During assessments, the probability of such violations has to be kept in mind.[9]

Practice point: For clinicians, it is worth remembering that the evaluation process is part of an engagement process with the person or the family. Many people with ASD need lifelong support from mental health professionals. Most families remember how the news of their ward's disability was conveyed and the attitude of the treating professional. An initial bad experience may have long-term impact on the family and the person, which may prevent them from seeking help again. Therefore, it merits repeated iterations that attitude of the professionals can and does have a lasting impact on the person and the family.

The genetics of autism spectrum disorder: A review of findings in the last decade (2015–2025).

Over the past decade, genetic research has transformed our understanding of ASD, revealing it as one of the most heritable psychiatric conditions, with estimates suggesting heritability between 70 and 90%.[10] This part synthesizes key findings from 2015 to 2025, emphasizing advances in gene discovery, the interplay of rare and common genetic variants, biological mechanisms, sex differences, and clinical implications for psychiatrists.

Practice point: For clinicians, an honest reality is that while the pace of discovery has been remarkable, translating these insights into practice remains a challenge. There is increasing availability of whole exome sequencing in India. Prudence needs to be exercised regarding use of these tests in clinical practice.

The past 10 years have solidified ASD as a genetically heterogeneous disorder, driven by a combination of rare, high-impact variants and common, low-effect variants.

Early optimism that the genome-wide association studies (GWAS) would pinpoint a handful of "autism genes" has given way to a more nuanced view: ASD arises from hundreds of genetic contributors interacting with environmental factors.

Rare Variants and De Novo Mutations

A landmark shift occurred with the widespread adoption of whole-exome sequencing (WES) and whole-genome sequencing (WGS), which detect rare variants not captured by earlier methods. Studies[11] have analyzed over 35,000 individuals, identifying 102 genes strongly associated with ASD, 60 of which were novel. These genes often harbor de novo mutations—spontaneous changes not inherited from parents—disrupting protein function. For instance, mutations in CHD8, a chromatin regulator, emerged as a recurring finding, linked to macrocephaly and severe ASD phenotypes.[12,13] Approximately 10–20% of ASD cases are now attributable to such rare variants, including copy-number variants (CNVs) such as 16p11.2 deletions and duplications.[14]

Common Variants and Polygenic Risk

While rare variants dominate in severe cases, common variants—small-effect polymorphisms shared across populations—collectively contribute to ASD risk. Grove et al.[15] have conducted the largest GWAS to date, involving 18,381 ASD cases, and identified five genome-wide significant loci. These findings introduced polygenic risk scores (PRS). PRS aggregate the effects of thousands of common variants to estimate an individual's genetic liability. Notably, children inheriting rare mutations alongside high PRS are more likely to develop ASD, even if their parents remain unaffected.[16] This supports the liability threshold model, suggesting a cumulative genetic burden tips individuals into the ASD phenotype.

Genetic Overlap with Other Psychiatric Disorders

One of the most paradigm-shifting revelations of the past decade (2015–2025) also has been the genetic overlap between ASD with other psychiatric disorders. Far from being an isolated condition, ASD shares substantial genetic architecture with schizophrenia, attention-deficit/hyperactivity disorder (ADHD), bipolar disorder, and major depressive disorder (MDD), among others. This convergence, elucidated through advanced genomic techniques, refutes the traditional diagnostic silos and emphasizes transdiagnostic approach in clinical practice. The genetic overlap provides us with a lens to rethink comorbidity, family history, and treatment strategies.

Whole-exome sequencing and WGS have pinpointed rare, high-impact variants that bridge ASD with psychiatric conditions. The autism sequencing consortium's landmark study by Satterstrom et al. identified 102 ASD-associated genes, with 30 also implicated in schizophrenia and ADHD.[11]

Genome-wide association studies also have illuminated the role of common variants, revealing a polygenic overlap that amplifies shared risk. Lee et al.[17] reported significant genetic correlations: 0.37 between ASD and schizophrenia, 0.40 with ADHD, 0.21 with bipolar disorder, and 0.22 with MDD. These and many other research findings suggest a diffuse genetic liability that spans diagnostic boundaries.

What are the Biological Mechanisms?

The genetic overlap ultimately converges on neurobiological pathways, for example, synaptic function. Genes such as *SHANK3* and *NLGN3*, critical for postsynaptic integrity, are disrupted in ASD and schizophrenia, impairing glutamatergic signaling.

Clinical Implications for Psychiatrists

This genetic intertwining has immediate relevance for psychiatric practice. Patients with ASD may face elevated risk for later psychiatric conditions—20–30% develop schizophrenia or psychosis by adulthood[18] particularly if carrying shared variants such as 22q11.2 or NRXN1 deletions. Conversely, an ADHD patient with high ASD PRS might exhibit subclinical social deficits, warranting screening.

Family history amplifies this: A parent with schizophrenia or bipolar disorder signals potential cross-disorder risk in an ASD child.[19]

Key Learning Points

- *Genetic complexity:* ASD is a mix of rare, high-impact variants (e.g., CHD8 mutations and 16p11.2 CNVs) and common, low-effect variants, interacting with environmental factors—no single "autism gene" exists.
- *Rare variants:* Whole-exome/genome sequencing revealed 102 ASD-linked genes, with 10–20% of cases tied to de novo mutations (e.g., CHD8 tied to macrocephaly) disrupting critical proteins.
- *Common variants:* Large GWAS studies (e.g., Grove et al.) found five key loci; PRS show how common variants pile up, increasing ASD risk, especially with rare mutations.
- *Psychiatric overlap:* ASD shares genes with schizophrenia, ADHD, bipolar, and depression (e.g., 30 of 102 ASD genes also link to schizophrenia/ADHD), pushing a transdiagnostic view.
- *Biological pathways:* Overlapping genes (e.g., SHANK3) affect synaptic function, such as glutamatergic signaling, tying ASD to other disorders biologically.
- *Clinical impact:* ASD patients may later develop psychosis (20–30% risk); family history (e.g., schizophrenia in parents) or high PRS in ADHD kids flags cross-disorder risks for screening.

Practice point: These findings emphasize the fact that psychiatrists should adopt a lifespan approach, for people with ASD. Monitoring for emergent symptoms (e.g., mood instability and attentional shifts) and tailoring interventions are frequently required for patients, who may have been well for variable periods in time.

Developmental Timing in Fetal Growth

Timing is critical. Sestan et al.[20] pinpointed mid-fetal prefrontal cortical development as a vulnerable period for many ASD risk genes. This aligns with findings from organoid models and induced pluripotent stem cells (iPSCs), which replicate ASD-related cellular deficits. These studies underscore that ASD's roots lie in early brain wiring, complicating later therapeutic correction.

The Female Protective Effect

Autism spectrum disorder's 4:1 male-to-female ratio has long puzzled researchers. Genetic studies over the past decade suggest a "female protective effect," where females require a higher genetic burden to manifest ASD. Gockley et al.[21] and Werling et al.[22] found females with ASD carry more rare mutations and higher PRS than males. WES data integration further revealed that females exhibit greater resilience to common variants, possibly due to hormonal or X-chromosome-linked factors.

Practice point: This has clinical implications—female patients may present with subtler symptoms, risking underdiagnosis. This necessitates a higher index of suspicion to detect ASD in women, and they warrant tailored assessment strategies.

Environmental Interactions

We definitely know a lot less about the environmental influences. What is known is that vaccines do not cause ASD. While genetics dominate ASD etiology, environmental factors probably amplify risk in genetically susceptible individuals. Pesticide exposure, for example, exacerbates behavioral deficits in CHD8 mutant rodents.[23] Maternal immune activation and prenatal stress also interact with genetic risk, though their specific contributions remain elusive due to methodological challenges.

Practice point: Psychiatrists should note that while counseling families on the cause of ASD, an overemphasis on genetic factors can lead to guilt, shame, and blame within families.

Clinical implications for psychiatrists: The genetic revolution in ASD offers practical insights, though direct therapeutic applications lag.

Diagnostic Utility of Genetic Advances

Chromosomal microarrays (CMAs) detect CNVs in 10–20% of ASD cases, while WES identifies single-gene mutations in 9–30%. Shen et al., 2014.[14] For patients with intellectual disability (ID), dysmorphic features, or family history, referral to clinical genetics can be made if the parents are considering having another child.

However, routine testing for all ASD cases lacks cost-effectiveness evidence,[24] a reality which psychiatrists must navigate amid patient expectations.

Counseling for Subsequent Pregnancy

The baseline prevalence of ASD in the general population is approximately 1–2%.[25] However, studies show that siblings of a child with ASD have a recurrence risk ranging from 7 to 20%, with variability depending on specific factors. A seminal study by Ozonoff et al. reported an overall recurrence risk of 18.7% in families with one affected child, based on a large prospective cohort.[26] This elevated risk underscores a strong familial component, likely driven by shared genetic and environmental influences.

Sex differences play a significant role in recurrence risk. ASD is diagnosed four times more frequently in males than females, suggesting a protective effect in females.[27] However, when the firstborn with ASD is female, the recurrence risk for subsequent siblings increases. Sandin et al.[28] found that families with an affected female proband had a 50% higher recurrence risk compared to those with an affected male, potentially due to a higher genetic load required for females to manifest ASD symptoms. This sex-linked pattern suggests that the underlying etiology may differ between males and females, impacting sibling risk.

The presence of ID in the firstborn also modifies recurrence risk. Approximately 30–50% of individuals with ASD have co-occurring ID.[28] When the firstborn has both ASD and ID, the likelihood of a second child being affected increases, as this combination often correlates with more severe genetic abnormalities. For instance, de novo mutations or copy-number variations identified in the firstborn, such as deletions in 16p11.2, are associated with higher recurrence risks if inherited or recurrent in the family.[29]

Genetic abnormalities further elevate risk. ASD has a strong heritable component, with monozygotic twins showing concordance rates of up to 90%. Seizure disorders, present in 20–30% of ASD cases, also signal a more complex phenotype. When the firstborn exhibits epilepsy alongside ASD, shared genetic factors such as SCN1A mutations may increase recurrence risk, particularly if these are inherited rather than de novo.[26]

Beyond numbers, counseling must address emotional and practical dimensions. Parents often seek certainty—"Will my next child have autism?"—but genetics offers probabilities, not promises. Psychiatrists can pivot to empowerment: "We can't predict everything, but we can watch for early signs and intervene sooner if needed. Your experience with your first child gives us a head start."

Highlighting the variability of ASD phenotypes is also critical. Even with a shared mutation, a second child might present milder symptoms or none at all due to sex differences, environmental factors, or modifier genes.[30] For instance, the female protective effect might lower risk or alter expression in a daughter, a nuance worth mentioning.

Key Learning Points

- *Genetic testing utility:* CMAs detect CNVs in 10–20% of ASD cases; WES finds single-gene mutations in 9–30%, especially useful with ID, dysmorphic features, or family history.
- *Not routine:* Routine genetic testing for all ASD cases is not cost-effective, though parents may expect it—psychiatrists must balance this reality.
- *Recurrence risk:* General ASD prevalence is 1–2%, but siblings of an affected child face a 7–20% risk (18.7% average as per Ozonoff et al.), driven by shared genetics and environment.

- *Sex differences:* ASD is 4× more common in males; if the firstborn with ASD is female, recurrence risk rises 50% hinting at higher genetic load in females as per Sandin et al.[28]
- *ID impact:* 30–50% of ASD cases have ID; firstborns with both ASD and ID increase recurrence risk, often tied to severe genetic issues such as 16p11.2 deletions.
- *Genetic and epilepsy factors:* Monozygotic twins show 90% ASD concordance; epilepsy (20–30% of cases) with genes like *SCN1A* raises recurrence risk if inherited.
- *Counseling focus:* Parents want certainty, but psychiatrists offer probabilities—emphasize early monitoring and intervention, leveraging prior experience.
- *Phenotype variability:* Even with shared mutations, a second child's symptoms may differ (milder or none) due to sex, environment, or modifier genes—e.g., female protective effect may reduce risk.

Practice point: Many parents have "broad autism phenotype". It refers to a set of subclinical traits and characteristics associated with ASD that are observed in individuals who do not meet the full diagnostic criteria for ASD. These traits include mild difficulties in social interaction, communication challenges, and a preference for routines or repetitive behaviors, often seen in close relatives of individuals with ASD. Broad autism phenotype (BAP) is considered a genetically influenced expression of autism-related features, suggesting a continuum of autism-like characteristics in the general population. For example, a parent might exhibit social aloofness or rigidity in thinking without significant impairment, reflecting BAP traits. Research indicates that BAP is more prevalent among first-degree relatives of individuals with ASD, with studies estimating that 20–30% of such relatives display these features.[31] Clinicians must account for these features when they are making provisions for family engagement or parent training programs.

In conclusion, psychiatrists should anticipate ethical and emotional fallout. Some parents fear stigma or regret overtesting; others fixate on recurrence odds, neglecting their current child's needs.

PSYCHOPHARMACOLOGICAL TREATMENT OF YOUNG PEOPLE WITH AUTISM SPECTRUM DISORDER

There are no, as yet, clinically proven or approved pharmacological treatments for the core symptoms of ASD. Yet, a survey of world literature reflects that majority children with ASD are on psychotropic or antiepileptic drugs.

The FDA has approved two drugs for treating irritability associated with autism in children: Risperidone and aripiprazole. Risperidone is approved for children between 5 and 16 years old, while aripiprazole is approved for children between 6 and 17 years old.

Research indicates that psychotropic medication use is common among young people with ASD, with rates varying 20–60% across different studies and countries.[32]

Psychotropic Medication Use

Commonly used psychotropic medications are:

- Stimulants, α-agonists, or atomoxetine
- Antipsychotics
- Antidepressants
- Melatonin
- ADHD medications

The medication use is higher with co-occurring conditions such as seizures, ADHD, OCD, bipolar disorder, or anxiety disorders. In many, there is polypharmacy because of the complexities of presentation.[32]

Practice point: There are several important issues which a psychiatrist must answer before starting any child with ASD on psychotropic medicines.

In our experience, the majority of children with ASD who come to psychiatry clinics probably require medication, at least in the short term. The most common questions which parents ask are what is it given for, what would be the side effects, and how long the medicine is going to be given. It is essential that psychiatrists are able to answer these questions with clarity, as majority of parents are wary of starting psychotropic medicines on their child.

The real challenge of psychopharmacological management of myriads of symptoms in a child with ASD is the management of comorbidities. Given the fact that children with autism may have difficulty communicating their experiences, it is challenging to identify side effects. This can lead to underreporting and potential delays in addressing adverse reactions.

In conclusion, it is prudent to be conservative about pharmacological management of children with ASD. Clinicians need to gain experience with 3–4 drugs initially and gain confidence, rather than start using a plethora of medicines before they have an adequate experience.

Gene-specific therapies remain aspirational, but discoveries inspire hope.

NONPHARMACOLOGICAL INTERVENTION STRATEGIES FOR AUTISM SPECTRUM DISORDER

This is the cornerstone of treatment for ASD. It is erroneous to believe that there is no treatment for ASD, as may be believed by many carers and practitioners. In last few decades, there have been some huge changes in the intervention processes and strategies for autism. With the advancement in understanding of autism, there have been some substantial growth and progress in the interventions, services, and supports for individuals with autism. With more and more self-advocates coming up and sharing their experiences, needs, and rights, the intervention methodology is going through constant changes, depending on the individual and contextual factors. Advances in the understanding are bringing change in the previous perception that one intervention strategy fits everyone and are providing actionable insight on "what works for whom and why". The knowledge about rights of the person with autism is being taken into consideration to make this intervention effective as well as respectful, which presume competence and does not restrict them into the preconceived notions. For example, a small but growing literature has focused on evaluating alignment between interventions based on applied behavior analysis (ABA) and the concepts that have developed within social models of disability and neurodiversity-affirming forums.[33-35] Rather than focusing on one mode of therapy, intervention plans currently surround around mainly three areas:

1. Supporting communication and social interaction needs
2. Supporting developing adaptive functioning skills and emotional regulation
3. Supporting learning needs

Slowly, it is being recognized that supporting the individual's sensory needs is also equally important and thus, interventions targeted this need are also emerging.

Here, we will discuss the evidence-based approaches of intervention techniques in ASD and also about a few emerging yet promising interventions that are based on humanitarian and naturalistic approaches and promote social integration.

Key Learning Points

- *Autism spectrum disorder is treatable:* The belief that there is no treatment for ASD is incorrect.
- *Intervention strategies are evolving:* Significant advancements in understanding ASD have led to substantial improvements in intervention processes and strategies.

- *Self-advocacy drives change:* Experiences and insights shared by self-advocates are crucial in shaping and adapting intervention methodologies.
- *Individualized approaches are essential:* The "one-size-fits-all" approach is outdated; interventions must be tailored to individual and contextual factors.
- *Respect for rights is paramount:* Interventions must be respectful, presume competence, and avoid preconceived notions, considering the rights of individuals with ASD.
- *Alignment with social models and neurodiversity is considered:* There is a growing focus on aligning interventions, particularly ABA, with social models of disability and neurodiversity-affirming principles.
- *Current intervention plans focus on three core areas:*
  1. Supporting communication and social interaction needs
  2. Supporting the development of adaptive functioning skills and emotional regulation
  3. Supporting learning needs
- *Sensory needs are increasingly recognized:* The importance of addressing sensory needs in ASD interventions is gaining recognition.
- *Evidence-based and emerging interventions are used:* Interventions include both evidence-based approaches and emerging, humanitarian, and naturalistic approaches that promote social integration.

Supporting Communication and Social Interaction Needs

Social interaction and communication differences have been the primary focus for any effective intervention.

Applied behavior analysis has been a primary intervention technique for developing not only the desired behavior but also language and communication. ABA has progressed over the past 60 years from the core principles established in the early Lovaas model and subsequent UCLA Young Autism Project into many comprehensive intervention models and focused intervention practices, methods, and teaching strategies, all of which aim to target deficits for children and youth with ASD across all levels of functioning, including cognition, language, social skills, problem behavior, and daily living skills.[36] The most cited foundational model of ABA is the *"Antecedent-Behavior-Consequence"* model which is often referred to as "A-B-C" principles; where manipulation of either or both the antecedent is done to bring desired changes in (social) behavior. There are also a number of ABA techniques that are worth noting, including reinforcement, extinction, prompting, video modeling, as well as the picture exchange communication system (PECS), though many of these are widely used in other intervention and education settings.[37-39] The analysis of verbal behavior or verbal behavior analysis (VBA) is concerned with the functions of language including requests, comments, and conversation. BF Skinner developed the verbal behavior classification system in 1957 and wrote about it in his book verbal behavior as he was concerned with expressive language as well. It is important to realize that verbal behavior is not an instructional methodology, but a framework for thinking about language development.

Alternative and augmentative communication (AAC): With the nonspeaking autistic individuals coming up with their experiences of the life-long deprivation from their rights to learn, grow, attend school, and having a regular mainstream life, and how the assumption that "nonspeaking means nonthinking" has contributed these deprivation in their life. This led to the reassessment and rethinking of the traditional communication intervention in autism. Thus, Didactic methods which are based on behaviorist theory take advantage of behavioral technologies such as massed trials, operant conditioning, shaping, and prompting are being reviewed. These approaches target the skills in a highly structured and isolated contexts, but currently more natural settings and interaction partners (e.g., mainstream classrooms and other children) are gradually integrated as a child demonstrates progress.

The traditional speech therapy is extending their realm to multimodal communication (gestures, signs, and alternative methods), and these are taking precedence as the speech drills alone are not sufficient when the child has apraxia of speech. The awareness and acceptance of AAC among professionals is improving. And it has created a huge difference in providing reliable means of communication through which they can fully participate in their educational or leisure activities. AAC is a solution to solve long-standing functional communication and education problems, by adapting to AAC devices based on their mental and physical condition. Therefore, it is essential to investigate an appropriate technology design fit for AAC to support effective social communication, plan individualized education plan (IEP), and increase classroom interaction quality. Be it the modest *picture exchange communication system (PECS)* or the hi-tech *Jellow or Avaz* app, AAC needs to be tailored according to the individual's needs.

For individuals who are nonverbal or verbal, but struggle to engage socially, naturalistic interventions are becoming increasingly popular. These approaches help them develop reciprocal communication, build real friendships, and navigate an ever-changing world. These interventions aim more toward relationship development and often are parent mediated. These works are guided by the developmental model of learning and works by child's growth-seeking drive to learn new skills. *Relationship development intervention (RDI), Floortime, and JASPER* are the intervention strategies that work on communication, emotional regulation, joint attention, declarative communication, social reciprocation, engagement, and building emotionally involved relationships through respectful guided participation and in a more natural way. RDI has a focus of increasing social awareness through the use of dynamic intelligence. RDI methods are used by the parents of the children in RDI therapy, since the general goal of the treatment is more natural and complete interactions among family members. The developer, Gutstein, calls RDI a "cognitive-developmental" parent training program. The program attempts to impact "experience sharing" and inflexibility in thinking. At the core of the program, parents learn how to perceive and scaffold opportunities for their child to respond in more flexible, thoughtful ways to new, challenging and unpredictable settings and problems. Parents are trained to incorporate these opportunities into their lifestyle, so that each day involves frequent, carefully framed opportunities presented seamlessly into the child's routine. Evidence shows that children who participated in RDI became significantly more socially related, engaged in more reciprocal communication, functioned in school settings with less adult participation, and also were perceived by parents as behaving in a dramatically more flexible and adaptive manner.

For teenagers, young adults or adults, social skills training is often found to be helpful where the individual has the agency over the strategies to be used and also gets to reflect on the different perspectives. A holistic approach by a psychologist or special educator is helpful in understanding the individual's need and working on it.

Key Learning Points

- *Communication and social interaction are primary intervention targets:* Addressing these areas is fundamental for effective ASD intervention.
- *Applied behavior analysis (ABA) is a core technique:*
  - It has evolved significantly from the Lovaas model.
  - It targets deficits across various domains, including language and social skills.
  - The A-B-C model (antecedent-behavior-consequence) is a foundational principle.
  - Various ABA techniques exist, such as reinforcement, prompting, and video modeling.
  - Verbal behavior analysis (VBA) focuses on the function of language.

- *AAC is crucial:*
  - It addresses the needs of nonspeaking individuals.
  - It challenges the assumption that "nonspeaking means nonthinking."
  - It involves multimodal communication (gestures, signs, and devices).
  - AAC devices, such as PECS, Jellow, and Avaz, should be tailored to individual needs.
- *Naturalistic interventions are gaining popularity:*
  - They emphasize relationship development and are often parent mediated.
  - They are guided by developmental models of learning.
  - Examples include relationship development intervention (RDI), Floortime, and JASPER.
  - RDI focuses on dynamic intelligence and experience sharing.
  - These interventions work on emotional regulation, joint attention, and social reciprocation.
- *Social skills training is beneficial for older individuals:*
  - It empowers individuals to use chosen strategies.
  - It encourages reflection on different perspectives.
  - A holistic approach by a psychologist or special educator is valuable.
- *Traditional speech therapy is evolving:*
  - It is expanding to include multimodal communication.
  - It recognizes that speech drills alone may be insufficient, especially for individuals with apraxia of speech.
- *The setting of intervention is shifting:*
  - A shift from highly structured and isolated context to more natural settings.

Supporting Developing Adaptive Functioning Skills and Emotional Regulation

The term "adaptive behavior" refers to general societal expectations about everyday functioning in socialization, communication, self-care, and life skills for personal independence and community living. Adaptive functioning is found to be an important determinant of outcome in individuals with ASD,[40] including educational attainment[41] and the level of independence that an individual can achieve in adulthood.[42] With more and more understanding of autism, the recent theories delve deeper into the "intention of behavior" and its association with the underlying emotional aspects. For example, learning the social skills required in a particular set up will need complete exploration of the environment, perception of the people in that environment (theory of mind) and also addressing the overwhelming emotions to address the unpredictability. Various intervention strategies try to target this unpredictability and the anxiety related to it which leads to difficulty learning adaptive functional skills.

Treatment and education of autistic-related communication-handicapped children (TEACCH) or the structured teaching process is believed to develop independence and self-esteem. Structured teaching contains strategies tailored to suit the strengths of people with autism. For example, the strong emphasis on visual strategies and predictability rests upon the assumption of a primarily visual and routine-based learning style. The developers of this model believed that interventions should help to balance the unique characteristics of the person with autism and the social conventions of the community. They coined the term "culture of autism" as a way of thinking about the characteristic patterns of behavior seen in individuals with autism and used this concept as the basis for interventions leading to the long-term goal of community participation.[43] The goal for the TEACCH practitioner is to support parents, educators, and others who work with persons with autism to see the world through their eyes, to understand the perspectives better. Those working with the person aim to teach them to function as independently as possible while making the environment more understandable, predictable and suited to the needs of the individual. TEACCH practitioners do not follow any standardized curriculum as they believe that each individual has his or her unique learning style and skills. However, all TEACCH programs include some key elements of structured teaching: Organization of the physical environment, visual information, task organization, and work systems. Visual information is intended to make tasks clear, meaningful, predictable, constant, and understandable for the learner. Common elements include instructions (i.e., verbal description of what a child has to do with the material provided for a task), a particular task organization (i.e., the separation and distribution of tasks into meaningful groups), and strategies to increase clarity (i.e., cues to what is the most important aspect of the task). TEACCH practitioners use visual information in lieu of verbal instructions owing to the limited receptive language ability in this population. Structured teaching may take many forms depending on the individual: from written checklists to visual schedules and actual objects. For example, visual schedules provide information about the order in which a series of tasks ought to be completed. Visual schedules help with transitions and can help the individual to become independent from the cues and prompts of others. Activity schedules have been shown to increase skill acquisition and on-task behavior while decreasing challenging behavior.

Social stories: A social story is a short, personalized story written in a specific style and format. Carol Gray created social stories in the early 90s, and since this time, they have been widely used to explain the complexities of various social situations to children and adults with autism. The theoretical foundation behind social story interventions is the concept of theory of mind (ToM), which is thought to be a core difficulty area in autism. The social impairments displayed by individuals on the autism spectrum can be explained by difficulties with ToM concepts such as understanding the perspective of others, making social situations seem unpredictable and incomprehensible. Therefore, the first approach to teaching a specific behavior that is expected in a social situation is creating an understanding of the social situation. Based on this enhanced understanding, social skills can be acquired. Social stories serve this function by describing the social situation and different perspectives included, and providing answers to the questions what, when, where, and why.

A social story is written to provide information on what people in a given situation are doing, thinking or feeling, the sequence of events, the identification of significant social cues and their meaning, and the script of what to do or say in that situation.[44] They are carefully designed to be written within the comprehension level of the child and directed toward dealing with one particular context only in a positive and patient way. Simple line drawings are often included to aid visualization of expected behaviors and automatically reduce anxiety. Social stories can help in situations which the child finds distressing or frustrating, and where the behavior may be associated with a social misunderstanding. They can also be particularly useful in preparation for a new event or potentially stressful event (e.g., going to the dentist) or when faced with a change to their usual routine (e.g., having a supply teacher). Also, when a new concept or skill has been mastered the story can be adapted to become one that praises the child for their achievement. It is recommended that at least half of all social stories praise or congratulate the child in order to increase self-confidence and self-esteem. Social stories are considered an evidence-based intervention for individuals with ASD,[45] and they are frequently used by teachers and professionals.

Cognitive behavior approach and therapy: People with ASD may have difficulties with cognitive processing such as differences in executive functioning, cognitive inflexibility, weak central coherence, and impaired theory of mind. Since these cognitive impairments are suggested to be intricately interlinked, interventions that directly address cognition as well as behavior may offer the opportunity for generalized improvement in adaptive functioning.[46] Thus, cognitive behavioral approaches are being used successfully to modify children's impulsive behaviors, to teach them academically relevant tasks, as well as to improve problem solving, and self-control abilities. Many studies on CBA interventions for adults with ASD reported promising results and some reported generalization of treatment gains, specifically, reduction in social anxiety and in the avoidance of social situations. Along with the comorbid mental health conditions, cognitive behavioral approaches target social communication differences and emotional dysregulation. While using CBT with autistic people, it often requires adaptation, so that this is better personalized to the needs and preferences of autistic individuals; for example, to accommodate fundamental autism traits, and impairments commonly associated with autism, such as alexithymia (difficulty identifying own emotions), and difficulties with perspective-taking and emotion regulation.[47,48] Adaptations often include: providing more sessions than is standard and slowing down the pace of the sessions; scaffolding the emotion recognition and regulation skills; focusing on wider skills development (e.g., social skills interventions, problem-solving strategies, and assertiveness training); making abstract constructs more concrete and explicit; using visual means to provide information; using more concrete and didactic methods; using social stories to explain complex scenarios and expectations; associating emotions with tangible objects (e.g., making a scrapbook of relevant pictures, creating drawings of relevant thoughts and emotions etc.; increased emphasis on coping strategies that do not involve much abstract language; use of alternative communication modes; giving more opportunity to exert their agency in problem solving; and involving parents or caregivers as cotherapists.[49,50]

Key Learning Points

- *Adaptive behavior is crucial for independence:*
  - It encompasses everyday functioning in socialization, communication, self-care, and life skills.
  - It significantly impacts educational attainment and adult independence.
- *Understanding the "intention of behavior" is essential:*
  - Recent theories focus on the emotional aspects underlying behaviors.
  - Addressing anxiety related to unpredictability is vital for learning adaptive skills.
- *TEACCH:*
  - It aims to develop independence and self-esteem.
  - It utilizes visual strategies and predictability, catering to visual and routine-based learning styles.
  - It emphasizes understanding the "culture of autism."
  - It focuses on making environments understandable and predictable.
  - It uses key elements such as organization of the physical environment, visual information, task organization, and work systems.
  - Visual schedules and activity schedules are used to promote independence and reduce challenging behaviors.
- *Social stories help explain social situations:*
  - They address difficulties with ToM.
  - They provide information about social situations, perspectives, and expected behaviors.
  - They use a specific format and style, tailored to the individual's comprehension.
  - They can prepare individuals for new or stressful events and changes in routine.
  - They are considered an evidence-based intervention.

- *Cognitive behavioral approaches (CBA) and cognitive behavioral therapy (CBT) are effective:*
  - They address cognitive processing difficulties, such as executive functioning and cognitive inflexibility.
  - They modify impulsive behaviors, improve problem-solving, and enhance self-control.
  - They target social anxiety, emotional dysregulation, and comorbid mental health conditions.
- *CBT for ASD often requires adaptations, including:*
  - Increased session duration and slower pace
  - Scaffolding emotion recognition and regulation skills
  - Focus on wider skills development
  - Making abstract concepts concrete
  - Using visual aids and concrete methods
  - Using social stories
  - Associating emotions with tangible objects
  - Emphasis on concrete coping strategies
  - Use of alternative communication modes
  - Increased agency in problem solving
  - Involving parents or caregivers

Comorbid psychological disorders are common in the ASD population, with anxiety disorders affecting almost 30–80% of them. The high frequency of anxiety disorders among individuals with ASD indicates that anxiety could be a vital treatment focus for many children on the autism spectrum. CBT has been used successfully to improve anxiety symptoms in children and adults with autism. CBT is a short-term, therapeutic process that focuses on the interconnection of thoughts, feelings, and behavior. The core components of treatment protocols include psychoeducation, cognitive restructuring (i.e., identifying and challenging maladaptive thinking), mindfulness techniques, and graded exposure. Parent reported outcomes for anxiety in autistic youth showed CBT as an efficacious treatment. Some characteristics of CBT, such as its highly structured, pragmatic focus on current problems may align with features of ASD such as increased need for structure and order, while other aspects such as reliance on verbal communication with the therapist, insight in one's own thoughts, feeling and actions, and recognition of emotions in oneself and others, may prove challenging for some clients with ASD. Thus, it is important to know the person and then adapt the CBT process according to the person's need. The evidence suggests that CBT generally leads to a moderate decrease in anxiety and an improvement in well-being in autism,[51] but the approach can be very resource intense due to the need for a trained therapist. Coping with the uncertainties in daily life is another important issue that is often addressed by CBT as well through relaxation techniques and cognitive restructuring, by using visual aids such as social stories.

Mindfulness-based therapies (MBT) might offer a productive alternative to standard CBT. Mindfulness refers to the ability to focus on present moment experiences, including sensations and feelings, and to accept them without judgement or reaction. MBT might be particularly useful for managing anxiety in autism by targeting the type of sensory processing difficulties and difficulties introspecting on own emotions that play such an important role in this group. Initial evidence indicates that practicing mindfulness reduces anxiety in autistic adults.[52] Moreover, the work by researchers at City, University of London, shows that online-based self-help mindfulness tools are effective in reducing anxiety in autistic adults,[53] suggesting that this approach may be scalable and flexibly adapted to different settings.

Key Learning Points

- *High prevalence of comorbid anxiety:*
  - Anxiety disorders are very common in individuals with ASD, affecting a significant portion of the population (30–80%).
  - This high frequency necessitates anxiety being a key treatment focus.
- *CBT is effective:*
  - CBT has demonstrated success in reducing anxiety symptoms in both children and adults with ASD.

  - CBT focuses on the interplay of thoughts, feelings, and behaviors.
- *Core components include:*
  - Psychoeducation
  - Cognitive restructuring (challenging maladaptive thinking)
  - Mindfulness techniques

Supporting Learning Needs

Decades of research indicate that inclusive education leads to positive academic and social emotional outcomes for all students, with and without disabilities. Students with disabilities have been viewed as having a problem that makes it difficult to participate in the normal curriculum of schools. A special education approach is informed by beliefs that highlight the problem (the disability) as a deficiency in the person and requires "treatment". "The assumption that children and young people who experience disability may be better placed in a 'special' education setting and the acceptance of the parallel systems of segregated 'special' and 'mainstream' education" is an example of how unquestioned ableist beliefs "subconsciously guide our thoughts, actions and social systems, with considerable implications for the legislation, policy, and practice that is consequently accepted".[54] Special placement in segregated settings for children with disabilities has resulted in a marginalized population that has been institutionalized, undereducated, socially rejected, segregated, and excluded from society. These types of outcomes are not the result of the disability but are the result of the social, economic, and political actions such as special education. It is clear that the model of special education has a historical basis highly supported by the beliefs and assumptions of the medical-based paradigm.

Decades of research indicate that inclusive education leads to positive academic and social emotional outcomes for all students, with and without disabilities. With the emphasis now on moving forward to an inclusive approach, educators need a positive attitude and inclusive values to support school practice. A focus on inclusion in education is based on a commitment to key values such as equity, justice, ethical integrity, an acceptance and appreciation of neurodiversity, and the importance of contributing to and benefiting from a deeper understanding of other cultures.

There is clear evidence that students who have a disability and who are educated in mainstream settings with nondisabled peers demonstrate better academic and vocational outcomes when compared to students educated in segregated special settings.[54,55] Developing an inclusive curriculum that will be accessible for all learners, including students on the autism spectrum, is a focus of an inclusive approach to education. This requires teachers and specialists to work together to implement a flexible curriculum and training to meet students' needs. Teachers who rely on a rigid approach to the curriculum and assessment will find it difficult to include all students in their classrooms. Cologon[54] highlights the importance to be aware of "micro-exclusion", "where a student is present within a 'mainstream' setting, but is separated from the group and the curriculum, often through the provision of 'inclusion support' that (usually intentionally) isolates the student educationally, socially, and even physically". Moving toward inclusion will also require educators to address exclusion wherever it occurs in policy and practice.

Social role valorization (SRV) explains that people with disabilities have been subjected to a systematic and possibly lifelong pattern of such negative experiences such as being perceived as deviant, being identified by their disabilities, being casted into negative roles such as "eternal child", "ill", "burden", "subhuman"; and continuously being rejected by the society; being put and kept at a social or physical distance, the latter most commonly by segregation. We all want the good things in life, such as belongingness, opportunities for participation, growth and development, self-actualization, dignity, respect, acceptance, education, acknowledgement, love, and so on; and it is same for people with disabilities as well. But historically, they have been imposed with the rejection and wounds and "bad things of life". SRV says that people are much more likely to experience the "good things in life" if they hold valued social roles than they do not. Thus, it is important to enhance the perceived value of the social roles of a person, a group, or an entire class of people, and doing so is called SRV. There are two major broad strategies for pursuing this goal for (devalued) people: (a) enhancement of people's social image in the Eyes of others, and (b) enhancement of their competencies, in the widest sense of the term. Image and competency form a feedback loop that can be both negative and positive. That is, a person who is competency-impaired is highly at risk of suffering image-impairment; a person who is impaired in image is pertinent to be responded to by others in ways that delimit or reduce the person's competency. But both processes work equally in the reverse direction as well. That is, a person whose social image is positive is apt to be provided with experiences, expectancies, and other life conditions which are likely to increase, or give scope to, his/her competencies; and a person who displays competencies is also apt to be imaged positively. And this social integration can happen when seeing the people with disabilities doing the typical things at typical places with typical people in typical ways as much as possible.

Thus, the valued role of a "learner" can bring in so many good things in an individual's life: belongingness, acceptance from other learners, dignity, opportunities to learn and grow and so on. To be in this role, everyone in the person's life needs to work on the competency enhancement of the person, by providing structured environment and other educational support but in as typical way as possible; so that the "micro-exclusion" can be avoided. These micro exclusions often build assumptions and negative role expectancies from the person leading to segregation in classrooms. SRV ideas work as a foundation, as a unifying theory of practice and every practice be it early intervention, inclusive education, employment, or residential services—all build on this foundation.

Key Learning Points

- *Inclusive education benefits all:*
  - Decades of research show inclusive education leads to positive academic and social-emotional outcomes for all students, regardless of disability.
  - It challenges the medical model's focus on disability as a "deficiency."
- *Challenging ableist beliefs:*
  - Segregated "special" education systems perpetuate marginalization, undereducation, and social rejection.
  - These negative outcomes are often a result of social, economic, and political actions, not the disability itself.
  - It is vital to challenge the subconscious ableist beliefs that guide social systems.
- *Values of inclusive education:*
  - Inclusive education is grounded in values such as equity, justice, ethical integrity, acceptance of neurodiversity, and intercultural understanding.
- *Benefits of mainstream settings:*
  - Students with disabilities educated in mainstream settings with nondisabled peers demonstrate better academic and vocational outcomes.
- *Inclusive curriculum and practices:*
  - Developing an accessible curriculum requires collaboration between teachers and specialists.
  - Flexible curriculum and training are crucial to meet diverse student needs.
  - Rigid curriculum and assessment approaches hinder inclusion.
- *Addressing micro-exclusion:*
  - "Micro-exclusion" (physical presence but social and educational isolation) must be addressed.
  - Educators must actively work to eliminate exclusion in all policies and practices.

- *SRV:*
  - SRV addresses the historical and ongoing devaluation of people with disabilities.
  - People with disabilities have often been subjected to negative experiences and roles.
  - SRV aims to enhance the perceived value of their social roles.
- *Strategies include:*
  - Enhancing social image.
  - Enhancing competencies.
- Social integration happens when people with disabilities are seen doing typical things, in typical places, with typical people, in typical ways.
- *The valued role of "learner":*
  - The role of "learner" brings belonging, acceptance, dignity, and opportunities for growth.
  - Competency enhancement through structured environments and educational support is essential.
- *SRV as a foundation:*
  - SRV provides a unifying theory of practice applicable to early intervention, inclusive education, employment, and residential services.

Analyzing the Barriers to Learning

When it comes to the child learning, there can be multifactorial aspects that can act as hindrance for the child's learning. Recognizing and providing support will need a holistic approach to understand the child and his or her needs first. Facilitating the child's learning may involve all or some of the above-mentioned intervention techniques such as structured teaching, AAC, social stories, cognitive behavioral approaches, and so on. But it is important to understand what is needed for the child to learn better. Asking the question "who is the person and what is the pressing need" should act like a guiding star to plan the intervention strategies. And having one focus person who understands the individual well can coordinate with other therapists and educators and work together.

Other Modalities of Treatment

Apart from the prior mentioned intervention techniques, there are a few more therapies which are showing promising results. Here, occupational therapy (OT) and sensory integration therapy (SIT) will be discussed briefly.

Occupational Therapy and Sensory Integration Therapy

In addition to the primary features, individuals with autism generally have sensory processing and sensory integration dysfunction, which affect adaptive behavior and participating daily activities. Many children with autism are unable to register many of the sensations from their environment. They struggle to integrate those sensations to form a clear perception of space. Atypical sensory registration and orientation can interfere with the processes of inhibition and facilitation in sensory systems. Some self-stimulatory behavior is the expression of a sensory need in children with autism. This sensory processing difficulty may be associated with challenging behavior such as aggression (e.g., to communicate discomfort with noise/touch), or additional "safe space" needs in the home. As far as motor functions are concerned, motor impairments have been reported in children with autism. The studies show that problems are observed in coordination, posture and balance control, locomotion, and motor preparation in individuals with autism. Sensory processing difficulties also pose significant challenges in main-stream education settings. Thus, interventions targeting sensory processing difficulties could result in development across behavioral, social, and educational aspects.

Occupational therapy has become an integral component of comprehensive interventions for children on the autism spectrum.[56] Occupational therapists enable individuals and communities to participate in daily life activities through engagement in occupations relevant to them, or by modifying the occupation or environment. OT interventions primarily address family-centered goals, including functional skills, performance and participation in activities of daily living, and quality of life. As with most complex rehabilitation interventions with heterogenous clinical conditions, therapists in pediatric OT for children on the autism spectrum often use a wide variety of treatment components and pieces of approaches rather than systematic whole interventions.[57,58] There are some commonly used OT interventions for autism such as sensory integration and sensory-based therapy, interactive relationship-based therapy, developmental skill-based therapy, etc.

Sensory integration therapy is a clinic-based approach that focuses on the therapist-child relationship and uses play-based sensory motor activities designed to improve sensation processing and integration. SIT aims to improve sensory processing abilities through structured sensory experiences, leveraging the brain's neuroplasticity to promote adaptive responses to sensory stimuli. SIT shows some potential as an effective therapy, but supporting evidence is limited. Ideally, the specific set of activities implemented in SIT is based upon an assessment of a child's sensory profile and follows the essential components of SIT described by Parham.[59] Specifically, SIT should involve: (a) Child safety; (b) opportunities to obtain tactile, vestibular, and/or proprioceptive sensory stimulation to support self-regulation, sensory awareness, or movement; (c) appropriate levels of participant alertness; (d) challenge to postural, ocular, oral, or bilateral motor control; (e) novel motor behaviors and efforts to organize movements in time and space; (f) preferences in the choice of activities and materials; (g) activities that are not too easy or too difficult; (h) activities in which the participant experiences success; (i) support for intrinsic desire to play; and (j) a therapeutic reliance. Though the results of various systematic reviews were that SIT had no consistently positive effect as a treatment for children with ASD. Given the lack of scientific evidence, it would seem alarming how often SIT is reported delivered to individuals with ASD.

These are the most commonly used and evidence-based intervention techniques for individuals with ASD. There are some more emerging practices coming up in this field which have a long way to go to prove their effectiveness. But it is very important to acknowledge that sometimes an autistic person's life revolves around different therapies, and he is casted into the role of "forever ill" or "forever diseased". Thus, when leisure activities such as music, dance, or horse riding take the form of therapy, then the person's life gets medicalized and is seen as a "client" of the medical system rather than an individual. Providing support and interventions to autistic individuals are very important, but equally important it is to understand them and that they have larger identity than being autistics.

Tarun Matthew Paul, a nonspeaking autistic young adult from Kochi, and a passionate self-advocate writes, *"Freedom to really just be me, that I value a lot. I like to be accepted as more than my autism and not be only included just for keeping up appearances."* This gives us a lot to think over.

Key Learning Points

Learning support:
- *Multifactorial hindrances:*
  - Learning difficulties in children with ASD can stem from various factors.
  - A holistic approach is essential to understand individual needs.
- *Tailored interventions:*
  - Intervention strategies such as structured teaching, AAC, social stories, and CBT should be selected based on individual needs.
  - The guiding principle should be "who is the person and what's the pressing need?"
- *Coordinated effort:*
  - A designated person should coordinate with therapists and educators for a unified approach.

OT and SIT:

- *Sensory processing issues:*
  - Individuals with ASD often experience sensory processing and integration dysfunction.
  - This can impact adaptive behavior and daily activities.
  - It can also impact motor skills and cause challenging behaviors.
- *OT's Role:*
  - OT helps individuals participate in daily life activities.
  - It addresses family-centered goals, including functional skills and quality of life.
  - OT interventions include sensory integration, relationship-based, and developmental skill-based therapies.
- *SIT's focus:*
  - SIT is a clinic-based approach that uses play-based sensory-motor activities.
  - It aims to improve sensory processing through structured sensory experiences.
  - The effectiveness of SIT is debated, and the supporting evidence is limited.
  - Proper SIT should follow the components described by Parham, including child safety and appropriate sensory stimulation.
  - Although SIT is widely used, evidence of its effectiveness is limited.
- *Motor impairments:*
  - Motor impairments are common in ASD, impacting coordination, posture, and balance.

Holistic understanding and considerations:

- *Medicalization of life:*
  - Excessive focus on therapies can medicalize an individual's life, reducing them to a "client" rather than a person.
  - Leisure activities should not always be turned into therapy.
- *Beyond autism:*
  - It is crucial to recognize individuals with ASD as having a broader identity than their diagnosis.
  - Acceptance of the person, outside of their diagnosis, is essential.
- *Self-advocacy:*
  - Self-advocates emphasize the importance of being accepted for who they are, not just for their autism.
  - Freedom to be oneself is highly valued.

Adult and Long-term Outcomes of Children with Autism Spectrum Conditions

The long-term trajectory for individuals with ASD varies widely and is extremely heterogenous due to the spectrum nature of the condition. It is influenced by factors such as intellectual ability, availability of early intervention, and societal support.

Early studies, such as those by Kanner in the 1940s, suggested poor prognoses, with many individuals institutionalized.[60] However, contemporary research indicates a broader range of outcomes, from severe dependency to substantial independence. A meta-analysis of longitudinal studies estimates that approximately 20% of adults with ASC achieve a "good" outcome—living independently, employed, and socially engaged—while 26.6% achieve a "fair" outcome with partial independence, and 49.3% experience a "poor" outcome marked by dependency and isolation.[61] These figures vary based on study definitions, sample characteristics, and support availability, but they highlight the spectrum of possibilities.

The key predictors of adult outcomes are:

- Intellectual ability, often measured by IQ, is a strong indicator, with higher IQ (above 70) linked to better employment and independence prospects.[62]
- Early language development is equally critical; children who acquire functional speech by age 5 or 6 tend to have improved social and vocational outcomes.[63] A longitudinal study found that childhood IQ and communication skills were significant predictors of adult adaptive functioning.[64]

Therefore, early intervention is crucial, keeping in mind the neuroplasticity of the brain decreases as age advances.

Social and environmental support also plays a key role. Higher maternal education and socioeconomic status often correlate with better outcomes, likely due to increased advocacy and resource access.[65] Conversely, lack of support can exacerbate challenges, increasing the likelihood of poor outcomes.[66]

Domains of Adult Life

Independent living: Achieving independent living is a key marker of success, yet fewer than half of adults with ASD accomplish this.[67] Adaptive skills, such as managing daily tasks, and the absence of ID improve the likelihood of independence. In India, most adults reside with family in the absence supported settings, which are commoner in some countries.[68]

Employment: Employment rates remain low, with estimates suggesting only 20–40% of autistic adults are employed, often in low-skill or part-time roles.[69] Individuals with higher cognitive abilities or specific talents (e.g., in technology) may secure competitive jobs, though social difficulties can impede success.[70] There are many vocational programs which show promise but face systemic barriers such as employer biases. In India, Keystone Foundation has started pioneering work in this domain of meaningful employment, although it is a small, very resource-intensive initiative.

Social relationships: Social integration is challenging, with many adults experiencing isolation. Childhood social impairment often predicts adult outcomes, though social skills training can help.[71] Individuals with milder symptoms report more success in forming relationships, although often distinct from neurotypical patterns.[72]

Mental health: Psychiatric comorbidities are common, and they further complicate outcomes. Most often they emerge in adolescence due to social pressures or unmet needs.[73] Access to autism friendly mental health services in India remains limited, exacerbating these challenges.

Quality of life: Well-being varies widely. Adults with independence and employment report higher satisfaction, though sensory issues and mental health challenges can detract from this.[74] For those with poor outcomes, quality of life is often diminished by dependency and isolation.[66]

Challenges and Barriers

One of the key challenges all over the world, including our country, is the transition to adulthood. It is fraught with obstacles. The "services cliff" at age 18 or 21, where educational and pediatric supports end, often disrupts progress.[75] Social misunderstandings can also lead to legal or interpersonal vulnerabilities, particularly for those undiagnosed or unsupported.[76] In the experience of the authors, many persons do come for assessments because of their inappropriate sexual or socially embarrassing behavior, only to be found out as having yet undiagnosed ASD.

Key Learning Points

- *Historical perspective:* Early studies (e.g., Kanner, 1940s) predicted poor outcomes, often institutionalization, but modern research shows more diverse possibilities.
- *Wide variability:* Outcomes for individuals with ASD vary greatly due to the condition's spectrum nature, ranging from severe dependency to substantial independence.
- *Influencing factors:* Intellectual ability, early intervention, and societal support heavily shape long-term outcomes.
- *Outcome statistics:* About 20% of adults with ASD achieve a "good" outcome (independent, employed, and socially engaged), 26.6% a "fair" outcome (partial independence), and 49.3% a "poor" outcome (dependency and isolation).
- *Key predictors:* Higher IQ (above 70) and early language development (by age 5–6) strongly predict better employment, independence, and social outcomes.

- *Early intervention:* Critical due to brain neuroplasticity, which decreases with age, making timely support essential.
- *Social support:* Higher maternal education and socioeconomic status improve outcomes by enhancing advocacy and resource access; lack of support worsens challenges.
- *Independent living:* Fewer than half of adults with ASD live independently; adaptive skills and no ID increase success, though many in India rely on family due to limited supported settings.
- *Employment:* Only 20–40% of autistic adults are employed, often in low-skill jobs; higher cognitive abilities help, but social barriers and employer biases persist.
- *Social relationships:* Social integration is tough, with isolation common; early social skills training and milder symptoms improve relationship success.
- *Mental health:* Psychiatric issues often arise in adolescence, worsened by limited autism-friendly services in places such as India.
- *Quality of life:* Independence and employment boost well-being, but sensory issues, mental health, and dependency can lower it for those with poor outcomes.

Practice point: A routine question which all clinicians will face from the carers is regarding the long-term outcome. It is obvious that there cannot be a one-size-fits-all kind of response. It is important to be sensitive, honest, and maintain hope. Focus should be on short-term gains in the beginning and give parents to come to terms with the diagnosis. Caution needs to be exercised against information overload regarding outcome and clinicians need to handhold carers during the first 1–2 years after a diagnosis is made. In the experience of the authors, most parents gradually figure out the journey ahead and may revisit the question regarding outcome and "what after us". It is always useful to direct them toward resources on the internet on guardianship, local support group and provide information regarding any new developments in the local areas or new government initiatives.

Psychiatric and Neurodevelopmental Comorbidities

In our opinion, the most challenging part of working with persons with ASD lies in teasing out the comorbidities and how they impact on clinical presentation. It is here, in this domain, the skill of the clinician is tested.

Presentation of ASD across the lifespan is far from uniform, with significant complexities arising from co-occurring psychiatric and neurodevelopmental comorbidities. These additional conditions influence symptom expression, functional outcomes, and intervention needs, making ASD a challenging condition to understand. Factors such as age, sex, intellectual ability, and the presence of comorbidities such as anxiety, depression, ADHD, epilepsy, and ID contribute to this variability.

In addition, the pathoplastic effect of environmental influences and frequent abuse, which many such persons face, makes the expression of the condition even more complex.

In early childhood, ASD often presents with core symptoms alongside developmental delays. However, comorbidities such as ADHD and anxiety can emerge, complicating the clinical picture. Lai et al.[77] highlight that up to 70% of children with ASD have at least one co-occurring psychiatric condition, with ADHD affecting 30–50% and anxiety disorders impacting 40%. These comorbidities can mask or exacerbate autism traits; for instance, hyperactivity may overshadow social deficits, delaying diagnosis. Neurodevelopmental issues such as epilepsy, present in 20–30% of cases, further diversify presentation, particularly when seizures start in toddlerhood, altering behavioral trajectories.[78]

As individuals with ASD transition into adolescence, psychiatric comorbidities often intensify. Puberty introduces greater self-awareness that can amplify anxiety and depression. OCD can emerge at any age. Simonoff et al.[73] found that 60% of adolescents with ASD experience clinically significant psychiatric symptoms, with mood disorders rising sharply. For those with co-occurring ID (affecting 30–50% of the ASD population), communication barriers heighten frustration, potentially manifesting as aggression or self-injury—behaviors often misattributed to autism alone. Neurodevelopmental comorbidities such as epilepsy may persist or worsen, with seizure frequency correlating with cognitive decline in some cases.[78] Sex differences also emerge: females with ASD are more likely to internalize symptoms (e.g., anxiety), while males may externalize (e.g., aggression), complicating identification and support.[77]

In adulthood, the presentation of ASD becomes even more intricate as societal expectations increase. Psychiatric conditions such as depression and schizophrenia spectrum disorders rise, with prevalence estimates of 20–30% for depression in autistic adults.[79] Chronic stress from social demands and unmet support needs often fuels these issues. For individuals without ID, "masking" of autistic traits—deliberately suppressing behaviors to fit in—can lead to burnout and delayed mental health diagnoses. Conversely, those with severe ID and epilepsy may face progressive functional decline, with comorbidities overshadowing autism itself. Neurodevelopmental trajectories diverge further; some adults develop late-onset epilepsy, while others stabilize, reflecting the unpredictable course of these co-occurring conditions.

The heterogeneity of ASD across the lifespan stems from the bidirectional influence of comorbidities. Psychiatric conditions can amplify autism traits (e.g., anxiety worsening social withdrawal), while autism's core deficits may predispose individuals to mental health challenges (e.g., communication struggles fostering isolation).

Eating disorders and gender dysphoria too are common in this population, which needs sensitive and respectful management.

Research consistently shows that comorbidity profiles evolve with age, necessitating longitudinal monitoring.[73]

Key Learning Points

- *Complexity of ASD:* The presentation of ASD varies significantly across the lifespan due to co-occurring psychiatric and neurodevelopmental comorbidities, making it challenging to diagnose and manage.
- *Prevalence of comorbidities:* Up to 70% of children with ASD have at least one co-occurring psychiatric condition, with ADHD and anxiety being particularly common.
- *ADHD in ASD:* ADHD affects 30–50% of children with ASD, often complicating the clinical picture by masking or exacerbating autism traits, especially when the child is very young.
- *Anxiety disorders:* Anxiety disorders impact about 40% of children and adults with ASD, potentially leading to increased symptom severity and psychosocial impairments.
- *Epilepsy:* Neurodevelopmental issues such as epilepsy are present in 20–30% of ASD cases, affecting behavioral trajectories, especially if seizures begin in early childhood.
- *ID:* ID affects 30–50% of the ASD population, complicating communication, and potentially leading to misattributed behaviors such as aggression or self-injury.
- *Adolescence:* During adolescence, psychiatric comorbidities intensify, with mood disorders rising sharply, and sex differences in symptom expression becoming more apparent.
- *Sex differences:* Females with ASD tend to internalize symptoms (e.g., anxiety), while males may externalize them (e.g., aggression), complicating diagnosis and support.
- *Adulthood:* In adulthood, psychiatric conditions such as depression and schizophrenia become more prevalent, with chronic stress from unmet support needs contributing to these issues. Transition from adolescence to adulthood is especially difficult period due to loss of support systems.
- *Masking in adulthood:* Autistic adults without ID may "mask" their traits, leading to delayed mental health diagnoses and burnout.

- *Eating disorders and gender dysphoria:* These conditions are more common than what we expect in ASD populations and require sensitive management.
- *Longitudinal monitoring:* Comorbidity profiles evolve with age, necessitating ongoing monitoring to provide appropriate support across the lifespan.

SUMMARY AND CONCLUSION

In our opinion, the dictum that "if you have seen one person with autism, you have seen 1 person with autism", as no 2 presentations are the same. In this chapter, the authors have tried to highlight some of the nuances of this truly fascinating human condition rather than present everything one needs to know about ASD, which can be found in any standard textbook.

REFERENCES

1. Taylor MJ, Rosenqvist MA, Larsson H, Gillberg C, D'Onofrio BM, Lichtenstein P, et al. Etiology of autism spectrum disorders and autistic traits over time. JAMA Psychiatry. 2020;77(9):936-43.
2. GBD 2019 Mental Disorders Collaborators. Global, regional, and national burden of 12 mental disorders in 204 countries and territories, 1990-2019: A systematic analysis for the Global Burden of Disease Study 2019. Lancet Psychiatry. 2022;9(2):137-50.
3. Zeidan J, Fombonne E, Scorah J, Ibrahim A, Durkin MS, Saxena S, et al. Global prevalence of autism: A systematic review update. Autism Res. 2022;15(5):778-90.
4. Hallmayer J, Cleveland S, Torres A, Phillips J, Cohen B, Torigoe T, et al. Genetic heritability and shared environmental factors among twin pairs with autism. Arch Gen Psychiatr. 2011;68(11):1095-102.
5. Russell G, Stapley S, Newlove-Delgado T, Salmon A, White R, Warren F, et al. Time trends in autism diagnosis over 20 years: A UK population-based cohort study. J Child Psychol Psychiatr. 2022;63(6):674-82.
6. Rahman MM, Carter SA, Lin JC, Chow T, Yu X, Martinez MP, et al. Associations of autism spectrum disorder with PM2.5 components: A comparative study using two different exposure models. Environ Sci Technol. 2023;57(1):405-14.
7. Polyak A, Kubina RM, Girirajan S. Comorbidity of intellectual disability confounds ascertainment of autism: Implications for genetic diagnosis. Am J Med Gene Part B: Neuropsychiatr Gen. 2015;168(7):600-8.
8. Hyman SL, Levy SE, Myers SM. Identification, evaluation, and management of children with autism spectrum disorder. Pediatrics. 2020;145(1):e20193447.
9. Jones L, Bellis MA, Wood S, Hughes K, McCoy E, Eckley L, et al. Prevalence and risk of violence against children with disabilities: A systematic review and meta-analysis of observational studies. Lancet. 2012;380(9845):899-907.
10. Tick B, Bolton P, Happé F, Rutter M, Rijsdijk F. Heritability of autism spectrum disorders: a meta-analysis of twin studies. J Child Psychol Psychiatry. 2016;57(5):585-95.
11. Satterstrom FK, Kosmicki JA, Wang J, Breen MS, De Rubeis S, An JY, et al. Large-scale exome sequencing study of autism. Cell. 2020;180(3):568-84.
12. Bernier R, Golzio C, Xiong B, Stessman HA, Coe BP, Penn O, et al. Disruptive CHD8 mutations define a subtype of autism early in development. Cell. 2014:158(2);263-76.
13. Platt RJ, Zhou Y, Slaymaker IM, Shetty AS, Weisbach NR, Kim JA, et al. Chd8 mutation leads to autistic-like behaviors and impaired striatal circuits. Cell Reports. 2017;19(2):335-50.
14. Shen MD. Cerebrospinal fluid and the early brain development of autism. J Neurodevelop Disord. 2018;10:39.
15. Grove J, Ripke S, Als TD, Mattheisen M, Walters RK, Won H, et al. Identification of common genetic risk variants for autism spectrum disorder. Nat Genet. 2019;51(3):431-44.
16. Weiner DJ, Liu L, Webb BT, Kajiwara Y, Kelsoe JR, Owen MJ, et al. The contributions of rare inherited and polygenic risk to ASD in multiplex families. Proc Natl Acad Sci U S A. 2023;120(31):e2215632120.
17. Lee PH, Feng YCA, Smoller JW. Pleiotropy and cross-disorder genetics among psychiatric disorders. Biological Psychiatry. 2021;89(1):20-31.

18. Jutla A, Foss-Feig J, Veenstra-VanderWeele J. Autism spectrum disorder and schizophrenia: An updated conceptual review. Aut Res. 2022;15(3): 384-412.
19. Sullivan PF, Magnusson C, Reichenberg A, Boman M, Dalman C, Davidson M, et al. Family history of schizophrenia and bipolar disorder as risk factors for autism. Arch Gen Psychiatry. 2012;69(11):1099-103.
20. Sestan N, State MW. Lost in translation: Traversing the complex path from genomics to therapeutics in autism spectrum disorder. Neuron. 2018;100(2): 406-23.
21. Gockley J, Willsey AJ, Dong S, Dougherty JD, Constantino JN, Sanders SJ. The female protective effect in autism spectrum disorder is not mediated by a single genetic locus. Molecular Autism. 2015; 6:25.
22. Werling DM, Brand H, An JY, Stone MR, Zhu L, Glessner JT, et al. An analytical framework for whole-genome sequence association studies and its implications for autism spectrum disorder. Nat Genet. 2018;50(5):727-36.
23. Modabbernia A, Velthorst E, Reichenberg A. Environmental risk factors for autism: An evidence-based review of systematic reviews and meta-analyses. Mol Autism. 2017;8:13.
24. Ziegler A, Rudolph-Rothfeld W, Vonthein R. Genetic testing for autism spectrum disorder is lacking evidence of cost-effectiveness: A systematic review. Methods Inf Med. 2017;56(3): 268-73.
25. Centers for Disease Control and Prevention. (2023). Autism spectrum disorder (ASD) data and statistics. [online] Available from https://www.cdc.gov/ncbddd/autism/data.html [Last accessed November, 2025].
26. Ozonoff S, Young GS, Carter A, Messinger D, Yirmiya N, Zwaigenbaum L, et al. Recurrence risk for autism spectrum disorders: A Baby Siblings Research Consortium study. Pediatrics. 2011; 128(3):e488-95.
27. Loomes R, Hull L, Mandy WPL. What is the male-to-female ratio in autism spectrum disorder? J Am Acad Child Adolesc Psychiatry. 2017;56(6):466-74.
28. Sandin S, Lichtenstein P, Kuja-Halkola R, Larsson H, Hultman CM, Reichenberg A, et al. The familial risk of autism. JAMA. 2014;311(17):1770-7.
29. Baio J, Wiggins L, Christensen DL, Maenner MJ, Daniels J, Warren Z, et al. Prevalence of autism spectrum disorder among children aged 8 years. MMWR Surveill Summ. 2018;67(6):1-23.
30. Wigdor EM, Weiner DJ, Grove J, Fu JM, Thompson WK, Carey CE, et al. The impact of rare protein coding variants on complex traits in autism spectrum disorder. Cell Genom. 2022;2(6):100134.
31. Sucksmith E, Roth I, Hoekstra RA. Autistic traits below the clinical threshold: re-examining the broader autism phenotype in the 21st century. J Autism Devel Dis. 2011;41(5):589-96.
32. Madden JM, Lakoma MD, Lynch FL, Rusinak D, Owen-Smith AA, Coleman KJ, et al. Psychotropic medication use among insured children with autism spectrum disorder. J Autism Dev Disord. 2017;47(1):144-54.
33. Schuck RK, Tagavi DM, Baiden KM P, Tagavi DM, Baiden KMP, Dwyer P, Williams ZJ, Osuna A, et al. Neurodiversity and autism intervention: Reconciling perspectives through a naturalistic developmental behavioral intervention framework. J Autism Dev Disord. 2022;52(10): 4625-45.
34. Wang M, Schuck R, Baiden KM. Naturalistic developmental behavioral interventions as value-based and culturally adapted EBPs for autistic individuals. In: Carotenuto M. Autism Spectrum Disorders—Recent Advances and New Perspectives. Intech Open; 2022.
35. Veneziano J, Shea S. They have a voice; are we listening? Behav Anal Pract. 2023;16(1):127-44.
36. Reichow B, Hume K, Barton EE, Boyd BA. Early intensive behavioral intervention (EIBI) for young children with autism spectrum disorders (ASD). Cochrane Database Systematic Rev. 2018;5(5):CD009260.
37. Granpeesheh D, Tarbox J, Dixon DR. Applied behavior analytic interventions for children with autism: A description and review of treatment research. Annals Clin Psychiatry. 2009;21(3): 162-73.
38. Sandbank M, Bottema-Beutel K, Crowley S, Cassidy M, Dunham K, Feldman JI, et al. Project AIM: Autism intervention meta-analysis for studies of young children. Psychol Bull. 2020; 146(1):1-29.

39. Stahmer AC, Collings NM, Palinkas LA. Early intervention practices for children with autism: Descriptions from community providers. Focus Autism Other Dev Disabil. 2005;20(2):66-79.
40. Farley MA, McMahon WM, Fombonne E, Jenson WR, Miller J, Gardner M, et al. Twenty-year outcome for individuals with autism and average or near-average cognitive abilities. Autism Res. 2009;2(2):109-18.
41. De Bildt A, Sytema S, Kraijer D, Sparrow S, Minderaa R. Adaptive functioning and behaviour problems in relation to level of education in children and adolescents with intellectual disability. J Intellect Disabil Res. 2005;49(9): 672-81.
42. Paul R, Miles S, Cicchetti D, Sparrow S, Klin A, Volkmar F, et al. Adaptive behavior in autism and pervasive developmental disorder-not otherwise specified: Microanalysis of scores on the Vineland adaptive behavior scales. J Autism Dev Disord. 2004;34(2):223-8.
43. Mesibov G, Shea V, Schopler E. The TEACCH Approach to Autism Spectrum Disorders. Springer; 2005.
44. Sansosti FJ, Powell-Smith KA, Kincaid D. A research synthesis of social story interventions for children with autism spectrum disorders. Focus Autism Other Dev Disabil. 2004;19(4):194-204.
45. National Autism Center. Findings and conclusions: National standards project, phase 2. Addressing the need for evidence-based practice guidelines for autism spectrum disorder. National Autism Center; 2015.
46. Klinger LG, Williams A. Cognitive-behavioral interventions for students with autism spectrum disorders. In Mayer MJ, Lochman JE, Van Acker R (Eds). Cognitive-Behavioral Interventions for Emotional and Behavioral Disorders: School-based Practice. Guilford Press; 2009. pp. 328-62.
47. Gaus VL. Cognitive-Behavioral Therapy for Adults with Autism Spectrum Disorder. Guilford Publications; 2018.
48. Stark E, Ali D, Ayre A, Schneider N, Parveen S, Marais K, et al. (2021). Psychological therapy for autistic adults: A curious approach to making adaptations. Authentistic UK. [online] Available from https://www.authentistic.uk/ [Last accessed November, 2025].
49. Kerns CM, Roux AM, Connell JE, Shattuck PT. Adapting cognitive behavioral techniques to address anxiety and depression in cognitively able emerging adults on the autism spectrum. Cognit Behav Pract. 2016;23(3):329-40.
50. Spain D, Happé F. How to optimise cognitive behaviour therapy (CBT) for people with autism spectrum disorders (ASD): A Delphi study. J Rational-Emotive Cognit-Behav Ther. 2020; 38(2):184-208.
51. Lang R, Regester A, Lauderdale S, Ashbaugh K, Haring A. Treatment of anxiety in autism spectrum disorders using cognitive behaviour therapy: A systematic review. Dev Neurorehabil. 2010;13(1):53-63.
52. Kiep M, Spek AA, Hoeben L. Mindfulness-based therapy in adults with an autism spectrum disorder: Do treatment effects last? Mindfulness. 2015;6(3):637-44.
53. Gaigg SB, Cornell ASF, Bird G. The psychophysiological mechanisms of alexithymia in autism spectrum disorder. Autism. 2018;22(2): 227-31.
54. Cologon K. Towards inclusive education: A necessary process of transformation. Children and Young People with Disability Australia; 2019.
55. Hehir T, Grindal T, Freeman B, Lamoreau R, Borquaye Y, Burke S. A summary of the evidence on inclusive education. Alana Institute; 2016.
56. Monz BU, Houghton R, Law K, Loss G. Treatment patterns in children with autism in the United States. Autism Res. 2019;12(4):517-26.
57. Van Stan JH, Whyte J, Duffy JR, Barkmeier-Kraemer JM, Doyle PB, Gherson S, et al. Rehabilitation Treatment Specification System: Methodology to identify and describe unique targets and ingredients. Arch Phys Med Rehabil. 2021;102(3):521-31.
58. Watling R, Daughton N. Current practices in OT for autistic clients: Alignment with evidence-based practice & practice guidelines. Am J Occup Ther. 2023;77(Suppl. 2):7711510337.
59. Parham LD, Roley SS, May-Benson TA, Koomar J, Brett-Green B, Burke JP, et al. Development of a fidelity measure for research on the effectiveness of the Ayres sensory integration intervention. Am J Occup Therapy. 2011;65(2):133-42.

60. Kanner L. Follow-up study of eleven autistic children originally reported in 1943. J Autism Child Schizophr. 1971;1(2):119-45.
61. Mason D, McConachie H, Garland D, Capp SJ, Stewart GR, Kempton MJ, Glaser K, Howlin P, et al. A meta-analysis of outcome studies of autistic adults: Quantifying effect size, quality, and meta-regression. J Autism Dev Disord. 2021;51(9): j3165-79.
62. Howlin P, Goode S, Hutton J, Rutter M. Adult outcome for children with autism. J Child Psychol Psychiatry. 2004;45(2):212-29.
63. Pickles A, McCauley JB, Pepa LA, Huerta M, Lord C. The adult outcome of children referred for autism: Typology and prediction from childhood. J Child Psychol Psychiatry. 2020;61(7):760-7.
64. Magiati I, Tay XW, Howlin P. Cognitive, language, social and behavioural outcomes in adults with autism spectrum disorders: A systematic review of longitudinal follow-up studies in adulthood. Clin Psychol Rev. 2014;34(1):73-86.
65. Fountain C, Winter AS, Bearman PS. Six developmental trajectories characterize children with autism. Pediatrics. 2012;129(5):e1112-20.
66. Billstedt E, Gillberg IC, Gillberg C. Aspects of quality of life in adults diagnosed with autism in childhood: A population-based study. Autism. 2011;15(1):7-20.
67. Henninger NA, Taylor JL. Outcomes in adults with autism spectrum disorders: A historical perspective. Autism. 2013;17(1):103-16.
68. Howlin P, Moss P. Adults with autism spectrum disorders. Canad J Psychiatr. 2012;57(5):275-83.
69. Roux AM, Shattuck PT, Cooper BP, Anderson KA, Wagner M, Narendorf SC. Postsecondary employment experiences among young adults with an autism spectrum disorder. J Am Acad Child Adolesc Psychiatry. 2013;52(9):931-9.
70. Lord C, McCauley JB, Pepa LA, Huerta M, Pickles A. Work, living, and the pursuit of happiness: Vocational and psychosocial outcomes for young adults with autism. Autism. 2020;24(7):1691-703.
71. Orsmond GI, Shattuck PT, Cooper BP, Sterzing PR, Anderson KA. Social participation among young adults with an autism spectrum disorder. J Autism Dev Disord. 2013;43(11):2710-9.
72. Howlin P, Moss P, Savage S, Rutter M. Social outcomes in mid- to later adulthood among individuals diagnosed with autism and average nonverbal IQ as children. J Am Acad Child Adolesc Psychiatry. 2013;52(6):572-81.
73. Simonoff E, Jones CRG, Baird G, Pickles A, Happé F, Charman T. The persistence and stability of psychiatric problems in adolescents with autism spectrum disorders. J Child Psychol Psychiatry. 2013;54(2):186-94.
74. Totsika V, Felce D, Kerr M, Hastings RP. Behavior problems, psychiatric symptoms, and quality of life for older adults with intellectual disability with and without autism. J Autism Dev Disord. 2010;40(9):1171-8.
75. Shattuck PT, Narendorf SC, Cooper B, Sterzing PR, Wagner M, Taylor JL. Postsecondary education and employment among youth with an autism spectrum disorder. Pediatrics. 2012;129(6): 1042-9.
76. Rava J, Shattuck P, Rast J, Roux A. The role of gender, age, and parental attachment in the adult transition experiences of young adults with autism. Autism. 2017;21(3):287-97.
77. Lai MC, Kassee C, Besney R, Bonato S, Hull L, Mandy W, et al. Prevalence of co-occurring mental health diagnoses in the autism population: A systematic review and meta-analysis. Lancet Psychiatry. 2019;6(10):819-29.
78. Hollocks MJ, Lerh JW, Magiati I, Meiser-Stedman R, Brugha TS, et al. Anxiety and depression in adults with autism spectrum disorder: A systematic review and meta-analysis. Psychol Med. 2019;49(4);559-72.
79. Croen LA, Zerbo O, Qian Y, Massolo ML, Rich S, Sidney S, et al. The health status of adults on the autism spectrum. Autism. 2015;19(7):814-23.

CHAPTER 9

Attention Deficit Hyperactivity Disorder

Prabhat Sitholey

INTRODUCTION

The Concept

In order to perform any task, a person is required to pay careful sustained attention to the task to understand it, make a suitable mental plan of action, make appropriate controlled movements to begin it, and persist in doing the task till it is completed. If there are any distractions, internal (in the form of thoughts or bodily needs) or external (say, a noise or a movement), one must ignore them and persist in doing the task at hand. But if a person is unable to do any one of the above, the task will not be accomplished.

The above applies to all our voluntary activities, at all stages of our lives, from childhood to adult life, be it the activities of daily living, play, studies, social interaction, or a job. Before initiating an activity, we normally consider the consequences of our actions, and if these are thought to be adverse, harmful, or painful, we prevent that activity. Such forethought has a protective effect.

In order to carry out an activity, it should be within a person's developmental and intellectual capacities. If a task is too difficult to understand, one will not be able to pay careful, sustained, and sufficient attention to it. If the ambient environment is full of distractions, paying attention will be difficult. If there are sensory impairments, for example, in hearing or vision, a motor weakness, or a distressing physical or mental disorder, one will be unable to do a desired activity. Lack of interest in or willingness to do an activity will have the same result.

It is also possible that a person is unable to keep his excessive voluntary movements (activity including speech) under control in situations that require calm and remaining seated, for example, during studies, in a classroom, while doing a job, or in social situations. Such excessive voluntary activity will make a person unable to persist and successfully complete the task. Besides, it will also have a disruptive effect upon others and if a joint group activity is to be done, as in a game or sport, it will be rendered incomplete. However, it must be noted that excessive activity can also be due to a physical disorder, for example, involuntary movements in chorea, or due to a mental disorder like mania.

If an activity is performed, upon an urge, internal or external, without planning or forethought of its consequences, it can have an adverse effect upon the doer and an intrusive or disruptive effect on others. Such an act will be called impulsive.

Normally, we can pay careful attention to a task, make voluntary movements to execute it, and not act impulsively. Occasionally, we may be inattentive, restless, or impulsive due to understandable reasons. This is normal. If lack of attention (inattention), excessive voluntary activity (hyperactivity), and thoughtless activity (impulsivity) are due to external environmental reasons or because of a physical or mental disorder, or else because of a medication or substance of abuse, these are then not a characteristic of a person. Such inattention, hyperactivity, and impulsivity will be transient, lasting as long as the above circumstances last.

However, there are persons in whom there is a persistent and pervasive pattern of inattention, hyperactivity and impulsivity (HI), not explained by the above factors. Such persons may be having a neurodevelopmental disorder (NDD), named attention-deficit/hyperactivity disorder (ADHD).

DEFINITION (DIAGNOSTIC REQUIREMENTS) OF ATTENTION-DEFICIT/HYPERACTIVITY DISORDER

A persistent pattern (over at least 6 months) of inattention symptoms and/or a combination of HI symptoms that are outside the limits of normal variation expected for age and level of intellectual development is required for diagnosis. Symptoms vary according to chronological age and disorder severity.[1] Several persistent symptoms of sufficient severity should be present that directly have a negative impact upon a person's academic, occupational, or social functioning[1] and on activities of daily living. The symptoms are from the domains of inattention and HI.[1]

Inattention

Several symptoms of inattention are present from the following symptom clusters:

- A difficulty in sustaining attention on tasks that are not highly stimulating or rewarding or require sustained mental effort; an inability to pay attention to detail, making careless mistakes in school or work assignments, and leaving tasks unfinished[1]
- Being easily distracted by extraneous stimuli or unrelated thoughts. Often does not listen when spoken to directly; often appears to be daydreaming or having mind elsewhere
- Losing things; forgetful in daily activities; forgetful of upcoming daily tasks or activities; difficulty in planning, organizing, and managing school or occupational tasks, and other normal activities.[1]

Hyperactivity–Impulsivity

Several symptoms of HI, most evident in structured situations that require behavioral self-control, are present from the following symptom clusters:

- Excessive motor activity; leaving seat when expected to remain still; often running about; fidgeting (younger children); inner restlessness and a discomfort with being quiet or sitting still (adolescents and adults)
- Difficulty in keeping quiet; overtalkative
- Blurting out answers in school or comments at work; difficulty awaiting one's turn in conversation or games
- A tendency to act in response to immediate stimuli without thinking of possible risks and consequences, e.g., physical injury, reckless driving, or impulsive decisions.[1]

Other Requirements

- Onset of significant inattention and HI symptoms before the age of 12 years. Adolescents and adults may come to clinical attention when they are unable to cope with increased demands upon them due to their ADHD symptoms.
- ADHD symptoms should be present across multiple settings, e.g., in school, home, at work, social situations.
- The symptoms are not explained by another physical or mental disorder.
- The symptoms are not due to medication (e.g., thyroxine, sympathomimetic broncho-dilators) or a substance[1] (e.g., withdrawal of benzodiazepines).

CLINICAL PRESENTATIONS OF ATTENTION-DEFICIT/ HYPERACTIVITY DISORDER

There can be three presentations of ADHD:

1. *Predominantly inattentive presentation:* Diagnostic requirements for inattention are met but not for HI.
2. *Predominantly HI presentation:* Diagnostic requirements for HI are met but not for inattention.
3. *Combined presentation:* Diagnostic requirements for both inattention and HI are met.

The prevalence of ADHD in children and adolescents (hereafter children unless specified) worldwide is between 5%[2] and 7%.[3] The male-female ratios in clinical samples are 4:1 and 2:1 in general population, respectively.[2] Low socioeconomic status predicts an increased probability of ADHD.[4] Genetic and environmental factors are considered significant in etiology. Psychobiological markers of ADHD are not specific enough for diagnosis which is made clinically.

ASSESSMENT

Information should be sought from multiple sources: Parents, siblings, or other caretakers, teachers at school and home, and peers. Information should be obtained about the child's behavior in different settings, for example, at home, school, play, and in social situations. All medical and school records should be obtained and carefully gone through.

Home environment should be explored to find out whether it is conducive for children's development and education. Similarly, the teachers' and other children's behavior toward the child should be found out. One should find out whether the child is a perpetrator or a victim of bullying and whether the teachers and other children ostracize the child or are sympathetic toward him.

A history of the child's appetite and food intake should be taken.

A history of ADHD, substance abuse, and psychiatric disorders in the family should be obtained.

A detailed physical examination should be done, and record of the child's height, weight, body mass index (BMI), pulse rate, and blood pressure should be kept and compared with the normative values. If there is a history of breathlessness on effort, and family history of early cardiac deaths, an assessment by a cardiologist is a must.

An unstructured clinical interview of the child and parents can be done but use of a semistructured interview schedule is preferable, e.g., Kiddie Schedule for Affective Disorders and Schizophrenia - Present and Lifetime Version.[5] This is applicable for children aged 6–18 years. The idea is to find out whether the child has ADHD or other comorbid psychiatric disorders. For preschool children, use of videos made at home and school in various activities can be made along with an unstructured interview. In all instances, both the children and parents should be interviewed and observed. For rating severity of ADHD symptoms, ADHD Rating Scale 5[6] are available, and these are updated and validated for DSM-5 and applicable to children aged 5–10 years and adolescents aged 11–17 years. Separate home and school versions are available for adolescents. Impairment due to inattention and HI can also be rated. The scale is sensitive to treatment changes.

For preschool children aged 3–5 years, ADHD Rating Scale IV: Preschool Version[7] is available. The items used are modifications of those in DSM-IV TR. The rating scale has sound psychometric properties.

Clinical Global Impression[8] rating scales can also be used. Although a number of tests are available, the above two are the easiest to use.

An assessment of intelligence, scholastic abilities, and speech and language development should also be done.

DIAGNOSIS AND DIFFERENTIAL DIAGNOSIS

It is very important to tell the child and his family that no psychological or physical investigations can give a diagnosis of ADHD. The diagnosis is made clinically by the psychiatrist after considering the presenting problems, history, physical examination, mental status examination, and the results of psychological and physical investigations, and therefore it is very important that the child and his family give their full cooperation to the psychiatrist.

The symptoms of ADHD should be inappropriately more when intelligence and development of the child are considered. The onset of at least some, if not all, impairing ADHD symptoms must have been in early childhood, say by the age of 7 years. A full picture must have emerged before the age of 12 years. The diagnostic criteria for ADHD must be fulfilled according to either DSM-5 TR[9] or CDDR for ICD-11 mental, behavioral, and NDDs.[1] Impairment due to ADHD symptoms must be present and the symptoms themselves must be present in two or more settings.

The symptoms would vary according to age. In preschool children, symptoms include very short play sequences of 3 minutes or less, incessant hyperactivity, children described as whirlwind, or those not listening when spoken to.

In school children, symptoms include overtalkativeness, being noisy, leaving a task unfinished in less than 10 minutes, inability to sit quietly when required to do so, fidgeting, running around, climbing up and down and talking out of turn, unable to await their turn, intruding upon conversation of others, and using things of others without taking their permission.

In adolescents (and adults), hyperactivity is replaced by a feeling of inner restlessness; they are uncomfortable in situations in which they are required to sit still and quiet. Their focus on a task lasts less than 30 minutes.

They make and break relationships very quickly, drive a vehicle fast and recklessly, break rules without thinking of consequences, experiment with substances of abuse, and are more likely to have road traffic accidents. They are forgetful, unmindful of time and appointments, and generally not good at academics.

Attention-deficit/hyperactivity disorder has high comorbidity rates. Oppositional defiant disorder (ODD), conduct disorder (CD), intellectual disability, learning disorders, language disorders, sleep disorders, enuresis, developmental motor coordination disorder, depression, anxiety disorders, tic disorders, and autism spectrum disorders are comorbid with ADHD. A meta-analysis found that children with ADHD are likely to have 10 times more ODD or CD and five times more anxiety disorders as compared to controls. There are no sex differences in comorbidity rates.

In adolescents with ADHD, eating disorders, substance-use disorders, bipolar disorders, and personality disorders are more frequent.[10]

The above comorbid disorders are also a differential diagnosis for ADHD because they may cause transient inattention and hyperactivity and apparent impulsivity. But in ADHD, the clinical picture is persistently and pervasively dominated by its core features while in the comorbid disorders their unique characteristic symptoms are predominant.

If inattention and HI symptoms occur only during the course of a comorbid disorder, for example, mania, then ADHD should not be diagnosed. But this rule will not work in persistent disorders with very early onset like intellectual disability and autism spectrum disorders which are comorbid with ADHD. Here, both these disorders can be comorbid and diagnosed on the basis of their characteristic clinical features.

If inattention and HI symptoms are of acute onset and short duration, then most likely ADHD is not the cause but is due to some other cause. Such cases should be carefully investigated. ADHD symptoms evolve gradually over a period of time and are persistent and pervasive, and impairment due to them is context dependent.

If inattention and HI symptoms appear for the first time after the age of 12 years, one should be very cautious in diagnosing ADHD. One should carefully investigate for the evidence of core ADHD symptoms in childhood before the age of 12 years. It is possible that the symptoms were present but mild, and there were no difficult, challenging contexts (in other words tasks faced by the child were easy for him) in which impairment would manifest. In this situation, the child would not be brought to clinical attention. But with the change in circumstances, difficult contexts, and lack of support and compensatory mechanisms, the symptoms and impairment caused by them would become obvious and the child may come to clinical attention.

A physical disorder or condition mimicking ADHD should be carefully ruled out.

MANAGEMENT PLAN

Rapport

The first task for the psychiatrist is to develop rapport with the child and his family. If the psychiatrist appears to the child and family as a person willing to listen patiently to their problems and who has developed an empathic understanding of them, and that he speaks to them in a language understandable to them in an unhurried manner, it is very likely that rapport will be formed. This should happen even before starting assessment. The psychiatrist should explain the need for assessment and why a particular assessment is being done and when the results are obtained discuss their significance with the child and his family.

Psychoeducation

The next step is to give the child and family the exact diagnosis of ADHD, and comorbid disorders, if any, in a nontechnical language they can understand. The child and the family should be asked about their understanding of the child's problems and of ADHD and comorbid disorders. Next, the child and family should be given correct factual information about ADHD and comorbid disorders again in a language they can follow. The impairment associated with the symptoms should also be explained.

This should be followed by telling them what all treatments are known to medical science and for which disorder. They should be informed about the medical and psychological treatments, and educational and social interventions. What treatments are locally and easily available, who will do them, the time and costs involved all should be discussed. A comparison of outcomes with treatment versus no treatment should be explained to the child and family.

Individualized Management and Therapeutic Alliance

A discussion about the child's and the family's needs in relation to the child's symptoms and his developmental and educational status should be done. This will mean considering the child's age, developmental level, and severity of his symptoms. The needs and how can they be met should be prioritized in collaboration with the child and his family. Consent of the family and assent of the child for the treatments mutually decided upon should be obtained. During the whole process, questions and doubts raised by the child and family should be openly and properly answered. This process leads to development of a therapeutic alliance between the child, his family, and the psychiatrist for management of ADHD and associated impairments. The idea is not to impose upon the child "one treatment that fits all" but treat him with an individualized plan specific to his current problems and needs. It is important to remember that the child's problems and needs may change over time necessitating a change in treatment plan.

In some cases, it is possible that a comorbid disorder may be the first priority for treatment. For example, if the child has a manic episode along with ADHD, management of mania will be the priority and ADHD can be treated only after the manic episode has remitted.

MANAGEMENT

The aim of management is to relieve the child's ADHD symptoms and associated impairments in educational, interpersonal, social, and health-related areas so that the child's development progresses. The risk factors, for example, financial constraints, child abuse, family disharmony, and psychiatric or substance-abuse disorders, in the family and bullying, scapegoating, humiliation, ostracism, and punishments in the school environment also need to be managed, as they adversely affect the child. The protective factors, for example, love, sympathy, understanding, support, facilitation of the child's organization and studies, and encouragement, have to be identified and promoted.

Medications like methylphenidate (MPH), atomoxetine, and clonidine act on inattention and HI, the core symptoms of ADHD. But there are a number of other problems associated with chronic ADHD. For example, with continuing long-term lack of success in studies and interpersonal and social interaction, children develop lack of confidence and social skills, feelings of inferiority, low self-esteem, anxiety and depression, procrastination and impulsive actions, and inability to manage time. These may not be at the level of a clinical disorder but are nevertheless enough to hinder a child's psychological development. These problems associated with ADHD have to be managed with nonpharmacological interventions.

For complete management, the comorbid physical and psychiatric disorders also need to be managed as per the standard of care for those disorders.

As mentioned earlier, the management would depend upon the child's chronological age, developmental and intellectual levels, symptoms and their severity, and impairments caused by them. In general, the younger the age, the greater the emphasis on psychological management, and the more severe the symptoms, the greater the reliance on pharmacological management. Except in preschool children, where most of the management is psychological, in all other children, a judicious combination of both psychological and pharmacological management along with family, social, and educational interventions is required.

Preschool Children

For preschool children, parent training is the main management. A number of parent training programs based on learning theory have been developed in Western countries. It is suggested that in India, we use an indigenously developed program.[11] Such programs are not specific for ADHD, but they help improve the behavioral problems of young children associated with ADHD and comorbid disorders. Similarly, teacher-given behavior therapy will be of help.

Medication is not advisable in preschool children unless hyperactivity is extreme. In them, benefits of medication may be offset by their side effects. A small dose of antipsychotics, for example, risperidone and aripiprazole, may be effective but one must be wary of their side effects. MPH can also be used.

School-age Children

Parent-training programs are useful in management. Medication is effective and can be used in the following order: MPH, atomoxetine, and clonidine. Classroom accommodations such as seating the child near and in front of the teacher, away from the window, giving small tasks and taking immediate feedback, encouragement, reducing distractions, and allowing a brief break of some physical activity may be helpful. Teacher-given behavior therapy will be useful.

The problem in India is that the number of children in a classroom is very large and usually it is not possible for the teachers to give individual attention to a child. Likewise, there are no or few special schools for children with ADHD.

Adolescents

Methylphenidate is the most effective medication for ADHD in adolescents followed by atomoxetine. If these do not work or cannot be used due to some reason, then clonidine may be used.

Cognitive behavior therapy (CBT) may be used for helping adolescents with ADHD, not with the core symptoms of ADHD, but with their low self-esteem, negative thinking, procrastination and impulsive actions, disorganization forgetfulness, lack of planning ahead, and depression.

Medications

Broadly, medications used for ADHD are psychostimulants and nonstimulants. A meta-analysis to compare the efficacy of medications for ADHD found that immediate-release (IR) psychostimulants had an effect size of 0.99 [95% confidence interval (CI) 0.88–1.1] whereas that for the extended-release ones was 0.95 (95% CI 0.85–1.1). The effect size for nonstimulants (atomoxetine, bupropion, modafinil, clonidine, and extended-release guanfacine) was 0.57 (95% CI 0.53–0.62). The effect sizes of IR and extended-release psychostimulants were similar, whereas those of nonstimulants were significantly lesser.[12]

Another meta-analysis[13] of studies for behavior therapy of ADHD found that most studies included were uncontrolled and none had used a double-blind design. Their standardized mean difference (SMD) was 0.67 (95% CI 0.54–0.80).[12] This is similar to SMD for nonstimulant medication and lessen than SMD for psychostimulants.

Methylphenidate

Methylphenidate (MPH) is currently the only psychostimulant available in India. It has lower addictive potential in comparison to amphetamine. It inhibits both dopaminergic and noradrenergic reuptake transporters. In children aged 6 years or more, the initial dose of MPH is 0.3 mg/kg/dose or 2.5–5 mg/dose before breakfast and lunch. The dose can be increased by 0.1 mg/kg/dose or 5–10 mg at weekly intervals. The maximum dose is 2 mg/kg/day[14] or 60 mg/day.

In India, MPH is available in IR, sustained-release (SR), and extended-release forms. The effect of IR form lasts for about 3–4 hours, that of SR form for about 6–8 hours, and that of extended-release form (Concerta, Addwize OD) for about 8–12 hours. Concerta comes as 18, 36, and 54 mg tablets. Addwize OD is available as 18 mg tablets. Multiple dosing will be required for IR and SR forms, whereas Addwize OD and Concerta can be given in a single-daily dose.

Methylphenidate improves the core symptoms of ADHD and also other problem behaviors associated with it, for example, road traffic accidents, low scholastic achievement, and criminality

Atomoxetine

Atomoxetine is a norepinephrine reuptake inhibitor. In the frontal areas of the brain, dopamine does not have its own reuptake transporter but shares the one with norepinephrine. Therefore, in the frontal areas of the brain, atomoxetine is a reuptake inhibitor for both epinephrine and dopamine. It is metabolized by CYP 2D6. Therefore, in those lacking in CYP 2D6, it must be given in small doses and very cautiously. Atomoxetine improves all the core symptoms of ADHD. It also improves anxiety and depression. Atomoxetine should be started with a small dose of 0.5 mg/kg/day for a week. If tolerated, one should start with the lowest therapeutic dose of 1.2 mg/kg/day for about 3–4 weeks. If there is no response, one could go up to 1.4 mg/kg/day and wait. A response may be obtained in the next 1–2 months. If no response is apparent, one can go up to unapproved 1.6 mg/kg/day or even higher dose. But this is for the specialists to do. The maximum dose of atomoxetine is 100 mg/day. For adolescents weighing 70 kg or more, one may begin with 40 mg/day and increase the dose to 80 mg/day after 1 week. Atomoxetine may be given in a single evening dose or in two divided doses.[14]

Clonidine

Clonidine is an alpha-2 adrenergic agonist. In a small randomized controlled trial (RCT) of young children with intellectual disability, clonidine IR in doses 4–8 µg/kg/day in two divided doses improved all the core symptoms of ADHD.[15] Clonidine extended release is approved by the Food and Drug Administration (FDA) for the treatment of ADHD.

Nonstimulants

Guanfacine extended release, bupropion, buspirone, modafinil, imipramine, haloperidol, risperidone, and aripiprazole have been used but, in view of the availability of MPH, atomoxetine, and clonidine IR, are not recommended unless the latter three medications are either ineffective or having unacceptable side effects.

Medication Side Effect

Side effects are a major reason for treatment discontinuation and therefore their management is necessary.

Methylphenidate: Its side effects of concern are insomnia, anorexia, growth retardation, anxiety, depression, hallucinations, psychosis, tics, seizures, tachycardia, and being frozen like a zombie. Insomnia can be managed by dosing early in evening or late in afternoon, reducing dose, and adding clonidine. Sleep hygiene should be practiced. Melatonin may be added. For anorexia, an appetizer can be added or else the dose reduced and/or administered after food. For growth retardation, height, weight, and BMI should be plotted on growth curves or else compared with age-appropriate norms. If growth retardation is definitely present, MPH will have to be stopped. For anxiety and depression, a dose reduction may be tried. If it does not work, MPH will have to be stopped and appropriate treatment started. MPH may be replaced by atomoxetine. If hallucinations and psychosis occur, MPH will have to be stopped. There is some evidence that MPH does not cause seizures or lower seizure threshold. But should this happen, MPH will have to be taken off. Likewise, MPH does not cause tics but if these appear for the first time or existing tics are exacerbated, first, being watchful, second, a dose reduction, and then stopping MPH will be required. Seizures will need to be investigated and anticonvulsants started, if required. For tics, MPH dose reduction should be tried, and clonidine or low-dose antipsychotic may be added. If the child becomes "frozen, like a zombie", dose reduction should help.

Atomoxetine: Hepatic toxicity is a major concern. If there is firm evidence of it, atomoxetine should be stopped and there should be no retrial. Another concern is development of suicidal ideation in the first few weeks of the treatment.

The parents should be cautioned about it and appropriate precautions taken. If this happens, the child should be closely monitored and if this is persistent atomoxetine should be taken off and appropriate treatment started. Reduction of appetite and insomnia should be managed as for MPH.

Clonidine: The main side effects are sedation and postural hypotension. Sedation wears off in the third or fourth week. For hypotension, the total daily dose should be lowered and administered in three or four doses and precautions taken.

Duration of and Discontinuation of Management

Attention-deficit/hyperactivity disorder is a lifespan disorder. Although hyperactivity is greatly reduced during adolescence and replaced by inner restlessness, inattention and impulsivity may persist with reduced or full severity. Approximately only 20% are completely free of ADHD as young adults. Approximately 60% have one or more impairing symptoms.[16] About 20% retain the full diagnosis of ADHD. In view of this, it is advisable to continue management as long as is required by the persistence of impairing ADHD symptoms.

INDIAN STUDIES

The overall pooled prevalence of ADHD was 63.2 (95% CI 49.2–77.1) in 1,000 children surveyed with significant heterogeneity in the systemic review.[17] Lower IQ scores, epileptiform EEG activity, not attending school, and male sex were found to be significantly associated with comorbid ADHD in children with epilepsy.[18] Literature highlights that a huge gap exists between global and Indian research in the area of children with ADHD, and there is a need for the development and efficacy testing of an indigenous intervention program in different areas of intervention for research and clinical practice in ADHD.[19] Adherence was found to be better in children with shorter duration of illness, lesser severity, absence of side effects, and stimulant prescription. It was also found that nonstimulant-based combination (40%) was more common as compared to stimulants (28%), with atomoxetine and risperidone being the most commonly prescribed medications in ADHD.[20] INDT-ADHD was found to be suitable for diagnosing ADHD in Indian children between the ages of 6–9 years.[21] There have been variable comorbidity rates of ADHD + BPD (borderline personality disorder) in different studies which are most likely due to differences in study setting, study sample, conceptualization of BPD, and assessment methods.[22] Neurological soft signs were found to be present in 84% of children and equally present in both the inattentive-hyperactive and impulsive-hyperactive types of ADHD.[23] Further studies with larger sample size and longer period of follow-up may be recommended in ADHD. Screening of school children for symptoms of ADHD is recommended for early diagnosis and treatment.[24] The ACTeRS has adequate psychometric properties for use in the Indian population for identifying ADHD.[25] There was a gap noted in research from India across the domains of biomarkers, course, and follow-up and nonpharmacological intervention. Studies from India on biomarkers, with prospective research design, larger sample size, and matched controls are further needed.[26]

GUIDELINES FOR ATTENTION-DEFICIT/HYPERACTIVITY DISORDER

The National Institute for Health and Care Excellence (NICE) Guidance, UK, covers recognizing, diagnosing, and managing ADHD in children, young people, and adults. The aim of the guideline is to improve recognition and diagnosis, as well as the quality of care and support for people with ADHD.[27] The AACAP Practice Parameter for the assessment and treatment of children and adolescents with ADHD discusses the clinical evaluation for ADHD, comorbid conditions associated with ADHD, research on the etiology of the disorder, and psychopharmacological and psychosocial interventions for ADHD.[28] Clinical Practice Guidelines for the assessment and management of ADHD provides a framework for its diagnosis and management in children and adolescents aged up to 18 years of age.[29]

NEUROSCIENCE AND ATTENTION-DEFICIT/HYPERACTIVITY DISORDER

The altered structural connectomes in those with ADHD provide significant signatures for prediction of symptoms and diagnostic classification. Literature further suggest that abnormalities in the structural connectome may be one of the neural underpinnings of ADHD psychopathology, and it shows potential for establishing imaging biomarkers in clinical evaluation.[30] ADHD is a highly polygenic NDD with a complex genetic architecture encompassing risk variants across the spectrum of allelic frequencies, which are implicated in neurobiological processes. The diagnosis of ADHD shares a large proportion of genetic risks with continuously distributed traits of ADHD in the population, with shared genetic risks also seen across development and sex. The genetic risks of ADHD are shared with those implicated in many other neurodevelopmental, psychiatric, and somatic phenotypes.[31] Disturbances in the monoamine interaction with clock genes in those with monoamine gene polymorphisms may regulate the susceptibility of ADHD and comorbid aggression/sleep disturbances.[32] Building models of neuronal processes is of key importance to fully understand disorders of the brain as it may provide a quantitative platform which is capable of binding multiple neurophysiological processes to phenotype profiles in ADHD.[33] Literature highlights that individuals with ADHD frequently have sleep disturbances, daytime sleepiness, and/or circadian rhythm abnormalities.[34]

ARTIFICIAL INTELLIGENCE AND ATTENTION-DEFICIT/HYPERACTIVITY DISORDER

The applications of artificial intelligence can be extended to multiple ADHD diagnostic tools, allowing for the development of a powerful clinical decision support pathway that can be used both in and out of the hospital.[35] The state-of-the-art diffusion processing and novel artificial intelligence approaches would be beneficial to fully understand the pathophysiology of ADHD.[36] The artificial intelligence algorithm model of ADHD children based on Parent Symptom Questionnaire (PSQ) scale has been found to have a high accuracy.[37] The machine learning model-based study supports the role of *DRD4*, *SNAP25*, and *ADGRL3* genes in outlining ADHD severity and a new prediction framework with potential clinical use.[38] Artificial intelligence models evaluating brain anatomy have highlighted changes in cortical thickness and the shape of the inferior frontal cortex, bilateral sensorimotor cortex, left temporal lobe, and insula in ADHD.[39]

SUMMARY AND CONCLUSION

Attention-deficit/hyperactivity disorder is a common lifespan NDD arising before the age of 12 years characterized by persistent, pervasive, and impairing symptoms of inattention and HI. Assessment requires gathering information from multiple informants and in multiple settings. Diagnosis is clinical. ADHD is a highly comorbid disorder (where oppositional defiant, conduct, and anxiety disorders are frequent). Individualized management is based on the child's current needs with appropriate integration of parent training, behavior therapy, CBT, and psychostimulant (or nonstimulant) medications, which may be required for long term till the impairing symptoms persist. For school-going children and adolescents, behavior therapy, social skills training, CBT, and medication may be used. For young schoolchildren, parent training should be used. Lastly, side effects of medications must be regularly checked and managed.

REFERENCES

1. World Health Organization. Clinical descriptors and diagnostic requirements for ICD - 11 mental, behavioural, and neurodevelopmental disorders. Geneva: World Health Organization; 2024.
2. Polanczyk G, Rohde LA. Epidemiology of attention deficit/hyperactivity disorder across the lifespan. Curr Opin Psychiatry. 2007;20(4):386-92.
3. Thomas R, Sanders S, Doust J, Beller E, Glasziou P. Prevalence of attention-deficit/hyperactivity disorder: a systematic review and meta-analysis. Pediatrics. 2015;135(4):e994-1001.
4. Larsson H, Sariaslan A, Langstrom N, D'Onofrio B, Lichtenstein P. Family income in early childhood and subsequent attention deficit. J Child Psychol Psychiatry. 2014;55(5):428-35.
5. Kaufman J, Schweder AE. The schedule for affective disorders and schizophrenia for school-age children: Present and lifetime version (K - SADS - PL). In: Hessen M (Ed). Comprehensive Handbook of Psychological Assessment, Vol. 2. New York: Wiley; 2004. pp. 247-55.
6. DuPaul GJ, Power TJ, Anastopoulos AD, Reid R. ADHD Rating Scale-5 for Children and Adolescents: Checklists, Norms, and Clinical Interpretation. New York: Guilford Press; 1998.
7. McGoey KE, DuPaul GJ, Haley E, Shelton TL. Parent and teacher ratings of attention-deficit/hyperactivity disorder in preschool: The ADHD rating scale IV preschool version. J Psychopathol Behavior Assess 2007;29:269-276.
8. Guy W. [Ed] ECDEU Assessment Manual for Psychopharmacology. Rockville, MD, U.S. Department of Health, Education, and Welfare; 1976.
9. American Psychiatric Association. Diagnostic and Statistical Manual of Mental Disorders, 5th edition. American Psychiatric Association; 2022.
10. De Freitas de Sousa A, Coimbra IM, Castanho JM, Polanczyk GV, Rohde LA. Attention deficit hyperactivity disorder. In: Rey JM, Martin A (Eds). JM Rey's IACAPAP e-Textbook of Child and Adolescent Mental Health. Geneva: International Association for Child and Adolescent Psychiatry and Allied Professions; 2020.
11. Shah R, Sharma A, Grover S, Sachdeva D, Chakrabarti S, Avasthi A. PGIMER Manual: Parent Skills Training for Families of Children with Attention-Deficit Hyperactivity Disorder, 2nd Edition, Department of Psychiatry, Postgraduate Institute of Medical Education and Research (PGIMER), Chandigarh, India, 2020.
12. Faraone SV. Using meta-analysis to compare the efficacy of medications for attention-deficit/hyperactivity disorder in youths. 2009;34(12):678-94.
13. Fabiano GA, Pelham WE Jr, Coles EK, Gnagy EM, Chronis-Tuscano A, O'Connor BC. A meta - analysis of behavioral treatments for attention - deficit / hyperactivity disorder. Clin Psychol Rev. 2009;29(2):129-40.
14. Fuller MA, Sajatavic M. Psychotropic Drug Information Handbook. Ohio: Lexi-Comp; 2005.
15. Agarwal V, Sitholey P, Kumar S, Prasad M. Double-blind, placebo-controlled trial of clonidine in hyperactive children with mental retardation. Mental Retard. 2001;39(4):259-67.
16. Kessler RC, Lenard AA, Barkley R, Biederman J, Conners CK, Faraoneet al. Patterns and prediction of attention deficit hyperactivity disorder persistence in adulthood: results from National Comorbidity Survey Replication. Biol Psychiatry. 2005;57:1442-51.
17. Chauhan A, Sahu JK, Singh M, Jaiswal N, Agarwal A, Bhanudeep S, et al. Burden of Attention Deficit Hyperactivity Disorder (ADHD) in Indian Children: A Systematic Review and Meta-Analysis. Indian J Pediatr. 2022;89(6):570-8.
18. Choudhary A, Gulati S, Sagar R, Sankhyan N, Sripada K. Childhood epilepsy and ADHD comorbidity in an Indian tertiary medical center outpatient population. Sci Rep. 2018;8(1):2670.
19. Satapathy S, Choudhary V, Sharma R, Sagar R. Nonpharmacological Interventions for Children with Attention Deficit Hyperactivity Disorder in India: A Comprehensive and Comparative Research Update. Indian J Psychol Med. 2016; 38(5):376-85.

20. Nayak AS, Nachane HB, Keshari P, Parkar SR, Saurabh KH, Arora M. Prescription patterns and medication adherence in preadolescent children with attention deficit hyperactivity disorder. Indian J Psychiatry. 2021;63(3):274-78.
21. Deshmukh V, Sagar R, Silberberg D, Bhutani VK, Pinto JM, Durkin M, et al.; INCLEN Study Group. INCLEN diagnostic tool for attention deficit hyperactivity disorder (INDT-ADHD): development and validation. Indian Pediatr. 2014;51(6):457-62.
22. Sivakumar T, Agarwal V, Sitholey P. Comorbidity of attention-deficit/hyperactivity disorder and bipolar disorder in North Indian clinic children and adolescents. Asian J Psychiatr. 2013;6(3):235-42.
23. Patankar VC, Sangle JP, Shah HR, Dave M, Kamath RM. Neurological soft signs in children with attention deficit hyperactivity disorder. Indian J Psychiatry. 2012;54(2):159-65.
24. Ajinkya S, Kaur D, Gursale A, Jadhav P. Prevalence of parent-rated attention deficit hyperactivity disorder and associated parent-related factors in primary school children of Navi Mumbai--a school based study. Indian J Pediatr. 2013;80(3):207-10.
25. Tsheringla S, Simon A, Russell PS, Shankar S, Russell S, Mammen P, et al. ADD-H-Comprehensive Teacher's Rating Scale (ACTeRS): a measure for attention deficit hyperactivity disorder among children with intellectual disability in India. Indian J Pediatr. 2014;81(Suppl 2):S161-4.
26. Kuppili PP, Manohar H, Pattanayak RD, Sagar R, Bharadwaj B, Kandasamy P. ADHD research in India: A narrative review. Asian J Psychiatr. 2017;30:11-25.
27. National Institute for Health and Care Excellence. Attention deficit hyperactivity disorder: diagnosis and management. [online] Available from https://www.nice.org.uk/guidance/ng87/resources/attention-deficit-hyperactivity-disorder-diagnosis-and-management-pdf-1837699732933 [Last accessed November, 2025]
28. Pliszka S; AACAP Work Group on Quality Issues. Practice parameter for the assessment and treatment of children and adolescents with attention-deficit/hyperactivity disorder. J Am Acad Child Adolesc Psychiatry. 2007;46(7):894-921.
29. Shah R, Grover S, Avasthi A. Clinical Practice Guidelines for the Assessment and Management of Attention-Deficit/Hyperactivity Disorder. Indian J Psychiatry. 2019;61(Suppl 2):176-93.
30. Bu X, Cao M, Huang X, He Y. The structural connectome in ADHD. Psychoradiology. 2021;1(4):257-71.
31. Brikell I, Burton C, Mota NR, Martin J. Insights into attention-deficit/hyperactivity disorder from recent genetic studies. Psychol Med. 2021;51(13):2274-86.
32. Mogavero F, Jager A, Glennon JC. Clock genes, ADHD and aggression. Neurosci Biobehav Rev. 2018;91:51-68.
33. Iravani B, Arshamian A, Fransson P, Kaboodvand N. Whole-brain modelling of resting state fMRI differentiates ADHD subtypes and facilitates stratified neuro-stimulation therapy. Neuroimage. 2021;231:117844.
34. Becker SP. ADHD and sleep: recent advances and future directions. Curr Opin Psychol. 2020;34:50-6.
35. Loh HW, Ooi CP, Barua PD, Palmer EE, Molinari F, Acharya UR. Automated detection of ADHD: Current trends and future perspective. Comput Biol Med. 2022;146:105525.
36. Gagnon A, Descoteaux M, Bocti C, Takser L. Better characterization of attention and hyperactivity/impulsivity in children with ADHD: The key to understanding the underlying white matter microstructure. Psychiatry Res Neuroimaging. 2022;327:111568.
37. Wang G, Li W, Huang S, Chen Z. A Prospective Study of an Early Prediction Model of Attention Deficit Hyperactivity Disorder Based on Artificial Intelligence. J Atten Disord. 2024;28(3):302-9.
38. Cervantes-Henríquez ML, Acosta-López JE, Martinez AF, Arcos-Burgos M, Puentes-Rozo PJ, Vélez JI. Machine Learning Prediction of ADHD Severity: Association and Linkage to *ADGRL3*, *DRD4*, and *SNAP25*. J Atten Disord. 2022;26(4):587-605.
39. Firouzabadi FD, Ramezanpour S, Firouzabadi MD, Yousem IJ, Puts NAJ, Yousem DM. Neuroimaging in Attention-Deficit/Hyperactivity Disorder: Recent Advances. AJR Am J Roentgenol. 2022;218(2):321-32.

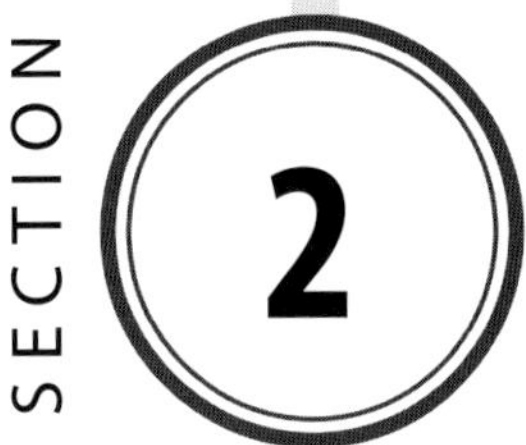

SECTION 2

Externalizing Disorders, Addictions, Mood, and Psychotic Disorders

CHAPTER 10

Disruptive Behavior, Dissocial Disorders, and Impulse Control Disorders

Chhitij Srivastava, Jyoti Singh

INTRODUCTION

Disruptive behavior, dissocial disorders, and impulse control disorders, as per DSM-5, are a group of psychiatric conditions characterized by persistent patterns of behavior that violate social norms and the rights of others.[1] The behaviors may range from excessive temper tantrums, defiance, and disobedience to more serious rule breaking, physical aggression, lying, and stealing. The boundaries between normal acceptable behavior at very young age to these group of disorders can appear blurred and have historically raised debates about their validity. People sometimes see these disorders as social constructs rather than true psychiatric conditions. However, as our biological understanding of these group of disorders has improved, the validity of these as psychiatric disorders has also improved.[2] These disorders often lead to significant impairments in social, academic, and occupational functioning. The primary disorders in this category include oppositional defiant disorder (ODD), conduct disorder (CD), and various impulse control disorders such as intermittent explosive disorder (IED) and pyromania.[3] They constitute one of the most common mental and behavioral problems in children and young people. In this chapter, we will cover ODD and CDs.

OPPOSITIONAL DEFIANT DISORDER AND CONDUCT DISORDERS

Classification Systems

10th revision of the International Classification of Diseases (ICD-10) classified ODD as a subtype of CDs thereby implying a continuum between ODD and CDs. DSM-5 has treated them as separate entities. This has reflected in an ongoing debate with some seeing the two disorders on a continuum while others choosing to see them as separate entities. ICD-11 is more in sync with DSM-5. This chapter will refer to the DSM-5 classification system as it has been in use for longer and people are familiar with it. However, we will point out the similarities and differences between DSM-5 and ICD-11.

Oppositional Defiant Disorder

Diagnostic criteria for ODD as per DSM-5 are as follows:

- A *persistent pattern* of defiant, disobedient, and antagonistic behavior
- For diagnosis, four or more of the following criteria must be present. It must not be limited to siblings only and should be present for >6 months. The symptoms can be separately clubbed in three subcategories as follows:
  1. *Angry/irritable mood:*
     - Often loses temper

- Often touchy or easily annoyed
- Often angry and resentful

2. *Argumentative/defiant behavior:*
   - Often argumentative with adults/ authority figures
   - Often defies or does not follow rules
   - Often deliberately annoys others
   - Often blames others
3. *Vindictiveness:* Spiteful or vindictive at least twice in last 6 months
   - For children <5 years, the above-mentioned behavior problems should occur on most days for 6 months while for those >5 years, behavior problems should occur at least once per week for 6 months.
   - DSM-5 also allows for severity to be specified as mild, moderate, or severe.
   - ICD-11 is similar overall. However, it also allows for symptom specifiers that can predict future trajectory as follows:
     - ODD can be diagnosed with chronic irritability and anger which has a higher chance of future depression.
     - ODD can be diagnosed without prosocial emotions (see section on CDs) which is more likely to develop into more severe CD and antisocial personality disorder (ASPD).

Conduct Disorder

Diagnostic criteria for CDs as per DSM-5 are as follows:

- A *repetitive and persistent* pattern of behavior in which basic rights of others or major age-appropriate societal norms or rules are violated.
- For diagnosis, three or more of the following 15 symptoms clubbed in four subcategories must be present in past 12 months, with at least one criterion present in past 6 months.[1]
  - *Aggression to people and animals:*
    - Often bullies, threatens, or intimidates others
    - Often initiates physical fights
    - Has used a weapon that can cause serious physical harm to others
    - Has been physically cruel to people
    - Has been physically cruel to animals
    - Has stolen while confronting a victim
    - Has forced someone into sexual activity
  - *Destruction of property:*
    - Has deliberately engaged in fire setting with the intention of causing serious damage
    - Has deliberately destroyed others' property (other than by fire setting)
  - *Deceitfulness or theft:*
    - Has broken into someone else's house, building, or car
    - Often lies to obtain goods or favors or to avoid obligations (i.e., "cons" others)
    - Has stolen items of nontrivial value without confronting a victim (e.g., shoplifting)
  - *Serious violations of rules:*
    - Often stays out at night despite parental prohibitions, beginning before age 13 years
    - Has run away from home overnight at least twice or once without returning for a lengthy period
    - Is often truant from school, beginning before age 13 years

Specifiers

Specifiers are based on:

- Onset of symptoms
- Severity
- Certain specific clinical characteristics
- These specifiers appear to carry prognostic value and help in predicting future trajectory.
- With respect to onset, one can specify if the symptoms have a *childhood, adolescence, or unspecified onset.*
  - ICD-11 has similar categories for onset of symptoms

    - There is evidence to suggest that childhood onset may predict a more persistent pattern of difficulties while adolescent onset symptoms may be more time limited. This was first brought out in the landmark Dunedin cohort study.[4] They found that in the early onset group, there was a significant risk of persistent antisocial behavior in adulthood. This group had a higher genetic loading that also reflected in poor childhood environment. In contrast, another group with adolescence onset had a much better outcome. While these two groups are largely accepted by the scientific community, there is also evidence that not all fit into these neat categories. In reality, there is a wider spectrum in that some early onset cases may be restricted to childhood only and some adolescent onset cases may persist into adulthood.
- The symptom specifier with respect to *prosocial emotions* carries significant *prognostic value,* and is present in both DSM-5 and ICD-11.
    - Those with limited prosocial emotions lack remorse or guilt, are callous (lack of empathy), show shallow or deficient effect, and are unconcerned about their performance.[1] Their aggression is more likely to be proactive than reactive.
    - It is important to note here that *reactive* aggression is characterized by emotional lability and impulsivity and is triggered by provocation.
    - On the other hand, proactive aggression tends to be driven by lack of emotional arousal and a motive to obtain benefits in the absence of provocation.[5]
    - This group with poor prosocial emotions has a significantly higher chance of persistence with poor prognosis into adulthood.
- DSM-5 also allows for specifying symptom severity into mild, moderate, and severe. ICD-11 does not have severity specifiers.

EPIDEMIOLOGY

If we consider ODD and CDs together, their prevalence is around 5–10% making them one of the most common psychiatric conditions of children and adolescents.[6,7] ODD symptoms typically decline after the age of 10 years and it is unlikely for someone to receive a new diagnosis after that age. On the other hand, CD is mostly diagnosed after the age of 5 years, typically during middle childhood or early adolescence. This is understandable as a number of symptoms listed for CD which are less likely to be fulfilled by young children. Male-to-female ratio is around 2:1 in younger kids with ODD.[8] It is much higher at 3:1–7:1 in older kids with CD.

ETIOLOGY (FIG. 1)

The risk factors for ODD and CDs are best seen as a combination of genetic and environmental factors.[9] However, there is also a lot of overlap between these factors. For example, antisocial parents confer the higher risk through both genetic and environmental factors like poor parenting. A lot of factors discussed below can be correlated with each other and are being discussed separately only for the ease of understanding. They should therefore not be seen in isolation. Genetic factors manifest through the child's early temperament. Neuropsychological and neurobiological findings are essentially correlates of the temperamental factors.[10] A lot of environmental factors may be simply a reflection of the genetic risk these children have. Environmental factors also interact with genes in multiple ways.

Genetics

The overall heritability is around 50% but there is a lot of heterogeneity. A number of risk genes for

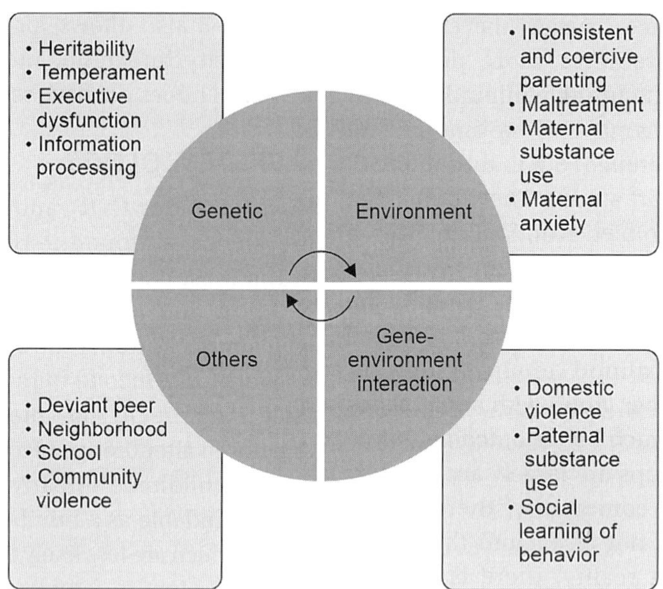

Fig. 1: Summary of etiological factors for oppositional defiant disorder (ODD) and conduct disorders (CDs).

ODD and CD may not be specific and instead are associated with attention-deficit/hyperactivity disorder (ADHD) and lower IQ.[11] There may be some specific genes related to negative emotionality and poor emotional regulation. Different genes may be relevant for rule breaking and overt aggression.[12]

Genetic factors are higher in males, in those with comorbid ADHD, poor prosocial emotions [callous-unemotional (CU) traits], physical aggression, and pervasive symptoms.[13]

Partly different genes may contribute to CD at different stages of the lifespan. This is understandable if we take into consideration that onset of symptoms at different ages have differing prognosis. Genetic contribution to conduct increases from childhood to adolescence which essentially means that if antisocial symptoms persist into adolescence, they are more likely to have a higher genetic contribution.

While some have suggested that ODD shares substantial genetic overlap with CD,[14] other studies have indicated unique effects for each.[15,16] In addition, it seems that genetic effects underlie the association between ODD and ADHD as well as between ODD and depressive disorder.[15,17] In a twin study of adolescents, self-reported irritability symptoms of ODD shared genetic effects with depressive symptoms, whereas "headstrong/hurtful" symptoms of ODD shared genetic risk with delinquent symptoms.[18]

Environmental Effects

Antenatal Environment and Childbirth

Environmental effects are important at all stages of life starting from the intrauterine period. Maternal use of alcohol, smoking, and other drugs during pregnancy along with psychosocial stress all contribute to the development of antisocial behavior.[19-21] These effects may be indirect though, by having a negative effect on the child's IQ. Fetal alcohol syndrome is a well-known complication of alcohol use during pregnancy. These children are more likely to have lower IQ and at a higher risk of developing conduct problems.[20] Environmental factors operating during pregnancy may also be an indirect effect of the genetic risk as mothers with high-genetic vulnerability are more likely to engage in using drugs and alcohol during pregnancy.

Effects of maternal stress during pregnancy on the development of the prefrontal cortex of the offspring might mediate the association of stress with conduct symptoms.[22] Maternal anxiety during the last trimester of pregnancy is associated with childhood-onset conduct problems.[23] Birth complications (through hypoxia) combined with early-life maternal rejection is linked to an increased risk of early-onset serious violence through negative effects on child's IQ. Family factors like low socioeconomic status, overcrowding, poor housing all appear to increase the risk. These factors reflect adverse family circumstances resulting in poor parenting practices which are an established risk factor for the development of conduct symptoms.

Parenting Practices

There are various parenting practices that are associated with conduct symptoms. *These include inconsistently enforced rules, unclear commands, parent–child conflict, harsh and coercive parenting, maltreatment, and abuse.*[24] Parenting factors become even more relevant if there is already a high genetic loading. When parents do not consistently enforce rules, it becomes difficult for children to comprehend which behavior is being punished, rewarded, or ignored. This inconsistent parenting is often due to the fluctuating emotional state of the parents. Children, therefore, do not develop an internal model of right and wrong and they instead try, and act based on the parental mood.

Paradoxical reward of challenging behavior is another concept that has to be understood carefully. In this scenario, parents ignore their child when he/she is playing quietly or behaving nicely. However, they respond critically when the child shows challenging behavior. Although it appears paradoxical, but getting punished actually reinforces the behavior in the context where positive behavior consistently gets ignored. Another mechanism that is at play here is when the parents unknowingly reward challenging behavior. In a typical scenario, child will make a request that the parent will ignore or respond negatively to. The child will escalate his/her demand into a tantrum, and the parent will give in and fulfill the child's demand. This teaches the child that by throwing a tantrum, he/she can get their way.

Harsh and coercive parenting operates through multiple possible ways.[25] Firstly, a child with conduct problems is more likely to evoke negative reactions in the parents thereby directly increasing the chances of parents being harsh and coercive. In this situation, coercive parenting practices may simply reflect the high genetic risk that has been passed on to the child. However, even if these factors are accounted for, harsh parenting does increase the chances of conduct problems independently especially if associated with aggression and child maltreatment.[26] Child abuse increases the chances of attachment problems which further increases the risk. Parental conflict further increases the risk. When children witness domestic violence, they are able to justify their own violent behavior. Social learning also plays an important part where the child learns to appraise situations incorrectly and resort to violence at the earliest. Also, through regular exposure to violence while growing up, these children get habituated to it and do not see it as a problem in their own relationships.[27] Institutional care also increases the risk through the same mechanisms discussed above.

Extrafamilial Factors

The environment beyond family also plays an extremely important role especially as the child grows older. Association with deviant peers and community violence contribute to the development of conduct symptoms.[28] However, the opposite is also be true in that children with conduct symptoms are more likely to choose deviant peers. Rejection by prosocial peers can further increase the risk. Schools also play an important role. However, the quality of schools that these children attend is confounded by other risk factors including low socioeconomic status and deprivation in the community. Children with conduct problems are therefore more likely to attend schools which have a higher percentage of deviant peers. However, schools that have fair policies and enforce rules consistently are more likely to be protective.

Temperament

Temperamental factors in toddlers such as irritability, impulsivity, and intensity of reactions to negative stimuli may contribute to the development of a pattern of oppositional and defiant behavior.[29] It is possible that ODD is arrived at through different temperamental routes that could serve to explain its comorbidity. Stringaris et al. (2010) showed that the comorbidity between ODD and internalizing disorders was more strongly associated with early temperamental emotionality, whereas the comorbidity between ODD and ADHD was better predicted by temperamental over activity.[30]

Gene-environment Interactions

Environmental factors (e.g., childhood maltreatment) can have a significant effect on a child's behavior based upon that child's genetic make-up.[31] In one of the landmark studies[32] by Caspi et al. (2002), a functional polymorphism in the promoter region of the gene that codes for the neurotransmitter-metabolizing enzyme monoamine oxidase A (MAO-A) was found to moderate the effect of child maltreatment on future conduct and antisocial problems,[32] although later studies did not find such an interaction.[33] Maltreated children with a genotype that leads to low levels of MAO-A activity more often displayed CD and antisocial behaviors at follow-up than children with a high-activity MAOA genotype.[32]

Hypothalamic-Pituitary-Adrenal Axis and Stress Response

Low levels of arousal have been reported in children with conduct problems which may make them more likely to engage in sensation seeking behaviors.[34,35] Low heart rate and skin conductance have been consistently reported. Adequate cortisol responses are necessary to correctly interpret the social situation. CU traits may be especially associated with low baseline cortisol levels and decreased cortisol secretion under stress.

Neuropsychological Findings

Low IQ, especially verbal, has been consistently reported in children with conduct problems.[36] Various mechanisms may be at work here. Poor verbal intelligence may make it more difficult to recall verbal instructions and interpret them properly. This would increase the chances of these children not complying to verbal instructions. They would also be less able to assert themselves using language and therefore more likely to act out physically on their impulses. These children would also struggle to use language to think through the consequences of their actions.[36,37]

Children with conduct problems are also more often found to have specific learning difficulties.[38] These difficulties may contribute to other risk factors at school like bullying, being rejected by prosocial peers and befriending deviant peers.[39] Educational struggles also make school less rewarding, which further increases the risk of developing conduct problems.

These children have poor executive functions which make it more difficult for them to stop themselves from acting out on their impulses, less likely to inhibit themselves due to fear of punishment and therefore engage in more risk-taking behavior.[40]

These children have poor social cognition. They often misinterpret neutral social cues and choose aggression to respond to situations that can be handled peacefully.[41]

Callous-unemotional traits may be characterized by poor recognition of emotion (particularly fear) in facial expression. Children with these traits have poor affective empathy.[42]

Neurobiological Findings

A lot of brain structural and functional imaging findings reported in ODD and CD are confounded by the comorbid presence of ADHD. However, some findings may be specific to ODD/CD. Lower amygdala volume and reduced right-sided insular volume have been reported in both early and adolescence onset ODD/CD.[43] Other implicated brain areas include anterior cingulate cortex, striatum, superior frontal gyrus, fusiform gyrus, and superior temporal gyrus. These findings predominantly relate to difficulties in emotional processing and are present even in those without CU traits. However, CU traits may be specifically related to amygdala hypofunction.

Executive dysfunction is most evident in those with comorbid ADHD. However, some executive dysfunction may be independent of ADHD. While ADHD is associated with "cool" executive functions (inhibitory, attention, and planning), ODD/CD is related to "hot" paralimbic system that regulated motivation and affect. These functions are correlated with lateral orbital and ventromedial prefrontal cortices, superior temporal lobes, and amygdala.[44]

ASSESSMENT

It is feasible to assess oppositional problems in children as young as 5 years of age.[45] A wide range of instruments is available to measure these symptoms to assist in the diagnostic process and monitoring. Clinicians should always bear in mind that diagnosis is based on their judgment and integration of the information gathered by *interviews, clinical examination, scales, and other means.*

Collecting Information from Varied Sources

- In an ideal scenario, the clinician should try and get information before seeing the child and family. Use of questionnaires to gather information is highly recommended ideally from the parent, teachers, and the child or young person.
- Strength and difficulty questionnaire (SDQ) is very helpful to get information from all the abovementioned sources.[46] It is free and quick and looks at a number of domains including emotional symptoms, conduct problems, hyperactivity symptoms, and peer problems. It also generates a prosocial score which helps look at the child's strengths.
- Other questionnaires include child behavior checklist,[47] Conners Child Behavior Checklist,[48] the Eyberg Child Behavior Inventory[49] but these are all paid.
- The Achenbach's child behavior checklist has an Indian adapted version known as childhood psychopathology measurement schedule (CPMS)[50] and is standardized on Indian children with good reliability.
- Questionnaires should be supplemented with information obtained qualitatively also from school and other agencies that the child may be engaged with.

Clinical Assessment

- The diagnosis relies on a thorough clinical assessment that includes detailed history and mental state examination.
- The child should be seen both together and separate from parents. Similarly, history should be obtained from parents without the

child being present in the room. This is to ensure that the parents feel comfortable in discussing about their concerns. It also gives parents the message of not discussing negative things about their child in front of her/him.

- A thorough assessment should include obtaining information on all the factors mentioned under etiology section of this chapter.
- A risk assessment, history of drug and alcohol use, and forensic history must always form a part of the comprehensive assessment.
- Particular focus should be given to the parenting practices especially in a younger child and stressors like bullying and deviant peer influence. These are potentially modifiable factors.
- As a part of the assessment process, structured diagnostic questionnaires can be applied. These include Diagnostic Interview Schedule for Children (DISC-5),[51] Schedule for Affective Disorders and Schizophrenia for School-age Children (K-SADS),[52] and Child and Adolescent Psychiatric Assessment (CAPA).[53]
- A psychometric assessment must be done where indicated given the high rate of learning disorders, both specific and generalized, in this group. This is also extremely relevant from a management point of view.

Considering Differential Diagnoses and Comorbidity

A number of conditions may present with conduct symptoms. They may be a *differential diagnosis* that have to be ruled out before making a diagnosis of ODD/CD. In some occasions, they may be a *comorbid diagnosis* that may have important implications for treatment.

- *ADHD* may present with conduct symptoms commonly. It may therefore be either a differential or a comorbid diagnosis. While any of the ADHD symptoms may be considered as that of CD, impulsivity is the most likely to be misinterpreted. Impulsivity in ADHD will be more generalized whereas when it is present in ODD/CD, it is more likely to be restricted to antisocial behaviors. Given that ADHD is a common comorbidity, it must be assessed in detail whenever an assessment for ODD/CD is done.
- *Mood disorders:* Both mania and depression can present with behavior disturbances such as irritability, defiance, and aggression which can mimic ODD/CD. However, there is a well-defined onset for mood disorders, and the ODD/CD symptoms will not be prominent in the premorbid state. Depression can often be a comorbidity, especially in ODD/CD with irritability and mood symptoms. However, if irritability is very marked, then a diagnosis of disruptive mood dysregulation disorder (DMDD) should be considered.
- *Adjustment disorders:* Psychosocial stressors can cause secondary behavioral problems which can mimic ODD/CD. Again, a well-defined onset and temporal relationship with the stressor should clarify the diagnosis.
- *Obsessive compulsive disorder (OCD):* Young people with OCD may present with oppositional and defiant symptoms if stopped from doing their compulsions. They may also be very rigid, which can come across as defiance. Again, a proper clinical history should clinch the diagnosis.
- *Autism spectrum disorder (ASD):* These may often present with aggression and tantrums which may be confused with ODD/CD. A detailed history of social communication difficulties along with rigid, repetitive behaviors should clarify the diagnosis. Their lack of social concern may be confused with CU traits. However, unlike CU traits, the apparent lack of empathy is due to poor understanding of social situations. If they are able to understand things, children and young people with ASD are better able to empathize.

- *Psychotic disorder:* These may present with excessive aggression. However, other clinical symptoms of psychosis and a clear onset of symptoms should be enough to clarify the diagnosis.
- *Phobias and other anxiety disorders:* Children with anxiety issues may exhibit excessive tantrums secondary to their anxiety.
- *Normal child:* Some apparently normally developing children may engage in occasional antisocial behavior in their adolescence but are not overtly aggressive or defiant. This is mostly transient and secondary to peer pressure. These young people should not be labeled with a diagnosis of ODD/CD. Similarly, temper tantrums are very common in young children and must not be confused with the more serious symptoms of ODD/CD.

Risk Assessment

- A detailed assessment of *actual or potential harm to others* should be done. This should include details of any convicted criminal offence or contact with the law agencies. Details of the offence should include the nature and seriousness of the offence, the characteristics of the targeted victim, motive, empathy toward the victim, and role in offence. It should be noted whether it is an isolated event or a repetitive pattern.
- Children with ODD/CD are impulsive and exposed to a number of psychosocial stressors. This also makes them at high risk of harm to self, and this should be assessed thoroughly.

CONTINUITY INTO ADULTHOOD/ OUTCOME (FLOWCHART 1)

- ODD and CD predict a varied range of disorders into adulthood. This continuity can be predicted based on the predominant symptoms and this variation in symptomatology has been built into the classification systems as described earlier.

Flowchart 1: Summary of trajectory of ODD and CDs.

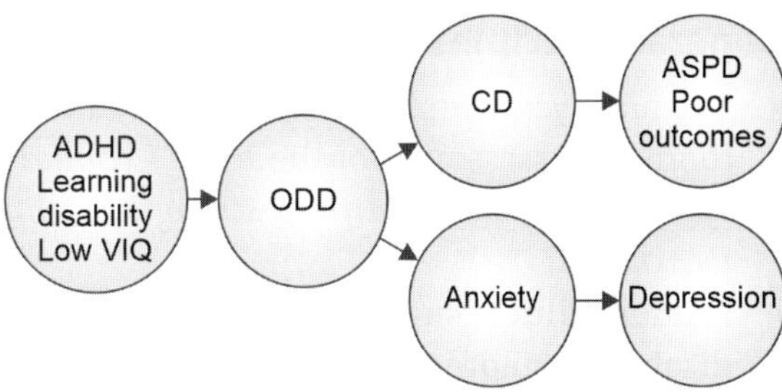

(ADHD: attention-deficit/hyperactivity disorder; ASPD: antisocial personality disorder; CD: conduct disorder; ODD: oppositional defiant disorder)

- Many children with ODD never meet full criteria for later CD and <50% of children with CD develop ASPD in adulthood.[4] However, most severe antisocial adults were antisocial in childhood.
- Apart from *homotypic* continuity, ODD/CD may also progress to a range of other disorders suggestive of *heterotypic* continuity as well.[54]
- In adolescence, CD is frequently associated with substance misuse which itself increases the risk of continuity.[54]
- ODD with more irritable characteristics is more likely to develop into anxiety and depressive disorders in adulthood. This may be more common in girls.
- ODD with more headstrong characteristics is more likely to follow a homotypic continuity into CD.[15]
- CU traits further increase the risk of these developing into more severe CD and ASPD into adulthood. This may be particularly true for the early onset group with risk factors such as high genetic loading, comorbid learning difficulties, ADHD, and social deprivation.[55]
- The adolescent onset group may grow out of it, but some develop a range of problems later on including anxiety, depression, and overall poor functional outcomes in adulthood.[56]

MANAGEMENT (BOX 1)

General Principles

- The management plan should be based on a thorough assessment of the child's *conduct symptoms, comorbidities, strengths, and weaknesses.*
- Comorbidities such as ADHD, learning disability, depression, and anxiety need proper treatment in their own right.
- The modifiable risk factors such as bullying, deviant peer relationship, and poor parenting practices should be especially addressed as part of the treatment package offered to the family.
- It should be communicated to the family that nonpharmacological treatments form a major part of the management plan. Medications are only used for comorbid conditions and to manage challenging behavior like aggression on a short-term basis.
- The most important and a critical initial step is engaging the family (see section on family therapy).

Nonpharmacological Treatments (Table 1)

Parent Management Training

- Parent management training is based on the principles of social learning and behavior theories and is key in the treatment of conduct symptoms, especially in younger children.
- Principles of social learning, particular in relation to operant conditioning (the role of reinforcement/consequences in altering behavior), have been found to be useful in modifying behavior in both parents and children.[57]
- Parent training also has a preventive role, and some uniform parental practices should be widely used by all parents.

BOX 1: Summary of management strategies.

- Family engagement
- *Personalized treatment plan:*
  - Identify comorbidities
  - Address modifiable risks
  - Work on both strengths and weaknesses
- *Parent management training (behavioral and social learning):*
  - The incredible years
  - Triple P (Positive Parenting Program)
- School-based interventions
- Family therapy
- Individual therapy [social skill training and cognitive-behavioral therapy (CBT)]
- Multimodal therapy
- Pharmacotherapy

TABLE 1: Summary of nonpharmacological treatments.

Nonpharmacological treatments	*Age groups*
Parent management training	3–11 years
School-based interventions	For school going children
Add individual therapy [cognitive-behavioral therapy (CBT) informed] including empathy-based individual training	>9 years
Family therapy	Any age but generally >9 years
Multimodal	>9 years, especially when there are more severe problems

Incredible years: One of the best validated parenting programs is Webster-Stratton's "Incredible Years", a behaviorally-based training program designed for use with parents,[58,59] teachers, and children.[58,60] The program has three components:

1. "Basic" for basic parenting skills
2. "Advanced" for parental relationship

3. "Partners" for building parent-teacher relationship

Triple P:

- Evidence-based parenting and family support program designed to prevent and manage behavior problems in preadolescent children by enhancing parenting skills and improving parent-child relationships.
- Triple P has been validated in a number of studies with a range of family types and cultural backgrounds.[61,62]
- The program comprises multiple levels:
  - Universal intervention designed to provide information on parenting issues for interested parents
  - Provision of advice for specific problem behaviors
  - Brief programs to provide advice and training parents dealing with minor behavior problems
  - More intensive programs comprising training in mood management strategies, coping skills, and partner support skills designed to address more persistent and pervasive behavior problems.
  - It is beyond the scope of this chapter to go into the details of these programs. However, we will discuss some basic strategies that these parenting programs use, as depicted in the parenting pyramid **(Fig. 2)**.
- Universal parenting practices are the most essential skills and need to be in place before other parenting skills can be effective. These include:
  - Child-directed play
  - Effective communication with the child
  - Giving attention to the child
  - Teaching problem solving.
- Child-directed play is the most important medium to teach the child. The idea is to

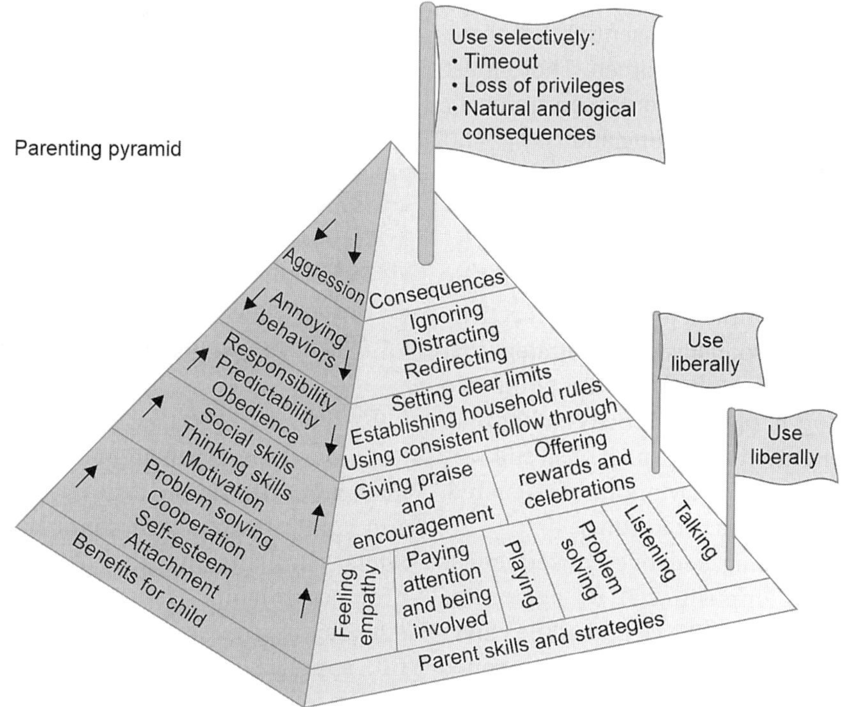

Fig. 2: Parenting pyramid.

let the child engage in play activities that he/she prefers. The parent provides the scaffolding and joins in while describing the various aspects of the interaction. This is called *"descriptive commentary."* Parents also learn to *describe the emotions* that the child experiences in these interactions thereby improving the child's emotional vocabulary.

- *Praising and giving reward* are combined with play and descriptive commentary. For it to be effective, *praise has to be very specific, instant, frequent, and not combined with negative statements*. Reward can be combined with a token economy system where the child earns points or other tokens for desirable behavior and these can be exchanged for tangible reward.
- Once the above parenting skills are in place then the other skills are taught. These include setting clear limits, enforcing rules and imposing consequences for certain behaviors.
- When setting rules, it is essential that these are fair and uniformly enforced. There must be certain rules that are enforced on every household member including adults, e.g., "no hitting, no abusing".
- *Consequences:*
  - Hyperactive behavior should never be punished. Instead, the child should be given an opportunity to use his/her activity levels more productively. The strategy that works here is to redirect the child into some sort of physical activity rather than asking him/her to stay quiet or sit still.
  - Minor irritating behaviors are best ignored. The same applies to tantrums.
  - When imposing negative consequences for actual oppositional or aggressive behavior, it should be clear that the child's physical activity should never be stopped especially in comorbid ADHD. That will only make the behavior problems worse. Consequences must be realistic and followed through. An example of negative consequence is restricting screen time.
  - Parents must never use hitting as a consequence. It can make the child fearful of parents and make him/her more secretive. It can also make the child more aggressive because of social learning.
  - Timeout is another strategy that can be used in place of actual consequences but is often difficult to impose in Indian settings where it may be difficult to find an isolated and quiet space for timeout.

School-based Interventions

Principles of social learning and behavior theories apply to school-based interventions similar to parenting programs. It is important to ensure consistency between home and school for behavior training to work. School-based interventions are also especially useful when the conduct problems are confined to or most prominent in the school setting. Moffitt and Scott (2008) have devised tools for teachers in four primary domains which are similar to parenting programs:[63]

- Promoting compliance and adherence to classroom rules and acceptable behaviors
- Developing problem-solving skills
- Preventing problem behavior
- Avoiding escalation of oppositional behavior

Individual Therapy

Cognitive-behavioral therapy (CBT) informed therapy has been found to be effective for children and young people with conduct problems.[64,65] Social skills training, anger management, problem solving, assertiveness training, and empathy-based training can be imparted using a CBT approach. The focus is on helping the young person to recognize the dysfunctional cognitions and correct them. This is then generalized to real-life situations that the young person is exposed to.

Family Therapy

Functional family therapy (FFT) was developed by James Alexander and colleagues and has a lot of good quality evidence for this population.[66] A lot of the techniques of FFT can be used in day-to-day work with these families even if formal family therapy may not be possible in our routine clinical settings. Some of the important principles of family therapy are summarized below:

- *Engagement:* The initial focus is on engaging the family and developing a good rapport. This allows to develop a good model for family functioning that the family members can emulate. The therapist must also avoid acting like an expert and instead be curious to learn about the family. Positive feedback must be given where appropriate which again becomes a model for social learning. Clinicians should not blame the child and parents for the child's problems. It is likely that the family has already faced a lot of blame from others and doing the same will surely make it difficult for them to engage.
- *Reframing:* The therapist must look at the child's difficulties in a positive way. For example, if parents are concerned about their son engaging in gang-based activities where he leads and manages the gang, positive skills like leadership and team-working should be highlighted. A parent who is seen as "nagging and controlling" by the young person, can be instead labeled as "caring and concerned" by the therapist. Families are encouraged to see themselves as doing the best to their abilities and what is possible under the given circumstances. Reframing also shows to the family that even if they have made mistakes, the therapist is willing to look at the positives.
- *Behavioral training:* A lot of principles that have been discussed under parenting are used here. The focus is on communicating with the child in a way that helps him/her get feedback and improve. The desirable behaviors should be discussed with the young person and targets should be set. Parents should avoid arguing in front of the young person and instead use social behaviors that they want the young person to emulate.
- *Generalization:* The goal is to help the young person to use his learnings in other settings beyond the family.

Multimodal Treatment

In late childhood and adolescence, especially with more severe conduct problems, various modalities need to be combined together for more holistic management. This includes integrating family strategies, behavioral strategies, and CBT.[67] The most established treatment model using this approach is multisystemic therapy.[68]

Multidimensional Treatment Foster Care is another approach for working with children and families who are in need of a high level of support due to high levels of abuse and neglect, severe mental health and behavioral problems, and problems with juvenile delinquency.[69]

Pharmacotherapy

Medications should not be used in ODD or CD on a routine basis as there is poor evidence to support that.

Pharmacotherapy is indicated especially when there is a comorbid disorder, e.g., ADHD.

Individuals with CD and high levels of reactive aggression and severe emotion dysregulation may be given antipsychotics if other nonpharmacological measures have not worked or to tide over an acute crisis.[70]

Risperidone has the best evidence base.[71] Antipsychotics may also be considered in comorbid intellectual disability where they may be more effective.[70] Whenever an antipsychotic is used, it must be on a short-term basis with a specific target symptom. Dosages must be kept on a low side to avoid side effects such as extrapyramidal and metabolic syndrome.

Stimulants like methylphenidate may be effective for comorbid ADHD. Overall methylphenidate and low-dose antipsychotics are the most commonly used medications in conduct problems in children with ADHD.[70]

There is some low-quality evidence for the use of atomoxetine, anticonvulsants (valproate or carbamazepine), selective serotonin reuptake inhibitors (SSRIs), lithium, clonidine, β-blockers in managing aggression.[2] They may be considered in individual cases if other measures have failed or to manage a specific comorbidity like depression where use of SSRI would be recommended.

SUMMARY AND CONCLUSION

Disruptive behavioral disorders are one of the most common mental health problems in children and adolescents. They are usually comorbid with other disorders like ADHD. Psychosocial and contextual factors play a key role in diagnosis and management and should be assessed thoroughly. Careful assessment of the disorder, comorbidities as well as prognostic factors should be done. Psychological treatment including psychoeducation, parent management training, and multisystemic therapy are the first choice of management. Pharmacological treatment is indicated in more severe cases and for the comorbid conditions.

REFERENCES

1. American Psychiatric Association (Ed). Diagnostic and Statistical Manual of Mental Disorders: DSM-5. 5th edition. Washington, DC, US: American Psychiatric Association; 2013.
2. Sagar R, Patra BN, Patil V. Clinical practice guidelines for the management of conduct disorder. Indian J Psychiatry. 2019;61:270-6.
3. Scott S. Oppositional and conduct disorders. In: Thapar A, Pine DS, Leckman JF, Scott S, Snowling MJ, Taylor E, (Eds). Rutter's Child and Adolescent Psychiatry. 6th edition. UK: John Wiley and Sons, Ltd; 2015.
4. Moffitt TE. Adolescence-limited and life-course-persistent antisocial behavior: a developmental taxonomy. Psychol Rev. 1993;100(4):674-701.
5. Poulin F, Boivin M. Reactive and proactive aggression: evidence of a two-factor model. Psychol Assess. 2000;12(2):115-22.
6. Meltzer H, Gatward R, Goodman R, Ford T. Mental health of children and adolescents in Great Britain. Int Rev Psychiatry. 2003;15(1-2):185-7.
7. Nock MK, Kazdin AE, Hiripi E, Kessler RC. Lifetime prevalence, correlates, and persistence of oppositional defiant disorder: results from the National Comorbidity Survey Replication. J Child Psychol Psychiatry. 2007;48(7):703-13.
8. Moore AA, Silberg JL, Roberson-Nay R, Mezuk B. Life course persistent and adolescence limited conduct disorder in a nationally representative US sample: prevalence, predictors, and outcomes. Soc Psychiatry Psychiatr Epidemiol. 2017;52(4):435-43.
9. Bornovalova MA, Hicks BM, Iacono WG, et al. Familial transmission and heritability of childhood disruptive disorders. Am J Psychiatry. 2010;167(9):1066-74.
10. Keenan K, Shaw D. Exploring the etiology of antisocial behaviour. In: Lahey BB, Moffitt TE, Caspi A (Eds). Causes of Conduct Disorder and Juvenile Delinquency. New York, NY: The Guilford Press; 2003. pp. 153-81.
11. Thapar A, Cooper M, Eyre O, Langley K. What have we learnt about the causes of ADHD?. J Child Psychol Psychiatry. 2013;54(1):3-16.
12. Burt SA. Are there meaningful etiological differences within antisocial behavior? Results of a meta-analysis. Clin Psychol Rev. 2009;29(2):163-78.
13. Viding E, Jones AP, Frick PJ, Moffitt TE, Plomin R. Heritability of antisocial behaviour at 9: do callous-unemotional traits matter? Dev Sci. 2008;11(1):17-22.

14. Kendler KS, Jacobson K, Myers JM, Eaves LJ. A genetically informative developmental study of the relationship between conduct disorder and peer deviance in males. Psychol Med. 2008;38(7): 1001-11.
15. Rowe R, Costello EJ, Angold A, Copeland WE, Maughan B. Developmental pathways in oppositional defiant disorder and conduct disorder. J Abnorm Psychol. 2010;119(4):726-38.
16. Dick DM, Aliev F, Krueger RF, Edwards A, Agrawal A, Lynskey M, et al. Genome-wide association study of conduct disorder symptomatology. Mol Psychiatry. 2011;16(8):800-8.
17. Hewitt JK, Silberg JL, Rutter M, Simonoff E, Meyer JM, Maes H, et al. Genetics and developmental psychopathology: 1. Phenotypic assessment in the Virginia Twin Study of Adolescent Behavioral Development. J Child Psychol Psychiatry. 1997;38(8):943-63.
18. Mikolajewski AJ, Taylor J, Iacono WG. Oppositional defiant disorder dimensions: genetic influences and risk for later psychopathology. J Child Psychol Psychiatry. 2017;58(6):702-10.
19. Gaysina D, Fergusson DM, Leve LD, Horwood J, Reiss D, Shaw DS, et al. Maternal smoking during pregnancy and offspring conduct problems: evidence from 3 independent genetically sensitive research designs. JAMA Psychiatry. 2013;70(9):956-63.
20. Popova S, Lange S, Shield K, Mihic A, Chudley AE, Mukherjee RAS, et al. Comorbidity of fetal alcohol spectrum disorder: a systematic review and meta-analysis. Lancet. 2016;387(10022):978-87.
21. Ruisch IH, Dietrich A, Glennon JC, Buitelaar JK, Hoekstra PJ. Maternal substance use during pregnancy and offspring conduct problems: A meta-analysis. Neurosci Biobehav Rev. 2018;84:325-36.
22. Sandman CA, Curran MM, Davis EP, Glynn LM, Head K, Baram TZ. Cortical Thinning and Neuropsychiatric Outcomes in Children Exposed to Prenatal Adversity: A Role for Placental CRH? Am J Psychiatry. 2018;175(5):471-9.
23. Raine A, Brennan P, Mednick SA. Interaction between birth complications and early maternal rejection in predisposing individuals to adult violence: specificity to serious, early-onset violence. Am J Psychiatry. 1997;154(9):1265-71.
24. Rutter M, Giller H, Hagell A. Antisocial Behaviour by Young People. Cambridge: Cambridge University Press; 1998.
25. Jaffee SR, Strait LB, Odgers CL. From correlates to causes: can quasi-experimental studies and statistical innovations bring us closer to identifying the causes of antisocial behavior? Psychol Bull. 2012;138(2):272-95.
26. Kim-Cohen J, Caspi A, Taylor A, Williams B, Newcombe R, Craig IW, et al. MAOA, maltreatment, and gene-environment interaction predicting children's mental health: new evidence and a meta-analysis. Mol Psychiatry. 2006;11(10): 903-13.
27. Norman RE, Byambaa M, De R, Butchart A, Scott J, Vos T. The long-term health consequences of child physical abuse, emotional abuse, and neglect: a systematic review and meta-analysis. PLoS Med. 2012;9(11):e1001349.
28. Boivin M, Brendgen M, Vitaro F, Forget-Dubois N. Evidence of gene-environment correlation for peer difficulties: disruptive behaviors predict early peer relation difficulties in school through genetic effects. Dev Psychopathol. 2013;25(1):79-92.
29. Scott M. Conduct disorders. In: Rey JM (Ed). IACAPAP e-Textbook of Child and Adolescent Mental Health. Geneva: International Association for Child and Adolescent Psychiatry and Allied Professions; 2012.
30. Stringaris A, Maughan B, Goodman R. What's in a disruptive disorder? Temperamental antecedents of oppositional defiant disorder: findings from the Avon longitudinal study. J Am Acad Child Adolesc Psychiatry. 2010;49(5):474-83.
31. Rutter M, Moffitt TE, Caspi A. Gene-environment interplay and psychopathology: multiple varieties but real effects. J Child Psychol Psychiatry. 2006;47(3-4):226-61.
32. Caspi A, McClay J, Moffitt TE, Mill J, Martin J, Craig IW, et al. Role of genotype in the cycle of violence in maltreated children. Science. 2002;297(5582):851-4.
33. Fergusson DM, Boden JM, Horwood LJ, Miller AL, Kennedy MA. MAOA, abuse exposure and antisocial behaviour: 30-year longitudinal study. Br J Psychiatry. 2011;198(6):457-63.
34. Fairchild G, Baker E, Eaton S. Hypothalamic-Pituitary-Adrenal Axis Function in Children and

Adults with Severe Antisocial Behavior and the Impact of Early Adversity. Curr Psychiatry Rep. 2018;20(10):84.

35. Koss KJ, Gunnar MR. Annual Research Review: Early adversity, the hypothalamic-pituitary-adrenocortical axis, and child psychopathology. J Child Psychol Psychiatry. 2018;59(4):327-46.
36. Goodman R, Simonoff E, Stevenson J. The impact of child IQ, parent IQ and sibling IQ on child behavioural deviance scores. J Child Psychol Psychiatry. 1995;36(3):409-25.
37. Loeber R, Menting B, Lynam DR, Moffitt TE, Stouthamer-Loeber M, Stallings R, et al. Findings from the Pittsburgh Youth Study: cognitive impulsivity and intelligence as predictors of the age-crime curve. J Am Acad Child Adolesc Psychiatry. 2012;51(11):1136-49.
38. Petersen IT, Bates JE, D'Onofrio BM, Coyne CA, Lansford JE, Dodge KA, et al. Language ability predicts the development of behavior problems in children. J Abnorm Psychol. 2013;122(2):542-57.
39. Murray J, Farrington DP. Risk factors for conduct disorder and delinquency: key findings from longitudinal studies. Can J Psychiatry. 2010;55(10):633-42.
40. Ogilvie JM, Stewart AL, Chan RCK, DHK. Neuropsychological measures of executive function and antisocial behavior: A meta-analysis. Criminology. 2011;49:1063-107.
41. Fontaine RG, Tanha M, Yang C, Dodge KA, Bates JE, Pettit GS. Does response evaluation and decision (RED) mediate the relation between hostile attributional style and antisocial behavior in adolescence? J Abnorm Child Psychol. 2010;38(5):615-26.
42. Fontaine NMG, McCrory EJP, Boivin M, Moffitt TE, Viding E. Predictors and outcomes of joint trajectories of callous-unemotional traits and conduct problems in childhood. J Abnorm Psychol. 2011;120(3):730-42.
43. Fairchild G, Passamonti L, Hurford G, Hagan CC, von dem Hagen EA, van Goozen SH, et al. Brain structure abnormalities in early-onset and adolescent-onset conduct disorder. Am J Psychiatry. 2011;168(6):624-33.
44. Hobson CW, Scott S, Rubia K. Investigation of cool and hot executive function in ODD/CD independently of ADHD. J Child Psychol Psychiatry. 2011;52(10):1035-43.
45. Kim-Cohen J, Arseneault L, Caspi A, Tomás MP, Taylor A, Moffitt TE. Validity of DSM-IV conduct disorder in 41/2-5-year-old children: a longitudinal epidemiological study. Am J Psychiatry. 2005;162(6):1108-17.
46. Goodman R. The Strengths and Difficulties Questionnaire: a research note. J Child Psychol Psychiatry. 1997;38(5):581-6.
47. Achenbach TM, Edelbrock C. Manual for the child behavior checklist and revised child behavior profile. Burlington: University of Vermont, Department of Psychiatry; 1983.
48. Conners CK, Barkley RA. Rating scales and checklists for child psychopharmacology. Psychopharmacology Bulletin. 1985;21:809-43.
49. Sorsa J, Fontell T, Laajasalo T, Aronen ET. Eyberg Child Behavior Inventory (ECBI): Normative data, psychometric properties, and associations with socioeconomic status in Finnish children. Scand J Psychol. 2019;60(5):430-9.
50. Malhotra S, Varma VK, Verma SK, Malhotra A. Childhood psychopathology meausrement schedule: development and standardization. Indian J Psychiatry. 1988;30(4):325-31.
51. Shaffer D, Fisher P, Lucas C. The Diagnostic Interview Schedule for Children (DISC). In: Hilsenroth MJ, Segal DL (Eds). Comprehensive Handbook of Psychological Assessment. Personality Assessment. Canada, New Jersey: John Wiley and Sons, 2004. pp. 256-70.
52. Kaufman J, Birmaher B, Brent D, Rao U, Flynn C, Moreci P, et al. Schedule for Affective Disorders and Schizophrenia for School-Age Children-Present and Lifetime Version (K-SADS-PL): initial reliability and validity data. J Am Acad Child Adolesc Psychiatry. 1997;36(7):980-8.
53. Angold A, Prendergast M, Cox A, Harrington R, Simonoff E, Rutter M. The Child and Adolescent Psychiatric Assessment (CAPA). Psychol Med. 1995;25(4):739-53.
54. Snyder HR, Young JF, Hankin BL. Strong Homotypic Continuity in Common Psychopathology-, Internalizing-, and Externalizing-Specific Factors Over Time in Adolescents. Clin Psychol Sci. 2017;5(1):98-110.

55. Fergusson DM, Horwood LJ, Ridder EM. Show me the child at seven: the consequences of conduct problems in childhood for psychosocial functioning in adulthood. J Child Psychol Psychiatry. 2005;46(8):837-49.
56. Olino TM, Seeley JR, Lewinsohn PM. Conduct disorder and psychosocial outcomes at age 30: early adult psychopathology as a potential mediator. J Abnorm Child Psychol. 2010;38(8): 1139-49.
57. Kazdin AE, Glick A, Pope J, Kaptchuk TJ, Lecza B, Carrubba E, et al. Parent management training for conduct problems in children: Enhancing treatment to improve therapeutic change. Int J Clin Health Psychol. 2018;18(2):91-101.
58. Webster-Stratton C, Hammond M. Treating children with early-onset conduct problems: a comparison of child and parent training interventions. J Consult Clin Psychol. 1997;65(1): 93-109.
59. Webster-Stratton C, Rinaldi J, Jamila MR. Long-Term Outcomes of Incredible Years Parenting Program: Predictors of Adolescent Adjustment. Child Adolesc Ment Health. 2011;16(1):38-46.
60. Scott S, Spender Q, Doolan M, Jacobs B, Aspland H. Multicentre controlled trial of parenting groups for childhood antisocial behaviour in clinical practice. BMJ. 2001;323(7306):194-8.
61. de Graaf I, Speetjens P, Smit F, de Wolff M, Tavecchio L. Effectiveness of the Triple P Positive Parenting Program on behavioral problems in children: a meta-analysis. Behav Modif. 2008;32(5):714-35.
62. Bor W, Sanders MR, Markie-Dadds C. The effects of the Triple P-Positive Parenting Program on preschool children with co-occurring disruptive behavior and attentional/hyperactive difficulties. J Abnorm Child Psychol. 2002;30(6):571-87.
63. Scott S. An update on interventions for conduct disorder. Adv Psychiatr Treat. 2008;14(1):61-70.
64. Lochman J, Magee TN, Pardini DA. Cognitive-behavioral interventions for children with conduct problems. In: Reinecke MA, Clarck DA (Eds). Cognitive Therapy Across the Lifespan: Evidence and Practice. Cambridge: Cambridge University Press; 2003.
65. Lochman JE, Boxmeyer CL, Kassing FL, Powell NP, Stromeyer SL. Cognitive Behavioral Intervention for Youth at Risk for Conduct Problems: Future Directions. J Clin Child Adolesc Psychol. 2019;48(5):799-810.
66. Alexander JF, Pugh C, Parsons BV, Sexton TL. Functional family therapy. In: Elliott DS (Eds). Blueprints for Violence Prevention (Book 3), 2nd edition. Boulder, CO: Center for the Study and Prevention of Violence, Institute of Behavioral Science, University of Colorad; 2000.
67. Garland AF, Hawley KM, Brookman-Frazee L, Hurlburt MS. Identifying common elements of evidence-based psychosocial treatments for children's disruptive behavior problems. J Am Acad Child Adolesc Psychiatry. 2008;47(5): 505-14.
68. Huey SJ Jr, Henggeler SW, Brondino MJ, Pickrel SG. Mechanisms of change in multisystemic therapy: reducing delinquent behavior through therapist adherence and improved family and peer functioning. J Consult Clin Psychol. 2000;68(3):451-67.
69. Chamberlain P. The Oregon Multidimensional Treatment Foster Care model: Features, outcomes, and progress in dissemination. Cogn Behav. Pract. 2003;10(4):303-12.
70. Fairchild G, Hawes DJ, Frick PJ, Copeland WE, Odgers CL, Franke B, et al. Conduct disorder. Nat Rev Dis Primers. 2019;5(1):43.
71. Loy JH, Merry SN, Hetrick SE, Stasiak K. Atypical antipsychotics for disruptive behaviour disorders in children and youths. Cochrane Database Syst Rev. 2017;8(8):CD008559.

CHAPTER 11

Mood Disorders, Affect Dysregulation, and Related Conditions

Preeti Kandasamy, Rajeev Jairam, Janardhan Reddy YC, Shoba Srinath

INTRODUCTION

Affect dysregulation in particular and mood disorders in general are a common and complex clinical issue in child and adolescent psychiatry and debate about their prevalence, diagnosis, and treatment approaches have existed over many decades.[1,2] Bipolar disorders (BDs) cover a wide range of clinical presentations among children and adolescents and are often underdiagnosed or misdiagnosed.[3] Apart from the complexity that the disorder poses, the developmental aspects can make it challenging to clinch the diagnosis and plan interventions.[3-5] Often symptoms do not fit classical descriptions of classificatory systems. It takes enormous effort in terms of serial observation and careful assessment to rule out close differential diagnosis to conclusively arrive at the final diagnosis and plan effective management.[6] Early identification of BD among youth has gained recognition, and there seems to be greater acceptance although there are some differences in recommendations provided by international guidelines.[7,8]

Early diagnosis and intervention are important for any child psychiatric disorder; however, planning interventions when mood symptoms are subsyndromal but still impairing is another challenge to the treating clinician and the child's care system. Pre-existing comorbid disorders can complicate matters further. Pharmacotherapies approved for children and adolescents are few and successful management of an episode and restoring functional gain is often a tough journey.[4] Early onset BD may affect key developmental skills, and it is important to understand the long-term outcome of the disorder.[8,9]

This chapter discusses some of the practical challenges that a (child) psychiatrist faces, current recommendations provided by practice guidelines, navigating unclear clinical situations, and processes involved in facilitating informed decision-making. Recommendations based on Indian studies are provided which could help clinicians and families understand the long-term outcome of BD and take a balanced approach to carefully weigh the risk-benefit of prophylactic interventions during critical developmental periods of young children.[10-14]

The main focus of this chapter is to cover BD and disruptive mood dysregulation disorder (DMDD) from an Indian perspective.

BIPOLAR DISORDER

Prevalence

Globally, the prevalence of pediatric BD is 1 in 200 and subthreshold BDs account for 4.3%. BD in the pediatric population is estimated to be 1.8%, and BD I accounts for 1.2%.[15-17] Indian studies report a prevalence of 2.1%.[18]

Reviews and narrative analyses have noted that the prevalence of pediatric BD has not increased.[19,20] However, there has been a significant increase in hospitalization over the years,[21] possibly because of greater awareness.

Phenomenology and Developmental Perspective

Bipolar disorder among youth presents with more mixed features, is more impairing, and has a poorer prognosis compared to adult BD.[19] Diagnosing mood disorders among children and adolescents essentially follows the same criteria with some exceptions provided for irritable mood and weight loss.[12] Diagnostic evaluation can be challenging when young children present with mood dysregulation, as current diagnostic classifications are not developmentally well-informed.[1]

Most common clinical symptoms include an (acute) onset of increased energy, irritability, mood lability, distractibility, goal-directed activity (72–79%), euphoria or elated mood, pressured speech, hyperactivity, racing thoughts, poor judgment (61–64%), grandiosity, inappropriate laughter, decreased need for sleep, and flight of ideas (54–57%).[22,23] Highly specific symptoms include elated mood and a decreased need for sleep; nonspecific symptoms include irritability, distractibility, and poor judgment.[22]

Studies from India have reported pressure of speech, irritability, elation, distractibility, increased self-esteem, expansive mood, flight of ideas, and grandiose delusions.[11] Other common presentations may include psychomotor agitation, anger, aggression, temper tantrums, reduced concentration, reduced sleep, defiance, and hyperactivity.[11]

Clinical Assessment and Diagnosis

Typical symptoms occur in later episodes; attenuated mood symptoms and sleep disturbance are often the common early symptom presentations.[2,6] A detailed history, inquiry about symptoms, their evolution, episodicity, early development, temperament, comorbid attention-deficit/hyperactivity disorder (ADHD), anxiety, family history, longitudinal course, and medication used if any and responses preferably from multiple informants supported with serial mental status examinations and observation should be conducted in a developmentally sensitive approach.[19,22,24]

In young children, elated mood, grandiosity, and racing thoughts help differentiate early-onset bipolar from ADHD.[25] When in doubt structured instruments such as K-SADS have been found more useful to differentiate clinically relevant symptoms compared to rating scales.[25,26]

Comorbid medical disorders, organicity, and substance use disorders need to be ruled out. Baseline investigations should include BMI, thyroid function test, renal function test, liver function test, complete hemogram, and ECG as indicated. Imaging, EEG, and neurological workup may be completed when organicity is suspected, especially in a child with very early onset of illness, atypical features, and in the absence of a family history of mood disorder.

Structured interviews and scales may assist in establishing the diagnosis and assess severity and functional impairment.[27] Commonly used instruments include:

- Mini-International Neuropsychiatric Interview for Children and Adolescents (MINI KID)[28]
- Kiddie Schedule for Affective Disorders and Schizophrenia-Present and Lifetime Version (K-SADS-PL)[26]
- Young Mania Rating Scale for children 5–17 years[29]
- Child Mania Rating Scale-Parent Version[30,31]
- Children's Depression Inventory (CDI)[32]
- Children's Depression Rating Scale (CDRS)[33]
- Center for Epidemiological Studies for Depression Scale for Children (CES-DC)[34]

Family history and past history should be elicited in detail to avoid misdiagnosis and drug-induced switch. Families should be explained the importance of these clinical details in deciding the choice of medication, and they should be given adequate time to bring up any relevant history on more than one occasion. Taking history independently from parents may help as they may be apprehensive to admit.

Understanding family pathology and dynamics is an important aspect of assessment. Instruments such as the North Carolina Family Assessment Scale, Psychosocial Schedule for School-Age Children–Revised, or WHO-Parent Interview schedule may be used.[35-37] Family history of ADHD, anxiety, mood disorder, and expressed emotions need to be explored, and potentially modifiable risk factors should be addressed.

Comorbidities

Co-occurring disorders are high among youth with BD and include ADHD, disruptive behavior disorders (DBD), anxiety disorders, obsessive-compulsive disorder (OCD), autism spectrum disorders, and substance use disorders.[38] Comorbid ADHD or anxiety is associated with more severe mood symptoms with impairment in neurocognitive and global functioning and an unfavorable clinical outcome.[11,17] Those with comorbid ADHD and DBD have an earlier age at onset and tend to remain ill for a longer duration.[39]

Course and Outcome

Geller et al. examined the continuity of child bipolar into adulthood over 8 years of follow-up and found that 44.4% had manic episodes after 18 years of age. Later episodes were similar to the initial episode with the presence of psychosis and ultradian cycling; however, it was relatively shorter than the first episode.[40]

Long-term outcome studies throw light on the trajectory of the illness.[8,9] The Longitudinal Assessment of Manic Symptoms (LAMS) study found that manic symptoms decreased over 24 months.[41] The Course and Outcome of Bipolar Youth Study (COBY) found that 82% recovered from their index mood episode after 2.5 years; 63% experienced recurrence 1.5 years after recovery.[42] BD-II and BD-NOS may be less stable across the lifespan; 25% of BD-II may later develop BD-I, 38% with BD-NOS later convert to BD-I or II over the course of 4 years.[42]

Early onset, longer symptom duration, lower socioeconomic status, BD-NOS, and the presence of psychotic symptoms predicted poor outcomes.[43] Compared to adults, adolescents with BD-I are more symptomatic and have mixed and cycling episodes with switch in polarity.[43] The presence of severe depression, suicidality, poor quality of life, and minority race among adolescents predicted a more symptomatic course.[44]

Prospective Indian studies conducted over 4–5 years with 30 subjects found 100% recovery from the index episode with low chronicity.[2] High rates of recurrence in the first 2 years were observed, with 72.4% of relapses occurring while on medication.[8,45] Similar observations were made in a retrospective review of 139 subjects; of the 35% who relapsed 89% occurred in the first 2 years.[13]

Interventions

Pharmacotherapy for Acute Mania

Monotherapy with second-generation antipsychotics (SGA) is effective for acute management of Mania.[45] Lithium and atypical antipsychotics are generally safe and effective for short-term management and FDA has approved risperidone, aripiprazole, quetiapine for children and adolescents 10–17 years, olanzapine for those 13–17 years, and lithium for children >12 years.[22,46] Meta-analyses show greater efficacy of SGAs compared to mood stabilizers. Increased weight and prolactin levels are associated with risperidone.[47] Olanzapine although efficacious has safety concerns.[48]

Pharmacotherapy for Maintenance

According to international guidelines for BD lithium, quetiapine, divalproex, lamotrigine, asenapine, aripiprazole, and quetiapine/aripiprazole in combination with lithium or divalproex are considered first-line treatment for maintenance therapy. Second-line treatments include risperidone, olanzapine, carbamazepine, paliperidone, and lurasidone/ziprasidone in combination with lithium or divalproex.[48]

Prospective follow-up studies from India support early prophylaxis with lithium.[2,8] In a systematic chart review from a tertiary care child psychiatry center, 90% of children with pediatric BD were started on thymoleptics following the index episode.[9] Lithium was among the most commonly prescribed in 85%, followed by valproate in 18% and 13% required a combination of mood stabilizers; 68% were on antipsychotics either alone or in combination with mood stabilizers.[9] Nearly 100% recovery from index episode was noted.[9,13] In another Indian study on early-onset BD, 51% were on lithium; 27.6% on valproate, 9.2% on risperidone, and 8.5% on carbamazepine.[49] Aripiprazole is approved for maintenance, and divalproex is not superior to lithium during the maintenance phase and should be used with caution among adolescent girls.[4] **Box 1** lists the various psychotropics that can be used in management of mood disorders in children and adolescents. **Box 2** provides the dosage and serum levels of the mood stabilizers.

Given high rates of relapse during crucial developmental periods, long-term maintenance needs to be discussed with the family soon after the first episode.[2] A thorough risk-benefit assessment and facilitation of informed decision-making by the parents is advised.[2,6,41]

BOX 1: List of various psychotropics used in mood disorders.[18,22,48]

For manic/mixed episodes:
- Lithium
- Valproate
- Risperidone
- Olanzapine
- Quetiapine
- Aripiprazole
- Ziprasidone
- Asenapine

For bipolar depression:
- Lithium
- Valproate
- Lamotrigine
- Quetiapine
- Lurasidone with lithium/valproate

For maintenance:
- Aripiprazole
- Lithium
- Valproate
- Lamotrigine

BOX 2: Dosage and serum levels of common mood stabilizers.[18,22,50]

- *Lithium:* 10–30 mg/kg/day
  - *Ser lithium:* 0.6–1.0 mmol/L
  - Steady state in 4–5 days
- *Valproate:* 15–30 mg/kg/day
  - *Serum valproate:* 50–125 mg/L (<100)
  - Steady state in 2–3 days
  - *ER:* Sample to be taken just before next dose (21–24 hours)

Pharmacotherapy for Bipolar Depression

Lithium, valproate, lamotrigine, and quetiapine are recommended as the first line, and lurasidone in combination with lithium or valproate as the second line.[17,48] Quetiapine has less evidence among depressed children compared to adults.[51] Aripiprazole has been shown to be ineffective as a monotherapy for bipolar depression.[48] For adolescents with partial response, a combination of lamotrigine and lithium may be considered.[18]

Pharmacotherapy for Comorbid Attention-deficit/Hyperactivity Disorder

In the presence of comorbid ADHD, mood disorder takes precedence in management.

If ADHD persists anti-ADHD preferably clonidine may be considered in the dose range of 3–7 μg/kg body weight/day in divided doses. Stimulants are best avoided to prevent manic induction.[52] Once manic/mixed symptoms are treated, under the cover of mood stabilizes and antipsychotics stimulants can be cautiously considered. Comorbid anxiety disorder or OCD is best treated with cognitive-behavior therapy. A subset of children may require selective serotonin reuptake inhibitor (SSRI) under the cover of a mood stabilizer/atypical antipsychotic when symptoms are severe or nonpharmacological interventions do not help. Children with ASD and ADHD have a greater risk for mood disorders with increasing age. Careful screening and observation are necessary to elicit mood disorders in children with neurodevelopmental disorders.

Psychosocial Management

More can be done in routine clinical practice to educate the young person and family about the nature of the disorder, the need for compliance with medication, and early recognition of changes in mood. Evidence supports the effectiveness of psychosocial interventions both in acute and maintenance treatment of early-onset BD.[22,53] It has been shown to reduce recurrence risk by 15%.[48]

The following are the evidence-based psychosocial interventions:[4]

- Psychoeducation about the risk of recurrence[48]
- Family-focused therapy—to improve functioning and decrease recurrence[54]
- Cognitive behavior therapy to enhance coping skills[55]
- Interpersonal and social rhythm therapy[56]

Electroconvulsive Therapy

Electroconvulsive therapy is considered for adolescents with severe and refractory symptoms.[45] The most common indication is the presence of catatonic symptoms.[57,58] It is recommended that the child be evaluated by two psychiatrists.[57] As per guidelines provided by the Mental Health Care Act, 2017, prior permission from the Mental Health Review Board is needed before planning modified ECT for minors.[58]

Duration of Treatment

The risk of recurrence is high in children and adolescents diagnosed with BD. Therefore, long-term maintenance treatment should be considered after the first bipolar episode. Since treatment adherence is central to favorable long-term outcomes, long-term maintenance treatment should be a negotiated decision with parents and the young person.

CASE VIGNETTE 1

A 14-year-old male child presented with complaints of reduced sleep, anxiety about the upcoming board examination, and crying spells. The child had normal development, no significant past history with family history of BD in paternal aunt. On mental status examination, he had anxious preoccupation about exams, ideas of hopelessness, active self-harm ideas, and depressed mood. A diagnosis of major depressive disorder made, pharmacotherapy was planned along with psychotherapy. The risk of a manic switch with SSRI in view of positive family history was discussed with the family. As there was also no clear indication to consider an antipsychotic or mood stabilizer for the current episode, weighing the risk-benefit ratio the child was started on low-dose SSRI (sertraline) under close monitoring after discussion with the family with the plan to consider lamotrigine or lithium in the event of any adverse behavioral side effects.[59]

The child tolerated low-dose SSRI and parents were advised to monitor closely with weekly follow-ups to monitor for behavioral activation/switch. The child improved at follow-up, therapy was continued, and follow-up was gradually spaced with advice to monitor early signs of hypomania/mania.

Six months later at follow-up, the child was noted to have complaints of increased activity, excessive grooming, posting inappropriate videos, reduced need for sleep, expressing expansive ideas, and lack of fear regarding the upcoming board examinations. On examination, psychomotor activity was increased, with flight of ideas, grandiose ideas, and elated mood. The diagnosis was revised to BD; SSRI was stopped and the child was started on lithium 300 mg and titrated to 750 mg with ser lithium of 0.8 mmol/L along with risperidone 4 mg/day and trihexyphenidyl 2 mg/day. Risperidone and trihexyphenidyl were tapered after the acute phase, and child was maintained on lithium for prophylaxis. The child improved and successfully completed his board examinations. The need for medication adherence was emphasized as the risk of recurrence is high and as the developmental age coincided with crucial academic years for the child. Interpersonal and social rhythm therapy was planned at the follow-up.

CASE VIGNETTE 2

A 9-year-old female child presented with increased activity, distractibility, anger outbursts, aggression, and reduced need for sleep. The child had history of reduced attention span, intrusive and impulsive behavior since early childhood. She was diagnosed to have ADHD and was on methylphenidate since 5 years of age and had shown improvement with it. There was no significant past or family history. On further clarification, there was a recent worsening in activity levels, frequent change in mood, anger outbursts, aggressive behavior with mood lability.

Child was also found to have racing thoughts and ideas about being a superhero and saving the world. She dressed like a superwomen and often engaged in high-risk behavior such as jumping from heights saying she could fly. Although child was known to talk excessively and watch superhero cartoons, these behaviors were not noted in the past. Child was also reported to be abusive and disrespectful toward teachers at school which was unlike her usual self. On mental status examination, child's psychomotor activity increased, there was flight of ideas, easy distractibility, and elated mood with grandiose ideas. Child was diagnosed with ADHD and BD. Risk of recurrence and benefit of mood stabilizers were explained. Family was apprehensive about considering mood stabilizer and preferred a trial of antipsychotic before taking a call on mood stabilizer. Methylphenidate was withheld, and aripiprazole was started considering child's high BMI and given its efficacy as maintenance therapy. Child started showing improvement with aripiprazole 7.5 mg. The plan was to consider reassessing need for anti-ADHD (clonidine/methylphenidate) at follow-up after adequately addressing mood symptoms. Family-focused therapy was also planned.

DISRUPTIVE MOOD DYSREGULATION DISORDER

Introduction

Emotional dysregulation is defined as an intense and rapid increase in emotionality with a low threshold and slow normalization.[60] While introduced for the first time in DSM-5, DMDD appears to share many characteristics of the earlier established "mixed disorders of emotions and conduct" (ICD 10).[61-63] Children manifest irritability, low frustration tolerance, and hyperarousal, and this is considered a prodrome for many mental disorders including mood disorders.[60] Long-term follow-up has shown an increased risk of unipolar depression, generalized anxiety disorder, ADHD, and greater socioacademic impairment, and less likelihood of having a parent diagnosed with BD and most do not convert to BD.[60,64] DMDD has significant overlap with BD and ODD, and it is important to rule out BD even if symptoms of DMDD are prominent.[25]

Prevalence

Disruptive mood dysregulation disorder is considered a childhood-onset depressive spectrum disorder characterized by persistent irritability and severe temper outbursts.[64,65] Prevalence of DMDD is estimated to range from 2.5 to 8.2% with the prevalence higher among preschool children compared to adolescents.[64]

Clinical Assessment and Diagnosis

There is currently a lack of evidence-based assessments to differentiate DMDD from other mood disorders.[24] Clinical presentation includes persistent irritability and frequent extreme behavioral dyscontrol. Nonepisodic irritability as against characteristic episodic mood swings in BD is the hallmark of DMDD.[64] Chronic irritability in the absence of manic symptoms shall not qualify for BD.[24]

Nearly 60% of children have a co-occurring behavioral or emotional disorder.[55] Indian studies have reported co-occurring conduct disorder, ADHD, anxiety, and academic decline among children with DMDD.[66,67] A diagnosis of DMDD cannot coexist with ODD, BD, and intermittent explosive disorder.

Studies have reported comorbid ADHD in 72%, ODD in 36%, CD in 27%, and anxiety disorder in about 50%.[65] It is likely that temperamental difficulties in children may complicate the clinical presentation of mood disorders. This is well known among adults with a personality disorder and inquiry into depressive symptoms and its equivalents is warranted.

Interventions

Comorbidities in DMDD often determine pharmacotherapy. Studies have noted that prescription rates for ADHD medications, antipsychotics, and antidepressants were higher among children with DMDD.[65] Nearly 60% of children with DMDD received ADHD medications compared to 34% among the BD group.[65] Parental training for young children and cognitive behavior therapy for adolescents is recommended[64] although it is challenging to implement in the presence of acute symptoms. More research data is needed on the course and outcome of DMDD.

CASE VIGNETTE 3

A 9-year-old boy presented with history of increased irritability, excessive engagement in gadget use, and school refusal for the past year with progressive worsening over the past month. The child also had episodes of intense anger outbursts and aggression with prolonged dysregulation when his demands were not met. On further clarification, the child had persistent irritability, delayed sleep onset, decreased appetite, and reduced interest in personal care. There was no history of elated mood, grandiosity, or pervasive low mood and the course was nonepisodic. He was developmentally normal and temperamentally difficult. A family history of mood disorder was reported in the father, but details regarding his past treatment were not available. The child was not cooperative for formal evaluation and displayed a similar episode of intense and prolonged anger outburst. The child was admitted for evaluation and management, a diagnosis of DMDD was made, and he was started on antipsychotics along with a short trial of low-dose benzodiazepine. Irritability and biological functions improved over the next few days. The child had significant anxiety related to school return. On further assessment, comorbid anxiety disorder was established, and CBT was planned for anxiety.

CASE VIGNETTE 4

A 7-year-old female child presented with irritability, crying spells, anger outbursts, and sleep disturbance over the past year with progressive worsening over the past 3 months. Anger episodes were severely characterized by head banging and hitting with prolonged dysregulation. The child had a background of speech delay and hyperactivity in the past which had improved with therapy. There was a family history of OCD in the father. A trial of low-dose antipsychotics was started in divided doses. Parental counseling was done regarding the nature of the problem, and inputs on parent training were provided for improving functioning of the child. The child's sleep improved; however, her irritable mood, crying and anger persisted, and the family was distressed. After a discussion with the family, the child was started on low-dose SSRI with weekly monitoring. The child started showing improvement over the next 2 weeks with 2.5 mg of escitalopram.

Discussion: Behavioral interventions should be considered first-line in any young child with mild-moderate severity of symptoms. An adequate trial of behavioral therapy for 8–12 weeks should be considered before considering pharmacotherapy. When symptoms are intense and severe, pharmacotherapy may be indicated along with behavioral interventions. Although the risk of behavioral activation and switch is <2% with SSRI, there is apprehension among clinicians and families regarding this, in an already dysregulated child.68 However, when done with careful evaluation, slow titration, close monitoring, and adequate discussion with family, young children with DMDD may benefit from SSRI.

SUMMARY AND CONCLUSION

Typical symptoms of BD occur in later episodes. Detailed history and inquiry for specific symptoms, serial mental status examinations, and observation are needed to ascertain the diagnosis, and comorbid conditions. Common comorbidities include ADHD and anxiety disorders. Past history and family history need careful elicitation and often help in preventing misdiagnosis. Risperidone, aripiprazole, quetiapine, and olanzapine are among the SGA approved for older children and adolescents. Aripiprazole is approved for maintenance. For bipolar depression, lithium, valproate, lamotrigine, quetiapine, and lurasidone in combination with lithium or valproate are recommended. Quetiapine has less evidence for effectiveness among children. Evidence supports the effectiveness of psychosocial interventions both in acute and maintenance treatment of early-onset BD and has been shown to reduce recurrence risk. The risk of recurrence is high in children and adolescents diagnosed with BD. Therefore, long-term maintenance treatment should be considered after first bipolar episode. Since treatment adherence is central to favorable long-term outcomes, long-term maintenance treatment should be a negotiated decision with parents. In the presence of comorbid ADHD, BD takes precedence in management. When indicated clonidine may be preferred over other medications for ADHD. Stimulants can be given cautiously under cover of mood stabilizers and antipsychotics. DMDD is characterized by chronic irritability and extreme temper outbursts. Comorbidities determine pharmacotherapy. Common comorbid conditions include ADHD, conduct disorders, major depression, and anxiety disorders. A diagnosis of DMDD cannot coexist with ODD, BD, and intermittent explosive disorder. Long-term outcome studies report a greater prevalence of depression, anxiety disorder, and ADHD among children with DMDD. Children with neurodevelopmental disorders also have a greater risk for mood disorders with increasing age. Accurate diagnosis is essential to initiate specific interventions and improve long-term outcomes among children and adolescents with mood disorders.

Early diagnosis is essential to initiate specific interventions and improve long-term outcomes in mood disorders among children and adolescents. Developmentally sensitive approach to evaluation and management is the key. While this chapter may address some of the common challenges, there may still be situations that remain unaddressed and require the knowledge and wisdom of the treating physician to choose what applies best to the individual child with parental consent. In very young children with complex clinical presentation referral/discussion with a child psychiatrist regarding management may be planned whenever feasible. Research data on early onset BD is still limited in the Indian context and need a larger focus to address many of the currently unanswered clinical questions for effective early diagnosis and management.

REFERENCES

1. Malhi GS, Jadidi M, Bell E. The diagnosis of bipolar disorder in children and adolescents: Past, present and future. Bipolar Disord. 2023;25(6):469-77.
2. Srinath S, Reddy YCJ, Girimaji SR, Seshadri SP, Subbakrishna DK. A prospective study of bipolar disorder in children and adolescents from India. Acta Psychiatr Scand. 1998:98;437-42.
3. Reddy Y, Shoba S. Review article: Juvenile bipolar disorder. Acta psychiatrica Scandinavica. 2000;102:162-70.
4. Jairam R, Prabhuswamy M, Dullur P. Do We Really Know How to Treat a Child with Bipolar Disorder or One with Severe Mood Dysregulation? Is There a Magic Bullet? Depress Res Treat. 2012:967302.
5. Chakrabarti S. Bipolar disorder in the International Classification of Diseases-Eleventh version: A review of the changes, their basis, and usefulness. World J Psychiatry. 2022;12(12):1335-55.
6. Preeti K, Jairam R, Srinath S. Affective Disorders—Current Status and Controversies. In: Malhotra S, Santosh P (Eds). Child and Adolescent Psychiatry. Springer, New Delhi; 2016. pp. 51-62.
7. Cahill C, Hanstock T, Jairam R, Hazell P, Walter G, Malhi GS. Comparison of diagnostic guidelines for juvenile bipolar disorder. Aust N Z J Psychiatry. 2007;41(6):479-84.
8. Jairam R, Hanstock T, Cahill C, Hazell PL, Walter GJ, Malhi GS. The changing face of bipolar disorder: adolescence to adulthood. Minerva Pediatrica. 2008;60(1):59-68.
9. Jairam R, Andreson R, Redwin R. "Paediatric Bipolar Disorder; Perspectives on Course and Outcome for the book, "New Developments in Mania Research". Nova Science Publishers NY; 2006.
10. Reddy YCJ, Srinath S, Jairam R. Paediatric bipolar disorder - from the perspective of India. In: Diler RS (Ed). Paediatric Bipolar Disorder - A global perspective. New York: Nova Science Publishers; 2007. pp. 91-107.
11. Reddy YCJ, Girimaji S, Shoba S. Clinical Profile of Mania in Children and Adolescents from the Indian Subcontinent. Canadian journal of psychiatry. Revue Canadienne de Psychiatrie. 1997;42:841-6.
12. Jairam R, Srinath S, Girimaji SC, Seshadri SP. A prospective 4-5 year follow-up of juvenile onset bipolar disorder. Bipolar Disord. 2004;6(5):386-94.
13. Rajeev J, Srinath S, Girimaji S, Seshadri SP, Singh P. A systematic chart review of the naturalistic course and treatment of early-onset bipolar disorder in a child and adolescent psychiatry center. Compr Psychiatry. 2004;45(2):148-54.
14. Pravin D, Rajkumar RP, Prabhuswamy, Srinath S, Girimaji S, Seshadri SP. Course and outcome of bipolar affective disorder in children. J. Indian Assoc. Child Adolesc Mental Health. 2005;1:15-23.
15. Van Meter AR, Moreira AL, Youngstrom EA. Meta-analysis of epidemiologic studies of pediatric bipolar disorder. J Clin Psychiatry. 2011;72:1250-6.
16. Cichoń L, Janas-Kozik M, Siwiec A, Rybakowski JK. Clinical picture and treatment of bipolar

affective disorder in children and adolescents. Psychiatr Pol. 2020;54(1):35-50.
17. Findling RL, Stepanova E, Youngstrom EA, Young AS. Progress in diagnosis and treatment of bipolar disorder among children and adolescents: an international perspective. Evid Based Ment Health. 2018;21:177-81.
18. Gautam S, Jain A, Gautam M, Gautam A, Jagawat T. Clinical Practice Guidelines for Bipolar Affective Disorder (BPAD) in Children and Adolescents. Indian J Psychiatry. 2019;61(S2):294-305.
19. Goldstein BI, Birmaher B. Prevalence, clinical presentation and differential diagnosis of pediatric bipolar disorder. Isr J Psychiatry Relat Sci. 2012;49(1):3-14.
20. Parry P, Allison S, Bastiampillai T. 'Pediatric Bipolar Disorder' rates are still lower than claimed: a re-examination of eight epidemiological surveys used by an updated meta-analysis. Int J Bipolar Disord. 2021;9(1):21.
21. Harpaz-Rotem I, Leslie D, Martin A, Rosenheck RA. Changes in child and adolescent inpatient psychiatric admission diagnoses between 1995 and 2000. Soc Psychiatry Psychiatr Epidemiol. 2005;40(8):642-27.
22. Findling RL, Jo B, Frazier TW, Youngstrom EA, Demeter CA, Fristad MA, et al. The 24-month course of manic symptoms in children. Bipolar Disord. 2013;15(6):669-79.
23. Youngstrom EA, Findling RL, Youngstrom JK, Calabrese JR. Toward an evidence-based assessment of pediatric bipolar disorder. J Clin Child Adolesc Psychol. 2005;34(3):433-48.
24. Goldstein B, Birmaher B, Carlson G, DelBello MP, Findling RL, Fristad M, et al. The International Society for Bipolar Disorders Task Force report on pediatric bipolar disorder: Knowledge to date and directions for future research. Bipolar Disord. 2017;19:524-43.
25. Geller B, Williams M, Zimerman B, Frazier J, Beringer L, Warner KL. Prepubertal and early adolescent bipolarity differentiate from ADHD by manic symptoms, grandiose delusions, ultra-rapid or ultradian cycling. J Affect Disord. 1998;51(2):81-91.
26. Kaufman J, Birmaher B, Brent D, Rao U, Flynn C, Moreci P, et al. Schedule for Affective Disorders and Schizophrenia for School-Age Children-Present and Lifetime Version (K-SADS-PL): initial reliability and validity data. J Am Acad Child Adolesc Psychiatry. 1997;36(7):980-8.
27. Youngstrom EA, Freeman AJ, Jenkins MM. The assessment of children and adolescents with bipolar disorder. Child Adolesc Psychiatr Clin N Am. 2009;18(2):353-90.
28. Sheehan DV, Sheehan KH, Shytle RD, Janavs J, Bannon Y, Rogers JE, et al. Reliability and validity of the Mini International Neuropsychiatric Interview for Children and Adolescents (MINI-KID). J Clin Psychiatry. 2010;71(3):313-26.
29. Youngstrom EA, Danielson CK, Findling RL, Gracious BL, Calabrese JR. Factor structure of the Young Mania Rating Scale for use with youths ages 5 to 17 years. J Clin Child Adolesc Psychol. 2002;31(4):567-72.
30. Pavuluri MN, Henry DB, Devineni B, Carbray JA, Birmaher B. Child mania rating scale: development, reliability, and validity. J Am Acad Child Adolesc Psychiatry. 2006;45(5):550-60.
31. Fristad MA, Weller EB, Weller RA. The Mania Rating Scale: Can It Be Used in Children? A Preliminary Report. J Am Acad Child Adolesc Psychiatry. 1992;31(2):252-7.
32. Kovacs M. Rating scales to assess depression in school-aged children. Acta Paedopsychiatr Int J Child Adolesc Psychiatry. 1981;46(5-6):305-15.
33. Mayes, TL, Bernstein IH, Haley CL, Kennard BD, Emslie GJ. Psychometric properties of the children's depression rating scale–revised in adolescents. J Child Adolesc Psychopharmacol. 2010;20(6):513-16.
34. Weissman MM, Orvaschel H, Padian N. Children's Symptom and Social Functioning Self-Report Scales Comparison of Mothers' and Children's Reports. J Nerv Ment Dis. 1980;168(12):736-40.
35. Reed-Ashcraft K, Kirk RS, Fraser MW. The reliability and validity of the North Carolina Family Assessment Scale. Res Soc Work Pract. 2001;11(4):503-20.
36. Puig-Antich J, Lukens E, Brent D. Psychosocial Schedule for School Age Children–Revised in 1986 and 1987. Pittsburgh, PA: Western Psychiatric Institute and Clinic; 1986.
37. Janca A, Chandrasekar CR. Parent Interview Schedule. In catalogue of assessment instruments used in the studies coordinated by the WHO

mental health programme. World Health Organization, Geneva; 1993.

38. Sesso G, Brancati GE, Masi G. Comorbidities in Youth with Bipolar Disorder: Clinical Features and Pharmacological Management. Curr Neuropharmacol. 2023;21(4):911-34.
39. Jaideep T, Reddy Y, Shoba S. Comorbidity of attention deficit hyperactivity disorder in juvenile bipolar disorder. Bipolar Disord. 2006;8:182-7.
40. Geller B, Tillman R, Bolhofner K, Zimerman B. Child Bipolar I Disorder: Prospective Continuity With Adult Bipolar I Disorder; Characteristics of Second and Third Episodes; Predictors of 8-Year Outcome. Arch Gen Psychiatry. 2008;65(10):1125-33.
41. Selvarajan S, Manohar H, Das S, Sakkarabani P, Kandasamy P. Lithium prophylaxis in early-onset Bipolar disorder: a descriptive study. Asian J Psychiatr. 2019;44:172-4.
42. Birmaher B, Axelson D, Goldstein B, Strober M, Gill MK, Hunt J, et al. Four-year longitudinal course of children and adolescents with bipolar spectrum disorders: the Course and Outcome of Bipolar Youth (COBY) study. Am J Psychiatry. 2009;166(7):795-804.
43. Birmaher B, Axelson D, Strober M, Gill MK, Valeri S, Chiappetta L, et al. Clinical course of children and adolescents with bipolar spectrum disorders. Arch Gen Psychiatry. 2006;63(2):175-83.
44. Weintraub MJ, Schneck CD, Axelson DA, Birmaher B, Kowatch RA, Miklowitz DJ. Classifying Mood Symptom Trajectories in Adolescents with Bipolar Disorder. J Am Acad Child Adolesc Psychiatry. 2020;59(3):381-90.
45. Hazell P, Jairam R. Acute treatment of mania in children and adolescents. Curr Opin Psychiatry. 2012;25(4):265-70.
46. Jairam R, Srinath S, Reddy YCJ, Shashikiran MG, Girimaji SC, Seshadri SP, et al. The index manic episode in juvenile onset Bipolar disorder: pattern of recovery. Can J Psychiatry. 2003:48;52-5.
47. Geller B, Luby JL, Joshi P, Wagner KD, Emslie G, Walkup JT, et al. A randomized controlled trial of risperidone, lithium, or divalproex sodium for initial treatment of bipolar I disorder, manic or mixed phase, in children and adolescents. Arch Gen Psychiatry. 2012;69:515-28.
48. Yatham LN, Kennedy SH, Parikh SV, Schaffer A, Bond DJ, Frey BN, et al. Canadian Network for Mood and Anxiety Treatments (CANMAT) and International Society for Bipolar Disorders (ISBD) 2018 guidelines for the management of patients with bipolar disorder. Bipolar Disord. 2018;20(2):97-170.
49. Selvarajan S, Srinivasan A, Sakkarabani P, Verma A, Rajendran P, Kandasamy P. Genetic polymorphisms influencing response to lithium in early-onset Bipolar disorder from south India. Asian J Psychiatr. 2022;70:103018.
50. Damegunta SR. Time Matters!: When is the Right Time to Estimate Serum Valproic Acid Levels? Indian J Psychol Med. 2014;36(3):349-50.
51. Srinivas S, Parvataneni T, Makani R, Patel RS. Efficacy and Safety of Quetiapine for Pediatric Bipolar Depression: A Systematic Review of Randomized Clinical Trials. Cureus. 2020;12(6):e8407.
52. Perugi G, Vannucchi G, Bedani F, Favaretto E. Use of Stimulants in Bipolar Disorder. Curr Psychiatry Rep. 2017;19(1):7.
53. Abrams Z. (2025). Diagnosing and treating bipolar spectrum disorders. American Psychological Association. [online] Available from https://www.apa.org/monitor/2022/01/ce-bipolar-spectrum [Last accessed 19 November, 2025].
54. Miklowitz DJ, Chung B. Family-Focused Therapy for Bipolar Disorder: Reflections on 30 Years of Research. Fam Process. 2016;55(3):483-99.
55. West AE, Weinstein SM, Peters AT, Katz AC, Henry DB, Cruz RA, et al. Child- and Family-Focused Cognitive-Behavioral Therapy for Pediatric Bipolar Disorder: A Randomized Clinical Trial. J Am Acad Child Adolesc Psychiatry. 2014;53(11):1168-78.
56. Hlastala SA, Kotler JS, McClellan JM, McCauley EA. Interpersonal and social rhythm therapy for adolescents with bipolar disorder: treatment development and results from an open trial. Depress Anxiety. 2010;27(5):457-64.
57. Jacob P, Gogi PK, Srinath S, Thirthalli J, Girimaji S, Seshadri S, et al. Review of electroconvulsive therapy practice from a tertiary Child and Adolescent Psychiatry Centre. Asian J Psychiatr. 2014;12:95-9.
58. Grover S, Vasthi A, Gautam S. Inpatient Care and Use of ECT in Children and Adolescents:

Aligning with Mental Health Care Act, 2017. Indian Psychiatric Society. [online] Available from https://indianpsychiatricsociety.org/wp-content/uploads/2020/01/mhca_childadol.pdf. [Last accessed 19 November, 2025].
59. Angal S, DelBello M, Zalpuri I, Singh MK. Clinical Conundrum: How do you treat youth with depression and a family history of bipolar disorder? Bipolar Disord. 2019;21(4):383-6.
60. Dougherty LR, Smith VC, Bufferd SJ, Kessel EM, Carlson GA, Klein DN. Disruptive mood dysregulation disorder at the age of 6 years and clinical and functional outcomes 3 years later. Psychol Med. 2016;46(5):1103-14.
61. Sagar-Ouriaghli I, Milavic G, Barton R, Heaney N, Fiori F, Lievesley K, et al. Comparing the DSM-5 construct of Disruptive Mood Dysregulation Disorder and ICD-10 Mixed Disorder of Emotion and Conduct in the UK Longitudinal Assessment of Manic Symptoms (UK-LAMS) Study. Eur Child Adolesc Psychiatry. 2018;27(9):1095-104.
62. American Psychiatric Association. Diagnostic and Statistical Manual of Mental Disorders, 5th edition. American Psychiatric Association; 2013.
63. World Health Organization. ICD-10: International Statistical Classification of Diseases and Related Health Problems: Tenth Revision, 2nd edition. World Health Organization; 2004.
64. Noller DT. Distinguishing disruptive mood dysregulation disorder from pediatric bipolar disorder. JAAPA. 2016;29(6):25-8.
65. Findling RL, Zhou X, George P, Chappell PB. Diagnostic Trends and Prescription Patterns in Disruptive Mood Dysregulation Disorder and Bipolar Disorder. J Am Acad Child Adolesc Psychiatry. 2022;61(3):434-45.
66. Tiwari R, Agarwal V, Arya A, Gupta PK, Mahour P. An exploratory clinical study of disruptive mood dysregulation disorder in children and adolescents from India. Asian J Psychiatr. 2016;21:37-40.
67. Sahu S, Saldanha D, Chaudhury S, Menon P, Marella S, Kalkat VS. Demographic and psychosocial profile of disruptive mood dysregulation disorder in Indian settings. Ind Psychiatry J. 2020;29(2):228-36.
68. Dwyer JB, Bloch MH. Antidepressants for Pediatric Patients. Curr Psychiatry. 2019;18(9):26-42F.

CHAPTER 12

Schizophrenia and Other Psychotic Disorders

Jasmin Garg, Nitin Gupta

INTRODUCTION

Psychosis is characterized by disruptions in cognition, perception, and behavior, leading to impaired reality testing. Psychosis is a distinctive feature of schizophrenia, but it can occur in many other neuropsychiatric conditions such as mood disorders, substance intoxication, delirium, neurological disorders, etc.[1-3]

Diagnostic criteria for schizophrenia and other psychotic disorders for children and adolescents are the same as for adults, as described in the Diagnostic and Statistical Manual of Mental Disorders (DSM-5) and the International Classification of Diseases (ICD-11). The primary psychotic disorders mainly include schizophrenia, schizoaffective disorder, schizotypal disorder, acute and transient psychotic disorder, delusional disorder, and other psychotic disorders.

The diagnosis of psychotic disorders is challenging in children and adolescents due to their unique developmental concerns. Misdiagnosis is very common. The onset of schizophrenia before 18 years of age is known as early onset schizophrenia (EOS), and before 13 years of age, it is known as childhood onset schizophrenia (COS).[4,5]

The prevalence of psychotic disorders in children and adolescents has been reported to be approximately 0.5%. The peak age of onset of schizophrenia is from 15 to 30 years.[4] EOS constitutes about 25% of cases of schizophrenia.[6] COS is extremely rare and data from Western countries have reported the approximate prevalence of COS as 0.04% with slight male preponderance.[3,5] The validity of the diagnosis of schizophrenia has not been established in children below 6 years of age.[3]

CHARACTERISTICS OF SCHIZOPHRENIA OF CHILDHOOD AND ADOLESCENT ONSET

The symptoms of EOS and COS identical with those of adult-onset schizophrenia, characterized by hallucinations, delusions, disorganized speech, disorganized behavior, and negative symptoms. However, hallucinations are more common in children and they may be multisensory. Delusions are less intricate and infrequent in children. Flat affect and disorganized speech are common, while catatonia is less reported.[1,4,5] These children may have subtle problems in their premorbid social and cognitive functioning. There can be an associated history of speech and developmental delay. Typically, at the onset of illness, the child becomes more withdrawn socially, his/her academic performance declines, and then there is expression of unusual thought content. Schizophrenia in this age, thus, generally has an insidious onset.[3,4,7] Here is an example of a case of typical childhood-onset schizophrenia **(Case Vignette 1)**.

CASE VIGNETTE 1

An 11-year-old boy was a student in the 5th class in 2022. He is a known case of cerebral palsy with weakness in the right side of his body. He was going to school regularly and doing well in studies. He had a few friends and occasionally played with them in the evening. In 2022, when the Ukraine-Russia war broke out, the child became increasingly engaged in watching news about the conflict. He would not go to play with peers as before. He would not interact much with parents, and when they tried to talk to him, he would mainly speak about the war, such as Putin said those things, sent fighter jets to Ukraine, and so many people were dead. After some months, they observed him talking to himself, smiling without apparent reason, and staring at the ceiling for extended periods. They also noted a decrease in his sleep, with episodes of smiling, talking, and gesturing throughout the night. When they asked the reason, he would say things like, "Someone is calling me, do not know who, may be Putin is calling me; Putin is standing outside the door; Zelensky is using abusive language; I can hear jets passing over us." He would also claim that he was seeing news reporters, dead bodies, and Putin's palace in his vision. When parents confronted him, he would become irritated and shout at them. The patient's school teacher also observed a noticeable decline in social interactions. He became increasingly withdrawn, often sitting alone at the back of the classroom. He exhibited self-muttering and self-smiling, appeared self-absorbed, and stared at the wall for extended periods. Additionally, there was a noticeable delay in his responses during class activities. Academically, his performance began to deteriorate. He became irregular in school attendance and faced difficulties in passing examinations. He would be so lost in muttering and gesturing that he would not listen to his parents. His parents had to call his name loudly and repeatedly, or they would clap loudly to bring his focus toward them. He would not agree to change clothes and take a bath. Afterward, the patient was taken to a psychiatrist and was prescribed tablet Olanzapine 2.5 mg/day. Over 6–8 months, the dosage was gradually increased to 15 mg. While there was some improvement in his sleep patterns, there was no significant amelioration of his other psychiatric symptoms. He would not go to school. He would also talk about hearing and seeing things he watched on TV news channels and YouTube videos. He would often start rocking while muttering and gesturing, saying that it was due to the effect of a ghost that he saw in a video.

In 2024, he was taken to another psychiatrist and was prescribed tablet Risperidone 2 mg/day gradually increased to 6 mg/day. The patient remained compliant with the prescribed medications, and his symptoms began to improve. He started going to school regularly, but did not study much. His self muttering and gesturing decreased. His parents did not have to clap to make him listen. He would comply with their requests to change clothes and take a bath. However, his speech became unclear with medicine due to extrapyramidal symptoms (EPS). So, after about 6 months of follow-up with this medication, the patient was taken to another psychiatrist who prescribed tablet Risperidone 4 mg/day. He was also given aripiprazole 5 mg/day. His magnetic resonance imaging (MRI) brain was done, and findings showed a paucity of white matter with areas of gliosis in the left periventricular/ peritrigonal region, suggestive of an old hypoxic insult. His Intelligence Quotient (IQ) on Malin's Intelligence Scale for Indian Children (MISIC) was 76, indicating borderline intellectual functioning. There was no improvement in his symptoms. He would exhibit occasional verbal aggression toward his parents. He would talk about hearing the voice of Prime Minister Narendra Modi and conflicts with China. Currently enrolled in the 7th grade (April 2025), he continues to sit at the back of the class, refrains from interacting with peers, and does not attend school for the entire duration of the school day. On mental status examination (MSE), he had continuous self-muttering, gesturing, and self-smiling. His speech was slurred due to EPS. His tone and reflexes were increased on the right side of body compared to the left. He also had a mild squint in the right eye. He was dressed appropriately to culture, weather, and situation. He did not make eye contact, and rapport could not be established. He would intermittently start rocking back and forth on the chair. The examiner had to repeat the interview questions several times to bring his focus to the present. He would begin answering a question and then get distracted and start self-muttering. Derailment was also evident in his thought process, as after speaking a sentence related to the question, he would jump to an entirely new topic, e.g., he was talking about seeing a ghost rocking in a chair, then he jumped to experiencing Akbar Birbal's court around him, and also told that he felt some power of the gurus within him. He also said he felt people were looking at him everywhere and talking about him. But he could not elaborate on it further. Auditory hallucinations were elicited for multiple persons. He said that Prime Minister Narendra Modi was saying, "Our nation is not free after so many years, it is time for a change, now there will be a revolution." He also said that a lady told him he should not study. If he studied, his parents would meet with an accident and they would fly in the air. Visual hallucinations were also elicited. He said he was seeing Putin's palace before his eyes. There were carpets in front of the palace. It was clearly visible to him. There was someone inside the palace looking at him. It was a scary doll moving around in the palace. He acknowledged that the palace was visible only to him, and no one else could see it. When asked if he could imagine visualizing something else, he said it was stuck in his eyes. He could not move it. In the assessment of cognitive functions, he could not cooperate much. He lacked insight into his illness.

This patient had florid psychotic symptoms. He would remain aloof and lost in his world. He had multi-sensory hallucinations and formal thought disorder. Children with schizophrenia mainly have hallucinations rather than delusions. He had cognitive decline, as previously he would get 90% marks, and now he had difficulty passing the exams. His symptoms did not improve with different antipsychotics. He also developed EPS with the medicines.

These children have more negative and cognitive symptoms compared to adult-onset schizophrenia. They exhibit a higher frequency of neurological soft signs involving frontal and temporal lobes compared to adolescent onset and adult-onset schizophrenia.[8] The majority of the patients with COS have impaired executive functioning, as demonstrated by neuropsychological testing. Their single-photon emission computed tomography (SPECT) scans reveal perfusion anomalies in the left frontal and temporal lobes, according to a study from North India.[9] They have lower N-acetyl aspartate (NAA) in the dorsolateral prefrontal cortex and hippocampus. Their brain atrophy is more marked and progressive compared to adult-onset schizophrenia.[10]

The clinical course usually involves the acute phase (with florid positive symptoms), recovery phase, and residual phase (with negative and cognitive symptoms). Children require long-term treatment with antipsychotics, and most of them develop moderate-to-severe disability across the lifespan. The earlier the onset of schizophrenia, the poorer the prognosis.[4,7,11] Compared to later age onset schizophrenia, patients with childhood-onset have poorer functioning, academic performance, lower intelligence quotients, florid phenomenology, and poorer response to treatment.[12]

PRODROME

A prodromal phase may precede the acute phase. There can be subthreshold psychotic symptoms during prodrome lasting weeks to years.[13] Prodrome may manifest as academic deterioration, social withdrawal, irritability, and depressive and anxiety symptoms.[1]

Since schizophrenia is a chronic, disabling mental condition, researchers have been trying to recognize those in prodrome or those with a high risk of developing schizophrenia so that its onset can be prevented. Different criteria for the identification of patients with a high risk for the development of psychosis have been made. These are of three subtypes: (1) Attenuated psychotic symptoms: occurrence of positive symptoms (delusions, hallucinations or formal thought disorder) at a lesser intensity than schizophrenia in the past 12 months. (2) Brief limited intermittent psychotic symptoms: fleeting positive psychotic symptoms that resolve spontaneously within a week. (3) Genetic risk: when there is a positive family history or traits of schizotypal disorder along with mild functional deterioration.[4,7,13]

Tools such as the Comprehensive Assessment of At Risk Mental States (CAARMS) and the Structured Interview for Psychosis-Risk Syndromes (SIPS) are used to identify young individuals in high-risk states.[5,7]

However, using these criteria, only 20% of identified individuals reportedly develop psychosis in the long term. Secondly, most research studies on identifying prodromal states recruited treatment-seeking young individuals for nonpsychotic problems. So, the identified individuals in prodromal states usually have other mental disorders such as anxiety disorders, mood disorders, or other behavioral disorders.[13]

Research is underway to predict at-risk states accurately and to find efficacious therapies to manage those in high-risk states. Antipsychotics have not proved efficacious so far. Omega 3 fatty acids have been tried with mixed results. Selective serotonin reuptake inhibitors (SSRIs) and nonpharmacological need-based therapies may be effective.[4,5]

DIFFERENTIAL DIAGNOSIS OF SCHIZOPHRENIA IN CHILDREN AND ADOLESCENTS

In this age group, often, it is challenging to establish a diagnosis of schizophrenia or psychotic disorders. The following case vignettes will demonstrate the elusiveness of diagnosing. Many times, it takes numerous sessions of history taking and mental status examination to reach a diagnosis. It is common for children to have a fear of ghosts during this phase of development. They have vivid imagination and fantasy **(Case Vignette 2)**.

CASE VIGNETTE 2

An 8-year-old boy, a student of class 3, was brought to psychiatry outpatient department (OPD) with the complaint of an episode of unresponsiveness in school. The boy was found lying unconscious on the school washroom floor the previous day. The latch of the washroom was open, and the boy was found lying fully clothed. There was no urinary incontinence or injury due to a sudden fall. There was no history of a tongue bite. There was no past history of seizures. There was no history of any complaints from the school regarding his behavior. He would play with his friends normally during his free time. The patient's mother reported that the child used to remain scared of ghosts at home. He would not go to the washroom alone at night for about 7–8 months. He was doing well in his studies.

His sleep and appetite were normal. During the mental status examination (MSE), the boy was cooperative and communicative and had a euthymic effect. He explained that he had gone to the school washroom and when he was alone, a headless man wearing black clothes suddenly appeared in front of him. The man tried to catch him and he got scared and fainted. The child also reported feeling scared and alone at home as his parents were working and his elder sibling was busy with her studies. He was scared to go to the school ground as he believed the see-saw and swings would sometimes start moving independently. The child was challenged that ghosts were not real. May be there was no one in the washroom, and probably the swings moved by wind. To all that, the child vehemently refused, said he was telling the truth, and actually saw what he described.

This boy accepted seeing ghosts with conviction. His parents also reported that he felt scared at home and refused to go to the washroom alone at night from 7 to 8 months. However, the child's socio-occupational function and biological functions were normal. There was no history of any academic decline. Even though the child seemed to have experienced visual hallucinations, he did not have schizophrenia.

The parents were suggested to spend quality time with the child. On follow-up, the child maintained well with psychosocial interventions. Many months later, he confessed that he had not seen any ghosts in the washroom and had made up the whole story.

Falsely held beliefs must be evaluated carefully in the context of developmental age. Up to 5% of normal children may report psychotic or psychotic-like symptoms.[1,5] Psychotic-like symptoms are also common in dissociative disorders in children **(Case Vignette 3)**.

CASE VIGNETTE 3

A 13-year-old male child, student of class 7, living in a joint family, resident of an urban area, belonging to a middle socioeconomic status, presented to the psychiatry outpatient department (OPD) with his mother and uncle with a psychiatric illness of approximate duration of 4 months. His birth and developmental history were uneventful.

As per the mother, his illness began with the complaint of pain in the abdomen, which was diffuse in nature and no associated symptom was found. He was taken to multiple doctors, but not much relief was reported. After 2 weeks, one day, he suddenly started saying, "Lord Hanuman is calling me. I have to meet him." The next day, the family took him to a temple, hoping he might recover. He visited the temple happily, and nothing unusual was noticed in his behavior. However, he started screaming on the way home, "There is Mata Rani (Goddess) in the car. She wants biscuits. She is calling me." The family took him to a faith healer, and he improved for some time. He continued to have similar symptoms periodically at home. He started remaining fearful at home and would keep clinging to his mother. He would say, "There is an old lady with long hair wearing white clothes, and I am scared of going outside." He also had anxiety and headaches off and on. The patient continued consulting faith healers. Meanwhile, the patient developed episodes of unresponsiveness with involuntary movements not associated with any tongue bite, injury due to falling or incontinence of urine. There was a history of 2–3 episodes/day in the beginning, which gradually increased in frequency. Due to this, the family avoided sending him to school. His sleep and appetite were normal. The family took him to different psychiatrists, and he was prescribed various psychotropics such as tablet aripiprazole 20 mg, tablet olanzapine 10 mg, tablet escitalopram 10 mg, tablet clonazepam 0.5 mg, tablet valproate chrono 300 mg BD, tablet sertraline 50 mg OD, and others. There was no improvement with medicines.

There was a history of conflicts within the family that increased with the patient's grandmother's death around 6 months ago. There were frequent fights between the parents, and since then, the father has been staying separately from the rest of the family.

The patient was admitted to the psychiatry ward for observation and diagnostic clarification. During mental status examinations (MSEs), he was found to be normally built and dressed appropriately. Psychomotor activity was normal in some MSEs; at other times, he would become unresponsive during interviews. He would become responsive again after sitting quietly without any intervention. The speech was coherent and comprehensible. In the thought content, he would say Hanuman ji and Mata Rani come to him. Suggestibility was evident in his behavior as he would say yes to most questions asked to elicit phenomenology. It could not be found explicitly whether he had thoughts, possessions, or hallucinations related to deities. Later, MSEs revealed worry related to himself and his family. During ward admission, it was observed that he would intermittently develop episodes of unresponsiveness, more so when the mother would forbid him from watching the smartphone. The patient was diagnosed according to ICD-10 as F44.4 (dissociative motor disorders). Psychosocial management was initiated.

It is common for normal children and adolescents to have imaginary friends. Younger children may have imaginary friends in the form of animals or birds. Imaginary friends may also be present in children with anxiety spectrum disorders **(Case Vignette 4)**.

CASE VIGNETTE 4

A 14-year-old female presented to psychiatry outpatient department (OPD) with complaints that she would smile too often for around 1 year. Also, she would communicate less with teachers and would not give answers to the questions asked in class. She was average in her studies and liked to draw in her free time. She was introvert by nature and would not talk much. During history taking, when the examiner was communicating with parents, the patient felt no one was looking at her, she was observed to be self-muttering. During mental state examination (MSE), the patient answered the greetings and sat comfortably in the chair. She was normally built and dressed according to social and weather situations. She was noticed smiling inappropriately when asked many questions during the interview. Eye-to-eye contact was maintained. Rapport was established. The mood was stated to be alright. But she appeared anxious in affect. She reported that whenever she would go to new surroundings or in front of teachers, whenever she felt nervous, she would not be able to control the smile on her face. She felt nervous while talking to teachers and unknown persons. When asked the reason for self-muttering, she reported that she had been hearing a voice coming from within herself. The voice was perceived as that of a girl who was her secret friend. She felt she lived by her side and came to talk to her whenever needed. Whenever she had something that she could not share with anyone, she would whisper it to that girl, and she would give a solution to the problem. The voice would talk only when the patient spoke first, and it was not distressing to her. Rather a pleasure for her.

This patient had psychotic-like experiences, yet her overall clinical picture did not fit with that of schizophrenia. She had self-muttering, but it was not due to true hallucinations. Also, children with schizophrenia usually have associated cognitive decline, which she lacked. Her inappropriate smiling and decreased communication were due to social anxiety.

Obsessive compulsive disorder (OCD) can be frequently misdiagnosed as schizophrenia in children and adolescents **(Case Vignette 5)**.

CASE VIGNETTE 5

A 16-year-old boy presented to psychiatry outpatient department (OPD) with a history dating back to when he was around 11 years of age and started becoming irritable with children coming for tuition from his mother. He expressed that they made fun of him. The intensity gradually increased through associated acts (fighting with them, avoiding sitting for studies during that time). Then, one day, he came home from school and said that a girl from his school lived in a cupboard at his house. He would not let anyone open it, citing that she would enter his body if done so. Over the next few days, he started reporting that he was seeing Mahatma Gandhi in his home and would avoid specific places where he would see him. After a period of a few months, he started expressing that another girl was sitting on one of the couches at home and would not go near it and not sit on that particular seat, saying she would enter his body, which he felt in the form of heaviness. He would then restrict himself to a bedsheet on the floor, not allowing it to be touched, changed, or cleaned. He also started scratching his face, causing visible lesions and scabs, citing that the girl's face was sticking to it.

Over the next few months, his self-care decreased. He started avoiding school with multiple days of absenteeism. He also started getting abusive and, at times, assaultive toward a stray dog in the locality, saying every time it barked, something would get into his brain, he felt irritated, and his head would get heavy. He would say that when it barked, some or other form of quarrel occurred at their house. Also, he started having repeated thoughts on seeing his housemaid that his day would be spoiled by looking at her. He would not be able to control the occurrence of this thought. He would ask his mother to fire her from her job. He had reassurance seeking in the form of confirming every information from the teacher and asking his mother to call his teacher in the evening and check if he had heard the things and homework correctly in school. He stopped using the tap in the bathroom, saying his uncle first went near the side of the sofa where he felt the girl sit, and then he touched the tap. So, she had now entered the bathroom (saying he saw a black shadow of the girl in the bathroom and that she would enter inside his body from there). He then started wearing some threads on his wrists and neck to protect himself from her. He also would avoid some specific roads from where his maid's son would come to their house, saying he would get repetitive thoughts that he had a bad eye on his mother, and these thoughts would be tough to control and cause him irritability. Then he was brought to the psychiatrist (after about 2 years of onset of illness), and at that time, it appeared that he had schizophrenia. He was started on tablet risperidone 2 mg, which was gradually increased to 8 mg over 3–4 months. There was an improvement in aggression with this. Later, 50 mg of tablet fluvoxamine was added, which was gradually increased to 200 mg. Skin picking, thoughts about the housemaid and her son, anger outbursts over the dog, and the visual and tactile phenomenon improved. He started attending school and participating in sports, winning 2 gold and a bronze medal. Academic interest and performance remained average.

Initially, the patient was diagnosed as having schizophrenia by the psychiatrist. He expressed that he would see a girl from his class sitting in his cupboard and Mahatma Gandhi, which were thought to be visual hallucinations. He also expressed that he would feel the girl entering her body and felt her on his face, which were believed to be somatic hallucinations. His illness was severe and functional impairment was also present. However, on reviewing the longitudinal history and case work-up, the diagnosis was revised to OCD with absent insight. The patient predominantly had obsessions throughout his course of illness, which he believed to be true. He had obsessional images of his classmate, Mahatma Gandhi, and magical thinking regarding the stray dog and the housemaid. He was very aggressive toward stray dogs, yet aggression is an inherent part of OCD. There was difficulty in eliciting obsessions initially, as whenever mental status examination (MSE) was done, he would affirmatively state that he would see that girl sitting there. This patient gradually improved, and the academic and functional decline was transient. There was no residual cognitive decline.

Sometimes, it becomes challenging to differentiate COS from autism spectrum disorder (ASD). Children with ASD have deficits in communication, poor socialization, restricted repetitive behaviors, sensory issues, speech delay, or loss of once-acquired speed. They may have associated intellectual disability, catatonia, hyperactivity, irritability, and aggressive outbursts. The communication problems and isolated play may resemble negative symptoms of schizophrenia. Stereotypic speech may be present in ASD, which may be confused with formal thought disorder.[1,4,5] Also, children with ASD may have self-talking behavior owing to auditory hyposensitivity. Self-talking may be confused with self-muttering due to hallucinations **(Case Vignette 6)**.

CASE VIGNETTE 6

Mr A, a 12-year-old male child, student of 6th class, resident of a rural area of North India, belonging to a lower socioeconomic status, presented to the psychiatry outpatient department (OPD) with his father with a continuous psychiatric illness of a total duration of 2–3 years.

His illness began when he was around 9–10 years old and was studying in the 4th grade. Family members started observing that he began to withdraw socially, spending hours alone, avoiding interaction with his family and friends, showing a delay in responding and decreasing academic performance. Around that time, he was also observed talking to himself and telling his family members that some people were always talking about him. Sometimes, he would cover his ears, and when asked why, he would say that he was hearing voices of people and wanted to block them. He occasionally displayed inappropriate emotional responses, such as laughing without apparent reason and becoming extremely anxious and fearful. He would not go to school regularly, and when he went, the teachers would observe him muttering to himself. He would not focus in the classroom or interact with other children. Teachers would also complain that when they tried to communicate with him, it was difficult for them to understand what he said. He had also started becoming irritable, shouting and hitting others for minor reasons. After around 1 year of onset, they visited a psychiatrist who prescribed him tablet risperidone 2 mg/day and valproate 250 mg/day. But he was not given the medicines regularly. He was taken to temples, where various poojas were performed. His symptoms kept on increasing in severity. He remained aloof and often said people were talking bad about him and wanted to harm him.

When some guests would visit their house, he would not tolerate them and tell them to go away or become aggressive towards them. His self-care deteriorated. He would not agree to take a bath or change clothes. He exhibited more physical aggression. He would bite family members when they asked him to take bath or any minor issue. He continued to have self-muttering, and when asked, he would say that he was hearing voices coming from speakers and batteries. Due to all these complaints, he was brought to psychiatry OPD again. He had attained all the developmental milestones for his age but delayed language milestones until he was 5 years old. He also had mild problems speaking from that age, as his father said that often, what he said would not be comprehensible to people other than his family. He would not play much with children of his age and used to talk less from the beginning. He was not good at studies, according to his father.

On mental status examination, he entered the doctor's room with his father, dressed appropriately for the culture, weather, and situation, but unkempt (clothes were dirty, hair not groomed or combed). Hallucinatory behavior was observed, including gesturing, muttering, and self-smiling. Eye contact was not sustained, and rapport was not established. The speech was low volume, at times incoherent and incomprehensible. Affect was indifferent. In content of thought, he expressed that people talked about him and wanted to harm him but did not elaborate. He said he heard voices from speakers and batteries but did not give details. In higher mental functions, he did not cooperate well on attention and concentration and memory testing, showed impaired abstract ability and judgment, poor fund of knowledge, and absent insight.

This child had childhood onset schizophrenia (COS) as he had positive symptoms in the form of auditory hallucinations and formal thought disorder. He had negative symptoms as he would remain withdrawn, had poor self-care, and had an indifferent affect. He also had a history of speech delay and subtle language problems. He was not much social from the beginning. History of premorbid cognitive, social, and language problems are often found in COS.[1,3] Children who develop COS can have lower intelligence quotients premorbidly, like this boy's father reported that he was not good in studies from the beginning.

He had mild dysfunction in the premorbid period. However, he did not have gross deficits in interaction or restricted repetitive behavior amounting to autism spectrum disorder (ASD).

Certain pointers help distinguish ASD from COS. First, in the case of COS, there is a history of a substantial period of grossly normal development. The onset of COS can be insidious, but it is distinct. Symptoms of ASD begin very early and a normal period of development may be absent or very brief. Secondly, there is a lack of positive symptoms (hallucinations and delusions) in children with ASD, although symptoms mimicking negative symptoms may be present. Thirdly, the premorbid dysfunction in COS is not as severe as in the case of ASD.[1,3] Still, the possibility of ASD comorbid with EOS should be kept in mind as up to 30% of children with ASD may develop psychosis.[5]

Mood disorders with psychotic symptoms are often misdiagnosed as schizophrenia in children. Mania with psychotic symptoms can be associated with florid delusions, hallucinations, and formal thought disorder. The social withdrawal of depression may be mistaken for negative symptoms. Depression with psychotic symptoms may present with mood-congruent or incongruent delusions. History taking should be done carefully and repeat interviews should be conducted in case of doubt in the diagnosis before initiating treatment.[1,3,5] EOS should also be differentiated from schizoaffective disorders **(Case Vignette 7)**.

CASE VIGNETTE 7

A 13-year-old female studying in 7th presented to psychiatry outpatient department (OPD) with her mother. The patient denied any complaints, while the mother reported decreased sleep for 15 days, fearfulness, crying episodes, and muttering to herself for around 7 days. The symptoms appeared around 3 weeks after menarche and progressed in intensity. No past psychiatry/medical/surgical history. She was an adopted child through some agency, so little is known about her biological family. On examination, she entered the room and started scanning around. Psychomotor activity was increased in the form of difficulty keeping seated, moving in and out of the chair, and also out of the room. Active hallucinatory behavior in the form of self-muttering and gesturing was noted. There was difficulty in sustaining eye-to-eye contact. Rapport could not be established. The mood was subjectively stated to be fine, but the effect was much anxious. She reported hearing voices of multiple persons. The voices talked about her, "She is a transgender." Voices commanded her to act like sitting up, standing up, moving there, etc. She said that she had to obey the voices. If she did not obey the people of the voices, she experienced pain in her head, and she would feel they were hitting her on the head. During the interview, she would start crying, saying she was being hit on the head when she was saying things that they were forbidding her to. During mental status examination (MSE), she suddenly ran out of the room, saying that a person wearing black clothes and a scary face had come to the doctor's room. She described the person vividly. Paranoid ideations could be elicited, but further thought content was difficult to elicit on the first MSE. The patient was started on risperidone 2 mg and gradually increased to 8 mg/day. With this dose, a partial remission was achieved in psychotic symptoms. During subsequent MSEs, she would continuously mutter to herself, and when asked any question, she would say, "See, now you know what I was thinking." She said that everybody knew what she was thinking. Her family also reported that there were incidents in which she would go and kiss some boys in public. The patient reported that she had to do that because she had to obey the voices. She went to school irregularly. Her academic performance was poor. After around 8 months of the onset of symptoms, she presented to the OPD with symptoms such as excessive grooming by using make-up, she would boast about herself that she was the most beautiful girl in the world, she would start talking to anyone she met, pressurized parents to buy a new car, there was decreased need for sleep and she would roam around excessively. She had elated mood, increased rate of speech, increased self-esteem and persistent auditory hallucinations auditory hallucinations were persistent. Oxcarbazepine 600 mg/day was added, which led to improvement in manic symptoms. However, other psychotic symptoms continued. Her academic performance kept deteriorating. Different antipsychotics were tried to control her hallucinations.

This patient had auditory hallucinations, visual hallucinations, and tactile hallucinations (multisensory) as psychotic symptoms. Auditory hallucinations persisted during most of the illness. She developed symptoms of a manic episode, which lasted around 1 month while auditory hallucinations were continuing. A diagnosis of schizoaffective disorder was considered but could not be made as it could not fulfill the ICD-10 or DSM-5 criteria for the same. According to DSM-5, mood symptoms should be persistent for most of the illness, yet in this patient, auditory hallucinations were present for most of the illness.

Literature reports that schizoaffective disorder is one of the most misdiagnosed disorders and has questionable reliability.[1,5] Transient manic symptoms can occur during the longitudinal course of schizophrenia.

Adolescents may also develop acute and transient psychotic disorders (ATPDs), which resemble schizophrenia.[14] Previous studies from India have also reported that the occurrence of ATPD is common in adolescents[15] **(Case Vignette 8)**.

CASE VIGNETTE 8

Mr X, a 14-year-old male child, student of class 9, resident of a rural area, belonging to a middle socioeconomic status, presented to the outpatient department of psychiatry with his parents with a history of psychiatric illness of 3 days. His birth and developmental history were uneventful.

As per the informant, his illness began 3 days back when his half-yearly exams were going on, and he suddenly became fearful and puzzled. He returned from school and said he was talking to someone during the exam, and the principal scolded him. He said that due to this, everyone at school was talking ill about him, and he was being made fun of. When his parents reassured him, he calmed down for some time but started saying these things again. He could not focus on his studies. His sleep and appetite decreased. He refused to go to school for the next exam, saying other students thought bad about him. He was reluctant to leave home, saying that people were talking bad about him and would harm him. The parents asked his school teachers and friends whether something odd had happened in school. But nothing relevant could be found.

On mental status examination (MSE), the patient entered the examiner's room and sat on the corner of the chair. He was looking anxious. He was dressed appropriately according to the weather and situation. Eye-to-eye contact was made but not sustained. His attitude was evasive and rapport could not be established. Psychomotor activity was normal. The speech was normal. Affect was perplexed. In thought content, he said, "I was talking to my friend and the principal came to the room. He scolded me and went back." When asked to explain more about the incident, he did not give details but said, "Others think wrong about me, but it is not so. I do not have a girlfriend, but they think so." He did not explain much again. When asked whether he felt scared of leaving home, he said that people would harm him, but no further relevant answer was given. The thought content was suggestive of primary delusions. No perceptual abnormality could be found. He did not cooperate much in the testing of higher mental functions. Insight was absent.

The patient was diagnosed with acute and transient psychotic disorders (ATPDs) and prescribed tablet risperidone 1 mg and tablet clonazepam 0.25 mg. He followed up after 1 week and reported that he was completely fine.

Psychotic symptoms can occur in the context of medical conditions in children such as epilepsy, neoplasms, autoimmune encephalitis, endocrine disorders, central nervous system (CNS) infections, genetic syndromes such as velocardiofacial syndrome, inborn errors of metabolism, Wilson's disease, delirium, and so forth.[1,3,5] One should carefully rule out medical conditions when there is an acute onset of psychosis associated with signs of organicity, such as focal neurological deficits, infection, seizures, confusion, or catatonia.[4]

Exposure to certain drugs, e.g., corticosteroids, dextromethorphan, anticholinergics, amphetamines, and antihistaminics can lead to the development of psychotic symptoms in children. Psychosis can also manifest after exposure to substances of abuse such as cannabis, inhalants, and stimulants. Acute psychosis due to drugs remits within days to weeks after stopping the causative drug. Cannabis use may lead to the development of schizophrenia ultimately.[1] Some common differential diagnosis are shown in **Box 1**.

There can be psychiatric comorbidities in children with EOS or COS, such as anxiety disorders, OCD, depression, etc. In children and adolescents, phenomenology evolves gradually, and the diagnosis may change longitudinally[3] **(Case Vignette 9)**.

BOX 1: Differential diagnosis of schizophrenia in children and adolescents.

- Normal fantasy
- Dissociative disorders
- Anxiety spectrum disorders
- Obsessive compulsive disorders
- Mood disorders
- Autism spectrum disorders
- Medical and surgical conditions
- Drugs and substance abuse
- Acute and transient psychotic disorder

CASE VIGNETTE 9

Ms X, a 20-year-old unmarried female, presented to the psychiatry outpatient department with her uncle with a continuous psychiatric illness of a total duration of 4–5 years. At the time of her birth, she was relinquished by her biological parents as they believed that keeping her would impede their chances of having a male child in the future. She was taken care of by her paternal aunt and uncle.

Her illness began when she was 16-year-old and was studying in class 9th. She had moved back to her parents' house. Initially, she started remaining irritable. After some months, she told her sister that she was getting repeated disturbing thoughts in her mind that she was having intercourse with God. She was very distressed due to these thoughts. Her symptoms escalated when she started having persistent thoughts that someone would reveal her secrets, contributing to increased anxiety and social withdrawal. When asked about the secret, she expressed fear that her nude video might have been leaked. Her academic performance also declined from before. Gradually, over 5 to 6 months, she started saying that people in the neighborhood were talking badly about her. She experienced auditory hallucinations occasionally, as if someone was calling her name. Her condition kept on deteriorating. She wouldn't go to school. Her self-care decreased, and her sleep was disturbed. Her parents took her to faith healers. She would suspect her parents that they had done black magic on her and she would remain very irritated with them. She came back to her paternal uncle's house within a year. She would often complain that someone had made her doll and was poking needles in the doll and she was feeling pain in her body because of that. She would also express that someone was controlling her mind and someone forced her to make a nude video of herself and share it online, which she did not want to do. She was taken to a psychiatrist by her paternal uncle. She was prescribed fluoxetine 20 mg, gradually increased to 60 mg/day and also aripiprazole 10 mg was added. She was on continuous treatment for about 2 years. Despite adherence to medications, only partial remission of symptoms was achieved. She could not continue her studies. She persistently believed that somebody was trying to control her, and she believed that she was made to sing songs at night as someone would move her lips, and she could not stop herself. She often said such things happened because her parents did black magic on her. She also had magical thinking. She would say that if I did not do things in a particular way, something bad would happen. She would advise her uncle to choose a particular route while going out. Otherwise, his trip would not be successful.

On current MSE, she had dressed appropriately for culture, weather, and situation. The speech was coherent and comprehensible. Affect was anxious. She expressed that some people, including her parents, were making her do things through a doll and she could not stop herself. She also expressed that she was getting repeated sexual thoughts in her mind that she should have intercourse with boys or talk to them. She said she knew she should not do so, but these thoughts were put in her mind through black magic. Her judgment was impaired and insight was absent.

This patient had obsessions in the beginning. Initially, the psychiatrist had prescribed fluoxetine for obsessions. However, during the course of her illness, psychotic symptoms became predominant. She had delusion of control, somatic hallucination, and thought insertion. So, this patient had OCD comorbid with EOS.

MANAGEMENT

Diagnostic assessments include history taking and physical and neurological examination. Those with suspected schizophrenia should be evaluated for comorbid medical conditions, substance abuse if any and level of functioning.[4] Diagnostic status should be reviewed over time as diagnosis tends to change in children and adolescents.[1] Certain diagnostic interview tools like the Kiddie Schedule for Affective Disorders and Schizophrenia (KSADS) may be used, which may aid in making the diagnosis.[4,5]

There are no diagnostic laboratory, psychological or neuroimaging tests for psychotic disorders. Cognitive assessment may be done for suspected comorbid intellectual disability and academic planning. Extensive investigations may be required in case of psychotic symptoms related to delirium or neurological illnesses. Neuroimaging and electroencephalogram (EEG) may be required in case of epilepsy.[1,4] Investigations should be done judiciously in children, as in previous research reports >98% of the time, the results of investigations are normal.[16] Routine investigations such as complete blood counts, liver function tests, fasting blood sugar, lipid profile, and electrocardiogram (ECG) may be done before starting antipsychotics for recording baseline levels.[5]

Antipsychotics are the primary treatment for the management of schizophrenia in children. The antipsychotics are of two types. The D2 antagonists (First-generation antipsychotics or FGA) and serotonin dopamine antagonists (SDA or second-generation antipsychotics). Studies from both adults and youth have demonstrated that no antipsychotic is superior in effect to another except clozapine.[1,5,7]

Long-term treatment spanning years is usually required in schizophrenia. An effort should be made to continue effective doses at minimum side effects. The FGAs are more often associated with extrapyramidal side effects than SGAs, which are more likely to produce metabolic side effects. Most guidelines suggest that lower doses should be started in children and slow up-titration should be done. Children are more sensitive to adverse effects of antipsychotics when compared to adults.[1,4]

SGAs have a comparatively favorable side effect profile, so they are usually started first in children.[4] All SGAs except asenapine and ziprasidone demonstrated efficacy in the management of schizophrenia in the young population.[3,5] However, most recommendations for antipsychotic use are based on adult studies as there are comparatively limited studies in the young population.[7]

While starting antipsychotics, the patient and family members should be explained about the options, possible side effects, the importance of adherence, and the need for monitoring. They should also be explained in terms of maintaining a healthy lifestyle, exercising, and taking dietary precautions.[4] There is limited research available to support the use of long-acting injectables for the management of schizophrenia in children. However, they may be considered in case there is history of nonadherence.[1,4] Positive symptoms have a good response to antipsychotics. Negative symptoms respond poorly. Cognitive symptoms have not been evaluated in children.[4]

Extra-pyramidal symptoms (EPS) can take the form of drug-induced Parkinsonism, neuroleptic malignant syndrome (NMS), dystonia, and akathisia. FGAs and high-potency SGAs produce more EPS. Acute EPS occurs in days to weeks. For Parkinsonism, the first step is to decrease the dose. If no improvement occurs with this, switch to some other antipsychotic. But if the drug cannot be changed, an anticholinergic agent can be added. In the case of acute dystonia, parenteral anticholinergic is given (promethazine). For severe akathisia, benzodiazepine or β-blocker can be added. When NMS develops, all antipsychotics should be stopped, and supportive management should be given. Antipsychotics can also cause hyperprolactinemia, more often due to FGAs. The first step is to decrease the dose and watch. If that is not possible, add bromocriptine or amantadine or aripiprazole.[4]

Monitor weight, lipid profile, and fasting blood sugar periodically for metabolic side effects. In case of a gain of 7% weight, the emergence of hyperlipidemia, hypertension, or hyperglycemia, the antipsychotic needs to be changed. If change is not possible, adding metformin or topiramate is to be considered. QTc prolongation may occur with high doses of haloperidol and quetiapine.[4] Adjunctive medicines such as mood stabilizers for manic symptoms and antidepressants for depression may be required.[1]

Treatment-resistant Schizophrenia

Clozapine is indicated for children who do not respond to a trial of two antipsychotics, each given for at least 6–8 weeks in adequate doses. Up to 50% of children may be treatment-resistant.[5,7] Clozapine is documented to be effective in improving positive symptoms of COS, as reported in data from Northern India. It did not produce any serious side effects in children with COS according to the same report.[17] According to most guidelines, weekly monitoring of absolute neutrophil count should be done for at least 6 months after starting clozapine.[1] However, recently, the FDA removed the mandatory requirement of weekly monitoring of neutrophil counts for clozapine administration as the benefits of clozapine far outweigh the risks. Weekly monitoring was cumbersome and many patients were deprived of its benefits.[18] Monitoring of metabolic parameters should be done once every 3 months.[1]

Electroconvulsive therapy (ECT) in adults is recommended for catatonia, refusal to eat, suicidality, affective symptoms, violence, rapid control of symptoms, good response in the past, and treatment resistance. For similar reasons, ECT can be considered in children. Mental Health Care Act (MHCA) 2017 prohibited the routine use of ECT for children. It can still be done after obtaining prior permission from Mental Health Review Boards (MHRB) and parental consent.[4]

Psychotherapeutic Interventions

Cognitive behavior therapy, family therapy, cognitive remediation, and social skills training have been found helpful in adults with schizophrenia. They are done with the goals of symptom reduction, improving social occupational functioning, and decreasing the risk of relapse. These interventions can be tried in children with similar goals.[1]

SUMMARY AND CONCLUSION

Early onset schizophrenia and COS present unique diagnostic and management challenges due to developmental complexities and the need to differentiate them from other conditions.

Early onset schizophrenia accounts for about 25% of cases of schizophrenia. It has some distinct features from adult-onset schizophrenia. Hallucinations are more common, while delusions are less so. There may be a history of minor deficits in premorbid language and cognitive development. EOS carries a relatively poorer prognosis. The diagnostic criteria for EOS are the same as those for adults. However, it is challenging to diagnose schizophrenia in children due to the complexities of developmental age. EOS has to be differentiated from autism spectrum disorders, mood disorders, and psychotic manifestations due to medical/surgical illnesses.

Despite the similarities in symptoms with adult-onset schizophrenia, children with EOS often have a poorer prognosis and require long-term antipsychotic treatment with careful dosing to manage adverse effects. Identifying high-risk individuals during the prodromal phase and employing psychotherapeutic interventions can improve outcomes. Comprehensive diagnostic assessments and tailored management strategies are essential for effectively treating schizophrenia in children and adolescents. Management of psychotic disorders in children goes in line with management of adults. Children and adolescents with EOS require life-long antipsychotic administration. Doses of antipsychotics are chosen carefully due to sensitivity to adverse effects.

ACKNOWLEDGMENTS

We sincerely thank Dr Priyanka Bansal, Dr Vinay, Dr Manpreet Kaur, and Dr Aditi Singla, resident doctors of the Department of Psychiatry, Government Medical College, Patiala, for their help in preparing the case vignettes. Written informed consent was obtained from all the patients and their guardians/parents to publish their case histories in this book chapter.

REFERENCES

1. McClellan J, Stock S; American Academy of Child and Adolescent Psychiatry (AACAP) Committee on Quality Issues (CQI). Practice parameter for the assessment and treatment of children and adolescents with schizophrenia. J Am Acad Child Adolesc Psychiatry. 2013;52(9):976-90.
2. Lachman A. New developments in diagnosis and treatment update: Schizophrenia/first episode psychosis in children and adolescents. J Child Adolesc Ment Health. 2014;26(2):109-24.
3. Sunshine A, McClellan J. Practitioner Review: Psychosis in children and adolescents. J Child Psychol Psychiatry. 2023;64(7):980-8.
4. Grover S, Avasthi A. Clinical practice guidelines for the management of schizophrenia in children and adolescents. Indian J Psychiatry. 2019;61: 277-93.
5. Khan BA, Mansuri Z, Qayyam Z. Psychotic disorders in children and adolescents. Int J Child Health Hum Dev. 2022;5:111-24.
6. Tor J, Dolz M, Sintes A, Muñoz D, Pardo M, de la Serna E, et al. Clinical high risk for psychosis in children and adolescents: a systematic review. Eur Child Adolesc Psychiatry. 2018;27:683-700.
7. Pattnaik JI, Panda UK, Chandran S, Padhy S, Ravan JR. Treatment resistant psychosis in children and adolescents and clozapine: Nuances. Front Psychiatry. 2023;14:1014540.
8. Biswas P, Malhotra S, Malhotra A, Gupta N. Comparative study of neurological soft signs in schizophrenia with onset in childhood, adolescence and adulthood. Acta Psychiatr Scand. 2007;115:295-303.
9. Malhotra S, Gupta N, Bhattacharya A, Kapoor M. Study of childhood onset schizophrenia (COS) using SPECT and neuropsychological assessment. Indian J Psychiatry. 2006;48:215-22.
10. Biswas P. Neurobiology of childhood-onset schizophrenia. J Indian Assoc Child Adolesc Mental Health. 2008;4:55-61.

11. Correll CU, Fusar-Poli P, Leucht S, Karow A, Maric N, Moreno C, et al. Treatment Approaches for First Episode and Early-Phase Schizophrenia in Adolescents and Young Adults: A Delphi Consensus Report from Europe. Neuropsychiatr Dis Treat. 2022;18:201-19.
12. Biswas P, Malhotra S, Malhotra A, Gupta N. A comparative study of clinical correlates in schizophrenia with onset in childhood, Adolescence and adulthood. J Indian Assoc for Child and Adolescent Mental Health. 2006;2:18-30.
13. Taylor JH, Huque ZM. Commentary: Schizophrenia prevention and prodromal psychosis in children and adolescents. J Child Psychol Psychiatry. 2021;62(5):674-6.
14. Malhotra S. Acute and transient psychosis: A paradigmatic approach. Indian J Psychiatry. 2007;49(4):233-43.
15. Grover S, Kathiravan S. Acute and transient psychotic disorders: A review of Indian research. Indian J Psychiatry. 2023;65(9):895-913.
16. Muhrer E, Moxam A, Dunn M, Rosen A, Taylor JH, Camacho P, et al. Acute medical workup for new-onset psychosis in children and adolescents: A retrospective cohort. J Hosp Med. 2022;17(11):907-11.
17. Malhotra S, Gupta N, Singh G. Clozapine in childhood-onset schizophrenia: A report of five cases. Clinical Child Psychology and Psychiatry. 2000;5:403-10.
18. U.S. Food and Drug Administration. Information on Clozapine. [Online] Available from https://www.fda.gov/drugs/postmarket-drug-safety-information-patients-and-providers/information-clozapine [Last accessed November, 2025].

CHAPTER 13

Alcohol and Substance Use Disorders

Gayatri Bhatia, Anju Dhawan

INTRODUCTION

Substance use among children and adolescents is a public health concern in several parts of the world. Onset of substance abuse during the formative years of life interferes with academic, social, and life skills development. Substance use among youth has a unique bidirectional association with psychiatric disorders, e.g., depressive disorders, anxiety disorders, attention-deficit/hyperactivity disorder (ADHD), and conduct disorders, each increasing the risk and worsening the prognosis of the other.[1] Substance use in adolescents is associated with other risky behaviors like unsafe sexual practices that may lead to sexually transmitted infections and teenage pregnancies, warranting a need for special attention in terms of prevention, recognition, and management.[2,3]

Earlier, substance use was seen as a problem associated mainly with street children but is now increasingly being seen across various subpopulations of children including school students and out-of-school children living at home with families.[4] The latest report from Monitoring the Future Survey, an ongoing study of behaviors, attitudes, and values of American adolescents, reported 10.9% of eighth graders, 19.8% of 10th graders, and 31.2% of 12th graders are using at least one illicit drug in 2023.[5] According to the recent national survey, Magnitude of Substance Use in India, 2019, the prevalence of current use among adolescents is 1.8% for opioids, 1.3% for alcohol, 1.17% for volatile solvents, and 0.9% for cannabis.[6] The fourth round of the Global Youth Tobacco Survey (GYTS-4), 2019, reported that 8.5% of Indian youth—9.6% males and 7.4% females used some form of tobacco; 7.3% smoked and 4.1% used smokeless tobacco. Another study conducted in 2015 by the National Commission for Protection of Child Rights (NCPCR), reported that the average age at initiation of substance use among adolescents was the lowest for tobacco (12.3 years) followed by inhalants (12.4 years), cannabis (13.4 years), and alcohol use (13.6 years). Opioids and pharmaceutical drugs were initiated at 14–15 years of age followed by injectable use (at 15.1 years). Street children were reported to initiate substance use approximately 1–1.5 years earlier as compared to those living at home.[7]

While studies on trajectories of substance use among adolescents are lacking in India, USA's National Comorbidity Survey-Adolescents (2001–2004), including children and adolescents in 3–18 years' age group, reported recreational use as the predominant pattern of substance use in a community setting, followed by harmful use and dependence. In a clinical setting, however, the predominant pattern observed is usually dependence with significant substance use related adverse consequences.[8] Adolescents are often brought for treatment by parents or guardians; sometimes by law enforcement authorities, and sometimes by social or child welfare organizations.

Substance use among adolescents is a multifaceted problem that requires understanding of various risk and proactive factors, bio-psycho-social considerations, and multiple aspects of management, which will be discuss in subsequent sections of this chapter.

RISK AND PROTECTIVE FACTORS FOR SUBSTANCE USE AMONG ADOLESCENTS

Involvement in substance use for any adolescent is usually determined by the interaction of individual vulnerabilities along with positive and negative social influences.[9,10] These factors can be divided into individual, family, and environmental factors, as summarized in **Table 1**.

- *Individual risk factors* encompass cognitive, personality, biological, and developmental factors like poor knowledge about risk of substance use, misconceptions about treatment, poor self-esteem, low assertiveness, impulsivity, rebelliousness, poor self-control, low social support, academic failures, poor coping skills, and psychiatric conditions like depressive and anxiety disorders, ADHD, conduct disorders, etc.
- *Family factors* include parenting practices, interpersonal dynamics, genetics, and behavior modeling.
- *Environmental factors* include risk factors encountered in the community, including laws and policies making substances easily available, media portrayal of violence and drug use, poverty, and neighborhoods lacking organization. On the other hand, engagement in prosocial activities like involvement in community service, religious groups, etc. is protective against substance use initiation.

CHALLENGES IN MANAGEMENT OF SUBSTANCE USE DISORDERS IN ADOLESCENTS

As mentioned earlier, substance use among adolescents has some unique distinctions from that in adult population. Adolescence is characterized by a natural curiosity to gain new experiences in addition to a low perception of harm. Biologically, significant neurodevelopmental changes occur at this age and any insult due to substance use may lead to far-reaching adverse neuropsychological consequences including attentional deficits, impaired working memory, poor executive

TABLE 1: Risk and protective factors for substance use among adolescents.

	Individual	*Familial*	*Environmental*
Risk factors	Rebelliousness, impulsivity, high sensation seeking, risk taking, low assertiveness, low self-esteem, academic failures, bullying, poor coping skills, ADHD, conduct disorders, early onset psychiatric disorders (schizophrenia, BPAD, anxiety disorders, etc.)	Poor family management, poor parenting and disciplining practices, conflicts, parental substance use, and unfavorable parental attitudes to problematic behaviors	Community disorganization, poor community involvement, housing and financial instability, easy availability of drugs, and acceptance of drug use by community
Protective factors	Conscientiousness, high harm avoidance, healthy self-esteem, good coping skills, self-regulation	Healthy bonding, open communication, supportiveness, and effective problem-solving approach	Prosocial activities, healthy engagement with community, having good role models and mentors, access to drug use prevention, and treatment initiatives

(ADHD: attention-deficit/hyperactivity disorder; BPAD: bipolar affective disorder)

control, emotional dysregulation, and impaired problem solving and decision-making.[11] These impairments may contribute to poor educational performance and socio-occupational difficulties.

Such adolescents are generally a hard-to-reach population due to poor involvement in school and community activities. They are more prone to long-term cognitive complications of using substances, including a higher risk of developing substance use disorders, psychiatric comorbidities such as depressive and anxiety disorders, along with physical complications including drug overdose.[3,12] Polysubstance use frequently complicates the presentation and management of these patients in emergency departments. In terms of treatment seeking, evidence reports that poor engagement with treatment and social services are frequently encountered while working with adolescents who use substances. These factors tend to worsen the disease prognosis in adolescents.

Another unique issue that needs careful consideration is confidentiality. A balance must be maintained between rapport with the adolescent and disclosure to parents or guardians. Confidentiality should be discussed at the first visit with the patient and parents. Limits to confidentiality, such as self-harm and criminal activity should be explained.

Adolescents have a higher risk of hazardous activities related to substance use, including having unplanned, unwanted, and unprotected sexual activity; driving while intoxicated; being a passenger in a car while the driver is intoxicated; self-injurious behavior, and suicide attempts.[9,13] Adolescents with substance use disorders are at an increased risk of being involved with the legal system. They are also at risk of their education being interrupted or negatively affected. Psychosocial risk factors often result in housing and financial instability, contributing to poor engagement in treatment. The complex interaction of physical, mental, legal, educational, and social issues among youth with substance abuse problems creates the potential for poor short-and long-term outcomes.[3,10,14]

CLINICAL PRESENTATION OF SUBSTANCE USE DISORDERS AMONG ADOLESCENTS

Substance use disorders in adolescents generally come with early warning signs which if unidentified, may progress to substance use disorders. Some early warning signs are as follows:

- Loss of interest in activities that were enjoyable earlier.
- Change in peer group
- Changes in disposition—anger, aggression, and dysphoria
- Changes in general physical health, sleep, and appetite patterns

Clinical features of substance use disorders among adolescents may be understood based on dysfunction or adverse consequences related to substance use in physical, behavioral, social, occupational, financial, and legal domains.

- *Physical:* Poor hygiene/change in appearance, glazed or bloodshot eyes, frequent runny nose or nosebleeds, paranoia, irritability, track marks on arms or legs (wearing long sleeves even in warm weather or extensive tattoos in an attempt to hide them), pupils larger or smaller than usual, cold or sweaty palms, tremors, sores on mouth, headaches, swollen face, extreme fatigue or extreme hyperactivity, and significant weight gain or loss.
- *Behavioral:* Difficulty staying focused, marked changes in mood ranging from euphoria to despondency, impatience, aggression, anxiety, fidgeting, avoiding eye contact, perceptual disturbances, cognitive impairments, guilt, regret, frequent lying and acting secretive, losing interest in hobbies or routine activities, continued use of substance

despite associated harms, seeking out reasons to use substances, impaired ability to control or reduce substance use, spending increasing amounts of time and resources to procure, use and recover from the effects of substances, high risk sexual behaviors with or without relation to substances.

- *Social:* Changing peer group, engagement with other substance using adolescents, isolation, frequent conflicts with family members, batch-mates and other social contacts resulting in strained relationships, and loss of respect in neighborhood and community.
- *Academic/occupational:* Frequent absences from school and work, academic decline, failures and expulsion from school, falling work performance, frequent changes of job, and unemployment.
- *Financial:* Increase in daily expenses, loss of savings, incurring debts, borrowing money, and selling household items to make money to procure substances.
- *Legal:* Engagement in illegal activities and drug-related crimes, frequent encounters with law enforcement agencies.

IDENTIFICATION OF SUBSTANCE USE DISORDERS IN ADOLESCENTS

Substance use during adolescence can be viewed along a developmental continuum that starts with experimental use, progressing to recreational use and ultimately substance use disorders. Although infrequent use of substances may not have immediate social, academic, psychological, or legal consequences, there is no known safe dose of psychoactive substances on the developing adolescent brain. It is thus imperative that clinicians are trained in early identification of substance use in adolescents.[15] Identifying substance use disorders in adolescents comprises of screening and detailed assessment.

SCREENING FOR SUBSTANCE USE DISORDERS

Screening aims to estimate an individual's level of risk toward developing a maladaptive substance use pattern or substance use disorder. The American Academy of Pediatrics (AAP) recommends annual screening for tobacco, alcohol, and other substance use, typically beginning at age 11 years, and suggests that pediatricians start discussing the unhealthy effects of alcohol, tobacco, and substance use as early as 9 years of age.[16]

Screening based on clinical history is usually supplemented with objective tools that increase the reliability and validity of the impression. Some screening questionnaires that may be used to screen adolescents for substance use related problems are briefly discussed below. A summary of common screening tools is presented in **Table 2**.

CRAFFT

The CRAFFT (Car, Relax, Alone, Forget, Family or Friends, Trouble) is a widely used screening tool that demonstrates high reliability and sensitivity in identifying adolescents with problematic substance use and a diagnosable substance use disorder. To administer the CRAFFT **(Fig. 1)**, the clinician begins by asking three questions to screen for the number of days of use during the past 12 months of alcohol, marijuana, and any other illegal or prescription medication for the purpose of getting high. If the patient reports zero days of use during the past 12 months for all three questions, the clinician follows up with the "Car" question only and provides appropriate affirmation or encouragement for continued abstinence. If the patient reports any days of use for any of the first three questions, then all six CRAFFT questions are administered **(Fig. 1)**. Each "yes" response is marked as a score of 1. Based on the responses, risk levels are defined and further actions are planned as shown in **Table 3**.[16]

TABLE 2: Screening tools for substance use among adolescents.

Name	*Population age (years)*	*Number of questions*	*Description*
CRAFFT (Car, Relax, Alone, Forget, Family or Friends, Trouble)	12–21	3–9 (depending on answers)	Screens for patients at risk of drug or alcohol problems; does not distinguish between alcohol and other drug use; does not screen for tobacco use or assess frequency of substance use
Brief Screener for Tobacco, Alcohol, and other Drugs (BSTAD)	12–17	6–38 (depending on answers)	Screens for frequency of alcohol, tobacco, cannabis, and other substance use in both respondents and their friends; asks about use in the past 30, 90, 365 days; does not ask specifically about hazardous use or symptoms of dependence
Screening to Brief Intervention (S2BI)	12–17	3–7 (depending on answers)	Screens for the frequency of alcohol, tobacco, cannabis, prescription, and other substance use in the past year; does not ask specifically about hazardous use or symptoms of dependence
Alcohol Use Disorders Identification Test (AUDIT)	18+	10	Screens for quantity and frequency of alcohol consumption, symptoms of dependence, and associated risky behaviors; does not screen for tobacco or other substance use
Drug Abuse Screening Test (DAST)	18+	10, 20, or 28 (depending on version)	Asks about consequences associated with drug use in the past 12 months; does not screen for alcohol or tobacco use
Tobacco, Alcohol, Prescription medication, other Substance use (TAPS)	18+	4 in part 1; 9–27 in part 2 (depending on answers)	*Two-part tool:* Part 1 asks about tobacco, alcohol, illicit substance use, and medication misuse in the past year; Part 2 assesses quantity of use, difficulties with control, and concerns by others over the past 3 months

Source: Quiggle AR, Burke CW, Wilens T. (2023). Substance Use Among Adolescents and Young Adults. [online] Available from https://www.psychiatrictimes.com/view/substance-use-among-adolescents-and-young-adults [Last accessed November, 2025].

S2BI

The Screening to Brief Intervention (S2BI) instrument **(Fig. 2 and Flowchart 1)** is also validated for use with adolescents and has demonstrated high sensitivity and specificity in identifying substance use disorders. The instrument begins by asking a patient about his or her frequency of use of tobacco, alcohol, and/or marijuana in the past year (never, once or twice, monthly, weekly, or more). If the patient endorses use of any of the three substances, then follow-up questions are posed to target use of prescription drugs, illegal drugs, inhalants, herbs, or synthetic drugs. The frequency of use reported is strongly correlated with the likelihood of having a substance use disorder. Adolescents who report using "once or twice" in the past year are very unlikely to have a substance use disorder. Those who endorse "monthly" use will generally meet criteria for a mild or moderate substance use disorder, and those who report "weekly" use are likely to have a severe risk of substance use disorder. Each of these is managed accordingly. Use once or twice in the past year

Part A

During the PAST 12 MONTHS, on how many days did you:

1. Drink more than a few sips of beer, wine, or any drink containing alcohol? Say "0" if none.	☐ # of days
2. Use any marijuana (weed, oil, or hash, by smoking, vaping, or in food) or "synthetic marijuana" (like "K2," "Spice") or "vaping" THC oil? Put "0" if none.	☐ # of days
3. Use anything else to get high (like other illegal drugs, prescription or over-the-counter medications, and things that you sniff, huff, or vape)? Say "0" if none.	☐ # of days

Did the patient answer "0" for all questions in Part A?

Yes ☐ → **Ask CAR question only, then stop**

No ☐ → **Ask all six CRAFFT questions below**

Part B

		No	Yes
C	Have you ever ridden in a CAR driven by someone (including yourself) who was "high" or had been using alcohol or drugs?	☐	☐
R	Do you ever use alcohol or drugs to RELAX, feel better about yourself, or fit in?	☐	☐
A	Do you ever use alcohol or drugs while you are by yourself, or ALONE?	☐	☐
F	Do you ever FORGET things you did while using alcohol or drugs?	☐	☐
F	Do your FAMILY or FRIENDS ever tell you that you should cut down on your drinking or drug use?	☐	☐
T	Have you ever gotten into TROUBLE while you were using alcohol or drugs?	☐	☐

Fig. 1: The CRAFFT (Car, Relax, Alone, Forget, Family or Friends, Trouble) questionnaire.

TABLE 3: Risk levels based on CRAFFT questionnaire.

Risk	*CRAFFT score*	*Action*
Low	0 No use in past 12 months	Psychoeducation
Medium	≤2 Yes to "car" question only	Psychoeducation with follow-up plan
High	>2 Use in past 12 months	Psychoeducation, brief advice, follow-up, and refer to specialized services

(CRAFFT: Car, Relax, Alone, Forget, Family or Friends, Trouble)

can be managed with brief advice. Monthly use is managed with motivational enhancement and advice on reducing risky behavior. Motivational enhancement, advice on risky behaviors, and referral to specialized services are recommended for weekly use.

TAPS

Developed by McNeely et al. in 2016, the TAPS (Tobacco, Alcohol, Prescription medication, other Substance Use Tool) combines screening and brief assessment for commonly used

The following questions will ask about your use, if any, of alcohol, tobacco, and other drugs. Please answer every question by checking the box next to your choice.

In the past year, how many times have you used:

Tobacco?

- Never
- Once or twice
- Monthly
- Weekly or more

Alcohol?

- Never
- Once or twice
- Monthly
- Weekly or more

Marijuana?

- Never
- Once or twice
- Monthly
- Weekly or more

Prescription drugs that were not prescribed for you (such as pain medication or Adderall)?

- Never
- Once or twice
- Monthly
- Weekly or more

Illegal drugs (such as cocaine or Ecstasy)?

- Never
- Once or twice
- Monthly
- Weekly or more

Inhalants (such as nitrous oxide)?

- Never
- Once or twice
- Monthly
- Weekly or more

Herbs or synthetic drugs (such as salvia, "K2", or bath salts)?

- Never
- Once or twice
- Monthly
- Weekly or more

Fig. 2: The Screening to Brief Intervention (S2BI) tool.

Flowchart 1: The Screening to Brief Intervention (S2BI) algorithm.

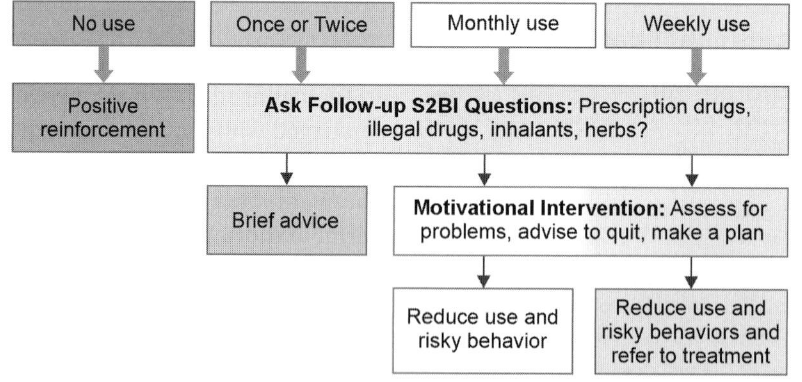

substances, eliminating the need for multiple screening and lengthy assessment tools (McNeely et al., 2016). The TAPS tool has two components. The first component (TAPS-1) is a 4-item screen for tobacco, alcohol, illicit drugs, and nonmedical use of prescription drugs. If an individual screens positive on TAPS-1 (i.e., reports other than "never"), the second component (TAPS-2) is applied, which consists of brief substance-specific assessment questions (TAPS-2) to arrive at a risk level for that substance. Clinicians are encouraged to provide positive feedback to patients who screen negative and support their choice to abstain from substances. For patients who have a positive screen on the TAPS-1, a brief assessment (TAPS-2) identifies the specific substance(s) use and risk level, ranging in severity from "problem use" to the more severe substance use disorder. Scores on these questions generate a risk level per substance endorsed, based on a range of possible scores per substance as shown in **Table 4**. For identifying DSM-5 substance use disorder at the recommended cut-off of 2+, the TAPS tool has adequate sensitivity (>70%) only for tobacco, alcohol, and marijuana. Further assessment should be conducted for patients with a score of 1+ for other substances. This assessment is a high priority for patients with a TAPS score of 2+, given its high positive predictive value for most substance classes.

Other screening tools such as AUDIT (Alcohol Use Disorders Identification Test), CAGE (Cut-down, Annoyed, Guilty, Eye-opening), ASSIST-Y (Alcohol, Smoking and Substance Involvement Screening Test-Youth) may also be used.

DETAILED ASSESSMENT

The aim of detailed assessment is to correctly elicit dysfunction in each domain of the adolescent's life caused due to drug use—physical, psychological, social, educational, occupational, familial, and legal **(Table 5)**. A thorough evaluation begins with quantitative information about what

TABLE 4: Interpretation of TAPS score.

TAPS score	*Risk category*
0	No use in past 3 months
1	Problem use
2+	Higher risk

(TAPS: Tobacco, Alcohol, Prescription medication, other Substance Use Tool)

TABLE 5: Components of a detailed assessment.

	Degree of impairment		
Risk factors	*Mild*	*Moderate*	*Severe*
Frequency of use	Monthly or less	Weekly	Daily or near daily
Intoxication/withdrawal	None/mild symptoms	Moderate symptoms	Severe/life threatening
Comorbid medical conditions	None/mild	Moderate/stable/controlled on treatment	Severe/unstable/ uncontrolled
Comorbid psychiatric conditions	None/mild	Moderate/stable/on treatment	Severe/uncontrolled symptoms/not on treatment
Motivation for treatment	High	Moderate	Low
Family/social environment	Supportive and stable	Mildly supportive, some conflict, and school difficulties	Homelessness, broken families, and out of school
Risk of relapse/overdose	Low and steady use pattern with single substance	Moderate, slight irregularities, and multiple substances	High, intravenous drug use, unstable pattern of use, and multiple substances

substances are being used, the frequency of use, as well as inquiring about any legal or functional difficulties. Although adolescents with substance use disorders are less likely than adults to present for treatment with medical complications and signs of withdrawal from their substance use, they are more likely to be misusing more than one primary substance. Adolescents are also more likely to hide or minimize their use compared to adults and tend to continue their use despite adverse legal or psychosocial consequences.[16,17] Collateral history from caregivers is also essential for this reason, given adolescents' possible reticence in being forthright in acknowledging their struggles.

It is also important to consider co-occurring physical health conditions. Many of these conditions can impact a patient's ability to safely receive treatment within an outpatient setting. Substances such as volatile solvents, alcohol, and opioids may also be associated with several physical harms, enumerated in **Table 6**, which also require thorough assessment and management.

Co-occurring psychiatric illnesses also pose additional safety risks for adolescents who are already at an increased risk of developing psychiatric illnesses by virtue of their substance use. Evaluating an adolescent's motivation for treatment is another dimension to consider, with the degree of motivation to change having been correlated with the success of treatment.[16]

Understanding and assessment of premorbid temperament is an integral component of assessment. Temperament in childhood is traditionally considered to include a narrower set of attributes than adult personality that are linked more directly to biological processes. Common attributes assessed are sociability, reactivity, and persistence. Studies have shown that children scoring high on sociability and reactivity, and low on persistence, are at a higher risk of early initiation of substance use.[18-20] A common tool used to assess temperament in adolescents is the temperament rating scale which assesses temperament under 10 headings—Intensity, activity levels, regularity, quality of mood, sensory sensitivity, adaptability, approach/withdrawal, distractibility, and persistence **(Table 7)**. Based on the responses, adolescents may have:

- *Easy-going temperament:* Regular bodily functions, a positive approach to new situations, adaptability, a positive mood, and a nonintense reaction to stimuli.

TABLE 6: Physical harms associated with substance use among adolescents.

Substance	*Associated physical harms*
Alcohol	Megaloblastic anemia, nutritional deficiencies, alcoholic myopathy, cardiac arrhythmias, Mallory–Weiss syndrome, aspiration pneumonia, gastritis, gastroesophageal reflux disease, acute tubular necrosis, acute renal failure, and alcohol-related liver disease
Volatile solvents	Chemical pneumonitis, neuropathies, convulsions, cerebral hypoxia, methemoglobinemia, megaloblastic anemia, cardiac arrhythmias, upper airway injuries and edema, and leukoencephalopathy
Opioids	Burns on fingers, thrombophlebitis, cellulitis, septicemia, anorexia, nutritional deficiencies, pulmonary hypertension, chronic bronchitis, chronic constipation, delayed ejaculation, viral hepatitis (B and C), and HIV infection
Cannabis	Respiratory tract irritation, bronchoconstriction, pneumonia, decreased intraocular pressure, ptosis, nystagmus, photophobia, and hypotension

TABLE 7: Temperament assessment scale.

Component	*Scoring*
Activity level: Ability to sit at a stretch while studying or engaged in an activity	High to low activity (score 1 to 5)
Regularity: Maintaining routine of sleep, meals, and other routine activities	Regular to irregular (Score 5 to 1)
Adaptability: Adjustment to new situations	Quick to slow (Score 5 to 1)
Approach/withdrawal: Initial reaction to new situations	Approach to withdrawal (Score 5 to 1)
Sensitivity: Reaction to changes in environment	Low to high sensitivity (Score 1 to 5)
Intensity of reaction: Strength of emotional reactions (joy, anger, sadness, and violence)	High to low intensity (Score 1 to 5)
Distractibility: Ease and frequency of distraction from task with external stimuli	High to low distractibility (Score 1 to 5)
Positive or negative mood: Predominant mood state	Positive to negative mood (Score 5 to 1)
Persistence: Continuing an activity in the face of difficulty	Long to short attention span (Score 5 to 1)

- *Difficult temperament:* Irregular bodily functions, withdrawal from new situations, slow adaptability, negative mood, and intense reactions.
- *Slow to warm up:* Low activity level and low intensity of reaction, a tendency to withdraw from new situations, slow adaptability, and somewhat negative mood.

It is important to note that the premorbid temperament should be assessed prior to the development of not just substance use disorder but also before any other chronic medical or psychiatric conditions.

DIAGNOSIS OF SUBSTANCE USE DISORDERS IN ADOLESCENTS

Clinical diagnosis: A detailed clinical interview comprising detailed history and examination is the mainstay of diagnosis. It is important to consider that adolescents may try to hide or minimize their substance use out of fear of consequences. Thus, maintaining a nonthreatening, nonjudgmental environment during interview is essential. More than one interview may be taken to elicit details of history. It is desirable to gather history from multiple sources, viz., parents, siblings, peers, teachers, and other close contacts of the adolescent.

- *History:* Details of substance use—age of initiation, route, preparation, expenditure, frequency, progression, adverse effects of substance use on multiple domains of life, abstinence attempts, reasons of relapse, treatment history, family history, relevant developmental history, and premorbid personality.
- *Physical examination:* A thorough head-to-toe general physical examination including tell-tale signs of substance use (conjunctival suffusion, stained teeth, burns on fingers, characteristic smell emanating from clothes, nasal bridge perforation, track marks from injection use, sclerosed veins, and punched out lesions on skin) along with other physical findings like cuts on wrists and inner thighs, other signs of health damage specific to the substance used, e.g., peripheral neuropathy in inhalant users.
- *Mental status examination:* General appearance and behavior, rapport, speech, mood, thought content, and perceptual abnormalities along with higher cognitive functions and motivation to seek treatment (desirable to record speech sample and decide the stage of motivation—precontemplation, contemplation, preparation, change, maintenance, and relapse).

BOX 1: ICD-11 diagnostic criteria for substance dependence.

- Substance dependence is a disorder of regulation of substance use arising from repeated or continuous use of the substance
- The characteristic feature is a strong internal drive to use the substance, which is manifested by impaired ability to control use, increasing priority given to use over other activities and persistence of use despite harm or negative consequences. These experiences are often accompanied by a subjective sensation of urge or craving to use the substance
- Physiological features of dependence may also be present, including tolerance to its effects, withdrawal symptoms following cessation or reduction in use of the substance, or repeated use of the substance or pharmacologically similar substances to prevent or alleviate withdrawal symptoms
- The features of dependence are usually evident over a period of at least 12 months, but the diagnosis may be made if use is continuous (daily or almost daily) for at least 3 months

Diagnostic criteria for mental and behavioral disorders due to use of substance as mentioned in ICD-11 **(Box 1)** may be used to aid in forming a diagnosis (06C40-49).

Laboratory investigations: While no laboratory investigations are considered essential for forming a diagnosis of substance use disorder, it is advisable to get baseline investigations like complete blood count, liver function tests, renal function tests including serum electrolytes and viral markers [hepatitis B surface antigen (HBsAg), hepatitis C virus (HCV), and human immunodeficiency virus (HIV)]. Urine drug screening has an important role in confirming drug use at the first visit and assessing effectiveness of treatment during follow-up visits.

GENERAL CONSIDERATIONS FOR MANAGEMENT OF SUBSTANCE USE IN ADOLESCENTS

Individual assessment is followed by the development of a treatment plan, which includes deciding the locus (inpatient and outpatient); focus (target points of treatment), and modus (method of service delivery) of treatment in accordance with the adolescent's treatment needs and expected outcomes. General principles of adolescent substance use management to consider are listed below:

- Addressing any substance use, even if it does not qualify as a disorder, should be a primary goal of all providers who work with adolescents.
- No single treatment or combination of evidenced-based treatments will be appropriate for all adolescents.
- Treatment is primarily based on psychological interventions. However, medications are warranted in opioid dependence, nonresponse to psychosocial interventions in tobacco use, and for alcohol dependence.
- Concomitant treatment of comorbid psychiatric disorders yields better outcomes.
- Substance dependence should be considered as a chronic illness with relapsing and remitting features in which individuals may oscillate between different levels of care.
- Effective treatment takes time. The longer the duration of treatment, the more sustained and positive the outcomes tend to be, and retention in care is associated with improved treatment outcomes.
- Since adolescents are often brought in treatment by their parents/guardians, it is important to engage them in treatment as well in order to ensure retention.
- Relapse is an opportunity for additional support to be put in place and/or indicates that the current level of care might not match the need.

PHARMACOLOGICAL MANAGEMENT OF SUBSTANCE USE IN ADOLESCENTS

As mentioned earlier, psychotherapies are central to managing substance use among adolescents, but medications are often essential in some substance use disorders, especially tobacco, alcohol, and opioids. Medications not only prevent complications during detoxification phase but also have good evidence for prolongation of abstinence by reducing craving and mitigation of withdrawal symptoms. **Table 8** provides an overview of major pharmacological agents used for managing substance use disorders in young adults along with levels of evidence. Specific medications are discussed under treatment of specific substances in the following section.

MANAGEMENT OF SPECIFIC SUBSTANCE USE DISORDERS IN ADOLESCENTS

In this segment, specific treatment for tobacco, alcohol, cannabis, opioids, and volatile solvent cannabis use among adolescents will be discussed. Levels of evidence for pharmacotherapeutic agents for these disorders in adolescents have been presented in **Table 8**. There are no definitive guidelines on long-term pharmacotherapies for these disorders, and the mainstay of treatment remains behavioral and family interventions.

TABLE 8: Pharmacotherapeutic agents for substance use disorders in adolescents.

Substance use disorder	*Target*			*Level of evidence*
	Withdrawal/ detoxification	*Maintenance or cessation aids*	*Overdose prevention*	
Opioids	BPN BPN-N	BPN BPN-N		Level 2
	Methadone	Methadone		Level 3
	Clonidine			Level 2
		Naltrexone		Level 3
			Naloxone	Level 3
Alcohol	Benzodiazepines			Level 3
		Naltrexone		Level 3
		Disulfiram		Level 3
		Topiramate		Level 3
		Ondansetron		Level 3
Tobacco		Nicotine replacement therapy		Level 2 for patch and level 3 for others
		Bupropion		Level 2
		Varenicline		Level 2
Cannabis	Gabapentin	Gabapentin		Level 2
		N-acetylcysteine		Level 3

Notes:
Level 1: Evidence from a systematic review or meta-analysis of all relevant randomized controlled trials (RCTs)
Level 2: Evidence from at least one well-designed RCT (e.g., large multisite RCT)
Level 3: Evidence from a single well-designed controlled trials without randomization (aka quasi-experimental studies) or a systematic review of a complete BOE (integrative review of higher and lower evidence) or mixed methods intervention studies
Level 4: Evidence from well-designed case–control or cohort studies
Level 5: Evidence from systematic reviews of descriptive and qualitative studies (meta-synthesis)
Level 6: Evidence from a single descriptive or qualitative study, EBP, EBQI, and QI projects
Level 7: Evidence from the opinion of authorities and/or reports of expert committees, reports from committees of experts and narrative and literature reviews
(BNP: B-type natriuretic peptide)

Pharmacotherapy for Tobacco Use

No smoking cessation medications are currently Food and Drug Administration (FDA) approved for use in children or adolescents (younger than 18 years). There are limited studies on nicotine replacement therapy (NRT) and bupropion among adolescent population. NRT with behavioral interventions are recommended in the National Institute for Health and Care Excellence (NICE) guidelines for patients with nicotine dependence beginning at age 12 years. The NICE guidelines state to avoid varenicline and bupropion in patients younger than 18 years. They recommend that a careful consideration of risks and benefits should be employed by the provider and explained to the patient and the legal guardian.

Table 9 presents the research trials conducted for pharmacotherapeutic agents for tobacco cessation among adolescents. Among NRTs, nicotine gums, patches, and nasal spray have been reported to be associated with small to moderate reduction in smoking rates among adolescents. Bupropion was noted to perform worse than placebo in conjunction with NRT and only a small difference without NRT. A trial of bupropion SR and contingency management (CM), bupropion alone, placebo plus CM, and placebo favored combination treatment with medication and therapy.[21] Some of the poor response in the trials reviewed may be explained by poor adherence to therapy, concomitant psychiatric diagnoses, other substance abuse disorders, high baseline smoking rates, and inadequate duration of therapy (i.e., <12 weeks). The lack of pharmacokinetic data for these smoking cessation medications in the adolescent population and, therefore, lack of accurate dosing, may also lead to poor response.[16] Additionally, many of the subjects in the NRT and bupropion trials lived in homes with other smokers, started smoking at young ages, and had other barriers to successfully quitting. Thus, the current consensus favors NRT along with behavioral interventions.

Pharmacotherapy for Alcohol Use

Alcohol withdrawal syndrome (AWS) is rare in adolescents. Presenting symptoms may include anxiety, tremor, diaphoresis, elevated blood pressure, nausea, vomiting, headache, auditory or visual hallucinations, or in rare cases in adolescents, seizures. To date, very few studies have examined pharmacotherapy interventions for AWS in adolescents.

Clinical guidelines for AWS in youth are modeled after best practices in adults. Benzodiazepines are currently the first line of pharmacotherapy for treatment of AWS in adults. Consensus guidelines suggest that adolescents

TABLE 9: Evidence for medications for tobacco cessation in adolescents.

Treatment	*Study (sample size)*	*Follow-up period*	*Tobacco cessation rates*
Nicotine patch	Smith et al., 1996 (*n* = 22)	8 weeks and 6 months	13.6% and 4.5%
	Hurt et al., 2000 (*n* = 101)	6 weeks and 6 months	10.9% and 5%
	Hanson et al., 2003 (*n* = 100)	10 weeks	28% (patch) and 24% (placebo)
Nasal spray	Rubinstein et al., 2008 (*n* = 35)	12 weeks	0% (patch) and 11% (counseling)
Bupropion 150 mg	Muramoto et al., 2007 (*n* = 312)	6 weeks	27% (OD dosing) 34% (BD dosing) 20% (placebo)
	Niederhofer et al., 2004 (*n* = 22)	90 days	55% (bupropion) and 18% (placebo)
NRT + Bupropion	Killen et al., 2004 (*n* = 211)	8 weeks NRT + Bupropion	23% (NRT + Bupropion) and 28% (placebo)

(NRT: nicotine replacement therapy)

with severe alcohol use disorder (AUD) who present with moderate-to-severe AWS should be treated with benzodiazepines in inpatient setting.[22]

Advancement of pharmacotherapies for AUD in adults has expanded the treatment options beyond behavioral therapy. In adults, naltrexone, acamprosate, and disulfiram are FDA-approved for the treatment of AUD.

While no studies exist on the use of long-acting injectable naltrexone in adolescent AUD, two small clinical studies of 4 and 6 weeks respectively have examined the effects of oral short-acting naltrexone, reporting reduction in drinks per day, binge drinking episodes, and alcohol-related thoughts/obsessions.[23,24] Naltrexone was fairly well-tolerated in usual doses of 25–50 mg in both studies.

Disulfiram is an aversive agent that irreversibly binds to the enzyme aldehyde dehydrogenase, resulting in accumulation of acetaldehyde when alcohol is consumed and producing aversive symptoms. One study has been completed in adolescents; a 90-day double-blind placebo-controlled study compared disulfiram (250 mg/day) to placebo in 26 adolescents receiving AUD outpatient treatment. The study results indicated that disulfiram was well-tolerated and not associated with adverse events. Compared to the group receiving placebo, the disulfiram group had more cumulative days of abstinence and higher rates of sustained abstinence.[25] However, this medication should be used with caution, given the potential severity of the disulfiram reaction when combined with alcohol. The coerced administration of this medication to individuals under the age of 18 years also raises potential ethical concerns.

Acamprosate is hypothesized to promote balance in excitatory-inhibitory neurotransmission by altering γ-aminobutyric acid (GABA) and glutamatergic activity and, in doing so, to reduce "protracted" withdrawal symptoms and cravings. It has not been systematically studied in adolescents as yet.

Ondansetron and topiramate also have preliminary evidence for reduction in heavy drinking days among adolescents with mild to moderated AUDs.

Pharmacotherapy for Cannabis Use

There are no FDA-approved medications for the treatment of cannabis use disorder (CUD) in adolescents at this time. As cannabis use modulates glutamatergic and GABAergic activity in the brain, pharmacotherapies that target these systems have shown promise as agents that aid with cannabis cessation.

There has been one open-label and one RCT examining N-acetylcysteine (NAC) in adolescents and young adults, which suggested that NAC was well-tolerated and was associated with cannabis use reduction when combined with CM.[26]

Topiramate in conjunction with motivational interviewing (MI) tried in an open-label study had significant drop-out rates due to adverse effects.[27] Considering the poor tolerability and inconsistent effect on cannabis use outcome measures, topiramate likely does not have a role in the treatment of adolescent CUDs.

Gabapentin modulates the GABAergic system and represents a potential medication for CUD, studies in adults showed some promise in reduction of withdrawal symptoms and craving but no systematic research in adolescent population has been carried out as yet.

Pharmacotherapy for Opioid Use

Opioid withdrawal (OW) is the only acute withdrawal syndrome for which controlled studies have been completed in adolescent samples. This syndrome is often accompanied by anxiety, restlessness, bone or joint aches, lacrimation (tearing), rhinorrhea (runny nose), mydriasis (dilated pupils), yawning, tremor, abdominal cramping, diarrhea, tachycardia (elevated heart rate), and diaphoresis (sweating).

The onset and duration of symptoms depend on the half-life of the opioid. For short-acting opioids such as heroin, symptoms often peak within 48–72 hours and resolve within 7 days. However, some symptoms such as insomnia and irritability may persist beyond this time period.

Buprenorphine-naloxone, a μ-opioid receptor partial agonist, has been shown to effectively reduce OW symptoms across three controlled studies in adolescents. The USFDA approved buprenorphine for adolescents (≥16 years) in 2003. Clonidine, an α-2-agonist and nonopioid detoxification medication, has also been shown to be effective at reducing OW symptoms. Efficacy of clonidine and buprenorphine were compared as part of a 28-day outpatient opioid detoxification protocol, in a double-blind, randomized controlled trial. Clonidine and buprenorphine were both effective at reducing OW symptoms, but compared to the clonidine group, youth in the buprenorphine arm had fewer opioid-positive urines and were more likely to remain in treatment and initiate a nonagonist maintenance treatment.[28,29]

Given these findings, buprenorphine is the detoxification agent of choice in youth with moderate-to-severe OUD and has shown to be effective in outpatient and inpatient settings. Clonidine might be the drug of choice for youth and families of youth with less severe OUD or those that are interested in nonopioid detoxification medications,[30] but preferably should be used in inpatient setting only. Lofexidine is another FDA-approved nonopioid medication that can be used for management of OW symptoms in adults but evidence in children and adolescents is lacking.

Three medications are currently indicated for long-term pharmacological treatment of moderate to severe opioid use disorder: methadone, naltrexone, and buprenorphine. Methadone, a full opioid agonist with a long half-life that can ameliorate the cycle of intense euphoria followed by intense withdrawal associated with opioid use, has long been established as an effective treatment of opioid addiction, although federal regulations prohibit most methadone programs from admitting patients younger than 18 years.[17]

Naltrexone, an opioid antagonist with high affinity for the opioid receptor, has also proven to be an effective treatment of opioid addiction. Oral naltrexone has been FDA-approved for adults (≥18 years) since 1984, and FDA approved a long-acting injectable formulation in 2010.[31] Unlike opioid agonists, naltrexone has a very limited potential for misuse or diversion. The extended-release formulation may improve patient adherence. Although there is no rigorous research support yet for efficacy in adolescents, growing experience and anecdotal reports support it as a promising practice.[17] Naltrexone, which also reduces alcohol cravings, may be a good therapeutic option for adolescents and young adults with co-occurring AUD, as well as those living in unstable or unsupervised housing.[32]

Buprenorphine is also suitable for long-term pharmacotherapy for opioid use disorders in adolescents under the rubric of medication-assisted treatment or opioid substitution therapy. Controlled trials have found that continued buprenorphine compliance is associated with an increase in treatment retention and can help adolescents to achieve long-term sobriety. In general, youth have lower rates of treatment retention compared with adults, underscoring the need to deliver developmentally appropriate treatment to achieve best outcomes.[33,34] Current consensus is thus clear on providing long-term medication-assisted treatment with buprenorphine along with behavioral interventions for adolescents with opioid use disorders. The dose and duration of buprenorphine administration varies from case to case. The principle to be followed is as much as the adolescent needs for as long as the adolescent needs. It is to be noted that evidence for buprenorphine-naloxone fixed dose combination for adolescent age group is still insufficient to form a definitive consensus. Buprenorphine mono-product is generally administered in a daily dispensing manner in adults. Take-home doses with brief intervals of follow-ups may be considered for adolescents under strict supervision of parents and guardians to minimize risk of diversion and improper use. **Table 10** provides an overview of evidence for long-term pharmacotherapy for opioid use disorders in adolescents.

Pharmacotherapy for Volatile Solvent Use

Emergency medical attention for volatile solvent use is usually sought in acute intoxication only when there are serious injuries or other threats to life. No medications currently available can reverse acute inhalant intoxication. Fortunately, the intoxications resolve spontaneously with supportive treatment. A patient suspected to be in acute intoxication needs to be monitored in a clinical setting, in close observation, for approximately 2–4 hours.[35] They should not be left alone for up to 24 hours,

TABLE 10: Overview of evidence for long-term pharmacotherapy for opioid use disorders in adolescents.

Drug	*Reference*	*Study design*	*Sample*	*Dose*	*Results*
Methadone	Mattick et al. (2009)	Systematic review	9 studies, (*n* = 6,263)	Oral, flexible dosing, for up to 6-month maintenance	Methadone more effective than nonpharmacological approaches in suppression of heroin use (RR = 0.66 95% CI: 0.56–0.78)
	Smyth et al. (2018)	Retrospective cohort study	(*n* = 88)	Outpatient methadone maintenance treatment	Heroin abstinence was 21% (CI: 9–36) at 3 months and 46% (95% CI: 30–63) at 12 months
Buprenorphine	Woody et al. (2008)	Randomized controlled trial	Outpatient, treatment-seeking youth (*n* = 152)	• Detox group—buprenorphine at 14 mg/day, tapering doses for 14 days • Maintenance group-up to 24 mg/day for 12 weeks	Maintenance group reported less opioid use (χ^2 (1) = 8.45, p > 0.001) and less injecting opioids (χ^2 (1) = 6.00, p = 0.01) till 12 weeks, no difference at week 52
	Mutlu et al. (2016)	Prospective cohort study	Adolescents between ages 12–18 years (*n* = 112)	Inpatient unit oral, flexible dosing, 12–month retention program	Retention on buprenorphine maintenance was 69.6% at day 30 and 16.1% at 1 year. Rates of abstinence were 69.0% at day 30 and 10.3% at 1 year
Extended-release naltrexone injection	Fishman et al. (2010)	Retrospective, chart review	Outpatient, treatment-seeking, adolescents, (*n* = 16)	XR-naltrexone, IM, 380 mg every 4 weeks	63% were retained in treatment for at least 4 months and nine of 16 56% reported decreased opioid use

(1) stands for degree of freedom.
(CI: confidence interval; RR: relative risk)

even if there are no serious symptoms, and for a longer period if symptoms like seizures or impaired consciousness are present.

During withdrawal phase, benzodiazepines may be used for management of anxiety or minor agitation. Induced psychosis mandates special attention to patient safety. Severe agitation will require cautious control with either haloperidol, risperidone, or carbamazepine which have been reported to be effective in management of induced paranoid psychosis.[36]

Isolated studies and case-series during post-withdrawal phase provide preliminary support for the use of baclofen, started at 10 mg/day and gradually increased to 50 mg/day over 1 week, to be beneficial in the management of craving and withdrawal and possibly in relapse prevention in patients with dependence.[37] An isolated report suggested that buspirone, at 40 mg per day for 2 months, was effective in relieving craving for inhalants.[38] Isolated case studies suggest potential role of lamotrigine and vigabatrin in dependence.[39] Risperidone 1 mg twice daily was found to reduce both craving for inhalants and paranoid ideation, and to maintain abstinence for 12 weeks.[36]

BEHAVIORAL INTERVENTIONS FOR SUBSTANCE USE IN ADOLESCENTS

Over the last two decades, several behavioral therapies have emerged with a strong evidence base as effective interventions for management of adolescents with substance use. Some of these interventions will be touched upon briefly in this section.

Family Therapies

Substance use often affects the family as a whole. For this reason, family therapy approaches involve family members along with the identified patient. This theoretical approach, based on Bronfenbrenner's integration of social ecological and life-span human development theories, assumes that children's development is influenced by a number of interacting systems across time. It places the child first and most centrally in the developmental ecology of the family because of the foundational role that families play across child and adolescent development. While individual genetic, personality, and cognitive factors are important in understanding adolescent behavior, emphasis is laid on contextual factors over individual factors because of their well-established role as central risk and protective factors. Since the family is viewed as a system of different parts, the underlying assumption is that a change in one part of the system will create changes in the other parts. The key components of family intervention are parental monitoring and behavioral management (both general and drug-specific parenting strategies), promoting positive relationships, encouraging self-regulation and stress management. This includes focus on the development of coping and communication skills. The process includes educating parents about drug use, process of treatment and recovery, engagement in the treatment process, identifying one or more parents who will be involved in the treatment process and monitoring. Family therapy sessions may include discussions of family concerns, how people are feeling, what problems need to be addressed, and what changes have been happening. The family also plays an important role in supporting the patient to handle high-risk situations, facilitating pursuing recreational interests and academic goals or develop vocational skills. Examples of family approaches supported by one or more randomized controlled trials include brief strategic family therapy (BSFT), functional family therapy (FFT), family behavior therapy (FBT), and multisystemic therapy (MST). Multiple meta-analyses and randomized controlled trials on each different type of family therapy have proved effectiveness in reduction in frequency of substance use by adolescents as compared to adolescents who were not provided with family interventions.[40,41]

Motivational Interviewing

Motivational interviewing approaches are typically brief and limited to interventions in screening situations, such as primary care offices, emergency departments, or school health centers. A single session is often used to help youth resolve ambivalent feelings about change and commit to participation in a treatment program. Five major principles of MI include expressing empathy through reflective listening, developing discrepancy between a patient's behavior and goals, dealing with resistance by avoiding confrontation, supporting self-efficacy to change, and developing autonomy.[42] Where indicated, MI may also be used to enhance the commitment to participation in a treatment program. While meta-analyses show small effect sizes, in a review of 39 studies on MI in adolescents, 67% reported statistically significant improved substance use outcomes.[43]

The basic principles of MI are represented by the acronym OARS. Using each of these components helps to make the discussion more successful in encouraging change.

- *Open-ended questions:* Asking questions that cannot be answered with yes/no.
- *Affirmations:* Recognizing and encouraging client's strengths.
- *Reflections:* Responses that emphasize careful listening and understanding on the therapist's part. This also allows the listener to express "empathy," the ability to see the world through another's eyes and share in their feelings and experiences. This can make the other person feel heard and understood.
- *Summarize:* Summaries allow the listener to "recap" what has been discussed. The summary can highlight the other person's strengths and reasons for change.

Cognitive Behavior Therapy

Cognitive behavior therapy (CBT) refers to a variety of interventions that focus on the present and goal-directed behavior change. The clinician is seen as a collaborator with the patient and uses strategies based on classical conditioning, operant conditioning, and social learning perspectives while taking contextual factors into account. MI techniques have been combined with CBT to form brief outpatient treatment interventions in specialty addiction treatment programs.[3,42] These are often known as motivational enhancement therapy and CBT, with evidence pointing toward improved treatment outcomes in small, single-center comparative studies.[14,42,44]

Contingency Management

In an operant behavioral approach, CM involves providing patients with tangible reward to reinforce positive behaviors (e.g., abstinence). One way in which this can be achieved is by providing incentive programs (e.g., vouchers or "fishbowl") where youth earns prizes that escalate in value for consecutive weeks of negative urine test findings. A major concern is that if CM prizes end, abstinence may end as well; however, results of studies examining this concern are mixed, with some research showing maintenance of effect over post-treatment follow-up and others showing drug use rebounding. For example, the punchbowl method reward negative screens for drug use with the opportunity to draw a prize from a "punchbowl." Most prizes have low monetary value (e.g., $1), but the inclusions of rarer large prizes (e.g., $50) both save money while offering a successful inducement for abstinence. CM procedures may use either stable or escalating reinforcement schedules, in which reinforcer value increases as duration of abstinence increases. In addition to contingencies linked to negative drug screens (e.g., from swab or urine toxicology screens), adaptive behaviors ranging from attendance to medication adherence have been successfully modified with CM approaches.

Despite research support, CM has not been as widely disseminated in practice as many of the other models discussed, and this may be due to concerns that providers or parents object to the idea of "paying youth to be abstinent." On the other hand, CM increases positive feedback for desirable behaviors which may reduce feelings of ambivalence about change and eventually outweigh the reward perceived with substance use.[45-47]

12-Step Facilitation Programs

A variety of 12-step programs exist for adults and adolescents who struggle with addiction and their families (e.g., Cocaine Anonymous, Marijuana Anonymous, Gamblers Anonymous, Al-Anon, Alateen, etc.). These community-based recovery support programs are peer-led; nonprofessional fellowships whose primary purpose is mutual help. 12-step programs are free of cost and are available in 180 countries. Grounded in the philosophy that people with addiction have lost the ability to control their substance use, the 12-step philosophy defines recovery as abstinence from substances and includes the personality changes and spiritual growth that result from practicing the 12 steps and assimilating the 12-step principles (like integrity, courage, hope, and other-focus) into one's value system. The emphasis of 12-step meetings is sharing recovery narratives. Sharing reduces members' sense of isolation, teaches practical skills for living a substance free life, and produces hope and a sense of belonging.[20,48] Existence of programs in India for adolescents is limited.

Relapse Prevention

Recovery support is essential to help adolescents make healthy choices and mature physically and emotionally, whether or not they are beginning a lifelong cycle of substance use, treatment, and relapse. Recovery capital refers to the internal and external resources that individuals can access to initiate and sustain recovery and consists of multiple facets **(Table 11)**. Research has found that individuals who engage in meaningful activities have significantly higher quality of life than those who do not. Individuals in treatment who report abstinence and engagement in meaningful activity report the highest quality of life. Participation in meaningful activities can create opportunities for developing personal recovery capital such as self-esteem and self-efficacy, provide ways to extend networks of prorecovery people, and facilitate access to community resources.[14,16,49]

TABLE 11: Types of recovery capital.

Personal	Physical health, financial health, educational/vocational skills, problem-solving ability, self-efficacy to manage high-risk situations, and interpersonal skills
Family/social	Relationships with partners, family, and other supportive of recovery
Community	Community efforts to reduce stigma, the availability of addiction treatment and mutual aid resources, the accessibility of sustained recovery support, and the availability of culturally appropriate recovery support

Adolescent Community Reinforcement Approach

Adolescent Community Reinforcement Approach (A-CRA) is one behavioral treatment for adolescent substance use disorders that has earned strong research support and is based on building new and pleasurable prosocial behaviors to increase recovery capital.[50] According to the concrete-representational-abstract (CRA) model, successful treatment begins with first listening to each patient in order to learn as much as possible about what their (nonusing) reinforcers and potential sources of recovery capital are. The more therapists learn from listening, the more effective they can be in helping patients access these reinforcers. Improving family/ social recovery capital by increasing positive communication with family and other important individuals and problem-solving through guided practice and feedback are often major reinforcers for patients and their significant others. The therapist next obtains a thorough understanding of the pleasurable as well as the negative consequences of substance use. This forms the future basis for illustrating the relationship between positive consequences of substance use and finding substitute positive reinforcers in new activities. After, the therapist has the patient rate their personal satisfaction with major areas of their community life (e.g., school, work, romantic relationships, family and peer relationships, emotional, economic, and other areas).

This self-assessment allows the therapist to support the patient in developing short-term, achievable goals and recovery capital in life/health areas that would increase positive reinforcement derived from a variety of interpersonal, social, vocational, educational, and family relationships. Five published randomized clinical trials of A-CRA demonstrated significant pre- and post-treatment improvements in number of days of abstinence and percentage of adolescents in recovery during the 12-month follow-up period. A-CRA was cost-effective and was a good choice of intervention for homeless, street children, youth with juvenile justice involvement, and as a continuing care approach for adolescents after residential treatment.[51,52] Secondary evaluation studies suggest that A-CRA shows potential to be an effective treatment for adolescents with co-occurring psychiatric disorders and youth with opioid use problems.[50,53]

Brief Interventions

As already mentioned, recreational and harmful use are commonly encountered patterns of substance use in a community setting. Brief intervention directed toward early intervention and behavior change is an ideal format for such a population and setting. These are nonstructured conversations that focus on promoting healthy choices and reducing high-risk behaviors among target population, include clear and pointed advice for adolescents to reduce substance use and succinct mention of the potential negative health effects of alcohol and drugs. For those who are using substances more heavily or frequently, BIs involve the use of MI strategies to help adolescents compare the benefits of continued use with the potential benefits of behavior change (cutting back and stopping) to empower them to make decisions that support their health, safety, and achievement of personal goals. Brief intervention includes education and concise session of counseling aimed at prevention of progression of substance use, risk identification, and treatment-seeking among adolescents. Evidence of effectiveness has focused on alcohol use in adolescents, indicating cost-effectiveness and increase in treatment seeking among adolescents with harmful patterns of alcohol use.[54]

MANAGEMENT OF DUAL DIAGNOSIS AMONG ADOLESCENTS

Adolescents with mental health disorders are at increased risk for the development of problematic substance use. Results from the National Comorbidity Survey indicate that up to 67% of adolescents with substance abuse or dependence have experienced at least one prior mental health disorder.[55] Adolescents who use substances are more likely to develop new psychiatric disorders or exacerbate preexisting mental health symptoms.[56] In practice, the clinical picture may be difficult to interpret, with substance use (or withdrawal from substances) potentially creating specific psychiatric symptoms, such as the sensation of panic, anxiety, or anhedonia. The term "co-occurring disorders" refers to conditions that exist at the same time, such as an AUD and a concurrent diagnosis of generalized anxiety disorder (GAD). A synonymous term that is often used is "dual diagnosis." Common conditions that occur as psychiatric comorbidities are depressive disorders (30%), anxiety disorders (40–45%), bipolar disorders (38–47%), psychosis, and ADHD.[57]

Treatment of co-occurring mental health disorders is especially important due to their detrimental influence on substance use. Even untreated mental health symptoms not meeting full diagnostic criteria for a disorder can negatively impact the course of treatment for substance use. In these cases, treatment planning can be difficult due to the unidentified etiology of existing mental health symptoms. Symptoms of substance use often mimic mental health disorders, with practitioners having historically voiced their inability to effectively diagnose a co-occurring mental health condition prior to the achievement of full abstinence. As a result, the treatment field focused on achieving full abstinence prior to treatment initiation for any co-occurring mental health symptoms. However, delaying treatment for a co-occurring mental health condition could impede successful substance use disorder recovery. For this reason, it is now more common, and strongly advised, to treat co-occurring conditions along with substance use disorders in a collaborative care setting.

SPECIALIZED TREATMENT SERVICES AVAILABLE IN INDIA

The Mental Healthcare Act, 2017, provides procedures and minimum standards of care for adolescents with mental health conditions including substance use disorders, considering them as minors until attainment of 18 years of age. Such adolescents may be admitted in hospital after due approval from competent mental healthcare providers, accompanied by a female caregiver, in developmentally appropriate facilities, with stipulated reporting procedures. Specialized treatment services for adolescents with substance use disorders are available in selected Government medical institutes and hospitals in India. The National Drug Dependence Treatment Center, All India Institute of Medical Sciences, New Delhi; Postgraduate Institute of Medical Education and Research, Chandigarh, Child and Adolescent Mental Health Clinic at National Institute of Mental Health and Neurosciences, Bengaluru have dedicated outpatient and inpatient department services for adolescents.

In 2020, Ministry of Social Justice and Empowerment, Government of India introduced Community Based Peer-Led intervention (CPLI), which is an outreach-based initiative, aiming at preventing and reducing the substance use among vulnerable children and early adolescents (10–18 years of age). The key elements of the program are peer educators who focus on primary activities among at-risk adolescents through educational sessions on life skills among children and side effects of substance use; and program officers who deliver specific interventions to adolescents in need and ensure linkage to treatment and rehabilitation services (For more details, readers are referred to https://grants-msje.gov.in/omrunningcpli).

Outreach programs need to be supplemented by empowering teachers, school authorities, and community leaders to identify substance use and related problems in adolescents and referral to appropriate services, along with maintenance of long-term contacts with such adolescents, facilitating a continuum of care.

SUMMARY AND CONCLUSION

Prevention for substance use disorders among adolescents is very important considering its deleterious consequences. Efforts toward early identification need to be made by screening in school, community, and healthcare settings. Interventions tailored to the needs of adolescents should be provided. Much of the literature on adolescent substance use is based on psychosocial interventions and these have been found to be effective. Further research needs to focus on pharmacological interventions as well. Longitudinal outcome studies would further our understanding of factors that are associated with improved prognosis.

REFERENCES

1. Dhawan A, Mandal P. Preventive strategies for substance use. Indian J Soc Psychiatry. 2017;33(2):108.
2. Nadkarni A, Tu A, Garg A, Gupta D, Gupta S, Bhatia U, et al. Alcohol use among adolescents in India: a systematic review. Glob Ment Health (Camb). 2022;9:1-25.
3. Gray KM, Squeglia LM. Research Review: What have we learned about adolescent substance use? J Child Psychol Psychiatry. 2018;59(6): 618-27.
4. Sivagurunathan C, Umadevi R, Rama R, Gopalakrishnan S. Adolescent Health: Present Status and Its Related Programmes in India. Are We in the Right Direction? J Clin Diagn Res JCDR. 2015;9(3):LE01-6.
5. NIDA. (2023). Reported drug use among adolescents continued to hold below pre-pandemic levels in 2023. [online] Available from https://nida.nih.gov/news-events/news-releases/2023/12/reported-drug-use-among-adolescents-continued-to-hold-below-pre-pandemic-levels-in-2023 [Last accessed November, 2023].
6. Ministry of Social Justice and Empowerment, Government of India. (2019). Magnitude of Substance Use in India. [online] Available from https://online.fliphtml5.com/ljdmb/aacc/#p=1 [Last accessed November, 2023].
7. Dhawan A, Pattanayak RD, Chopra A, Tikoo VK, Kumar R. Pattern and profile of children using substances in India: Insights and recommendations. Natl Med J India. 2017;30(4):224-9.
8. Kessler RC, Avenevoli S, Costello EJ, Green JG, Gruber MJ, Heeringa S, et al. National comorbidity survey replication adolescent supplement (NCS-A): II. Overview and design. J Am Acad Child Adolesc Psychiatry. 2009;48(4):380-5.
9. Leslie K. Youth substance use and abuse: challenges and strategies for identification and intervention. CMAJ Can Med Assoc J. 2008;178(2):145-8.
10. Nath A, Choudhari SG, Dakhode SU, Rannaware A, Gaidhane AM. Substance Abuse Amongst Adolescents: An Issue of Public Health Significance. Cureus. 2022;14(11):e31193.
11. Hamidullah S, Thorpe HHA, Frie JA, Mccurdy RD, Khokhar JY. Adolescent Substance Use and the Brain: Behavioral, Cognitive and Neuroimaging Correlates. Front Hum Neurosci. 2020;14:298.
12. Winters KC, Arria A. Adolescent Brain Development and Drugs. Prev Res. 2011;18(2):21-4.
13. Dhawan A, Balhara YPS, Natasha. Adolescent Substance Abuse and Suicide. J Indian Assoc Child Adolesc Ment Health. 2007;3(2):34-42.
14. Fadus MC, Squeglia LM, Valadez EA, Tomko RL, Bryant BE, Gray KM. Adolescent Substance Use Disorder Treatment: An Update on Evidence-Based Strategies. Curr Psychiatry Rep. 2019;21(10):96.
15. Scheier LM (Ed). Handbook of adolescent drug use prevention: Research, intervention strategies, and practice. Washington DC, US: American Psychological Association; 2015.
16. Welsh JW, Hadland SE (Eds). Treating Adolescent Substance Use: A Clinician's Guide. Cham: Springer International Publishing; 2019.
17. Hadland SE, Aalsma MC, Akgül S, Alinsky RH, Bruner A, Chadi N, et al. Medication for Adolescents and Young Adults with Opioid Use Disorder. J Adolesc Health Off Publ Soc Adolesc Med. 2021;68(3):632-6.
18. Willem L, Bijttebier P, Claes L, Sools J, Vandenbussche I, Nigg J. Temperamental characteristics of adolescents with substance abuse and/or dependence: A case-control study. Pers Individ Differ. 2011;50:1094-8.

19. Strickhouser J, Terracciano A, Sutin A. Parent-reported childhood temperament and adolescent self-reported substance use initiation. Addict Behav. 2020;110:106503.
20. Thatcher DL, Clark DB. Adolescents at Risk for Substance Use Disorders. Alcohol Res Health. 2008;31(2):168-76.
21. Karpinski JP, Timpe EM, Lubsch L. Smoking Cessation Treatment for Adolescents. J Pediatr Pharmacol Ther JPPT. 2010;15(4):249-63.
22. Das JK, Salam RA, Arshad A, Finkelstein Y, Bhutta ZA. Interventions for Adolescent Substance Abuse: An Overview of Systematic Reviews. J Adolesc Health. 2016;59(4):S61-75.
23. Deas D, May MPHK, Randall C, Johnson N, Anton R. Naltrexone treatment of adolescent alcoholics: an open-label pilot study. J Child Adolesc Psychopharmacol. 2005;15(5):723-8.
24. Miranda R, Ray L, Blanchard A, Reynolds EK, Monti PM, Chun T, et al. Effects of naltrexone on adolescent alcohol cue reactivity and sensitivity: an initial randomized trial. Addict Biol. 2014; 19(5):941-54.
25. Niederhofer H, Staffen W. Comparison of disulfiram and placebo in treatment of alcohol dependence of adolescents. Drug Alcohol Rev. 2003;22(3):295-7.
26. Gray KM, Carpenter MJ, Baker NL, DeSantis SM, Kryway E, Hartwell KJ, et al. A double-blind randomized controlled trial of N-acetylcysteine in cannabis-dependent adolescents. Am J Psychiatry. 2012;169(8):805-12.
27. Miranda R, Treloar H, Blanchard A, Justus A, Monti PM, Chun T, et al. Topiramate and motivational enhancement therapy for cannabis use among youth: a randomized placebo-controlled pilot study. Addict Biol. 2017;22(3):779-90.
28. Marsch LA, Bickel WK, Badger GJ, Stothart ME, Quesnel KJ, Stanger C, et al. Comparison of pharmacological treatments for opioid-dependent adolescents: a randomized controlled trial. Arch Gen Psychiatry. 2005;62(10):1157-64.
29. Marsch LA, Moore SK, Borodovsky JT, Solhkhah R, Badger GJ, Semino S, et al. A randomized controlled trial of buprenorphine taper duration among opioid-dependent adolescents and young adults. Addict Abingdon Engl. 2016;111(8):1406-15.
30. AAP Committee on Substance use and Prevention. Medication-Assisted Treatment of Adolescents With Opioid Use Disorders. Pediatrics. 2016;138(3):e20161893.
31. Bruneau J, Ahamad K, Goyer MÈ, Poulin G, Selby P, Fischer B, et al. Management of opioid use disorders: a national clinical practice guideline. CMAJ. 2018;190(9):E247-57.
32. Carney BL, Hadland SE, Bagley SM. Medication Treatment of Adolescent Opioid Use Disorder in Primary Care. Pediatr Rev. 2018;39(1):43-5.
33. Matson SC, Hobson G, Abdel-Rasoul M, Bonny AE. A retrospective study of retention of opioid-dependent adolescents and young adults in an outpatient buprenorphine/naloxone clinic. J Addict Med. 2014;8(3):176-82.
34. Oliveira JR, Oliveira RA de, Lima SFC, Filho ASS, Cunha RM, Espindola GF, et al. Stress generated by remote exams during the Covid-19 crisis and its relationship to physical activity: a cross-sectional study among medicine students. Res Soc Dev. 2022;11(7):e42511729456.
35. Cavanagh JJ, Smith TY. Inhalant (Alkyl Nitrites, Nitrous Oxide, Hydrocarbons) Intoxication AKA: Poppers | SpringerLink. In: Quick Guide to Psychiatric Emergencies: Tools for Behavioral and Toxicological Situations. Berlin: Springer International Publishing; 2018. pp. 183-6.
36. Hernandez-Avila CA, Ortega-Soto HA, Jasso A, Hasfura-Buenaga CA, Kranzler HR. Treatment of inhalant-induced psychotic disorder with carbamazepine versus haloperidol. Psychiatr Serv Wash DC. 1998;49(6):812-5.
37. Muralidharan K, Rajkumar RP, Mulla U, Nayak RB, Benegal V. Baclofen in the Management of Inhalant Withdrawal: A Case Series. Prim Care Companion J Clin Psychiatry. 2008;10(1): 48-51.
38. Niederhofer H. Treating inhalant abuse with buspirone. Am J Addict. 2007;16(1):69.
39. Menon PG, Rani A, Ts J. Solvent Use and its Management - An Overview. Kerala J Psychiatry. 2015;28(1):42-51.
40. Horigian VE, Anderson AR, Szapocznik J. Family-based Treatments for Adolescent Substance Use. Child Adolesc Psychiatr Clin N Am. 2016; 25(4):603-28.

41. Skeer MR, Sabelli RA, Rancaño KM, Lee-Bravatti M, Ryan EC, Eliasziw M, et al. Randomized controlled trial to test the efficacy of a brief, communication-based, substance use preventive intervention for parents of adolescents: Protocol for the SUPPER Project (Substance Use Prevention Promoted by Eating family meals Regularly). PLoS One. 2022;17(2):e0263016.
42. Winters KC. TIP 32: Treatment of Adolescents with Substance Use Disorders: Treatment Improvement Protocol (TIP) Series 32. 1999;207.
43. Barnett E, Sussman S, Smith C, Rohrbach LA, Spruijt-Metz D. Motivational Interviewing for adolescent substance use: a review of the literature. Addict Behav. 2012;37(12):1325-34.
44. McHugh RK, Hearon BA, Otto MW. Cognitive-Behavioral Therapy for Substance Use Disorders. Psychiatr Clin North Am. 2010;33(3):511-25.
45. Johnson S, Rains LS, Marwaha S, Strang J, Craig T, Weaver T, et al. A contingency management intervention to reduce cannabis use and time to relapse in early psychosis: the CIRCLE RCT. Health Technol Assess Winch Engl. 2019;23(45):1-108.
46. Stanger C, Budney AJ. Contingency Management Approaches for Adolescent Substance Use Disorders. Child Adolesc Psychiatr Clin N Am. 2010;19(3):547-62.
47. Stanger C, Lansing AH, Budney AJ. Contingency Management Approaches for Adolescent Substance Use Disorders. Child Adolesc Psychiatr Clin N Am. 2016;25(4):645.
48. Nash AJ. The Twelve Steps and Adolescent Recovery: A Concise Review. Subst Abuse Res Treat. 2020;14:1178221820904397.
49. Van der Westhuizen MA. Relapse prevention for chemically addicted adolescents in recovery: so which model works? J Evid-Inf Soc Work. 2015;12(4):400-11.
50. Godley SH, Smith JE, Passetti LL, Subramaniam G. The Adolescent Community Reinforcement Approach (A-CRA) as a Model Paradigm for the Management of Adolescents With Substance Use Disorders and Co-Occurring Psychiatric Disorders. Subst Abuse. 2014;35(4):352-63.
51. Garner BR, Godley SH, Funk RR, Dennis ML, Smith JE, Godley MD. Exposure to Adolescent Community Reinforcement Approach treatment procedures as a mediator of the relationship between adolescent substance abuse treatment retention and outcome. J Subst Abuse Treat. 2009;36(3):252-64.
52. Meyers RJ, Roozen HG, Smith JE. The Community Reinforcement Approach. Alcohol Res Health. 2011;33(4):380-8.
53. Godley SH, Smith JE, Meyers RJ, Godley MD. Adolescent Community Reinforcement Approach (A-CRA). In: Springer DW, Rubin A (Eds). Substance Abuse Treatment for Youth and Adults: Clinician's guide to evidence-base practice. Hoboken, NJ, US: John Wiley & Sons Inc; 2009. pp. 109-201.
54. Mattoo SK, Prasad S, Ghosh A. Brief intervention in substance use disorders. Indian J Psychiatry. 2018;60(Suppl 4):S466-72.
55. Conway KP, Swendsen J, Husky MM, He JP, Merikangas KR. Association of Lifetime Mental Disorders and Subsequent Alcohol and Illicit Drug Use: Results From the National Comorbidity Survey-Adolescent Supplement. J Am Acad Child Adolesc Psychiatry. 2016;55(4):280-8.
56. Deas D, Brown ES. Adolescent substance abuse and psychiatric comorbidities. J Clin Psychiatry. 2006;67(7):e02.
57. Welsh JW, Knight JR, Hou SSY, Malowney M, Schram P, Sherritt L, et al. Association Between Substance Use Diagnoses and Psychiatric Disorders in an Adolescent and Young Adult Clinic-Based Population. J Adolesc Health Off Publ Soc Adolesc Med. 2017;60(6):648-52.

Digital Media/Internet Overuse and Behavioral Addictions

Debasish Basu, Shalini Naik, Harpreet Singh Dhillon

INTRODUCTION

The American Society of Addiction Medicine (ASAM) defined addiction as a treatable, chronic medical disease involving complex interactions among brain circuits, genetics, environment, and an individual's life experiences. In 2019, the ASAM framed addiction as encompassing not only substance use disorders but also engagement in nonsubstance-related behaviors, expanding its scope to recognize various activities such as gambling, shopping, gaming, food, exercise, and phenomenologically distinct Internet-enabled behavior such as online video gaming, social media interactions, and diverse forms of sexual behavior.[1] These behavioral addictions share common characteristics with substance dependence, including salience, compulsive use (loss of control), mood modification, and the alleviation of distress, tolerance, withdrawal, and continued use despite adverse consequences. This chapter delves into the nature of digital media overuse in children and adolescents, explores the mechanisms that make them particularly vulnerable, and guides psychiatrists in assessing clinical presentation and adapting effective treatment strategies to address digital media overuse. A brief note on other behavioral addictions is included at the end.

What is Internet addiction?

Digital media is any content stored in a digital format that can be shared electronically, while the Internet is the global network that enables the transmission and access to digital media. Digital technology has transformed communication, breaking down geographical barriers and connecting people through email, instant messaging, video calls, and real-time multimedia sharing. Kimberly Young et al. proposed internet addiction (IA) as an impulse-control disorder by modifying the DSM-IV criteria for pathological gambling for inclusion in DSM-IV TR.[2]

- Initial emphasis had been on the "duration" of use. It was challenged as internet use has risen extraordinarily due to the pervasive nature of digital space in our daily activities.
- Currently, the focus has shifted to the "quality" of usage, whether it is used for "productive or essential" purposes and "detrimental effects" on an individual's physical, mental, social, or emotional well-being.
- The internet is a medium, and individuals are addicted to specific features of the Internet (for instance, gaming, sexual activity, etc.); hence, there is a recommendation to change IA to "addictions to the specific Internet-related activities[3] or internet-use related disorder".
- The nonessential engagement with the internet has to be rewarding (psychological or monetary, or equivalent gains), and the reward must be immediate.
- Both inherently rewarding aspects of internet use and the consequences of engagement in these behaviors (escapism, socializing, etc.) act as reinforcers.

- Most importantly, one's prediction of experiencing reward has to be uncertain to have enhanced dopamine sensitization,[4] thereby invigorating salience.[5]
- Emerging neuroimaging evidence demonstrated activation of the brain's reward system to behavioral cues related to gambling[6] and gaming,[7] much comparable to substance use.
- Digital media/Internet overuse falls under the behavioral addiction category,[8] and the psychiatric implications of digital media/ Internet overuse go beyond mere excessive usage, often leading to disruptions in social, academic, and occupational functioning.
- Today, IA is best understood on a spectrum of healthy use, hazardous use, problematic/ pathological use, and addiction, much similar to the spectrum of substance use **(Fig. 1)**.
- In Hazardous use, there is internet overuse for nonessential purposes, which might pose a risk of deleterious effects. In problematic/ pathological internet use (PIU), individuals are continuing to use despite harmful effects; while in addiction affected people experience salience (preoccupation with digital media), loss of control (inability to regulate use), mood modification (emotional reliance on digital engagement), tolerance and withdrawal (increased use required for gratification, distress when stopped) and continued use despite harm (impact on academics, social life, and health).

What are the subtypes of Internet addiction?

Based on specific media or content used excessively, IA has many subcategories, such as:

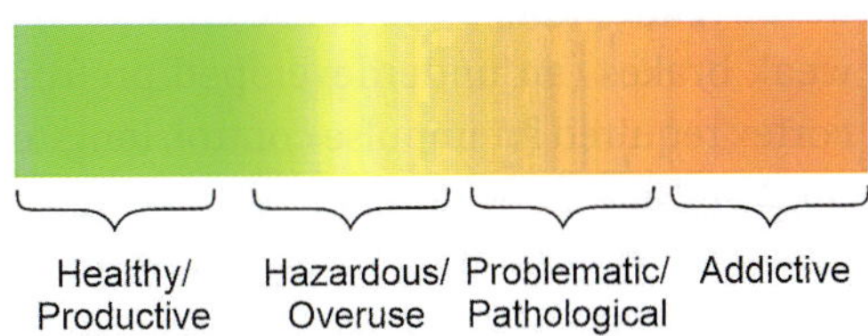

Fig. 1: Spectrum of Internet use-related disorder.

- *Gaming disorder (GD):* Excessive gaming, leading to impairment.
- *Compulsive sexual behavior disorder (CSBD)/ pornography addiction:* Uncontrolled online sexual content consumption.
- *Social media addiction (SMA):* Compulsive social media use.
- *Online shopping addiction:* Impulsive online purchases.
- *Cyberchondria:* Excessive online health-related searches.
- *Streaming addiction:* Binge-watching, leading to neglect of responsibilities.
- *Cyberbullying:* Engaging in or experiencing digital harassment.
- *Nomophobia:* The fear of being without a mobile phone or internet connection, leading to anxiety and distress when separated from digital devices.
- *Digital hoarding:* Excessive accumulation of digital material such as emails, files, media, and software.

Why is Internet overuse in children and adolescents a concern?

- Digital media use is an integral part of growing children, providing them with immersive learning experiences and creativity from the early stages of development,[9] and mediating better academic performance in school children.[10]
- They have unprecedented access to digital media through smartphones, tablets, computers, and gaming consoles for every aspect of life, from education and communication to social interaction and entertainment.
- While digital technology/use enhances education, business, entertainment, public services, and social needs, it also poses the risk of overuse and addiction for several reasons, such as easy accessibility, multisensory stimulation, and immediate gratification.

- In growing children, digital media hinders learning, inhibiting impulsive responses, emotional resilience, and reducing opportunities to develop prosocial skills, such as empathy, communication, and conflict resolution with peers **(Fig. 2)**.
- *Addictive attributes of digital space—ACE model:*[11]
  - "Anonymity" to conceal one's true identity.
  - "Convenience" to shop or watch online without leaving home.
  - A swift "escape" from the real world's challenges into a virtual environment with immediate gratification.
- *Risk for addiction:*
  - Neurobiologically, addiction begins with the brain's learning of rewarding experiences through dopamine-based positive reinforcement, regardless of the stimulus (e.g., "use" of a drug or social networking media).
  - Over a period of continuous use, this process activates antireward mechanisms, creating negative reinforcement that perpetuates compulsive behaviors.[12]

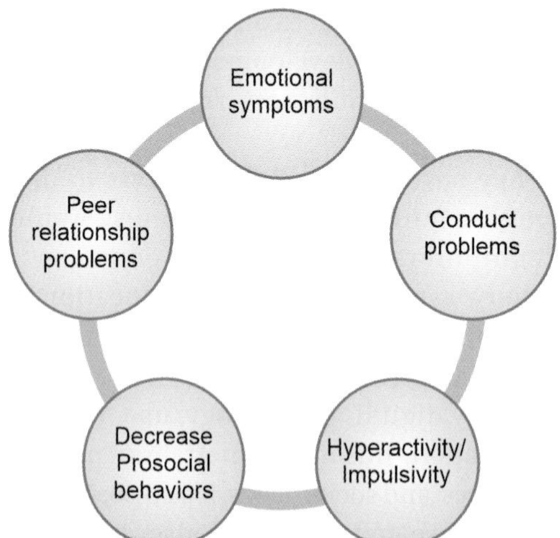

Fig. 2: Problems associated with digital media use in growing children.

  - Children are particularly at higher risk of overuse and addiction due to inherently poor regulation of rewarding behaviors.
  - Unlike adults, their maturing brains are more susceptible to digital space's rewarding and deeply engaging features, thereby quickly spiraling from healthy use to hazardous use to problematic or PIU and culminating into a dysregulated use, called IA **(Fig. 1)**.
  - A meta-analysis of 317,443 adolescents from 52 countries found the prevalence of heavy use of the Internet (defined as nonessential use of the Internet for more than 2 hours per day) was 60.3%, 30.7% and 9% in those who were first exposed to the Internet at age of ≤9 years, 10–12 years and ≥13 years of age, indicating early internet exposure is associated with heavy Internet use.[13]
- Besides addiction, two alarming internet-use-related harms are cyberbullying and unwanted sexual solicitation from the internet among children.[14]
- It is essential to carry out early identification for timely intervention, preventing the progression of digital media overuse into more severe behavioral addictions (Warning signs for parents, teachers, and clinicians in **Figure 3**).

Metaphorical example on the developing brain and risk for addiction

- The brain of children and adolescents is compared to a car with a strong accelerator (reward-seeking in terms of sensation, thrill, novelty, attention, and intense emotions) but weak brakes (an underdeveloped prefrontal cortex required for impulse control, long-term thinking, and decision-making).
- Children experience powerful impulses or urges (as a result of a fully active accelerator) but have limited control, increasing the

Parents	Teachers	Clinicians
• Excessive screen time • Distracted during screen use • Neglect of academic responsibilities • Social withdrawal • Irritability and aggression • Sleep disruptions • Irregularities in food intake • Loss of interest in hobbies • Secrecy and deception • Neglecting physical health • Compulsive spending on digital content	• Inattention and distractibility • Incomplete assignments • Drowsy or less alert in the class • Academic decline • Social isolation at school • Agitation when disconnected • Obsessive talk about gaming/social media • Impulsivity and risky behavior • Cyberbullying • Physical symptoms	• Preoccupation with digital activities • Mood changes linked to digital use • Loss of control over usage • Sleep and appetite disturbances • Tolerance of internet use • Withdrawal symptoms • Compulsive internet spending/gambling • Psychosocial and family conflict • Self-harm or suicidal ideation • Negative impact on functioning

Fig. 3: Warning signs for internet use-related disorder in children and adolescents.

risk of poor judgment, which translates to engagement in problematic behaviors, sensitivity to peer pressure, and seeking rewards.

- The transition isn't a sudden shift from all acceleration to all brakes; instead, adolescents gradually learn to manage both, gaining better control over their actions.
- Those with attention-deficit/hyperactivity disorder (ADHD), anxiety, and adverse childhood experiences would have a more hyperactive limbic system and an underperforming prefrontal cortex.
- Acceleration with poor brakes is a risk for the uninhibited use of any rewarding substance or behavior.

NOSOLOGY

Behavioral addictions related to digital media/internet are not yet universally classified as distinct disorders in the DSM-5 and ICD-11. In May 2013, internet gaming disorder (IGD), a subcategory of internet addiction disorder (IAD), was listed in Section III of DSM-5 as a "condition for further study" to validate the diagnosis, increase public awareness, and develop treatment.[15] In 2019, ICD-11 recognized only two subtypes of IA, i.e., GD and CSBD, as disordered. As most research has focused on IGD or GD, which has observed commonalities between GD and Substance use disorder in terms of cue-reactivity, attentional biases, impaired decision-making, and stimulus-specific poor inhibitory control, ICD-11 lists GD **(Table 1)** under the category of "addictive disorders." Unlike DSM-5, ICD-11 illustrated "hazardous gaming (HG)."

ICD-11 mentioned CSBD under "impulse-control disorders" in response to the growing functional impairment related to excessive pornographic viewing.[16] IGD/GD is a useful framework for understanding digital media-related behavioral addictions.

Hazardous Gaming (Coded as QE22 in International Classification of Diseases, 11th Revision)

A pattern of gaming, either online or offline, that appreciably increases the risk of harmful physical or mental health consequences to the individual or others around the individual.[17] It comprises either risky gaming behavior (neglect of other activities and priorities and adverse consequences of gaming at school/home/work), excessive gaming (gaming time and frequency), or a combination of both. Gaming Disorder and Hazardous Gaming Scale (GDHGS) is the only assessment scale to distinguish between HG and GD.[18]

TABLE 1: Diagnostic criteria for gaming disorder in DSM-5 TR and ICD-11.

DSM-5 TR	*ICD-11*
Termed internet gaming disorder (IGD)	***Termed gaming disorder (GD)***
Persistent and recurrent use of the Internet to engage in games, often with other players, leading to clinically significant impairment or distress as indicated by *five (or more)* of the following in a *12-month period* • *Preoccupation* with gaming (thinks about previous gaming activity or anticipating playing the next game) • *Withdrawal* symptoms when gaming is taken away or not possible (sadness, anxiety, and irritability) • *Tolerance*—need to spend more time gaming to satisfy the urge • *Loss of control:* Inability to reduce playing, unsuccessful attempts to quit gaming • *Loss of interest in previously enjoyed activities* due to gaming, giving up other activities • *Use despite harm:* Continuing to play the game despite knowledge of psychosocial problems • *Deceptiveness:* Deceiving family members or therapists, or others about the amount of time spent on gaming • *Escape/relief from negative mood:* Use of gaming to relieve negative moods, such as guilt or hopelessness • *Adverse consequences*—having jeopardized opportunities or losing a job or relationship due to gaming	A persistent pattern of gaming behavior (digital gaming or videogaming), which may be predominantly online (i.e., over the internet or similar electronic networks) or offline, manifested by *all* of the following: • *Impaired control* over gaming behavior (e.g., onset, frequency, intensity, duration, termination, and context) • *Salience:* Increasing priority given to gaming behavior to the extent that gaming takes precedence over other life interests and daily activities • *Continuation or escalation of gaming behavior despite negative consequences* (e.g., family conflict due to gaming behavior, poor scholastic performance, and negative impact on health) • Pattern of gaming behavior results in *significant distress or impairment* in personal, family, social, educational, occupational, or other important areas of functioning • Pattern of gaming behavior may be *continuous or episodic and recurrent,* but is manifested over an *extended period of time* (e.g., 12 months)
This can include gaming on the internet with others or alone	If symptoms and consequences of gaming behavior are severe (e.g., gaming behaviors persist for days at a time without respite or have major effects on functioning or health) and all other diagnostic requirements are met, *GD can be diagnosed for a period briefer than 12 months (e.g., 6 months)*
Specifier: Severity, mild, moderate, and severe, depending on the degree of disruption of normal activities	*Specifier:* Online (6C51.0) and Offline (6C51.1)

Gaming Disorder (Coded as 6C51 in International Classification of Diseases, 11th Revision)

A pattern of gaming behavior ("digital gaming" or "video gaming") online (over the internet) or offline. Both ICD-11 and DSM-5 essential diagnostic features are illustrated in **Table 1**.

Besides, ICD-11 advises exploring the following additional features of GD in the clinical history.

- Numerous unsuccessful efforts to control gaming behavior, either self-initiated or imposed by others.
- Duration or frequency of gaming behavior increases over time or experiences a need to engage in games of increasing levels of complexity or requiring increasing skills or strategy to maintain or exceed previous levels of excitement or to avoid boredom.

- Experiences urge or cravings to engage in gaming during other activities.
- Experience dysphoria and exhibit adversarial behavior or verbal or physical aggression on cessation/reduction of gaming behavior, often imposed by others.
- Exhibits substantial disruptions in diet, sleep, exercise, nutrition, and other health-related behaviors that can result in negative physical and mental health outcomes, particularly if there are very extended periods of gaming.
- Explore for depression, anxiety, attention-deficit/hyperactivity disorder, financial loss, academic decline, and poor quality of life.

Raising the Number of Internet Use-related Conditions in Children

Internet users are nearly 67% of the world's total population, i.e., 5.4 billion people as of April 2024.[19] The coronavirus disease 2019 (COVID-19) lockdowns necessitated the widespread use of internet-enabled devices such as smartphones to maintain the continuity of educational activities for school children in urban and rural settings alike.[20]

- Meng et al. in their meta-analytic review, reported global pooled prevalence estimates of 27%, 17.4%, 8.2% and 6% for smartphone addiction, social media addiction, cybersex addiction, and gaming addiction, respectively.[21,22]
- The Entertainment Software Association (ESA) reported that 18% of video gamers are people under 18 years of age and observed a dramatic rise to 76% in their 2023 report.[23]
- The prevalence of IGD is 1% and 4.6% in adults and adolescents, respectively, suggesting younger ages are at greater risk for disordered gaming.[24]
- A plethora of psychosocial risk factors, such as male gender, single-parent household, concurrent diagnoses of depression and anxiety, heightened stress, and interpersonal challenges.[25]
- Social isolation increased digital media screen time during the COVID-19 pandemic.[21]

Cooccurring Psychiatric Disorders

- *Anxiety and depression:*
  - Excessive social media use leads to anxiety due to social comparison, cyberbullying, and FOMO (fear of missing out).[26]
  - Adolescents feel pressure to present an idealized life online, causing loneliness and inadequacy.
  - High screen time is associated with increased depression, replacing real-life interactions with online engagement.[27]
  - Depression and IGD have a reciprocal relationship.[28]
- *Attention deficit and hyperactivity:*
  - ADHD is a risk factor for IAD.[29]
  - Prolonged exposure to fast-paced digital content weakens attention span, especially in academic settings.
  - Adolescents with ADHD are more vulnerable to distraction and worsened symptoms due to digital overuse.
  - Instant gratification from gaming and social media reinforces dopamine-driven behavior, reducing focus on long-term tasks.
  - Constant digital stimulation shortens attention spans and makes it harder to concentrate on sustained tasks.
- *Disruptive mood dysregulation disorder (DMDD):* IGD increases the risk of DMDD in adolescents, especially those with ADHD.[30]
- *Sleep disorders:*
  - Excessive screen use, especially at night, leads to sleep disturbances.[31]
  - Blue light exposure suppresses melatonin, affecting sleep quality and causing daytime fatigue.

- Poor sleep worsens anxiety, depression, and mood disorders.

Cooccurring Physical Problems

- *Obesity:*
  - The sedentary nature of gaming, social media, and video consumption leads to reduced physical activity.
  - Lack of physical activity, combined with unhealthy eating habits often associated with screen time (e.g., snacking during gaming or streaming sessions).
  - A study found a positive correlation between IAD severity and body mass index.[32]
  - It can potentially contribute to the rising rates of childhood obesity, cardiovascular problems, and poor physical health overall.
- *Digital eye strain:* Prolonged screen time is associated with eye strain, characterized by headaches, blurred vision, dry eyes, and discomfort.[33]
- *Postural problems:* Children are prone to developing poor postural curvatures from sitting in front of screens for long periods, which can result in chronic back and neck pain.

EVALUATION AND ASSESSMENT

When evaluating digital media overuse and behavioral addictions in children and adolescents, psychiatrists must conduct a thorough assessment that includes the following components:

- *Clinical interview:*
  - The clinician should gather a detailed history of the child or adolescent's digital media habits, including the time spent on various devices, the nature of the activities (e.g., gaming, social media, and streaming), and how these behaviors affect daily life **(Table 2)**.
  - Interviews with parents or caregivers can provide insight into how children's or adolescents' digital habits impact family dynamics and academic performance **(Box 1)**.

TABLE 2: Difference in clinical manifestation between children and adolescents.

Aspect	*Children (<12 years)*	*Adolescents (12–18 years)*
Media access	More reliant on parents for access	More autonomy and higher personal media ownership
Preoccupation with media	Expressed as frequent or persistent requests to parents to access media	Experienced as intrusive thoughts about gaming
Response to limits	Strong resistance to parental limits on media use	May recognize problematic media use but still struggle to regulate
Impact on home life	Causes sibling conflict, disrupts family routines, and leads to parent-child conflict	Can still cause family conflict, but with more self-awareness of impact
Impact on school life	Delays or avoids schoolwork for media use	May recognize disruption but struggle with control
Impact on social development	May interfere with face-to-face peer interaction, affecting social competence	More aware of how media use affects their social life
Awareness of media impact	Unaware of how media use affects their daily life	More self-reflective and able to report disruptions
Preferred reporters	Parents, teachers, and other caregivers	Adolescents themselves can provide self-reports

BOX 1: History-taking and clinical assessment.

- Detailed history taking
- Use of screening instruments if there are initial hints of the presence of excessive internet use
- Detailed assessment of those found positive on initial screening
- Assessment of the early development period, including the prenatal, perinatal, and postnatal phases
- A thorough physical examination should be conducted after the developmental assessment to look for any soft neurological signs
- Assessment of the child/adolescent's digital media use, including the time spent on various devices, and the nature of the activities (e.g., gaming, social media, and streaming). Relevant scales may be utilized
- Interviews with parents or caregivers can provide additional insight into how the child/adolescent's digital habits impact family dynamics and academic performance
- Assess for parenting styles/child abuse/neglect
- Establishing the diagnosis as per the current diagnostic criteria
- *Evaluation for comorbidities:* ADHD, anxiety, depression, and autism
- Assessment for substance use
- Assessment of suicidal behavior
- Assessment of family environment as well as resources
- Dysfunction in terms of the impact of the symptoms on the educational attainment/performance, regularity in school/school refusal/inability to go to school
- Relevant physical (malnutrition, obesity, vision, posture), biochemical, psychological (cyberbullying), and neuroimaging (e.g., mass lesion in the brain) testing should be done to correlate clinically

    - In adolescents, excessive internet use is associated with a high prevalence of comorbid depressive and anxiety disorders and low reports of substance use; it might be an epiphenomenon of underlying psychiatric disorders.
- *Functional impairment analysis:*
    - Evaluating how digital media use affects the child's or adolescent's functioning in key domains, such as school, home, and peer relationships, is crucial.
    - Functional impairment is considered to be a more reliable indicator of IA than the amount of screen time.
- *Standardized assessment tools:* The following are standardized, widely used assessment instruments for screening problematic use or addiction. No diagnostic instrument tool has been developed yet; hence, the final diagnosis must involve a clinical assessment, and the broader context of the children's behavior and its impact on their lives.
    - *Internet addiction test (IAT):* The oldest, widely used, 20-item self-report tool to measure the severity of compulsive, nonwork-related use of the Internet in six factors: (1) Salience, (2) excessive Internet use, (3) neglecting work, (4) anticipation, (5) lack of control, and (6) neglecting social life, with a total score ranging from 20 to 100. This test helps understand Internet use on a continuum, where scores 20–39 represent normal users with adequate control of their Internet use, scores 40–69 represent PIU, and scores 70–100 represent IAD.[34]
    - *IGD-9 short form (IGDS9) SF:* DSM-5 nine diagnostic criteria-based self-report, 5-point Likert scale. A cut-off score >25 and 36 indicates problematic gaming, disordered gaming (GD) in children and adolescents, respectively.[35]
    - *Bergen Social Media Addiction Scale (BSMAS):* A 6-item self-report tool designed to assess addiction-like symptoms related to social media use over the past year.[36] A score of 19 or higher suggests problematic use of social media.
    - *Problematic media use measure (PMUM):* A 27-item parent-report instrument specifically developed to evaluate problematic

media use in children. A 9-item, parent-report short form of PMUM (PMUM-SF) is validated; a cut-off of 20 or more denotes problematic screen media use.[37]

MANAGEMENT

Guiding Principles

- There is a consensus that total abstinence from the Internet is not a realistic goal of any intervention.
- Abstinence from problematic applications and well-regulated Internet usage should be achieved.
- Effective treatment for digital media overuse and behavioral addictions requires a panoramic approach combining cognitive behavioral, family- and mindfulness-based interventions with pharmacotherapy.[38]
- Parents play a critical role in managing children's digital media use because younger children lack awareness and self-regulation.
  - *Children <12 years:* Parent-based intervention
  - *Children >12 years:* Individual and parent or family-based intervention

Pharmacotherapy

- There is no evidence-based pharmacological intervention available for PIU/IAD and its subtypes.
- However, there is emerging evidence for antidepressants such as Selective serotonin reuptake inhibitors (SSRIs), in cases where digital media overuse cooccurs with psychiatric conditions such as anxiety and depression.
- Anti-ADHD medications can help manage underlying attention disorders.
- Treatment of psychiatric comorbidities reduces the compulsive need for digital escape.

Cognitive Behavioral Therapy for Internet Addiction

- Young developed cognitive behavioral therapy for internet addiction (CBT-IA) for individuals with IAD,[39] and later, it was adapted to a group format for adolescents.[40]
- Both have shown some efficacy in reducing screen time and slowly rekindled offline relationships over time.
- In the context of digital media overuse, CBT helps adolescents identify the thoughts and triggers that lead to compulsive online behavior.
- The focus is on developing healthier coping mechanisms, managing emotional triggers, and implementing time management strategies to reduce screen time **(Box 2)**.
- Cognitive restructuring is particularly important in addressing the distorted beliefs that may underlie social media addiction, such as unrealistic social comparisons or the need for constant approval.

Parental Guidance and Media Monitoring

Parents play a critical role in managing their children's screen time. The Expert Committee of

BOX 2: Behavioral strategies to reduce internet-use related disorder.

- Practice the opposite time of Internet use (discover the child's patterns of Internet use and disrupt these patterns by suggesting new schedules)
- Use external stoppers (actual events or activities prompting the patient to log off)
- Set goals (about the amount of time)
- Abstain from a particular application (that the child/adolescent is unable to control)
- Use reminder cards [cues that remind the child of the costs of internet addiction disorder (IAD) and the benefits of breaking it]
- Develop a personal inventory (shows all the activities that the child used to engage in or can't find the time due to IAD)

the Indian Academy of Pediatrics (IAP) framed guidelines on screen time and digital wellness in infants, children, and adolescents in March 2021.[41] The key components of successful intervention are educating them on the potential dangers of excessive screen time and healthy digital media practices **(Box 3)**.

Family Therapy and Parental Involvement

- Given that children and adolescents live within a family system, it is essential to involve parents in the treatment process and also to address relational problems in the family.
- If conflicts between parents and children hinder the effective implementation of healthy digital media practices, then family-based interventions can help parents set appropriate boundaries around screen time, implement media-free zones in the home (e.g., at the dinner table), and encourage nondigital activities that promote family bonding.[42]
- A functional magnetic resonance imaging (fMRI) study found greater activation of the Caudate in response to images depicting parental love following family therapy intervention, and this was inversely correlated with gaming time. This highlights that family cohesion is one of the key factors in recovery from IGD.[43]

BOX 3: Guidance for parents on healthy digital media practices.

- *Screen time restriction:*
  - *Children <2 years:* No exposure to any screen.
  - *Children 2–5 years:* Up to one hour under parental supervision
  - *Children 5–10 years of age:* <2 h/day
- *Essential activities* for a child's overall health and growth are outdoor physical exercise, reading, sleep, interaction with family (family meals, quality time) and peers, academic work, and skill development
- *Screen time should not replace essential activities*
- Families should provide a *warm, supportive, fun, and secure home environment*
- They should monitor their children's screen usage to ensure the *content is educational, age-appropriate, and nonviolent*
- Alert them for *signs of cyberbullying or media addiction*
- Educate on how to *model healthy digital behavior*, as children are likely to mimic their parents' screen habits

Digital Detox and Time Management

- A gradual reduction in screen time, or a digital detox, is often recommended to break the cycle of compulsive media use.
- Adolescents may be encouraged to set daily limits on screen time, turn off notifications, and establish tech-free times (e.g., before bed or during meals).
- Adolescents should be encouraged to engage in alternative activities that foster creativity, physical health, and social engagement, such as sports, hobbies, or volunteer work.

Mindfulness and Stress Reduction Techniques

- Teaching adolescents' mindfulness and stress management techniques can help them become more aware of online behaviors and reduce impulsive, emotionally driven digital use.
- Mindfulness practices, such as deep breathing, meditation, and body scanning, can promote emotional regulation and reduce anxiety.

School-based Interventions

- Schools can play a key role in promoting healthy digital habits by incorporating media literacy education into the curriculum.
- Educating students about the responsible use of technology, online safety, and the risks of overuse can empower young people to make informed choices about their digital behavior.
- Schools should also set guidelines for screen time in the classroom and encourage physical activity and social engagement through extracurricular programs.

INTERVIEW AND COUNSELING STRATEGIES FOR WORKING WITH ADOLESCENTS

Building a therapeutic alliance with adolescents is quite challenging due to their developmental stage of forming individual identities, emotional volatility, and mistrust in adults and authority figures. Hence, working with them requires flexibility, creativity, and an understanding of their developmental needs. Mental health professionals must work on building trust and rapport, using developmentally appropriate communication, and promoting positive self-esteem **(Fig. 4)**.[44]

CLINICAL CASE-BASED LEARNING

CASE VIGNETTE 1: ADOLESCENT WITH GAMING DISORDER

Case History

Rithvik (pseudonym), a 17-year-old boy with below-average academics, is temperamentally slow to warm up. His parents adopted him at 5 years of age after a decade of marriage and several failed assisted reproductive treatments. His father, often absent due to work, indulged him with expensive gadgets and unlimited credit card access, while his anxious mother was strict about studies, frequently comparing him to his peers.

At 14 years of age, Rithvik received an expensive smartphone, which he used for gaming and social networking. At 15 years of age, in 11th grade, he struggled with social interactions, self-consciousness, and academic pressure in the junior college. He experienced anxiety symptoms, including tremors and palpitations, particularly during exams. A severe bout of gastroenteritis led him to skip exams. During this break, he discovered a "First Person Shooter" game. He enjoyed the interactive nature but was soon introduced to a "Role-Playing Game" (RPG), which captivated him.

He became deeply immersed in the RPG, enjoying teamwork and strategic domination. His gaming escalated to overnight sessions, affecting his hygiene, meals, classes, and family interactions. His mother criticized him as "lazy" and "irresponsible." Their relationship was further strained after she complained to his college principal, who advised limiting his screen time. R became increasingly irritable whenever ineffective attempts to restrict his time were made and were preoccupied with gaming. After 3 days of restriction, he mocked his parents and threatened suicide if his access was cut. Over a year, his screen time rose to 16–18 hours daily. He excelled in a massively multiplayer online role-playing game (MMORPG), spending over ₹10 lakhs from his father's credit card to buy in-game advantages. His hygiene and health deteriorated. When his father blocked credit access, he became distressed, self-harmed with hesitation cuts, and showed them to his father. Brought for consultation, Rithvik was initially withdrawn but opened up about his gaming addiction. He described feeling powerful when dominating online matches, enjoying validation from coplayers while feeling criticized by real-life peers and family. He recognized his excessive gaming but felt compelled to continue.

Case Evaluation

Understand contextual factors, patterns of gaming, and co-occurring physical and psychiatric conditions:

- *Contextual factors:*
    - Adopted at age 5 after parents faced infertility struggles.

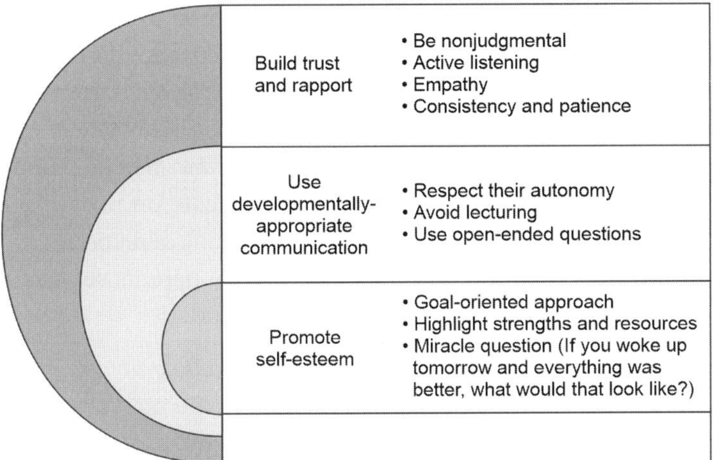

Fig. 4: Key techniques for counseling adolescents.

- *Father's role:* Frequently absent, compensates with expensive gifts and unlimited credit access.
- *Mother's role:* Anxious, strict about academics, and frequently compares him to peers.
- Below-average academic performance.
- Temperamentally slow-to-warm-up.
- Struggled with social interactions and self-consciousness in junior college.
- Experienced academic pressure and exam-related anxiety

▪ *Onset and progression of gaming addiction:*
  - *At 14 years of age*: Received an expensive smartphone; started gaming and social networking.
  - *At 15 years of age*: Developed exam anxiety, leading to avoidance behaviors.
  - *Gaming escalated*: 16–18 hours daily, playing overnight, spent over ₹10 lakhs for in-game purchases, neglecting hygiene, meals, academics, and strained interactions with parents.
  - Attempts to limit gaming resulted in irritability, self-harm attempts, and threats.

Case Management

Intervene at three stages: (1) Immediate, (2) short-term, and (3) long-term.

Immediate intervention:

▪ *Risk assessment:*
  - Assess suicidal risk (due to previous threats and self-harm).
  - Evaluate the severity of the gaming disorder (impact on daily functioning, withdrawal symptoms)
  - Screen for coexisting mental health conditions (anxiety, depression, and low self-esteem).

▪ *Emergency support and family counseling:*
  - Ensure safety planning for suicide risk.
  - Educate parents on supportive and structured intervention instead of punishment.
  - Encourage father's active involvement to balance indulgence and discipline.

Short-term intervention:

With the adolescent:

▪ *Cognitive behavioral therapy (CBT):*
  - Address maladaptive thought patterns (e.g., self-worth tied to gaming).
  - Develop alternative coping strategies for stress and anxiety.
  - Teach impulse control and time management strategies.

▪ *Gradual digital detox and screen time management*:

- Implement a structured reduction plan instead of abrupt restrictions.
- Introduce healthy screen use habits (time-limited gaming, alternative activities).

- *Social skills training and real-life engagement:*
  - Help rebuild peer relationships through offline activities.
  - Encourage team sports or hobby-based groups for social exposure.
- *Pharmacological treatment (if necessary):*
  - If severe anxiety, depression, or ADHD-like symptoms persist, appropriate medical treatment may be considered.

With parents:

- *Parental guidance on gaming and digital media practices:*
  - Father to transition from financial indulgence to active emotional involvement.
  - Mother to replace criticism with constructive reinforcement.
  - Encourage structured family bonding activities outside of screen time.
- *Psychoeducation on GD:*
  - Educate on reward-seeking behaviors in gaming addiction.
  - Help parents set firm but compassionate boundaries.

Long-term follow-up and monitoring:

- Regular therapy sessions to track progress and prevent relapse.
- Monitor school performance and real-world engagement.
- Assess risk of alternative addictive behaviors.
- Encourage vocational guidance to build self-confidence beyond gaming.

CASE VIGNETTE 2: A CHILD WITH EXCESSIVE SCREEN MEDIA USE

Case History

Manoj (pseudonym), an 8-year-old boy, was born to working parents. By age 2, he showed motoric hyperactivity—throwing things, pulling clothes and hair, and hitting when not attended to. He was fussy with food, smearing it around and demanding meals at irregular times.

At 2 years of age, he started watching cartoon videos on his father's phone during feeding time, which kept him engaged and tantrum-free. His parents continued this practice, noticing that he mimicked cartoon voices and dialogues. However, he lost interest in social interactions at prenursery, preferring people with phones. He threw inconsolable tantrums until he was given a phone. To manage this, parents restricted his phone access at home, but he then switched to watching cartoons on TV for 3–5 hours after school until they returned.

At home, he was inattentive, barely responding when called. Teachers noted he could not sit still like his classmates, often climbing on benches, pulling clothes, and laughing at his peers. He frequently forgot homework, left assignments incomplete, and struggled with notetaking. At home, he insisted on watching TV before doing schoolwork. When disciplined, he reacted by breaking belongings.

Over time, parents found it difficult to make him sit still unless watching TV or using a phone. He struggled with interactive play and was labeled mischievous and difficult by teachers, family, and neighbors. His academic performance remained below average.

Concerned about his behavior, inattention, and reliance on screens, his parents sought medical consultation.

Case Evaluation

Assess for underlying neurodevelopmental disorder, its dynamic interaction with screen media use, and the impact of developmental trajectory.

Developmental history:

- *Early signs of hyperactivity (age 2 years):*
  - *Motoric hyperactivity:* Throwing objects, pulling hair/clothes, and hitting when ignored.
  - *Fussy eating habits:* Food smearing and irregular meal demands.
- *Early screen exposure (Age 2 onward):*
  - Introduced to cartoons on his father's phone to keep him calm during meals.
  - Became fixated on-screen content, mimicking cartoon voices.
  - Lost interest in social interactions, preferred individuals with phones.
  - Severe tantrums when denied phone access.

Behavioral and academic concerns:

- *Screen dependence and tantrums:*
  - *At home:* Inconsolable tantrums without phone or TV.
  - Switched to watching TV for 3–5 hours daily after school.
- *Assess for ADHD:*
  - Inattentive at home, unresponsive when called.
  - *At school:*
    - Cannot sit still like peers; frequently climbing on benches.
    - Disruptive behavior (pulling clothes, laughing inappropriately).
    - Incomplete homework, struggling with notetaking.
  - *At home:*
    - Insisted on watching TV before schoolwork.
    - Reacted aggressively (breaking objects) when disciplined.
- *Social and academic difficulties:*
  - Could only sit still while using screens.
  - Struggled with interactive play, limited peer relationships.
  - Labeled "mischievous and difficult" by teachers, family, and neighbors.
  - Academically below average.

Screen addiction assessment:

- Evaluate dependency on digital media (withdrawal symptoms and excessive use).
- Assess impact on cognitive, social, and emotional development.

Psychosocial and family assessment:

- Parental screen habits (to model healthier behavior).
- Home discipline strategies and reinforcement techniques.

Case Management

Parent-based intervention is critical as the child is young and under their direct supervision.

Pharmacological treatment: Medical treatment for ADHD depends on the severity.

Parent management training (PMT):

- Educate parents on positive reinforcement instead of screen pacification.
- Teach consistent discipline strategies for tantrums.
- Set structured meals and sleep routines without screens
- Gradual reduction of screen exposure (not abrupt removal).
- Introducing alternative engagement activities (books, storytelling, and hands-on learning).
- Encourage structured playtime and physical activity.
  - Fixed schedules for meals, study, play, and sleep.
  - Encourage outdoor play and sports to improve attention and social skills.

- Increase parent-child interaction without screens:
  - Engage in screen-free family bonding activities (games and outdoor activities).
  - *Parental modeling*: Limit own screen use to set an example.
- *Alternative rewards and coping strategies:*
  - Replace screen-based rewards with nondigital incentives (stickers, praise, and outings).
  - Teach healthy coping mechanisms for frustration (breathing exercises and mindfulness).

School-based interventions:

- Individualized support for attention and learning difficulties.
- Encourage structured classroom behavior strategies (visual schedules and reward systems).
- Collaborate with the teacher to modify teaching approaches.

OTHER NOTABLE BEHAVIORAL ADDICTIONS

Gambling disorder and compulsive sexual behavior disorder are identified as behavioral addictions in ICD-11. Gambling disorder is the quintessential behavioral addiction model that establishes similarities in the neurobiological mechanisms between chemical and behavioral addiction. The diagnostic criteria for gaming disorder **(Table 1)** were adapted from the gambling disorder.

Gambling Disorder

It was formerly known as pathological gambling (F63) under "Habit and Impulse disorders" in ICD-10. It is recognized as a disorder (6C50) and clustered under "Addictive disorders" in ICD-11.

It is characterized by a pattern of persistent or recurrent gambling behavior, which may be online (i.e., over the internet) or offline, manifested by:

- Impaired control over gambling (e.g., onset, frequency, intensity, duration, termination, and context).
- Increasing priority given to gambling to the extent that gambling takes precedence over other life interests and daily activities.
- Continuation or escalation of gambling despite the occurrence of negative consequences.

The pattern of gambling behavior may be continuous or episodic and recurrent and results in significant distress or impairment in personal, family, social, educational, occupational, or other important areas of functioning over a period of at least 12 months. It has a specifier of Online and offline, similar to IGD. Gambling conducted over the internet is classified as Online Gambling Disorder. Indulgence in excessive gambling is termed "at-risk gambling," and when that leads to adverse consequences to gamblers, their close ones, or the community, it is considered to be "problem gambling." DSM-5 categorizes gambling disorder as mild, moderate, and severe. The Gambling Disorder Identification Test (GDIT) is a 14-item self-report that explores gambling behavior, gambling symptoms, and their negative consequences. GDIT cut-off scores indicate severity, such as at-risk (10–14), problem gambling (15–19), mild (20–24), moderate (25–29), and severe (≥30) gambling disorder.[45] Prevalence is observed across all age groups, but it is typically late teens to mid-30s, and highest in young adults (18–24 years). Men are about 3.4 times more likely to engage in problem gambling than women.[46] There is no approved pharmacotherapy. Management strategies are similar to IAD.

Compulsive Sexual Behavior Disorder

It was formerly considered as "excessive sexual drive" (F52.7) under "Sexual disorders" in ICD-10. It is classified under "Impulse control disorders" (Code 6C72) in ICD-11. It is characterized by persistent failure to control intense, repetitive sexual urges or impulses resulting in repetitive sexual behavior manifested by one or more of the following essential features for a period of 6 months or more.

- Engaging in repetitive sexual behavior has become a central focus of the individual's life to the point of neglecting health and personal care or other interests, activities, and responsibilities.
- The individual has made numerous unsuccessful efforts to control or significantly reduce repetitive sexual behavior.
- The individual continues to engage in repetitive sexual behavior despite adverse consequences (e.g., marital conflict due to sexual behavior, financial or legal consequences, negative impact on health).
- The person continues to engage in repetitive sexual behavior even when the individual derives little or no satisfaction from it

Sexual behavior includes masturbation, pornography viewing, cybersex (internet sex), telephone sex, and partnered sex. CSBD-19 is a 19-item scale developed to measure the frequency and intensity of compulsive sexual behaviors, as well as the associated emotional distress and functional impairment.[47] Global prevalence of CSBD is 3–10% in men and 2–7% in women.[48] There is no approved treatment for CSBD. SSRI and Naltrexone have shown some preliminary efficacy. Androgen receptor blockers may be indicated for comorbid paraphilic disorders.[49]

SUMMARY AND CONCLUSION

The widespread availability of digital devices, combined with the unique developmental vulnerabilities of youth, has led to a rise in mental health, social, and physical health concerns related to excessive screen time. Despite the debate about which component of Internet use is a person "addicted" to, however, PIU/IAD needs clinical attention and a nuanced approach. It is imperative to screen all children and adolescents in both clinical and nonclinical settings.

Early Internet exposure is associated with heavy Internet use. Functional impairment is considered to be a more reliable indicator than screen time. Psychiatric comorbidity is very common. Treatment of psychiatric comorbidities reduces IA. Treatment modalities lack evidence; hence, psychiatrists must employ cognitive behavioral therapy, family therapy, and mindfulness training. Parental engagement is essential for promoting healthier relationships with digital technology and fostering mental well-being in children and adolescents, since younger children have limited awareness and struggle with self-regulation.

REFERENCES

1. American Society of Addiction Medicine. (2024). ASAM-2019-Definition-of-Addiction. [Online] Available from https://www.asam.org/docs/default-source/quality-science/asam's-2019-definition-of-addiction-(1).pdf?sfvrsn=b8b64fc2_2 [Last accessed 16 November, 2025].
2. Young K. Internet Addiction: Diagnosis and Treatment Considerations. J Contemp Psychother. 2009;39(4):241-6.
3. Starcevic V, Aboujaoude E. Internet addiction: reappraisal of an increasingly inadequate concept. CNS Spectr. 2017;22(1):7-13.
4. Zack M, St George R, Clark L. Dopaminergic signaling of uncertainty and the aetiology of gambling addiction. Prog Neuropsychopharmacol Biol Psychiatry. 2020;99:109853.
5. Bromberg-Martin ES, Matsumoto M, Hikosaka O. Dopamine in motivational control: rewarding, aversive, and alerting. Neuron. 2010;68(5):815-34.
6. Fauth-Bühler M, Mann K, Potenza MN. Pathological gambling: a review of the neurobiological evidence relevant for its classification as an addictive disorder. Addict Biol. 2017;22(4):885-97.

7. Niu X, Gao X, Zhang M, Yang Z, Yu M, Wang W, et al. Meta-analysis of structural and functional brain alterations in internet gaming disorder. Front Psychiatry. 2022;13:1029344.
8. Dalal PK, Basu D. Twenty years of Internet addiction ... Quo Vadis? Indian J Psychiatry. 2016; 58(1):6-11.
9. Anshari M, Almunawar MN, Shahrill M, Wicaksono DK, Huda M. Smartphones usage in the classrooms: Learning aid or interference? Educ Inf Technol. 2017;22(6):3063-79.
10. Wang JC, Hsieh CY, Kung SH. The impact of smartphone use on learning effectiveness: A case study of primary school students. Educ Inf Technol. 2023;28(6):6287-320.
11. Young KS, Griffin-Shelley E, Cooper A, O'mara J, Buchanan J. Online infidelity: A new dimension in couple relationships with implications for evaluation and treatment. Sexual Addic Compuls. 2000;7(1-2):59-74.
12. Lüscher C, Robbins TW, Everitt BJ. The transition to compulsion in addiction. Nat Rev Neurosci. 2020;21(5):247-63.
13. López-Bueno R, Koyanagi A, López-Sánchez GF, Firth J, Smith L. Association between age of first exposure and heavy internet use in a representative sample of 317,443 adolescents from 52 countries. Eur Child Adolesc Psychiatry. 2023;32(3):395-403.
14. Guan SSA, Subrahmanyam K. Youth Internet use: risks and opportunities. Curr Opin Psychiatry. 2009;22(4):351-6.
15. American Psychiatric Association. Diagnostic and Statistical Manual of Mental Disorders, 5th edition. Arlington, VA: American Psychiatric Association; 2013.
16. Brand M, Rumpf HJ, Demetrovics Z, Müller A, Stark R, King DL, et al. Which conditions should be considered as disorders in the International Classification of Diseases (ICD-11) designation of "other specified disorders due to addictive behaviors"? J Behav Addict. 2020;11(2):150-9.
17. World Health Organization. (2019). QE22 Hazardous gaming. International Classification of Diseases. 11th Revision. [Online] Available from https://icd.who.int/browse/2024-01/mms/en#1586542716 [Last accessed November, 2025].
18. Balhara YPS, Singh S, Saini R, Kattula D, Chukkali S, Bhargava R. Development and validation of gaming disorder and hazardous gaming scale (GDHGS) based on the WHO framework (ICD-11 criteria) of disordered gaming. Asian J Psychiatr. 2020;54:102348.
19. Digital Around the World. DataReportal - Global Digital Insights. [Online] Available from https://datareportal.com/global-digital-overview [Last accessed 16 November, 2025].
20. Jonnatan L, Seaton CL, Rush KL, Li EPH, Hasan K. Mobile Device Usage before and during the COVID-19 Pandemic among Rural and Urban Adults. Int J Environ Res Public Health. 2022;19(14):8231.
21. Zarco-Alpuente A, Ciudad-Fernández V, Ballester-Arnal R, Billieux J, Gil-Llario MD, King DL, et al. Problematic internet use prior to and during the COVID-19 pandemic. Cyberpsychology. 2021; 15(4).
22. Meng SQ, Cheng JL, Li YY, Yang XQ, Zheng JW, et al. Global prevalence of digital addiction in general population: A systematic review and meta-analysis. Clin Psychol Rev. 2022;92:102128.
23. Entertainment Software Association. 2023 Essential Facts About the U.S. Video Game Industry. the ESA. [Online] Available from https://www.theesa.com/resources/essential-facts-about-the-us-video-game-industry/2023-2/ [Last accessed 16 November, 2025].
24. Darvesh N, Radhakrishnan A, Lachance CC, Nincic V, Sharpe JP, Ghassemi M, et al. Exploring the prevalence of gaming disorder and Internet gaming disorder: a rapid scoping review. Syst Rev. 2020;9(1):68.
25. Tadpatrikar A, Sharma MK, Amudhan S, Desai G. The Prevalence and Correlates of Internet Addiction in India as Assessed by Young's Internet Addiction Test: A Systematic Review and Meta-analysis. Indian Journal of Psychological Medicine. 2024;46(6):511-20.
26. Franchina V, Vanden Abeele M, van Rooij AJ, Lo Coco G, De Marez L. Fear of Missing Out as a Predictor of Problematic Social Media Use and Phubbing Behavior among Flemish Adolescents. Int J Environ Res Public Health. 2018;15(10):2319.
27. Li L, Zhang Q, Zhu L, Zeng G, Huang H, Zhuge J, et al. Screen time and depression risk: A

meta-analysis of cohort studies. Front Psychiatry. 2022;13:1058572.

28. Jeong H, Yim HW, Lee SY, Lee HK, Ptenza MN, Jo SN, et al. Reciprocal relationship between depression and Internet gaming disorder in children: A 12-month follow-up of the iCURE study using cross-lagged path analysis. J Behav Addict. 2019;8(4):725-32.
29. Yoo HJ, Cho SC, Ha J, Yune SK, Kim SJ, Hwang J, et al. Attention deficit hyperactivity symptoms and internet addiction. Psychiatry Clin Neurosci. 2004;58(5):487-94.
30. Tzang RF, Chang CH, Chang YC. Structural Equation Modeling (SEM): Gaming Disorder Leading Untreated Attention-Deficit/ Hyperactivity Disorder to Disruptive Mood Dysregulation. Int J Environ Res Public Health. 2022;19(11):6648.
31. Arshad D, Joyia UM, Fatima S, Khalid N, Rishi AI, Rahim NUA, et al. The adverse impact of excessive smartphone screen-time on sleep quality among young adults: A prospective cohort. Sleep Sci. 2021;14(4):337-41.
32. Bozkurt H, Özer S, Şahin S, Sönmezgöz E. Internet use patterns and Internet addiction in children and adolescents with obesity. Pediatric Obesity. 2018;13(5):301-6.
33. Mylona I, Deres ES, Dere GDS, Tsinopoulos I, Glynatsis M. The Impact of Internet and Videogaming Addiction on Adolescent Vision: A Review of the Literature. Front Public Health. 2020;8:63.
34. Young KS. Internet Addiction: The Emergence of a New Clinical Disorder. CyberPsychology Behav. 1998;1(3):237-44.
35. Pontes HM, Griffiths MD. Measuring DSM-5 internet gaming disorder: Development and validation of a short psychometric scale. Computers in Human Behavior. 2015;45:137-43.
36. Andreassen CS, Billieux J, Griffiths MD, Kuss DJ, Demetrovics Z, Mazzoni E, et al. The relationship between addictive use of social media and video games and symptoms of psychiatric disorders: A large-scale cross-sectional study. Psychol Addict Behav. 2016;30(2):252-62.
37. Domoff SE, Harrison K, Gearhardt AN, Gentile DA, Lumeng JC, Miller AL. Development and Validation of the Problematic Media Use Measure: A Parent Report Measure of Screen Media "Addiction" in Children. Psychol Pop Media Cult. 2019;8(1):2-11.
38. Chang CH, Chang YC, Yang L, Tzang RF. The Comparative Efficacy of Treatments for Children and Young Adults with Internet Addiction/ Internet Gaming Disorder: An Updated Meta-Analysis. International Journal of Environmental Research and Public Health. 2022;19(5):2612.
39. Young KS. Treatment outcomes using CBT-IA with Internet-addicted patients. J Behav Addict. 2013;2(4):209-15.
40. Du Y song, Jiang W, Vance A. Longer term effect of randomized, controlled group cognitive behavioural therapy for Internet addiction in adolescent students in Shanghai. Aust N Z J Psychiatry. 2010;44(2):129-34.
41. Gupta P, Shah D, Bedi N, Galagali P, Dalwai S, Agrawal S, et al. Indian Academy of Pediatrics Guidelines on Screen Time and Digital Wellness in Infants, Children and Adolescents. Indian Pediatr. 2022;59(3):235-44.
42. Liu QX, Fang XY, Yan N, Zhou ZK, Yuan XJ, Lan J, et al. Multi-family group therapy for adolescent Internet addiction: exploring the underlying mechanisms. Addict Behav. 2015; 42:1-8.
43. Han DH, Kim SM, Lee YS, Renshaw PF. The effect of family therapy on the changes in the severity of on-line game play and brain activity in adolescents with on-line game addiction. Psychiatry Res. 2012;202(2):126-31.
44. Bhide A, Chakraborty K. General Principles for Psychotherapeutic Interventions in Children and Adolescents. Indian J Psychiatry. 2020;62(Suppl 2):S299-318.
45. Molander O, Wennberg P, Berman AH. The Gambling Disorders Identification Test (GDIT): Psychometric Evaluation of a New Comprehensive Measure for Gambling Disorder and Problem Gambling. Assessment. 2023;30(1):225-37.
46. Dellosa G, Browne M. The influence of age on gambling problems worldwide: A systematic review and meta-analysis of risk among younger, middle-aged, and older adults. J Behav Addict. 2024;13(3):702-15.
47. Bőthe B, Potenza MN, Griffiths MD, Kraus SW, Klein V, Fuss J, et al. The development

of the Compulsive Sexual Behavior Disorder Scale (CSBD-19): An ICD-11 based screening measure across three languages. J Behav Addict. 2020;9(2):247-58.

48. Böthe B, Koós M, Nagy L, Kraus SW, Demetrovics Z, Potenza MN, et al. Compulsive sexual behavior disorder in 42 countries: Insights from the International Sex Survey and introduction of standardized assessment tools. J Behav Addict. 2023;12(2):393-407.

49. Turner D, Briken P, Grubbs J, Malandain L, Mestre-Bach G, Potenza MN, et al. The World Federation of Societies of Biological Psychiatry guidelines on the assessment and pharmacological treatment of compulsive sexual behaviour disorder. Dialogues Clin Neurosci. 2022;24(1):10-69.

Internalizing Disorders, Stress, and Trauma

Childhood Depression and Related Conditions

N Prasanna Kumar, Lakshmi Sravanti

INTRODUCTION

Depressive disorders are among the most common psychological disorders seen in children and adolescents. They are particularly important because they can impair cognitive and academic functioning in children. It is a pervasive disorder of emotion leading to impairment in functioning and must be differentiated from normal and brief emotional reactions common in adolescent life. Depression presents with sadness or irritability and is associated with a loss of interest in pleasurable activities, somatic complaints, changes in psychomotor activity. In preschool children, depression manifests as a loss of interest in play and reduced interaction with family members. In adolescents, the evaluation and management of depression are especially crucial due to the potential for suicidal thoughts during this developmental stage.

The prevalence of depression increases with age, but studies suggest a prevalence of up to 2% in even in preschool children.[1] Its prevalence is 1.1% in the age group of 10–14 years, and 2.8% in the age group of 15–19 years.[2] According to the National Comorbidity Survey, the lifetime prevalence of major depressive disorder or dysthymia is 15.9% for females and 7.7% for males.[3] The National Mental Health Survey reports a prevalence of depressive episodes and dysthymia of 1.6% in adolescents.[4] The prevalence has been increasing in recent years and is a significant concern. The coronavirus disease 2019 (COVID-19) pandemic has also been a contributor to the recent trends with a prevalence ratio of 2.54 following the pandemic.[5]

Depression in children and adolescents can be conceptualized from different perspectives, and the biopsychosocial model provides a better understanding, as discussed in **Table 1**.

TABLE 1: Etiological aspects of depressive disorders in children and adolescents.

Biological factors	*Psychological*	*Social factors*
• Family history • Medical illness • Medication • Substance use • Temperament-negative affectivity • Impaired self-regulation	• Negative coping styles • Insecure attachment • Hopelessness and helplessness • Faulty mentalization • Suicidal ideation	• Family conflicts • Strained interpersonal relationships • Parental discord • Faulty parenting styles • Grief • Abuse • Adverse childhood experiences • Poverty • Discrimination/bullying • Academic pressure • Parental substance use

CLINICAL FEATURES OF DEPRESSION IN CHILDREN AND ADOLESCENTS

Depression in children and adolescents presents with a diverse range of emotional, behavioral, cognitive, and physical symptoms, often differing from the typical sadness seen in adults. Younger children may exhibit increased irritability, somatic complaints, or social withdrawal, whereas adolescents may display withdrawn behavior, academic decline, hopelessness, risk-taking behaviors, and self-harm or substance use, which can sometimes be mistaken for typical teenage rebellion. In very young children, clinginess and irritability are common, while cognitive symptoms may be less apparent. Additionally, cultural and individual differences influence symptom expression, with some children struggling to verbalize their emotions, leading to underreporting of depressive symptoms. **Table 2** outlines signs of childhood depression. Recognizing these signs can help caregivers, educators, and healthcare professionals in starting timely support and intervention.

Besides the nature of the presentation posing challenges for the diagnosis of depression in children and adolescents, the presence of additional conditions can further complicate the clinical picture, making it harder to distinguish depressive symptoms from those of the coexisting disorder. In neurodevelopmental conditions such as autism spectrum disorder and intellectual disability, communication difficulties, and challenges in articulating emotions may mask underlying depressive symptoms, making self-reporting unreliable. In attention-deficit/hyperactivity disorder (ADHD) and oppositional defiant disorder (ODD), irritability, or defiance may be misinterpreted by clinicians as primary symptoms of these conditions, leading to missed identification of coexisting depression. Excessive worry, restlessness, or physical symptoms

TABLE 2: Signs and symptoms of depression in children and adolescents.

Category	*Signs and symptoms of depression in children and adolescents*
Emotional	• Frequent and unexplained tantrums • Irritability • Excessive fears or separation anxiety • Increased irritability or anger outbursts • Persistent sadness or low mood • Frequent and unexplained crying spells • Increased irritability or frustration • Feeling unloved or unwanted • Feelings of hopelessness or worthlessness • Excessive guilt or self-blame
Behavioral	• Clinginess or separation anxiety • Loss of interest in play, school, or hobbies • Withdrawal from family, friends, or activities • Frequent complaints of boredom or fatigue • Regression of previously attained milestones (e.g., bedwetting in a child who attained bladder control) • Risk-taking behaviors or self-harm
Cognitive	• Difficulty in concentrating or making decisions • Decline in academic performance • Negative self-talk or preoccupation with failure • Increased sensitivity to criticism • Expressions of worthlessness or hopelessness • Expressing thoughts of death or suicide
Social	• Decreased engagement in conversations • Difficulty in expressing feelings or thoughts • Avoidance of social situations • Increased conflicts with peers or family • Reluctance to attend school or social events
Physical	• Unexplained aches and pains (headaches and stomachaches) • Low energy or fatigue • Changes in appetite (increased or decreased) • Sleep disturbances (insomnia or excessive sleep) • Psychomotor agitation or slowing

(e.g., headaches and stomachaches) of anxiety disorders may overshadow underlying depressive symptoms. In children with learning disabilities, academic struggles and frustration may lead to low self-esteem and mood symptoms, which may be mistaken as purely educational difficulties. Substance use may be a coping mechanism for undiagnosed depression, complicating symptom recognition. In children with post-traumatic symptom disorder (PTSD), they may also have depression due to emotional distress, feelings of helplessness, and disruptions in their sense of safety and trust resulting from the traumatic experience. Therefore, it is crucial to screen for depression in these children to ensure timely recognition and appropriate intervention. A high degree of clinical suspicion, comprehensive assessment, and careful differentiation of overlapping symptoms are essential to ensure the identification of depression in children and adolescents and appropriate intervention. **Box 1** provide tips for clinicians with practical strategies to recognize early warning signs across emotional, behavioral, cognitive, and social domains.

BOX 1: Tips for clinicians to identify depression in children and adolescents early.

- Ensure a safe space for the interview
- Build rapport
- Have a nonjudgmental stance
- Pay attention to nonverbal cues
- Consider developmental context
- Explore academic and family stressors
- Screen for depression in children with attention-deficit hyperactivity disorder (ADHD), learning difficulties, anxiety, and trauma exposure that may mask the condition
- Use standard criteria and screening tools

ASSESSMENT AND DIAGNOSIS OF DEPRESSION IN CHILDREN AND ADOLESCENTS

While interviewing a child or adolescent, adequate care must be taken to preserve confidentiality and privacy, especially when discussing conflicts or stressors, except in cases where there is a risk of harm to self. Depression should be diagnosed according to the classification systems of the International Classification of Diseases, 11th Revision (ICD-11),[6] and the Diagnostic and Statistical Manual of Mental Disorders, Fifth Edition (DSM-5).[7] ICD-11 or DSM-5 mostly aligns with respect to major features. While the ICD-11 includes a specifier for psychosis in moderate depression, with symptoms including depressed mood, diminished interest in activities, decreased energy levels, concentration difficulties, feelings of hopelessness, worthlessness, guilt, and suicidal ideation, the DSM-5 also notes hypersomnia and increased appetite in addition to the rest of the symptomatology.

In the Indian context, while structured tools may be used in specialized or academic settings, clinical interviews remain the cornerstone of diagnosis, particularly in resource-limited environments. Assessments include clinical evaluation supplemented, when appropriate, by standardized screening tools such as the Patient Health Questionnaire-Adolescent (PHQ-A), Kiddie Schedule for Affective Disorders and Schizophrenia (KSADS), Child Depression Inventory (CDI-2), and the short or long mood and feelings questionnaire.[8] These tools may be helpful in structured settings or for monitoring severity and treatment response over time. The Children's Depression Rating Scale (CDRS)[9] and Reynolds Adolescent Depression Scale (RADS)[10] can assist in assessing the severity of depression when needed. Brief suicide screening tools, including "Ask Suicide Screening Questions" and the Columbia Suicide Severity Rating Scale (C-SSRS), may be useful in evaluating suicidality, particularly in moderate- to high-risk scenarios.[11]

STEPS FOR ESTABLISHING A DIAGNOSIS OF DEPRESSION

1. *Initial assessment:*
   - *Understanding the context:* Gather history from child, parents, caregivers, and teachers
   - Identify emotional, behavioral, cognitive, and physical symptoms
   - Screen for risk factors (family history, trauma, and chronic stressors) including psychosocial factors (family dynamics, peer relationships, school environment, and any significant life events)
   - Assessment of suicidality (suicidal thoughts, plans, behaviors, and risk factors) to ensure the safety and well-being
2. *Use standardized screening tools, when appropriate:*
   - Consider administering tools such as the CDI-2 or PHQ-A in moderate-to-severe or diagnostically uncertain cases, or for monitoring response over time.
   - Supplement clinical interviews with parent/teacher-report tools such as the Child Behavior Checklist (CBCL) or Strengths and Difficulties Questionnaire (SDQ), where feasible.
   - Note that these tools are not substitutes for clinical judgment but can aid in assessment and documentation.
3. *Evaluate for comorbid conditions:*
   - Assess for anxiety, ADHD, ASD, PTSD, learning disabilities, behavioral disorders.
   - Differentiate primary versus secondary symptoms (i.e., determine whether depression is the main condition or if it arises as a consequence of another disorder).
4. *Rule out medical conditions:*
   - Screen for hypothyroidism, anemia, nutritional deficiencies, and chronic illnesses
   - Assess medication side effects.
5. *Assess psychosocial stressors:*
   - Explore bullying, family conflicts, academic stress, and peer relationships
   - Identify trauma history, abuse, and neglect
6. *Confirm diagnosis based on DSM-5/ICD-10 criteria:*
   - Persistent low mood or irritability
   - Loss of interest/pleasure (anhedonia)
   - Accompanying symptoms (sleep/appetite changes, concentration issues, fatigue, self-worth decline, and suicidality)
   - Symptoms persist for at least 2 weeks and cause functional impairment.
7. *Develop management plan:*
   - Psychoeducation for child, parents, and teachers
   - Therapy options—cognitive behavior therapy (CBT), interpersonal therapy (IPT), and family therapy
   - Medications—for example, selective serotonin reuptake inhibitors (SSRIs) if indicated
   - Monitor for suicidality and implement crisis intervention if necessary.

The process of assessment and establishing the diagnosis is depicted by the **Flowchart 1.**

COURSE OF DEPRESSION

The majority of children will improve from depression with a good recovery rate. Compared to adults, children have a higher recovery rate but experience longer episodes and longer interepisode periods. A history of suicidality, conflicts or negative life events, and comorbidities may predict recurrent depressive episodes. Most depressive episodes improve within 9 months. However, recurrence is observed in 72% of cases

Flowchart 1: Flowchart for assessment and establishing diagnosis.

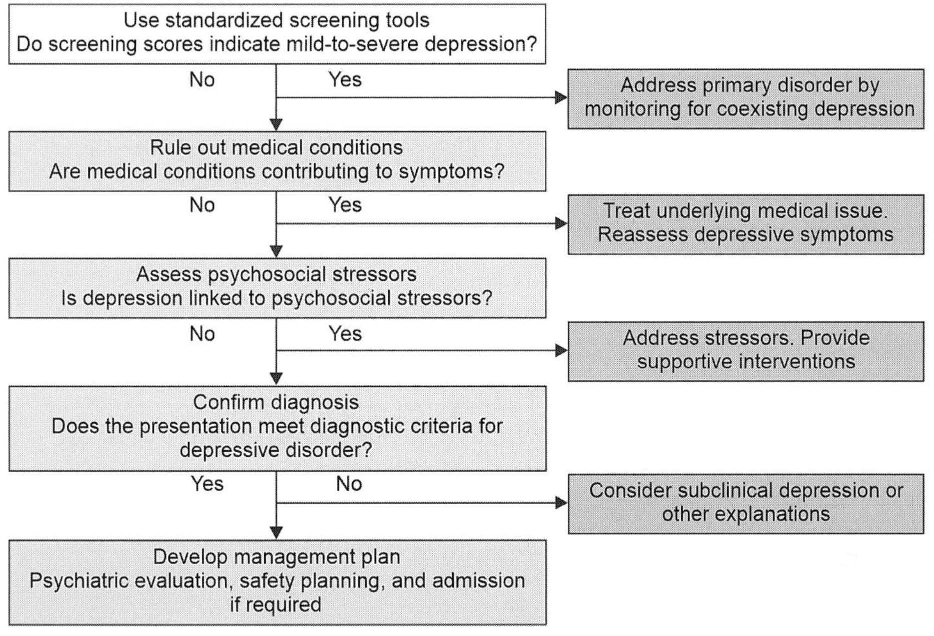

within 3–5 years after the first episode.[12] A relapse prevention trial carried out for 32 weeks with a fixed dosage of fluoxetine reported a relapse rate of 34%.[13] A 78-week trial reported a lower relapse rate with a combination of medication and CBT compared to medication alone (36 vs. 62%).[14] Anhedonia can be a negative prognostic indicator in adolescents with treatment-resistant depression.[15]

MANAGEMENT OF DEPRESSION IN CHILDREN AND ADOLESCENTS

Effective management of depression in children and adolescents requires a multimodal approach, integrating psychotherapy, pharmacotherapy, and environmental support. **Box 2** outlines the general guidelines to ensure proper intervention and long-term well-being while minimizing relapse risk. The Indian Psychiatric Society (IPS),[16] National Institute for Health and Care Excellence (NICE),[17] and American Academy of Child and Adolescent Psychiatry (AACAP)[18] provide evidence-based guidelines for the assessment and management of depression in children and adolescents. These guidelines **(Box 2)** emphasize a stepped-care approach, prioritizing psychotherapy as the first-line treatment, with pharmacotherapy reserved for moderate-to-severe cases or when psychotherapy alone is insufficient.

Some aspects of treatment are discussed below, considering developmental age appropriateness.

PARENTAL PSYCHOEDUCATION

Psychoeducation should focus on the causes, current risk factors, symptoms, course, treatment options, progress of the illness, warning signs, and the responsibility and role of family members in the child's improvement, as well as the possibility of suicidal behavior. Emphasis should also be placed on identifying family members who can provide support during a crisis, as well as close

BOX 2: General guidelines for management of depression in children and adolescents.

- Establish rapport with the child and family
- Provide psychoeducation about depression, its causes, and treatment options
- Emphasize the importance of early intervention
- Screen for suicidal thoughts/self-harm risk at each visit
- Treatment should include a combination of pharmacotherapy, family education, and supportive interventions at home and school
- When available, psychotherapy can be highly beneficial, complementing other treatment modalities and enhancing treatment outcomes
- Develop a safety plan and involve caregivers
- Address comorbid conditions
- Consider modifications in therapy approaches for children with autism or language difficulties
- Hospitalization if high suicidal risk, psychosis, or severe functional impairment is present
- Address stigma
- Engage teachers, school counselors, and peers in supporting the child's well-being
- Facilitate academic accommodations if needed (e.g., reduced workload and extra time for tasks)
- Reduce stressors like bullying, family conflict, or peer pressure
- Schedule regular follow-ups (weekly to biweekly initially)
- Assess treatment response and side effects
- Adjust therapy/medications as necessary
- Continue treatment for at least 6–12 months after symptom remission
- Gradual tapering of medications under supervision
- Teach relapse prevention strategies and ensure ongoing psychosocial support

friends or trusted individuals with whom the child can share their conflicts or feelings, and ensuring a safe environment. The evaluation of stressors at school and home and understanding conflicts from the child's perspective need to be highlighted. Activity scheduling, monitoring the child, and close supervision until the next follow-up should be discussed with family members or caregivers.

CLINICAL ACTION PLAN

Children and adolescents presenting with severe depressive symptoms with suicidality should be referred to emergency services for immediate intervention. Those with mild-to-moderate depression may be managed with a combination of SSRIs and CBT, by actively monitored on a weekly or fortnightly basis. In all cases, safety planning and crisis intervention strategies should be discussed with parents or caregivers.

PHARMACOLOGICAL MANAGEMENT

Selective serotonin reuptake inhibitors are the first-line pharmacological treatment for moderate-to-severe depression in children and adolescents, especially when psychotherapy alone is insufficient, or when there is significant functional impairment, suicidality, or treatment resistance. Start low and go slow, but aim to reach a therapeutic dose unless side effects limit titration. **Table 3** provides a clinical guide to prescribing SSRIs for children and adolescents with depression, including age indications, dosing, and key monitoring considerations.

If an adolescent fails to respond to two adequate SSRI trials, it is essential to re-evaluate the diagnosis, assess for comorbidities, treatment adherence, and psychosocial stressors, and review the adequacy of psychotherapy. Once these factors are addressed and nonresponse persists, the child or adolescent should be referred for consultation with a child and adolescent psychiatrist.

TABLE 3: Clinical guide to prescribing selective serotonin reuptake inhibitors (SSRIs) for children and adolescents with depression.

An overview of pharmacological management	
Choice of SSRI	
Fluoxetine	It is the most studied SSRI in adolescents and has the strongest evidence for efficacy and safety. It is approved for use from 8 years of age and is generally considered the first-line agent, particularly in typical presentations of adolescent depression[19-21]
Escitalopram	It is approved for use in adolescents ≥12 years, and may be considered when anxiety features are prominent or fluoxetine is not tolerated[19,21]
Sertraline	While not officially approved for depression in children, it has demonstrated effectiveness in clinical practice and trials, especially when there is comorbid anxiety, obsessive-compulsive features, or in cases where fluoxetine or escitalopram are not suitable. It is commonly used off-label in children from 6 to 7 years[19,21]
Other SSRIs	Other SSRIs like citalopram, paroxetine, and venlafaxine are not routinely recommended in this population due to limited evidence or higher risk of adverse effects (e.g., suicidality with paroxetine and venlafaxine)[19,21]
Tricyclic antidepressants	They are not recommended due to poor efficacy and higher risks (e.g., cardiotoxicity)
Special considerations	If there are signs of bipolar depression: early activation, treatment resistance, psychotic features, or family history of bipolar disorder, SSRIs may worsen symptoms. Alternatives include mood stabilizers or atypical antipsychotics like lurasidone or olanzapine-fluoxetine combination[22,23]
Starting dosage and titration	
Fluoxetine	Start at 5–10 mg/day, increase by 10 mg every 1–2 weeks; usual target dose is 20 mg/day. It can go up to 40 mg/day if needed[16-18]
Escitalopram	Start at 5 mg/day (age ≥12 years), increase to 10 mg/day after 1–2 weeks; maximum 20 mg/day[16-18]
Sertraline	Start at 25 mg/day, especially in younger children or those with anxiety; increase to 50 mg/day after 1–2 weeks. Usual range: 50–100 mg/day, with a maximum of 200 mg/day in adolescents if well-tolerated[16-18]
Monitoring and side effects	
Common side effects	• Gastrointestinal upset, insomnia or drowsiness, restlessness, and headaches. SSRIs can cause behavioral activation—manifesting as increased energy, impulsivity, or agitation, especially early in treatment[16,21] • Behavioral activation should be distinguished from a switch to mania, which presents with euphoria, decreased need for sleep, and grandiosity[16,21]
Monitoring for suicidal ideation	• Systematic monitoring for suicidal ideation, especially in the first 4–6 weeks, is essential • The Treatment for Adolescents with Depression Study (TADS) found suicidal events in fluoxetine therapy (14.7%), combination therapy (8.4%), and CBT alone (6.3%).[20] However, more recent data support that with careful monitoring, the benefits of SSRIs outweigh the risks
Parents should be counseled about side effects, the need for regular follow-up, and the importance of not discontinuing medication abruptly	

Contd...

Contd...

An overview of pharmacological management	
Duration of treatment	
Maintenance phase	• Continue the SSRI at an effective dose for 6–9 months[16-18] • In cases of recurrent depression, severe impairment, suicidality, or depression with psychotic features, maintenance treatment may be extended to 12 months or longer after full symptom remission
Long-term follow-up and monitoring	
Long-term monitoring	• Childhood depression carries a higher risk of switching to bipolar disorder than adult-onset cases • Children with psychotic features, a history of antidepressant-induced switching, or a family history of bipolar disorder should be closely monitored for polarity shifts during follow-up

NONPHARMACOLOGICAL INTERVENTIONS FOR DEPRESSION IN CHILDREN AND ADOLESCENTS

Nonpharmacological interventions form a crucial part of depression management in children and adolescents, especially in mild-to-moderate cases. These include psychotherapy, psychoeducation, lifestyle changes, and family support strategies. In India, access to specialized therapies may be limited, and general psychiatrists often manage care with limited resources.

Cognitive behavior therapy (CBT) and interpersonal therapy (IPT) have the most evidence,[16] but when trained therapists are not available, for children/adolescents with mild depression, general psychiatrists can:

- Provide basic psychoeducation to the child and family about depression.
- Teach simple behavioral activation techniques.
- Address parent-child interactions and stressors through supportive counseling.
- Encourage routine, sleep hygiene, and reduced screen time.
- Liaise with schools when feasible.

In moderate-to-severe depression, CBT combined with SSRIs has shown better outcomes than either alone. However, if CBT is unavailable, initiating fluoxetine with psychoeducation and regular follow-up is acceptable and effective.

Referral to a child and adolescent psychiatrist is recommended when:

- There is high suicidality, psychosis, or treatment resistance.
- Significant comorbidity (e.g., ASD, severe anxiety, or trauma) complicates management.
- Family dysfunction or abuse requires systemic intervention.

In preschool and younger children, psychotherapeutic interventions must be adapted to their developmental level. In resource-poor settings, developmentally appropriate methods such as play-based interactions, storytelling, and emotion identification through pictures or role-play can be effective. The focus should be on building emotional vocabulary, encouraging expression through play, and improving the parent-child relationship. Caregivers can be guided to adopt consistent routines, offer predictable emotional responses, and reduce harsh discipline. Even without formal therapy, these foundational strategies promote emotional regulation and coping in young children showing signs of depression.

ELECTROCONVULSIVE THERAPY AND NEUROMODULATION

Electroconvulsive therapy (ECT) is reserved for severe, treatment-resistant depression in adolescents, especially in the presence of psychotic features, catatonia, refusal to eat or drink, or high suicidality, where it may be life-saving. As per the Mental Healthcare Act (MHCA), 2017, ECT in minors requires informed guardian consent and prior approval from the Mental Health Review Board. Unmodified ECT is not permitted. ECT may also be considered earlier when medication trials are not feasible due to intolerance or clinical urgency.[16]

Neuromodulation may be considered for adolescents with moderate-to-severe depression who have not responded to at least two adequate trials of first-line pharmacological and psychotherapeutic interventions. In the Indian context, where access to neuromodulation services for children and adolescents is often limited, referrals should ideally be made to tertiary care centers with specialized expertise in child and adolescent mental health. Decisions regarding timing and suitability should be guided by documented treatment resistance, degree of functional impairment, and family readiness for advanced interventions.

Transcranial magnetic stimulation (TMS) has shown promising results in treatment-resistant depression in adolescents[24] and is generally considered safe, with side effects such as scalp discomfort, mood changes, itching, local redness, and headache.[25] Data on transcranial direct current stimulation (tDCS) in adolescents remain limited, though adult studies suggest potential benefit in depressive disorders.

Understanding the complexities of depression in children and adolescents requires attention to a related condition, disruptive mood dysregulation disorder (DMDD). DMDD presents unique challenges in diagnosis and treatment. This section will delve into the prevalence, characteristics, and treatment options for DMDD, highlighting its distinction from other related disorders.

DISRUPTIVE MOOD DYSREGULATION DISORDER

The prevalence rate of DMDD (3-month prevalence) was reported to be 0.8–3.3%. DMDD is seen in the age group of 6–18 years and is characterized by recurrent temper outbursts with chronic irritability at baseline over a span of 12 months. Unlike ODD, chronic irritability in DMDD is not related to outbursts. This disorder may progress to unipolar depression. Earlier, severe mood dysregulation (SMD) was reported, and the current DMDD shares some clinical features with SMD but without hyperarousal symptoms. DMDD is not diagnosed alongside ODD, intermittent explosive disorder, or bipolar affective disorder (BPAD).[6,26]

Understanding the characteristics of DMDD is crucial for accurate diagnosis and effective treatment planning in children and adolescents. This disorder often coexists with other conditions such as ADHD, necessitating a multifaceted treatment approach. Combining behavioral therapy with medication, particularly stimulants and risperidone, has shown significant efficacy in managing the symptoms and improving overall outcomes.

While pharmacological interventions may be helpful for children with severe irritability and comorbid conditions like ADHD, practitioners should be cautious when interpreting the evidence base. There are limited randomized controlled trials (RCTs) in children specifically diagnosed with DMDD, and many treatment recommendations are extrapolated from studies on related conditions such as ADHD, SMD, and aggression. Divalproex adjunctive to stimulants had a response rate of 57% in children with

ADHD and aggression.[27] The Treatment of Severe Childhood Aggression study examined the use of risperidone for children who are on stimulants and receiving parental training, reporting a medium effect size.[28] Optimizing stimulant medication leads to a significant decline in depressive symptoms, mood severity index scores, and ADHD symptoms with good tolerability.[29] An earlier meta-analysis revealed that psychostimulants had a moderate to large effect on oppositional behavior.[30] Risperidone was reported to be effective in reducing irritability in SMD with improvement in ADHD and depression.[31] The Multimodal Treatment Study of Children with ADHD (MTA) reported that the combination of behavioral treatment and stimulants was superior in treating irritability.[32] In practice, general psychiatrists should first optimize stimulant treatment and behavioral strategies before considering adjunctive antipsychotic medications. If symptoms remain severe or impairing, referral to a specialist in child and adolescent psychiatry is recommended for careful consideration of adjunctive agents like risperidone or mood stabilizers, while balancing risks and benefits.

SUMMARY AND CONCLUSION

In summary, assessment and treatment of depression in children and adolescents require a comprehensive and developmentally informed approach, considering psychosocial stressors, comorbidities, and family context. Early identification, psychoeducation, and a combination of pharmacological and psychotherapeutic strategies are essential for effective and sustained management. Comorbid conditions, especially ADHD and anxiety disorders, are common and can impact presentation, treatment choices, and outcomes, necessitating integrated care planning. DMDD adds to diagnostic complexity and requires careful differentiation and tailored interventions. Long-term follow-up in depression is vital to monitor progress, manage relapses, and to watch for the emergence of bipolar disorder or other psychiatric comorbidities. Finally, by adopting evidence-based and context-sensitive practices, clinicians can significantly improve outcomes for children and adolescents with depression.

REFERENCES

1. Whalen DJ, Sylvester CM, Luby JL, MD. Depression and Anxiety in Preschoolers: A Review of the Past 7 Years. Child Adolesc Psychiatr Clin North Am. 2017;26(3):503-22.
2. World Health Organisation. (2021). Mental health of adolescents: Key facts.. [online] Available from https://www.who.int/news-room/fact-sheets/detail/adolescent-mental-health [Last accessed 19 November, 2025].
3. Kathleen R, Jian-Ping H. Lifetime Prevalence of Mental Disorders in US Adolescents: Results from the National Comorbidity Study-Adolescent Supplement (NCS-A). J Am Acad Child Adolesc Psychiatry. 2010; 49(10):980-9.
4. Ministry of Health and Family Welfare Government of India. (2016). National Mental Health Survey of India, 2015-16, Prevalence, Pattern and Outcomes. [online] Available from https://indianmhs.nimhans.ac.in/phase1/Docs/Report2.pdf [Last accessed 19 November, 2025].
5. Wang S, Chen L. Depression and anxiety among children and adolescents pre and post COVID-19: A comparative meta-analysis. Front Psychiatry. 2022;13:917552.
6. American Psychiatric Association. Diagnostic and Statistical Manual of Mental Disorders, 5th edition. Washington, DC: American Psychiatric Association; 2013.
7. World Health Organization. International Classification of Diseases, Eleventh Revision (ICD-11). Geneva: World Health Organization; 2022.
8. Roseman M, Kloda LA, Saadat N, Riehm KE, Ickowicz A, Baltzer F, et al. Accuracy of Depression Screening Tools to Detect Major Depression in

Children and Adolescents: A Systematic Review. Can J Psychiatry. 2016;61(12):746-57.
9. Poznanski EO, Grossman JA, Buchsbaum Y, Banegas M, Freeman L, Gibbons R. Preliminary studies of the reliability and validity of the children's depression rating scale. J Am Acad Child Psychiatry. 1984;23(2):191-7.
10. Osman A, Gutierrez PM, Bagge CL, Fang Q, Emmerich A. Reynolds adolescent depression scale-second edition: a reliable and useful instrument. J Clin Psychol. 2010;66(12):1324-45.
11. Gipson PY, Agarwala P, Opperman KJ, Horwitz A, King CA. Columbia-suicide severity rating scale: predictive validity with adolescent psychiatric emergency patients. Pediatr Emerg Care. 2015;31(2):88-94.
12. Maria K, Scott O. The course of major depressive disorder from childhood to young adulthood: Recovery and recurrence in a longitudinal observational study. J Affect Disord. 2016;203:374-81.
13. Graham J, John H. Fluoxetine treatment for prevention of relapse of depression in children and adolescents: a double-blind, placebo-controlled study. J Am Acad Child Adolesc Psychiatry. 2004;43(11):1397-405.
14. Graham J, Betsy D. Continued Effectiveness of Relapse Prevention Cognitive-Behavioral Therapy Following Fluoxetine Treatment in Youth with Major Depressive Disorder. J Am Acad Child Adolesc Psychiatry. 2015;54(12):991-8.
15. McMakin DL, Olino TM, Porta G, Dietz LJ, Emslie G, Clarke G, et al. Anhedonia predicts poorer recovery among youth with selective serotonin reuptake inhibitor treatment-resistant depression. J Am Acad Child Adolesc Psychiatry. 2012;51(4):404-11.
16. Grover S, Avasthi A. Clinical Practice Guidelines for the management of depression in children and adolescents. Indian J Psychiatry. 2019;61(Suppl 2):226-40.
17. National Institute for Health and Care Excellence. (2019). Depression in Children and Young People: Identification and Management. [online] Available from https://www.nice.org.uk/guidance/ng134 [Last accessed 19 November, 2025].
18. Birmaher B, Brent D; AACAP Work Group on Quality Issues; Bernet W, Bukstein O, Walter H, et al. Practice parameter for the assessment and treatment of children and adolescents with depressive disorders. J Am Acad Child Adolesc Psychiatry. 2007;46(11):1503-26.
19. Cheung AH, Emslie GJ, Mayes TL. The use of antidepressants to treat depression in children and adolescents. CMAJ. 2006;174(2):193-200.
20. John S, Susan S. The Treatment for Adolescents With Depression Study (TADS): long-term effectiveness and safety outcomes. Arch Gen Psychiatry. 2007;64(10):1132-43.
21. Cipriani A, Zhou X, Del Giovane C, Hetrick SE, Qin B, Whittington C, et al. Comparative efficacy and tolerability of antidepressants for major depressive disorder in children and adolescents: a network meta-analysis. Lancet. 2016;388(10047):881-90.
22. Kishi T, Ikuta T, Matsuda Y, Sakuma K, Okuya M, Mishima K, et al. Mood stabilizers and/or antipsychotics for bipolar disorder in the maintenance phase: a systematic review and network meta-analysis of randomized controlled trials. Mol Psychiatry. 2021;26(8):4146-57.
23. Patel RS, Veluri N, Patel J, Patel R, Machado T, Diler R. Second-Generation Antipsychotics in Management of Acute Pediatric Bipolar Depression: A Systematic Review and Meta-analysis. J Child Adolesc Psychopharmacol. 2021;31(8):521-30.
24. Amy E, Michael S. Addressing the Needs of Adolescents with Treatment Resistant Depressive Disorders: A Systematic Review of rTMS. Brain Stimul. 2014;7(1):7-12.
25. Chandramouli K, Luciana S. Safety of Noninvasive Brain Stimulation in Children and Adolescents. Brain Stimul. 2015;8(1):76-87.
26. Copeland WE, Angold A, Costello EJ, Egger H. Prevalence, comorbidity, and correlates of DSM-5 proposed disruptive mood dysregulation disorder. Am J Psychiatry. 2013;170(2):173-9.
27. Blader JC, Schooler NR, Jensen PS, Pliszka SR, Kafantaris V. Adjunctive divalproex versus placebo for children with ADHD and aggression refractory to stimulant monotherapy. Am J Psychiatry. 2009;166(12):1392-401.
28. Barterian JA, Arnold LE, Brown NV, Farmer CA, Williams C, Findling RL, et al. Clinical Implications From the Treatment of Severe Childhood

Aggression (TOSCA) Study: A Re-Analysis and Integration of Findings. J Am Acad Child Adolesc Psychiatry. 2017;56(12):1026-33.
29. Baweja R, Belin PJ, Humphrey HH, Babocsai L, Pariseau ME, Waschbusch DA, et al. The Effectiveness and Tolerability of Central Nervous System Stimulants in School-Age Children with Attention-Deficit/Hyperactivity Disorder and Disruptive Mood Dysregulation Disorder Across Home and School. J Child Adolesc Psychopharmacol. 2016;26(2):154-63.
30. Pringsheim T, Hirsch L, Gardner D, Gorman DA. The pharmacological management of oppositional behaviour, conduct problems, and aggression in children and adolescents with attention-deficit hyperactivity disorder, oppositional defiant disorder, and conduct disorder: a systematic review and meta-analysis. Part 1: psychostimulants, alpha-2 agonists, and atomoxetine. Can J Psychiatry. 2015;60(2):42-51.
31. Krieger FV, Pheula GF, Coelho R, Zeni T, Tramontina S, Zeni CP, et al. An open-label trial of risperidone in children and adolescents with severe mood dysregulation. J Child Adolesc Psychopharmacol. 2011;21(3):237-43.
32. Fernández de la Cruz L, Simonoff E, McGough JJ, Halperin JM, Arnold LE, Stringaris A. Treatment of children with attention-deficit/hyperactivity disorder (ADHD) and irritability: results from the multimodal treatment study of children with ADHD (MTA). J Am Acad Child Adolesc Psychiatry. 2015;54(1):62-70.e3.

CHAPTER 16

Anxiety, Fear, Obsessive-Compulsive Disorder, and Related Conditions

Vivek Agarwal, Rashmi Shukla, Aditya Agrawal

INTRODUCTION

Anxiety disorders are the most common childhood-onset psychiatric disorders. These are associated with educational underachievement as well as functional impairments that may persist into adulthood.[1] Anxiety is characterized by the apprehension and anticipation of danger by external or internal stimuli. This response represents a fundamental emotion that emerges during infancy and persists into childhood, exhibiting a range of expressions from mild to severe along a continuum.[1] Anxiety might manifest as fear or worry, it can also provoke irritability and anger in children. In children, anxiety arises in several situations, which may be developmentally appropriate. Therefore, pathological anxiety at any stage can be defined by enduring or significant levels of anxiety and avoidance, coupled with subjective distress or impairment. Distinguishing between normal and pathological anxiety is notably challenging in children, given that fears and anxieties are common facets of typical development in childhood.[2,3] While these experiences can be intensely distressing, they are common occurrences in most children and usually transient. For instance, separation anxiety typically arises between 12 and 18 months, fears of thunder or lightning emerge around 2–4 years, and similar patterns follow. Such anxiety is prevalent in most children and typically resolves without lasting effects.[4]

The American Psychiatric Association's Diagnostic and Statistical Manual of Mental Disorders, 5th Edition (DSM-5), includes seven anxiety disorders seen in children.[5] The central characteristic of anxiety disorders is avoidance.[6] This often entails clear avoidance of particular situations, locations, or stimuli, but it can also manifest in subtler forms such as hesitation, uncertainty, withdrawal, or ritualistic behaviors. These patterns remain relatively consistent across different disorders, with the primary distinction lying in the specific triggers for avoidance. Alongside these cognitive aspects, anxious children often report various physical complaints indicative of heightened arousal; however, these symptoms are typically nonspecific to any particular disorder and thus not diagnostic. Common physical symptoms among anxious children include headaches, stomach aches, nausea, vomiting, diarrhea, and muscle tension. Distress and impairment in several domains of children life must be present to diagnose anxiety and related disorders.[5] Clinically, anxious children rarely meet criteria for only one disorder. Within treatment-seeking populations, around 80–90% meet criteria for more than one mental disorder. The majority, up to 75%, meet criteria for more than one anxiety disorder. A further 10–30% also meet criteria for an additional mood disorder.[7]

EPIDEMIOLOGY OF ANXIETY DISORDERS AND OBSESSIVE-COMPULSIVE AND RELATED DISORDERS

Table 1 shows the overview of the epidemiological factors associated with different anxiety disorders and obsessive-compulsive and related disorders.

TABLE 1: Overview of the epidemiological factors associated with different anxiety disorders and obsessive-compulsive and related disorders (OCRD).[5,8-16]

Disorder	*Prevalence*	*Development and course*	*Risk factors*	*Comorbidity*
Separation anxiety disorder	• 1.6–4% • 0.2%* • Clinical sample: M = F • Community sample: F > M	• Onset may be as early as preschool • Peak incidence between 7 and 9 years of age • Fluctuating course with periods of exacerbation and remission	• Environmental—life stress and loss • Genetic—heritability 73%	• Generalized anxiety disorder • Specific phobia
Selective mutism	0.03% and 1%	Onset is usually before age of 5 years	• Temperamental—neuroticism or behavioral inhibition • Environmental—overprotective parenting	Social anxiety disorder
Specific phobia	• 2.4–3.3% • 2.9%* • F > M (2:1)	Onset-early childhood <10 years	• Temperamental—neuroticism or behavioral inhibition • Environmental—overprotective parenting, negative, or traumatic encounters with the feared object or situation	Depression
Social anxiety disorder (Social phobia)	• 0.5–2% • 0.3%* • F > M	• Usual age of onset 8–15 years • Onset may follow a stressful or humiliating experience (e.g., being bullied, vomiting during a public speech) • It may be insidious, developing slowly	• Temperamental—behavioral inhibition and fear of negative evaluation • Environmental—childhood maltreatment and adversity • Genetic—first-degree relatives have a 2–6 times greater chance of having social anxiety disorder	• Depression • Substance use disorder • Other anxiety disorders

Contd…

Contd…

Disorder	*Prevalence*	*Development and course*	*Risk factors*	*Comorbidity*
Panic disorder	• 0.6–4.7% • 0.1%* • F > M (2:1) • The rates show a gradual increase during adolescence, particularly in females, and possibly following the onset of puberty • 36–63% of adolescence experience panic attack	• Childhood onset rare • Chronic waxing and waning course	• Temperamental—neuroticism and anxiety sensitivity • Environmental—childhood experiences of sexual and physical abuse and smoking • Genetic—first-degree relatives have higher risk	• Agoraphobia • Depression • Bipolar disorder • Alcohol use disorder • Medical conditions, e.g., cardiac arrhythmias, hyperthyroidism, asthma, chronic obstructive pulmonary disease (COPD), and irritable bowel syndrome
Agoraphobia	• 1.7–2.6% • 0.1%* • F > M (2:1)	• Childhood onset rare • Substantial incidence risk in late adolescence • Course is persistent and chronic	• Temperamental—neuroticism or behavioral inhibition and anxiety sensitivity • Environmental—negative events in childhood (e.g., separation and death of parent) • Genetic—heritability is 61%	• Other anxiety disorders • Depressive disorder • Post-traumatic stress disorder • Alcohol use disorder
Generalized anxiety disorder	• 0.5–7.1% • 0.3%* • F > M (2:1)	• Initially, this can present as anxious temperament • Mean age of onset 8–9 years • Chronic waxing and waning course	• Temperamental—neuroticism or behavioral inhibition and harm avoidance • Environmental—childhood adversity and overprotective parenting • Genetic—genetics contribute to approximately one-third of the likelihood of developing generalized anxiety disorder	• Other anxiety disorders • Depressive disorder

Contd…

Contd…

Disorder	*Prevalence*	*Development and course*	*Risk factors*	*Comorbidity*
Obsessive-compulsive and related disorders				
Obsessive compulsive disorder (OCD)	• 1.2% • 0.1%* • M > F • Earlier age of onset (<7 years) has a female preponderance and higher likelihood of positive family history • Nearly 25% of males have onset before age of 10 years	• The onset of symptoms is typically gradual. • Symptoms fluctuate in severity with time and may increase during stress • Chronic, waxing, and waning course	• Temperamental traits include heightened internalizing symptoms, increased negative emotionality, and tendencies toward behavioral inhibition • Environmental—physical and sexual abuse, stressful, or traumatic events • Genetic—Among first-degree relatives of individuals with onset of OCD in childhood or adolescence, the rate is increased to 10–20%	• Anxiety disorders • Depression • Bipolar disorder • Tic disorder—attention-deficit/hyperactivity disorder and disruptive behavior disorders
Body dysmorphic disorder (BDD)	• 1–2% • No significant gender differences	• Most common age of onset 12–13 years • Chronic course	• Environmental—childhood neglect and abuse • Genetic—high risk in first-degree relatives	• Depression • Social phobia • OCD • Substance use disorders
Hoarding disorder	• 2–6% • M > F	• Emergence of symptom as early as 11–15 years • Chronic course	• Temperamental—indecisiveness • Environmental—stressful traumatic event • Genetic—hoarding tendencies often run in families, with approximately 50% of individuals who hoard reporting that they have a relative who also exhibits hoarding behavior	• Mood disorder • Anxiety disorder
Trichotillomania (Hair pulling disorder)	• 1–2% • M = F	• Hair pulling typically begins during or after the onset of puberty • Chronic course	Genetic—the disorder is more prevalent among individuals with OCD and their immediate family members compared to the general population	• Depression • Skin picking disorder
Excoriation (skin-picking disorder)	• 2–4% • F > M	• Skin picking typically begins during adolescence, often coinciding with or following the onset of puberty • Chronic course	Genetics—excoriation disorder is more prevalent among individuals with OCD and their immediate family members compared to the general population	• OCD • Trichotillomania • Depression

*Indian data.

DISTINGUISHING FEATURES OF DIFFERENT ANXIETY DISORDERS[5,6]

Separation Anxiety Disorder

- Most common anxiety disorder in children <12 years of age.
- More common in childhood than preschool years or adolescence.
- Characterized by excessive inappropriate anxiety during real or imagined separation from parents or home.
- Worry that parents may be harmed or some unforeseen event may lead to separation from them.
- Refusal to go to school.
- Child may insist on sleeping with the primary attachment figure.
- Recurrent somatic symptoms like stomach-ache and headache are common that worsen at the time of going to school
- It should be distinguished from normal separation anxiety based on onset or increasing severity in school years, duration of symptoms, and degree of impairment.
- The symptoms should last at least 4 weeks, be impairing, and must be present before 18 years of age.

Specific Phobia

- Specific phobia is characterized by excessive and unreasonable fear on exposure to or anticipation of exposure to a specific object or situation.
- These objects or situations include animals, insects, blood, heights, or closed spaces, etc.
- Exposure to phobic stimuli may lead to a panic attack.
- Very young phobic children may cry a lot, scream, or avoid and seek comfort from parents on exposure to a specific situation or object.
- The symptoms should last at least 6 months and be associated with impairment.

Social Anxiety Disorder (Social Phobia)

- Specific fear of being scrutinized by people, especially unfamiliar ones, during social or performance situations.
- May be generalized in which an individual is anxious in different social situations or restricted to a specific situation like public speaking.
- Common fears include public speaking, participation in class, initiating conversations, attending social events and eating in front of others.
- Children with social phobia will appear extremely shy, blush a lot, and worry about doing or saying something wrong in public or peer group.
- Socially phobic children have test anxiety, avoid school or social settings, and have difficulty in making friends.
- The symptoms should last at least 6 months and be associated with impairment.

Panic Disorder

- Recurrent, unexpected, short lasting attacks of acute anxiety with feeling of impending doom.
- Commonly reported symptoms in panic disorder in children are tremors, dizziness, palpitation, nausea, breathlessness, and sweating.
- In the interval period, worry of another attack is present.
- In children, somatic symptoms are more prominent than cognitive symptoms.
- It is imperative to rule out physical conditions such as cardiac problems, hyperthyroidism, hyperparathyroidism, vestibular dysfunction, and seizure disorders.

Agoraphobia

- It involves fear and avoidance of several situations, commonly due to a fear of experiencing a panic attack in those situations.

- Common agoraphobic situations include places from which quick escape is difficult such as public transport, enclosed spaces cinemas, hairdressers, or heavy traffic.
- There is a common reliance on specific safety cues, commonly a safe attachment figure.

Generalized Anxiety Disorder

- Characterized by the presence of excessive worry that is difficult to control.
- Anxiety related to competence, approval, future events, and new or unfamiliar situations
- Frequently seek reassurance from others.
- Somatic symptoms, like headache, stomachache, muscle aches and pains, and sleeping difficulties are common.
- Inability to relax, irritability, and restlessness
- Appear overly sensitive and perfectionist, and have negative self-image.
- Often report first to pediatrician because of frequent somatic symptoms.
- Commonly associated with other disorders as well as childhood disorders (around 50%).
- It may lead to development of other anxiety disorders, substance abuse, depression or behavioral problems.

Selective Mutism

- Characterized by consistent failure to speak in specific social situations in which there is an expectation for speaking (e.g., at school) despite speaking in other situations.
- The disturbance is often marked by high social anxiety.
- Excessive shyness, fear of social embarrassment, social isolation and withdrawal, clinging, compulsive traits, negativism, temper tantrums, or mild oppositional behavior.
- It is important to establish that the inability to speak is not due to a lack of familiarity or proficiency with the necessary spoken language in the given social context.
- The symptoms should last at least 4 weeks and be associated with impairment.

Primary characteristics and associated features of obsessive-compulsive and related disorders are as follows:[5,15]

Obsessive-compulsive and related disorder:

- Characterized by the presence of obsessions and/or compulsion, pure obsessional illness is rare in children.
- Commonly reported obsessions are of contamination (most common), pathological doubts, aggression, symmetry, sex, religious, and somatic.
- Common compulsions reported are cleaning and washing, repeating, checking, ordering, counting, and hoarding.
- Insight and ego-dystonic nature of obsessions is not required to make diagnosis in children.
- Children are secretive and may not reveal their symptoms.
- May be brought for secondary problems such as temper tantrums, declining academic performance, depression, anxiety, changed eating pattern, etc.
- Comorbid psychiatric disorders are common in obsessive compulsive disorder (OCD) (in 50%)
- Common comorbid disorders are depressive disorders, other anxiety disorders, tic disorder, attention-deficit/hyperactivity disorder (ADHD), and disruptive behavior disorders.
- Symptoms fluctuate in severity with time and may increase during stress.
- Content and context of symptoms may also change with time.

Body dysmorphic disorder:

- Children with body dysmorphic disorder (BDD) are preoccupied by one or more perceived imperfections or flaws in their physical appearance which they perceive as ugly, unattractive, abnormal, or deformed.

- The perceived imperfections are either not observable or appear minor to others.
- Excessive repetitive behaviors or mental actions (such as constant comparing) are carried out in response to the preoccupation.

Hoarding disorder:

- The fundamental is the enduring struggle to discard or let go of possessions, irrespective of their actual worth.
- Indecisiveness, perfectionism, avoidance, procrastination, difficulty planning and organizing tasks, and distractibility

Trichotillomania (hair pulling disorder):

- Repetitive action of pulling out one's own hair
- The most common sites are the scalp, eyebrows, and eyelids.
- Hair pulling might be accompanied by various behaviors or rituals related to the hair (pulling specific texture/color hair and pulling hair in a specific way).
- Preceded or accompanied by various emotional states; it may be triggered by feelings of anxiety or boredom, may be preceded by an increasing sense of tension or may lead to gratification, pleasure, or a sense of relief when the hair is pulled out.

Excoriation (skin-picking disorder):

- Repeated picking at one's own skin.
- The most commonly picked sites are the face, arms, and hands.
- Skin picking might be accompanied by various behaviors or rituals related to the skin or scabs.

ASSESSMENT OF A CASE OF ANXIETY AND OBSESSIVE-COMPULSIVE AND RELATED DISORDER IN CHILDREN

- Any suspected case of anxiety and related disorders in children and adolescents should consist of detailed assessment using multiple informants such as parents, caregivers, teachers, friends, siblings and, other members of family.[6,17]
- Since anxiety can be developmentally appropriate, presence of anxiety is not sufficient to diagnose it as anxiety disorder. During assessment it becomes essential to differentiate this from pathological anxiety.
- Pathological anxiety presents as a pervasive and unrealistic anxiety and results in impairment of functioning. At times, even if anxiety is not causing any impairment, it should be treated if its causing significant distress to the patient.[18]
- Assessment for anxiety disorder should also be done in cases where somatic pains, crying spells, defiance behavior, argumentativeness, and disobedience of instructions have presented without other medical or psychiatric diagnosis.[6]
- Talking to children is essential in all cases. Initial interaction with a child having anxiety disorder should involve making the child comfortable and relaxed. After establishing rapport, detailed evaluation of the situations, thoughts or images that provoke anxiety should be asked for. Such questioning should be appropriate to the developmental level of the child. Particularly in cases of OCRD, children may not recognize the excessive nature of their thoughts or the unreasonable nature of compulsive behaviors.[19]
- Sometimes, anxious children may give socially desirable answers to "appear good", whereas anxious parents may exaggerate the symptoms in children. Children may also not recognize the excessive or unreasonable nature of their fear.[6]
- Due to high prevalence of comorbid conditions in children with anxiety disorder, each case should be evaluated for comorbid

conditions including other anxiety disorders, depression, OCRD, ADHD, and disruptive behavior disorders.[6,17]

- A broad assessment of various precipitating factors and maintaining factors is necessary to plan a psychological intervention in children. Focus on modifiable factors that maintain the illness, such factors can be parenting styles such as overprotection and intrusiveness, anxiety disorder in parents, troubled family environment, and cognitive biases and beliefs regarding threat and anxiety.[6]
- Specific assessments in cases of OCD should focus on assessing for level of insight, presence of sensory phenomenon, "getting it just right" feeling and comorbid conditions such as tic disorder, BDD, trichotillomania, and other anxiety disorders.[20,21]
- Evaluation of family should include assessing the dynamics with the patient, effect of symptoms on family and their understanding and response to anxious and compulsive behavior by the child, accommodation and proxy compulsions as these are more common in childhood onset OCD.[17,20]

Differential Diagnosis

- In few cases evaluation for a medical condition that may mimic anxiety disorders should be done. These include panic disorder where evaluation for cardiorespiratory condition should be considered as mentioned in **Table 1**.
- In cases of OCRD, infections involving respiratory or GI tract may present as "Pediatric Acute-onset Neuropsychiatric Syndrome (PANS)". This is particularly necessary as additional treatment with antibiotics improves response in such cases.[21]
- Drugs and medications can also cause anxiety like symptoms. Stimulants, sympathomimetics, steroids, caffeine and analogs, and thyroxine are such common medications. Intoxication with cannabinoids, withdrawal of alcohol, benzodiazepines and inhalants can produce anxiety as well.[17]
- Secondary anxiety symptoms are differentiated from primary anxiety disorder based on its characteristics as described in **Table 2**.
- Patients with suspected OCD must be assessed for subclinical phenomena that may be normal and not interfering with the functioning of the child. Also, anankastic personality traits

TABLE 2: Differentiating features of pathological anxiety disorder from developmental anxiety and secondary anxiety.[17,18]

Features	*Developmental anxiety*	*Pathological anxiety disorder*	*Secondary anxiety*
Physical symptoms	Less prominent	Present	More prominent than psychological symptoms
Psychological symptoms	Realistic and nonpervasive worrying	Pervasive and unrealistic worrying	Less common
Avoidance	Absent	Prominent	Absent
Presence of stressor	Absent	Present	Absent
Impairment	No impairment	Present	May be present
Response to medications	Poor	Good	Poor
Other features	Appropriate to age and environment	Somatic pains, argumentativeness, and disobedience may be seen	Presence of medical condition and substance use

TABLE 3: Rates of response with treatment in children and adolescents with social anxiety disorder (SAD), generalized anxiety disorder (GAD), and social phobia as found in the child–adolescent anxiety multimodal study.[26]

Modality of treatment	*Response rates (N = 488)*
Cognitive behavioral therapy only	60%
Sertraline only	55%
Combination	81%
Placebo	24%

may be present. Such children will have rigid routines, and need for orderliness that does not cause anxiety or subjective distress.[20]

ASSESSMENT SCALES

- Various instruments have been developed to diagnose anxiety disorders in children.
- The Multidimensional Anxiety Scale for Children (MASC) and Screen for Child Anxiety Related Emotional Disorders (SCARED) are the most commonly used screening tools.[17,22,23]
- Diagnostic schedules such as Kiddie Schedule for Affective Disorders and Schizophrenia—Present and Lifetime Version (KSADS-PL) is helpful for detailed evaluation but are time-consuming.[24]
- For OCRD, the Children's Yale–Brown Obsessive Compulsive Scale (CY–BOCS) is a widely used instrument.[25]

APPROACH TO TREATMENT

The primary goal of treatment should be functional recovery of child. Reduction in anxiety can come as a second goal. Comorbid conditions should be targeted from the beginning of treatment.

- Basic types of treatment include pharmacotherapy, psychotherapy, or a combination of these.
- For mild severity of disorder only psychological treatment is given. For moderate severity, treatment can be started with monotherapy with either psychological treatment or pharmacotherapy based on availability of resources and patient's choice. For severe disorder and partial responders to monotherapy, combined treatment is advised **(Table 3)**.

Psychological Treatments

When used as a single modality of intervention, psychological therapies have a higher rate of response compared to pharmacotherapy alone. For mild level of anxiety disorders, low-intensity intervention using psychoeducation material, self-help manuals with telephonic assistance or online therapy can be offered.[6] Majority of recommendations for therapy are based on evidence from adult population. Despite that the American Academy of Child and Adolescent Psychiatry recommends CBT for all patients with anxiety disorders aged 6–18 years. The general recommendations are mentioned in **Table 4**.

Cognitive behavioral therapy including exposure training remains the gold standard for treatment of childhood anxiety disorders and OCD. CBT is individualized as per patient, and their diagnosis and severity of disorder. The major components of CBT include psychoeducation, emotional awareness training, relaxation training, problem solving, cognitive restructuring, exposure training, and relapse prevention.

TABLE 4: Recommendations for psychological therapies based on various national and international guidelines.[6,27-29]

Disorder	*Recommended psychological therapies*	*Other therapies*
Separation anxiety disorder[30]	• Cognitive behavioral therapy (CBT) • Parental training	• Relaxation training • Contingency management
Selective mutism[17,31]	• Graded exposure therapy • Contingency management for speaking	CBT
Specific phobia[27]	Exposure training	• Systemic desensitization • Relaxation training • Applied tension (for blood/needle injury phobia)
Social anxiety disorder[17,27]	• Individual CBT • Exposure training	• Group CBT • Social skills training • Behavioral therapy
Panic disorder and agoraphobia[17,27]	• CBT • Exposure training	• Relaxation training • Supportive therapies
Generalized anxiety disorder[27]	CBT	• Relaxation training • Third-wave psychotherapies (Mindfulness based)
Obsessive compulsive disorder[28]	CBT with exposure and response prevention (ERP)	• Modeling • Relaxation training • Group CBT
Body dysmorphic disorder (BDD)[27,28]	CBT	
Trichotillomania[27,32]	Habit reversal therapy	• Dialectical behavioral therapy • Acceptance and commitment therapy
Excoriation disorder[27]	Habit reversal therapy	Acceptance and commitment therapy

Pharmacological Treatment

- Due to lack of resources for psychological treatments, pharmacotherapy remains first line in most cases in India. Pharmacological treatment cuts across the specific diagnosis of anxiety disorders and is majorly same even in OCRD except for a few additional drugs.
  - *Pharmacological considerations in prescribing in children:* Metabolic capacity and relative body fat are lower in children compared to adults. This results in accumulation of lipophilic medications and changes in pharmacokinetics. Metabolic activity of cytochrome enzymes also differs according to age and genetic variations.[33]
- Three major class of drugs are used in children [selective serotonin reuptake inhibitors (SSRIs), serotonin-norepinephrine reuptake inhibitors (SNRIs), and tricyclic antidepressants (TCAs)]. Similar drugs as used in adult patients are used for children. The Food and Drug Administration (FDA) approved drugs for anxiety disorder are given in **Table 5**.
- Duloxetine is the only FDA approved for GAD in children above 7 years, not all other drugs have been approved for pediatric anxiety

TABLE 5: Level of evidence for pharmacotherapy for anxiety disorders in children.[15,21,34,40]

Drugs	*Age group approved in*	*Initial dose*	*Target dose range*	*Strength of evidence*[a]
Fluoxetine	7–17	10 mg	10–80 mg/day	Level I
Escitalopram	12–17	5 mg	10–30 mg/day	Level I
Sertraline	6–17	25 mg	50–200 mg/day	Level I
Paroxetine	8–17	10 mg	10–60 mg/day	Level II
Fluvoxamine	7–17	25 mg	50–300 mg/day	Level II
Clomipramine	10–17	12.5 mg	50–200 mg/day	Level II
Duloxetine	7–17	30 mg	40–120 mg/day	Level V

[a]Level of recommendation by the American Academy of Child and Adolescent Psychiatry.

disorders. However, other SSRIs that are approved for depression and OCD in children are used and found to be effective for anxiety disorders in a number of trials.[34,35]

- Selective serotonin reuptake inhibitors show the highest effect size in terms of improvement in anxiety disorder when compared to other classes of medications in multiple meta-analyses.[36] Fluoxetine, sertraline, escitalopram, fluvoxamine, and paroxetine have been studied in children with anxiety disorders.
- Serotonin-norepinephrine reuptake inhibitors also reduce anxiety symptoms but the evidence is not consistent.[36] Venlafaxine and duloxetine have been tried for GAD and social anxiety disorder but their evidence is lesser than that of SSRIs.[33]
- Use of benzodiazepines although not approved can be done in severe cases. Clonazepam has been commonly used for this purpose. The use should be limited to not >8 weeks and only for severe anxiety symptoms due to concerns of dependence and other side effects.
- Other antianxiety drugs such as buspirone and β-blockers have little to no evidence for efficacy in children.[30,36]
- Clonidine can be used in children where there is an intense autonomic response with regular blood pressure monitoring.[15]

Dosing: When dosing SSRIs or TCAs in children, the general rule is to begin low and go slow with initial dose starting at half to one-fourth of adult dose and waiting for 2–4 weeks for response. The optimal duration of the SSRI trial in pediatric anxiety disorders is considered as 8 weeks.[26] In some cases, it may take up to 12–16 weeks of treatment to show response.[30,36]

Side effects: Common side effects of SSRIs in children include activation syndrome, drowsiness, abdominal discomfort, nausea, and headache.

- Activation side effects are more commonly seen with SSRIs than SNRIs. These constitute of hyperactivity, restlessness, disinhibition, impulsivity, insomnia, and irritability. One should lower the dose of AD drugs to manage it.[33]
- Rarely, patients may have hypomanic switch, increased suicidal ideations, apathy, or easy bleeding/bruising.[36,37] Educating about acute and self-resolving side effects is essential to improving adherence to treatment.
- In 2004, the FDA has given a black box warning for antidepressant use in children for the risk of increased suicidality.[34] However, recent meta-analyses have found no difference in suicidality among children receiving SSRIs.[38,39] It is still advisable to remain watchful for suicidality during the first month of treatment with antidepressants.

- Discontinuation symptoms are more common with SSRIs than SNRIs. Fluoxetine has the least overall discontinuation symptoms.

Duration of Treatment

In cases of anxiety disorder, such as separation anxiety disorder, it is recommended to continue pharmacotherapy for 6–9 months.[33] Some clinicians give SSRI treatment for at least 1 year after attaining remission,[6] following which joint decision to discontinue the drugs can be taken.

Discontinuation of Pharmacotherapy

Decision to discontinue pharmacotherapy should be taken in context of the patient's current psychosocial milieu. Discontinuation during vacation leaves, periods free from stress are preferred to reduce the risk of relapse.[33] Discontinuation should be slow and medications should be tapered over 4–8 weeks while remaining watchful of discontinuation symptoms or recurrent of illness.[37]

Risk of relapse remains high during the first 3 months of discontinuation during which, it is advisable to monitor for signs of relapse.[33]

MANAGEMENT OF TREATMENT-RESISTANT CASES

- All SSRIs are equally efficacious in anxiety disorders and OCD. Treatment resistance to one SSRI does not predict a resistance to another SSRI drug. Hence, after failure of one SSRI, one should consider using another SSRI drug. SNRIs have very limited evidence of efficacy in anxiety disorders. TCAs like clomipramine have high side-effect propensity and use of such drugs is reserved for cases where there is resistance to treatment with SSRIs.[30,36]
- Switching from one SSRI to another should not be delayed hoping for late response as most responders show signs of improvement within first 8 weeks.[33]

TABLE 6: Summary of recommendations for treatment of obsessive compulsive disorder (OCD).[15,21]

Type	*Recommendations*
Mild OCD	CBT
Moderate OCD	CBT or combination of CBT + SSRI
Severe OCD	CBT + SSRI
Remission	Maintenance of CBT or maintenance of SSRI for 12 months at same dose
Partial response	• Switch to another SSRI • Augment with CBT or atypical antipsychotic or clomipramine
Nonresponse	• Review diagnosis, comorbidities, compliance, and family accommodation • Switching to another SSRI • Augment with CBT or atypical antipsychotic or clomipramine • Clomipramine alone
Failure of two SSRIs	• Augmentation with CBT • Combination of SSRI + Clomipramine • Fluvoxamine + Clomipramine • Inpatient intensive CBT

(CBT: cognitive behavioral therapy; SSRIs: selective serotonin reuptake inhibitors)

In cases of OCD where partial response occurs, one can augment SSRI with use of low-dose atypical antipsychotics. Aripiprazole and risperidone are both effective and safe in children.[15,21] **Table 6** shows the recommendations for treatment of OCD in children and adolescents.

COURSE AND OUTCOME

Anxiety disorders and OCD in children and adolescents have a favorable outcome. Rates of response on different modalities of treatment found in the Child-adolescent Anxiety Multimodal Study (CAMS) are given in **Table 3**. These rates vary between 55 and 80%.[26] In studies done in India on pediatric anxiety disorder and OCD, significant improvement was reported at 12 weeks and by 24 weeks 58–65% of patients attained remission. The remission rates are lower for children with higher baseline severity of illness.[41,42] Social anxiety disorder had lesser rates of remission (51%) at 24 weeks.[42] Interestingly, the rates of remission did not differ among the modality of intervention given, i.e., groups receiving CBT, SSRIs and CBT + SSRIs had similar outcomes.[42] Longer follow-up periods of 3–4 years have shown recovery rates ranging from 80 to 96%, with lower rates seen in phobic and panic disorder (70%).[43,44] Specific subtypes of anxiety disorders also change as children age, with specific phobia being common in early childhood and GAD being the most common in adolescent age group.[45] Anxiety symptoms in early childhood do not predict anxiety later in life, but the presence of phobia and separation anxiety in middle childhood predicts increased risk of GAD in adolescence.[45] Adolescent anxiety disorders predict a two- to threefold increased risk of anxiety disorders, substance abuse, and suicide in adulthood.[44]

In children with OCD, subclinical or no symptoms at 3 months following treatment initiation has been reported in 54% of patients in an Indian study.[46] By the onset of adulthood, about 42% of adolescents attain remission of OCD.[47]

SUMMARY AND CONCLUSION

Anxiety disorders are one of the most common childhood onset psychiatric disorders which include separation anxiety, generalized anxiety, social anxiety, phobias, panic disorder, and selective mutism. The OCD is also common and its related conditions (including body dysmorphic disorder, hoarding disorder, trichotillomania and excoriation disorder) can be present in children. Diagnosing these disorders is difficult as anxiety also presents during the normal developmental period, and phenomenology in children is different from adults.

Children may present with irritability and argumentative behavior rather than anxiety and they may not recognize the excessive nature of their anxiety or irrational nature of their obsessions. Comorbidity is a rule rather than an exception in children and causes a significant impact on functioning and development of children. A detailed assessment focusing on ruling out medical conditions and substance abuse should be done. Assessment should include multiple sources including psychosocial factors. One must try to differentiate developmental anxiety, primary anxiety disorder, and secondary anxiety due to other causes.

Psychological intervention, particularly CBT, is the first line in all cases of anxiety disorders and OCD. Additional exposure training in phobias, ERP in OCD and habit reversal training in trichotillomania can be added to CBT.

Medications for anxiety disorders should be started in severe cases, when CBT is not feasible or when there is no response to it. SSRIs remain the first-line agents and benzodiazepines can be used for a short course. SNRIs and TCAs can be used with caution in treatment-resistant cases. For OCD, in cases of partial response SSRIs can be augmented with low dose of antipsychotics. Clomipramine is also effective in childhood-onset OCD.

REFERENCES

1. Beesdo K, Knappe S, Pine DS. Anxiety and Anxiety Disorders in Children and Adolescents: Developmental Issues and Implications for DSM-V. Psychiatr Clin North Am. 2009;32(3): 483-524.
2. Morris R, Kratochwill T. Childhood fears and phobias. In: Kratochwill T, Morris R (Eds). The Practice of Child Therapy, 2nd edition. United Kingdom: Pregamon Press; 1991. pp. 76-114.
3. Muris P, Merckelbach H, Mayer B, Meesters C. Common fears and their relationship to anxiety

disorders symptomatology in normal children. Personal Individ Differ. 1998;24(4):575-8.

4. Campbell MA, Rapee RM, Spence SH. Developmental changes in the interpretation of rating format on a questionnaire measure of worry. Clin Psychol. 2001;5(2):49-59.
5. American Psychiatric Association. (2013). Diagnostic and Statistical Manual of Mental Disorders: DSM-5, 5th edition. [online] Available from https://psychiatryonline.org/doi/book/10.1176/appi.books.9780890425596. [Last accessed 15 November, 2025].
6. Raphe RM. Anxiety disorders in Children and adolescents: Nature, development, treatment and prevention. In: Rey J (Ed). IACAPAP E-Textbook of Child and Adolescent Mental Health. Geneva, Switzerland: International Association for Child and Adolescent Psychiatry and Allied Professions; 2018.
7. Costello EJ, Mustillo S, Erkanli A, Keeler G, Angold A. Prevalence and Development of Psychiatric Disorders in Childhood and Adolescence. Arch Gen Psychiatry. 2003;60(8):837.
8. Warner EN, Ammerman RT, Glauser TA, Pestian JP, Agasthya G, Strawn JR. Developmental Epidemiology of Pediatric Anxiety Disorders. Child Adolesc Psychiatr Clin North Am. 2023; 32(3):511-30.
9. Yap MBH, Pilkington PD, Ryan SM, Jorm AF. Parental factors associated with depression and anxiety in young people: A systematic review and meta-analysis. J Affect Disord. 2014;156:8-23.
10. Kessler RC, Berglund P, Demler O, Jin R, Merikangas KR, Walters EE. Lifetime Prevalence and Age-of-Onset Distributions of DSM-IV Disorders in the National Comorbidity Survey Replication. Arch Gen Psychiatry. 2005;62(6): 593.
11. Becker ES, Rinck M, Türke V, Kause P, Goodwin R, Neumer S, et al. Epidemiology of specific phobia subtypes: Findings from the Dresden Mental Health Study. Eur Psychiatry. 2007;22(2): 69-74.
12. Beesdo K, Bittner A, Pine DS, Stein MB, Höfler M, Lieb R, et al. Incidence of Social Anxiety Disorder and the Consistent Risk for Secondary Depression in the First Three Decades of Life. Arch Gen Psychiatry. 2007;64(8):903.
13. Manjunatha N, Jayasankar P, Suhas S, Rao GN, Gopalkrishna G, Varghese M, et al. Prevalence and its correlates of anxiety disorders from India's National Mental Health Survey 2016. Indian J Psychiatry. 2022;64(2):138.
14. Srinath S, Girimaji SC, Gururaj G, Seshadri S, Subbakrishna DK, Bhola P, et al. Epidemiological study of child & adolescent psychiatric disorders in urban and rural areas of Bangalore, India. Indian J Med Res. 2005;122(1):67-79.
15. de Alvarenga PG, Mastrorosa RS, do Rosário MC. Obsessive Compulsive Disorder in Children and Adolescents. In: Rey J (Ed). IACAPAP E-Textbook of Child and Adolescent Mental Health. Geneva, Switzerland: International Association for Child and Adolescent Psychiatry and Allied Professions; 2012.
16. Nazeer A, Latif F, Mondal A, Azeem MW, Greydanus DE. Obsessive-compulsive disorder in children and adolescents: epidemiology, diagnosis and management. Transl Pediatr. 2020; 9(S1):S76-S93.
17. Taylor JH, Lebowitz ER, Silverman WK. Anxiety disorders. In: Martin A, Bloch MH, Volkmar FR (Eds). Lewis's Child and Adolescent Psychiatry: A Comprehensive Textbook, 5th edition. Gurugram: Wolters Kluwer India Pvt Ltd; 2018.
18. Pine DS, Klein RG. Anxiety disorders. In: Thapar A, Pine DS, Leckman JF, Scott S, Snowling MJ, Taylor E, eds. Rutter's Child Anad Adolescent Psychiatry, 6th edition. United States: John Wiley & Sons Ltd; 2015.
19. Srinath S, Jacob P, Sharma E, Gautam A. Clinical practice guidelines for assessment of children and adolescents. Indian J Psychiatry. 2019; 61(8):158.
20. Towbin KE, Riddle MA. Obsessive-Compulsive disorder. In: Martin A, Bloch MH, Volkmar FR (Eds). Lewis's Child and Adolescent Psychiatry: A Comprehensive Textbook, 5th edition. Gurugram: Wolters Kluwer India Pvt Ltd; 2018.
21. Avasthi A, Sharma A, Grover S. Clinical practice guidelines for the management of obsessive-compulsive disorder in children and adolescents. Indian J Psychiatry. 2019;61(8):306.
22. Birmaher B, Khetarpal S, Brent D, Cully M, Balach L, Kaufman J, et al. The Screen for Child Anxiety Related Emotional Disorders

(SCARED): Scale Construction and Psychometric Characteristics. J Am Acad Child Adolesc Psychiatry. 1997;36(4):545-53.

23. March JS, Parker JDA, Sullivan K, Stallings P, Conners CK. The Multidimensional Anxiety Scale for Children (MASC): Factor Structure, Reliability, and Validity. J Am Acad Child Adolesc Psychiatry. 1997;36(4):554-65.
24. Kaufman J, Birmaher B, Brent DA, Ryan ND, Rao U. K-SADS-PL. J Am Acad Child Adolesc Psychiatry. 2000;39:1208.
25. Scahill L, Riddle MA, McSwiggin-Hardin M, Ort SI, King RA, Goodman WK, et al. Children's Yale-Brown Obsessive Compulsive Scale: Reliability and Validity. J Am Acad Child Adolesc Psychiatry. 1997;36(6):844-52.
26. Piacentini J, Bennett S, Compton SN, Kendall PC, Birmaher B, Albano AM, et al. 24- and 36-Week Outcomes for the Child/Adolescent Anxiety Multimodal Study (CAMS). J Am Acad Child Adolesc Psychiatry. 2014;53(3):297-310.
27. Reddy YCJ, Sudhir PM, Manjula M, Arumugham SS, Narayanaswamy JC. Clinical Practice Guidelines for Cognitive-Behavioral Therapies in Anxiety Disorders and Obsessive-Compulsive and Related Disorders. Indian J Psychiatry. 2020; 62(8):230.
28. NICE. (2005). Obsessive-compulsive disorder and body dysmorphic disorder: treatment—clinical guidelines. [online] Available from https://www.nice.org.uk/guidance/cg31/resources/obsessivecompulsive-disorder-and-body-dysmorphic-disorder-treatment-pdf-975381519301 [Last accessed 15 November, 2025].
29. Walter HJ, Bukstein OG, Abright AR, Keable H, Ramtekkar U, Ripperger-Suhler J, et al. Clinical Practice Guideline for the Assessment and Treatment of Children and Adolescents With Anxiety Disorders. J Am Acad Child Adolesc Psychiatry. 2020;59(10):1107-24.
30. Figueroa A, Soutullo C, Ono Y, Saito K. Separation anxiety. In: Rey J (Ed). IACAPAP E-Textbook of Child and Adolescent Mental Health. Geneva, Switzerland: International Association for Child and Adolescent Psychiatry and Allied Professions; 2012.
31. Oerbeck B, Manassis K, Overgaard KR, Kristensen H. Selective Mutism. In: Rey J (Ed). IACAPAP E-Textbook of Child and Adolescent Mental Health. Geneva, Switzerland: International Association for Child and Adolescent Psychiatry and Allied Professions; 2019.
32. Towbin KE. Trichotillomania and Excoriation disorder. In: Martin A, Bloch MH, Volkmar FR (Eds). Lewis's Child and Adolescent Psychiatry: A Comprehensive Textbook, 5th edition. Gurugram: Wolters Kluwer India Pvt Ltd; 2018.
33. Strawn JR, Vaughn S, Ramsey LB. Pediatric Psychopharmacology for Depressive and Anxiety Disorders. FOCUS. 2022;20(2):184-90.
34. Patel DR, Feucht C, Brown K, Ramsay J. Pharmacological treatment of anxiety disorders in children and adolescents: a review for practitioners. Transl Pediatr. 2018;7(1):23-55.
35. Garakani A, Murrough JW, Freire RC, Thom RP, Larkin K, Buono FD, et al. Pharmacotherapy of Anxiety Disorders: Current and Emerging Treatment Options. Front Psychiatry. 2020;11: 595584.
36. Nicotra CM, Strawn JR. Advances in Pharmacotherapy for Pediatric Anxiety Disorders. Child Adolesc Psychiatr Clin N Am. 2023;32(3): 573-587. doi:10.1016/j.chc.2023.02.006
37. Ferguson JM. SSRI Antidepressant Medications: Adverse Effects and Tolerability. Prim Care Companion J Clin Psychiatry. 2001;3(01):22-7.
38. Strawn JR, Welge JA, Wehry AM, Keeshin B, Rynn MA. Efficacy and Tolerability of Antidepressants in Pediatric Anxiety Disorders: A Systematic Review and Meta-Analysis: Research Article: Pediatric Anxiety Meta-Analysis. Depress Anxiety. 2015;32(3):149-57.
39. Mills JA, Strawn JR. Antidepressant Tolerability in Pediatric Anxiety and Obsessive-Compulsive Disorders: A Bayesian Hierarchical Modeling Meta-analysis. J Am Acad Child Adolesc Psychiatry. 2020;59(11):1240-51.
40. Lorberg B, Davico C, Martsenkovskyi D, Vitiello B. Principles in using psychotropic medication in children and adolescents. In: Rey J (Ed). IACAPAP E-Textbook of Child and Adolescent Mental Health. Geneva, Switzerland: International Association for Child and Adolescent Psychiatry and Allied Professions; 2019.
41. Vitiello B. Searching for Moderators and Mediators of Pharmacological Treatment Effects in Children and Adolescents With Anxiety

Disorders. J Am Acad Child Adolesc Psychiatry. 2003;42(1):13-21.
42. Kandasamy P, Girimaji SC, Seshadri SP, Srinath S, Kommu JVS. Favourable short-term course and outcome of pediatric anxiety spectrum disorders: a prospective study from India. Child Adolesc Psychiatry Ment Health. 2019;13(1):11.
43. Last CG, Perrin S, Hersen M, Kazdin AE. A Prospective Study of Childhood Anxiety Disorders. J Am Acad Child Adolesc Psychiatry. 1996;35(11):1502-10.
44. Vallance AK, Fernandez V. Anxiety disorders in children and adolescents: aetiology, diagnosis and treatment. BJPsych Adv. 2016;22(5):335-44.
45. Steinsbekk S, Ranum B, Wichstrøm L. Prevalence and course of anxiety disorders and symptoms from preschool to adolescence: a 6-wave community study. J Child Psychol Psychiatry. 2022;63(5):527-34.
46. Deepthi K, Sagar Kommu J, Smitha M, Reddy YJ. Clinical profile and outcome in a large sample of children and adolescents with obsessive-compulsive disorder: A chart review from a tertiary care center in India. Indian J Psychiatry. 2018;60(2):205.
47. Palermo SD, Bloch MH, Craiglow B, Landeros-Weisenberger A, Dombrowski PA, Panza K, et al. Predictors of early adulthood quality of life in children with obsessive-compulsive disorder. Soc Psychiatry Psychiatr Epidemiol. 2011;46(4):291-7.

CHAPTER 17

Dissociative Disorder in Children and Adolescents

Rachna Bhargava, Bichitra Nanda Patra, Ummul Fatima

INTRODUCTION

"Dissociative disorder (DD)" is one of the most culturally nuanced psychological conditions with significant implications for its manifestation, etiology, and treatment. The expression of dissociative symptoms often varies across cultural contexts with phenomena such as possession states, trance experiences, or identity alterations being interpreted through culturally specific lenses. For instance, in Western contexts, they are more likely to be diagnosed as "dissociative identity disorder (DID)" or depersonalization whereas in many non-Western societies, dissociative experiences may be framed as spiritual possession or divine intervention (controlled by deity). Thus, dissociative convulsions are more commonly observed in India, whereas dissociative identity disorder and fugue are more frequently reported in Western countries.[1]

Dissociative disorders are characterized by a disruption of and/or discontinuity in the normal integration of consciousness, motor control, memory, perception, emotion, identity, body representation, and behavior (DSM-5). Although differences exist in the nomenclature and classification systems of the DSM-5[2] and ICD-11,[3] "dissociative neurological symptom disorder (DNSD)" is categorized as a distinct entity under DDs in the ICD-11, whereas in the DSM-5, the equivalent condition—functional neurological symptom disorder—is classified within the broader category of "somatic symptom" and related disorders. Throughout this paper, the term "dissociative disorder" will be used for the ease of understanding.

SYMPTOM MANIFESTATIONS AND PREVALENCE

In India, cases of DD are commonly encountered in psychiatric practice. Initially called as "hysteria", DD has been found to be prevalent in 31% of inpatients and 15% of outpatients within a predominantly postpubertal patient sample.[4,5] Considerable variability has been noted in the prevalence of DD among children and adolescents, ranging from as low as 0.5% to as high as 17%[6] globally. In clinical setting, dissociative motor disorder is the most common presentation seen in Indian children and adolescents followed by an approximately equal prevalence of dissociative convulsion in both in-patient and out-patient settings.[4] An Indian study reported that in children and adolescents, dissociative stupor (37.3%) was the most common type of presentation followed by dissociative convulsions (21.6%).[7] Young children having history of trauma may present with symptoms such as trans like states, perplexity, forgetfulness, and behavioral and emotional fluctuations. They may also present with regressive behavior. They may show disruptive behavior and flashes of anger that appear out of context to what is going on around them. Adolescents' symptom pattern becomes more like those of adults. The symptoms usually include frequency of self-destructive behavior, acting out and unstable relationships.[8]

Case vignette 1 is a typical illustration of how symptom-related distress can be deeply traumatizing for families, often leading to emergency presentations even when there is no actual threat to life.

CASE VIGNETTE 1

A 16-year-old girl was brought to an emergency department in an unresponsive state by her parents. On examination by the emergency team, no significant clinical findings were found on general and systemic examination though she would not respond when called or any instructions given, e.g., to show the tongue. Her pulse and blood pressure were within normal limits. The routine investigations, e.g., hemogram, liver and kidney function tests, serum electrolytes, and ECG were found to be within normal limit. Unresponsiveness lasted for 25 minutes after which she recovered fully. As per parents reporting, the child was having these symptoms since last 3 months with each episode of 15–20 minutes duration or till the family members sprinkled water over her face. After the spells, she would be completely aware about the surroundings immediately. During the spells, sometimes she would have involuntary movements, e.g., opisthotonus movement of whole body, forcibly closing her eyes associated with grunting sounds. She did not have any tongue bite/frothing from mouth/uprolling of eyeballs/urinary or fecal incontinence. And after exploring the semiology of her movements, she was discharged from emergency as she recovered in half an hour. The family was advised to come to "Neurology OPD" the next day. During neurology consultation, she was advised for CT scan of head and EEG. And these investigations came out to be within normal limits. Then, she was referred to "Psychiatry OPD".

In the detailed history examination by the Psychiatry team, it was clear that, during the spells of unresponsiveness, there was no loss of consciousness (LOC). The girl remained aware about the surroundings, though she did not speak or respond to her name when called. The history elicited that all previous episodes had occurred at home and in the presence of a family member. She had never been injured or had any fall due to her unresponsive spells. And it had never occurred during sleep.

Apparently, the episodes had an acute onset and a detailed history indicated a temporal association with declaration of examination results. Though she had passed but a gradual decline in the performance was evident. She was scolded by her father and often compared with her elder sister who was pursuing a professional course. She also had a younger brother who was pampered due to history of epileptic fits.

Since the onset of her illness, the patient received considerable attention from parents and was made to skip school. Since the course has been insidious and progressive, the parents had taken her to various doctors. However, the prescription of antiepileptic drugs by the local practitioner yielded no change in her frequency of episodes. The clinical interview with the patient suggested depressive features with disturbed sleep and appetite along with frequent arguments with sibling and mother.

The diagnosis of dissociative motor disorder along with depressive symptoms was made and seizure disorders was ruled out due to the following points in history and examinations:

- *No general tonic-clonic movement but opisthotonus movement of body not of any pattern indicative of seizure disorder*
- *No history of frothing/tongue bite/incontinence*
- *No postictal confusion*
- *Never had a fall/injury due to the involuntary spell*
- *CT scan of head and EEG investigations within normal limit*

TABLE 1: Points for differential diagnosis.

Conversion disorder: • Absence of tonic-clonic pattern of movement and, if present, the patient usually does not suffer from any injury • Seizure would usually occur in the presence of other family members • No tongue bite, frothing of mouth, urinary/fecal incontinence • Lack of occurrence during sleep • Awareness of the episode along with responsiveness during the episode • Absence of fall/injury due to fall • EEG/Video EEG confirmatory	*Seizure disorder:* • Frequent tongue bite, frothing of mouth, urinary/fecal incontinence • Lack of awareness and memory of episode • Nonresponsive to external stimulation • May occur during sleep • Frequent losing of balance/injury due to fall
Dissociative disorder: • Symptoms are not intentional in nature • The primary/secondary gains are neither intentional nor apparent to the patient	*Factitious disorder and malingering:* • Symptoms are intentionally produced to assume a sick role • There is psychological gain either by the patient or the caregiver • Malingering involves fabrication of symptoms to obtain an incentive, money, or some other material gain, or to avoid a disliked responsibility or punishment

The presentation of dissociative symptoms is often mistaken for physical illness, leading to misdiagnosis. However, mere exclusion of organic pathology does not necessarily indicate DD and needs a careful assessment of the situational context and close observation during the clinical interview for accurate differentiation.[9] **Table 1** provides some points in ruling in/out the differential diagnoses.

Though the DD symptoms can be a part of other psychiatric disorders, e.g., anxiety disorder or depressive disorder, a comorbid diagnosis may be made if the signs/symptoms warrants. Many times, the child may have both: Epileptic fits along with pseudo seizures leading to diagnostic confusion for psychiatrist as well as neurologist. For example, in *Case vignette 2*, the girl had past history of epileptic fits but for the presenting symptoms, diagnosis of DD was made as there were no significant clinical indications on MRI or CT scan along with absence of any significant evidence for risk of injury to self. The detailed historical presentation of symptoms was atypical and could not be explained organically.

CASE VIGNETTE 2

A 15-year-old girl belonging to an upper middle status who apparently suffered a paralytic attack and lost the ability to walk and speech was brought in emergency. She was conscious but could produce meaningless sounds only. She was eventually admitted in neurology department and was examined by neurologists and later by psychiatrists. There was a history of two episodes of seizures in early childhood that had been adequately treated and had remained asymptomatic over the last 12 years. Except for mild abnormality in EEG, there were no other significant findings on CT or MRI. After several consultations by psychiatrists and discussions with neurologists, the case was referred for psychological evaluation, but a consensus could not be reached even after 3 months as the child could not speak or walk.

Based on several family and individual sessions with each family member, diagnosis of DD was made. Apparently, initially the child started showing aversion to having any interaction with father and would refuse to talk to father. Gradually, the girl started avoiding social interactions where father would be present like family meals or social functions, etc. before she exhibited having seizures lasting for 2–3 days during which she could not walk or talk. The episodes were progressive and increased in frequency to 1–2 times per month and the girl had not been going to school for over 8 months.

The patient was seen at outpatient level and initially any attempt to have direct conversation were unsuccessful. The direct enquiry about stressors was stopped and frequent sessions were aimed in building rapport by exploring patients' interest and past achievements. She was continued on antidepressants and the effort was made to initiate activities, decrease solo meals, increase frequency of food (patient had lost significant weight in the past 1 year), and exposure to outdoor activities. A study routine was developed eventually which was gradually increased in time with the help of home tutors. Every activity was introduced with the concurrence of patient and minute details were discussed with the parents to avoid any possibility of triggers.

Separate sessions with each parent gave an insight to not only family relationships but also helped in building empathetic relationship with mother who would usually accompany the patient.

The parents were psychoeducated regarding the nature of illness that also ensured treatment adherence and lowered the expectation of the family for immediate positive outcome. The fact that psychotherapy was the only mode of treatment took several sessions for acceptance even though the family was educated and had already consulted several hospitals and health professionals (medicine, pediatrician, neurologist, and psychiatrist).

In absence of any apparent stressor that could have been elicited through interviews, projective tests (TAT, Draw a Person Test and Sentence Completion Test) were applied on the patient once she became cooperative and had regained hand movements and speech. The findings across tests showed that the patient had fear of losing father due to his relationships outside marriage besides having difficulty in coping with academic pressure. Based on the findings, the sessions with mother were held and patient was encouraged to ventilate. The component of confidentiality was reiterated with mother as well along with the emphasis on the need to resolve relationship issues as they have induced stress and conflict in the children. The mother who was already stressed due to spouse extramarital relationship became proactive in bringing harmonious atmosphere at home and the father was provided a platform for reflecting upon his actions and its impact on children well-being, mental health, and values they are imbibing in their growing up process.

ETIOLOGY AND CULTURE

The etiology of DDs is also deeply embedded in cultural narratives around trauma, identity, and social norms. Cultural context shapes not only how these disorders develop but also how they are understood and addressed within a given society. While dissociation is often rooted in exposure to overwhelming stress or trauma—particularly during early developmental stages—the way such trauma is experienced, interpreted, and processed is deeply mediated by cultural norms and values. In cultures where open discussion of trauma or emotional distress is discouraged, individuals may unconsciously channel their psychological pain into dissociative symptoms, which are more socially or spiritually acceptable. However, in many cultures, physical symptoms are considered more acceptable as an expression of distress, while psychological symptoms may be stigmatized. Additionally, psychological distress is often dismissed or misunderstood due to poor awareness, or psychological help may be unavailable. Hence, distress may seek forcible expression through physical symptoms perceived as deserving attention and assistance.[10]

Dissociative disorders do not emerge in isolation; rather, they reflect a dynamic interaction between brain functioning, temperamental styles, personality, stressors, and life experiences impacting the processing of emotions, cognition, and memory.[11] All biopsychosocial factors converge to determine the trajectory of DD. Factors unique to certain cultures, such as patriarchal or hierarchical social order, low literacy levels, and lack of empowerment, may make certain demographic groups (e.g., rural populations, underprivileged castes/sections, and women) more vulnerable to DDs.[12]

Girls are twice more likely to have DD than boys, this can be attributed to the culture of discrimination in India and the consequent experience of loss of control. The Indian landscape of power dynamic, patriarchy, educational disparity, and autonomy constraints exposes adolescent girls to a range of chronic stressors such as hindrances to opportunities, excessive criticism, being mocked for gender-related concerns and emotional concerns related to gender disparity.[13] Given the anticipated negative consequences of openly expressing emotional distress, many girls suppress their feelings, leading to the somatic manifestation of psychological distress as a socially and culturally sanctioned outlet.[10,14]

There is substantial evidence to support that up to 80% of the participants report traumatic events, with emotional and physical abuse being very common among children and adolescents. Harassing experience of sexual nature is frequently reported by adolescents who are currently experiencing symptoms of DD.[15] Exposure to adult sexual activity, even indirectly, can be profoundly disturbing for young children, potentially resulting in deep-seated psychological conflict and developmental disruptions as observed in *Case vignette 2*. Responses to traumatic experiences can range from mild detachment to severe disconnection from physical and emotional experiences and may be either transient or chronic in nature.

While one perspective emphasizes the strong association between adverse life events or trauma and dissociation, another highlights the roles of modeling, media influence, and suggestibility in the development of dissociative symptoms.[16] Children and adolescents with dissociative symptoms are often highly suggestible and prone to fantasy, making them more likely to imitate symptoms they have observed in mothers. For instance, a child may replicate a relative's paralysis when confronted with stressors, as a means of coping. Thus, understanding beliefs and family dynamics are important in identifying the processes involved in symptom manifestation. Family issues such as parental discord, sibling rivalry, and punitive parenting have been particularly documented in the Indian context as significant contributors to the development of DDs.[17]

Some of the common psychosocial factors have been listed in **Table 2**.

MANAGEMENT

The treatment of DD is as complex and multifaceted as the condition itself. Given the functional nature of the symptoms, the primary mode of treatment is typically nonpharmacological. A significant challenge in treating children with DD is the tendency for frequent doctor changes or "doctor shopping" by parents when immediate

TABLE 2: Common psychosocial factors.

Intrafamilial factors	*Extrafamilial factors*
Punitive parenting	Academic struggles (examination stress and pressure)
Family disharmony	Culture of discrimination
Financial difficulties	Irregular attendance
Parental marital discord	Peer conflicts/pressure
Violence between parent	Suggestibility
Sibling rivalry	Abuse (emotional, physical, and sexual)
Familial emotional over-involvement	Adverse/Traumatic experience
Emotional neglect	Bullying
Poor communication and criticism	Chronic illness

Note: A single case may have one or more risk factors/stressors; same risk factors may lead to completely different symptom presentation based on the unique psychosocial history of the patient.

improvement is not observed. To build the family's confidence in the treatment process and improve adherence, it becomes crucial to prioritize socio-occupational functioning—such as attending school and participating in household chores—over directly addressing dissociative symptoms, which may take longer to resolve.

Pharmacotherapy

Most medications (e.g., antidepressants and anxiolytics) are prescribed for comorbid anxiety and mood symptoms, but these medications do not specifically treat the dissociation. Atypical antipsychotics may be used for mood stabilization, overwhelming anxiety, and intrusive post-traumatic stress disorder (PTSD) symptoms in patients with DD. Other possible suggestions for pharmacological interventions for symptomatic management in DD include the use of prazosin in reducing nightmares, carbamazepine to reduce aggression, and naltrexone for amelioration of recurrent self-injurious behaviors.[18] Paroxetine and naloxone are the only pharmacological agents studied through randomized controlled trials (RCTs) and found to have modest evidence for controlling depersonalization symptoms and dissociative symptoms that are comorbid with PTSD and borderline personality disorder (BPD) though these findings should be interpreted with caution in view of high heterogeneity and scanty literature on RCTs on various subtypes of DD.[19]

Nonpharmacological Interventions

Dissociative symptoms are frequently linked to traumatic experiences, and evidence suggests that early intervention leads to better prognosis. However, there is a dearth of research on the treatment of DD in children and adolescents. Psychotherapy is the most recommended treatment modality, though there is no standardized framework.[20] The symptoms of DD often take a long time to resolve with treatment typically requiring twice-weekly sessions over a course of several years. However, in low-resource settings like India, this approach may not always be feasible. Therefore, a more pragmatic and adaptable treatment model is necessary to address DD within India's unique cultural landscape. To foster a strong therapeutic alliance while considering practical constraints, initial sessions—including assessment and psychoeducation—could be scheduled biweekly when possible, with session frequency gradually adjusted based on individual needs and contextual challenges.

THERAPEUTIC PROCESS

The psychotherapy process may usually be divided into initial phase, middle phase, and termination phase.

Initial Phase

In the initial phase, orientation to psychotherapy sessions vis-à-vis frequency and duration of sessions is given to the patient and the family members along with the psychoeducation regarding the psychogenic nature. The empathic relationships along with awareness about illness are the hallmark features that gradually help in building confidence and adherence to learning adaptive skills.

Therapeutic Alliance

As with any psychological disorder, the initial phase of therapy for DD in children and adolescents primarily centers on establishing a strong therapeutic alliance. This foundational step not only fosters trust but also enables the clinician to elicit a comprehensive understanding of the child's psychosocial environment and lived experiences, thereby unraveling the "why," "when," and "how" of the illness. Patient ratings of the therapeutic alliance have been shown to improve symptoms, support recovery, and predict better outcomes for patients with DD. Secure attachment with a therapist within an egalitarian relationship creates a safe and interpersonal space. This approach facilitates the child's acceptance of and adherence to follow-up and treatment strategies. For example, in the scenario of *Case vignette 2*, although the family was initially unaware of the underlying cause of the dissociative symptoms and there was no noticeable improvement, meaningful progress began only after a therapeutic alliance was established between the patient and the therapist. This relationship formed the foundation for the child's compliance with recommended behavioral changes, such as adjustments in daily routine.

In this context, emotional expression is neither condemned nor punished, but rather encouraged as an adaptive way of experiencing and expressing distress, this proves to be greatly therapeutic aiding both greater understanding and acceptance of the pathology as well as recovery from it.[21] Children and adolescents with DD have high suggestibility which can be used by therapist to induce adaptive responses (like attending school) instead of dissociative ones in the face of stressor/crisis. A strong therapeutic bond aids the process of suggestibility-induced functional behavior. In the Indian context, the *guru-chela* relationship serves as a foundational model for the therapeutic alliance, where the therapist assumes a higher-status, authoritative role while employing directive techniques.[22] This hierarchical dynamic aligns in therapy with Indian parenting practice and social structures, fostering adherence and compliance with prescribed psychotherapeutic interventions, thereby enhancing treatment effectiveness. Thus, it may become easier for the therapist to negotiate changes in parenting styles or initiating regularity in study timings.

Assessment

Once the nonorganic nature of underlying symptoms is confirmed by investigations or the physician, both psychiatric evaluation and structured assessments along with behavioral observation play a crucial role in making diagnosis of dissociation. Since the majority of referrals for DD originate from neurologists or medical doctors, it is essential to conduct a thorough evaluation of the child's medical history. This includes assessing the number of medical professionals the child has consulted, the duration and nature of prior neurological or medical assessments/ treatments, and the specific reasons that led to the referral to a mental health facility. Additionally, it is crucial to evaluate the extent to which both the child and their parents understand the psychogenic basis of the condition, as this knowledge can significantly influence engagement with psychological interventions and overall treatment outcomes.

The very essence of DD lies in the inaccessibility of stressors and distress at the conscious level, making assessment the key to identifying and addressing its underlying pathology. Few of the objective tests that can be used in assessment are—"16 Personality Factor (16PF), Child Behavior Checklist (CBCL), Family Assessment Device (FAD) and tests of Attachment such as MacArthur story stem battery (MSSB) or Attachment Story Completion Task (ASCT)." These tests may help clinicians to evaluate aspects of temperament, personality factors, attachment style, family functioning, and life stressors that are uniquely contributing to the development of the disorder. However, as a child's distress is often concealed behind the "smokescreen" of symptoms, projective or unstructured tests—such as the "Children's Apperception Test (CAT), Sentence Completion Test (SCT), Rorschach Inkblot Test (RIBT), and Raven's Controlled Projection Test (RCPT)"—can be more effective in uncovering core conflicts or hidden distress.

Following a thorough assessment and the confirmation of a diagnosis, one of the primary challenges encountered is the acceptance of its psychogenic, rather than neurological, origin—both by the child and their caregivers. The deeply ingrained stigma surrounding mental illness, coupled with a limited awareness of how neurological-appearing symptoms may lack identifiable organic pathology, often leads to skepticism and resistance. This stage is particularly fraught in families from lower socioeconomic backgrounds, where financial constraints and psychosocial stressors amplify frustration. In such contexts, there is an increased likelihood of parental hostility, blame, or accusations of symptom fabrication directed at the child. Consequently, the therapeutic alliance is at its most fragile, and treatment adherence may be compromised.

Confidentiality and Psychoeducation

To navigate this delicate juncture, a skilled therapist must tailor psychoeducation to the caregivers' level of education and psychological mindedness, presenting the disorder in a manner that is neither confrontational nor attributive of fault—whether to the child or the parents. Instead, the explanation should frame the illness as an attempt to adapt and cope with unique psychosocial, academic, or financial stressors. This is particularly challenging while dealing with families belonging to lower socioeconomic strata who usually expect pharmacotherapy and exhibit resistance to the idea of "psychological" origin of the "disease". In some cases, multivitamins are prescribed as a placebo to help to maintain family engagement in therapy though there is not much evidence for the same. Alternatively, a contract for a specific period for follow-up with carefully selected reinforcers may help in case verbal explanations may fail to convince parents.

A significant challenge in working with children and adolescents is navigating the ethical dilemma of maintaining confidentiality amidst parental pressure. In India, this challenge is particularly pronounced, as parents typically accompany the child, cover the session costs, and often expect full disclosure from the therapist. They may perceive it as the therapist's duty to share details of the sessions with them.[23] To address this, it is crucial to establish clear boundaries from the outset. The therapist should explicitly communicate—in the presence of both the child and the parents—that discussions within the therapeutic space will remain confidential and will not be disclosed without the child's consent (except in cases of risk to safety). Reinforcing this principle not only upholds ethical practice but also fosters a sense of trust and security, particularly for adolescents. When assured of confidentiality, they are more likely to engage openly, facilitating a more effective therapeutic process.

Goal Setting

Given the constraints of a low-resource setting like India, where long-term therapy may feel overwhelming for families and logistically unfeasible due to time and financial limitations, the treatment plan should be concise and structured. By streamlining treatment and focusing on practical, achievable goals, therapists can enhance engagement and improve outcomes within the available resources. Using contingency management techniques, short-term and long-term goals may be decided with the family. Thus, rather than the symptom removal, emphasis on social-occupational dysfunction as the immediate goal helps in inducing a feeling of improvement. This may also indirectly address underlying concerns perceived by the child or parents, even if these are not explicitly verbalized during therapy. For example, school absenteeism in an adolescent girl with borderline intelligence and partial paralysis (dissociative symptom) may actually be providing secondary gains, helping her escape from academic stress. Thus, a short-term immediate goal of regularity in school (this includes telephonic communication with school authorities regarding the nature of illness and need for regularity) along with planning of individual coaching would help in not only eliminating secondary gains but also would ensure positive coping with academic stress.

The egalitarian approach to goal-setting, often emphasized in Western therapeutic frameworks, may not apply as neatly in the Indian context, particularly in low-resource settings where the traditional *guru-chela* dynamic remains deeply ingrained. This inherently hierarchical socialization positions the therapist as an authoritative guide, setting goals for the child rather than collaboratively with them. Such an approach aligns with cultural norms and allows the therapist to exert greater influence over the child's progress and symptom resolution. Within this framework, the therapist (*guru*—teacher) assumes the role of a mentor, guiding the child (*chela*—disciple) toward psychological transformation in a relationship rooted in respect, trust, and deference to expertise.

However, when working with adolescents, a shift toward collaborative goal-setting is essential to accommodate their growing need for autonomy and independence. In such cases, fostering a sense of agency can enhance engagement and treatment adherence. Regardless of the therapeutic approach, it is crucial for the therapist to clearly define the nature of the therapeutic relationship, outlining role expectations and establishing firm boundaries. This includes introducing key psychotherapy concepts (confidentiality and nonjudgmental approach), emphasizing structured goal-setting, fostering realistic expectations, and framing therapy as an ongoing process rather than a quick-fix solution.

Middle Phase

During the middle phase of therapy, psychological strategies aim to reduce symptom intensity, alleviate distress, improve functionality, and address the underlying causes of dissociation. Effective treatment of DDs should follow a structured, phased approach—starting with symptom stabilization, addressing acute family crises, engaging the patient in individual psychotherapy, and ultimately incorporating family-based interventions.[5]

Behavior Therapy Techniques

Behavioral therapy techniques such as differential reinforcement, activity scheduling, relaxation, distraction, and environmental manipulation play a crucial role in reducing symptom frequency and enhancing functionality. One key approach used is *"Differential Reinforcement of Other Behavior (DRO)"* in which adaptive behavior (such as engaging in conversation with the therapist, painting, coloring, or playing with toys) is rewarded (attention) and maladaptive behaviors (dissociative episodes) are systematically ignored or not reinforced with active attention. The core principle of DRO is that by consistently rewarding the absence of maladaptive behavior, adaptive responses become more likely over time. Reinforcers used by parents should primarily be social, such as family outings and increased attention, rather than material rewards such as money, gifts, or new toys. Relying on material reinforcers is neither sustainable nor effective, as their impact diminishes over time, often requiring escalation to maintain the same effect. In *Case vignette 3*, DRO was implemented by instructing the father to withhold attention when the child exhibited dissociative symptoms or adopted a sick role, while the family was encouraged to offer praise and warmth when the child engaged in appropriate behaviors, such as attending school.

CASE VIGNETTE 3

Master C, a 10-year-old boy, presented to the OPD with a 2-year history of episodic hyperventilation followed by loss of consciousness (LOC). He was the second-born child of a nonconsanguineous union. His symptoms began soon after the family transitioned from a joint to a nuclear living arrangement due to his father's transfer to a new army base, which required the father to live separately. Initially, the episodes were characterized by brief hyperventilation lasting approximately 1 minute, followed by LOC. During these episodes, he remained partially responsive to verbal stimuli with no history of urinary or fecal incontinence, tongue biting, or injury. As the frequency of these episodes increased, concerns grew about his ability to cope in a school environment. The school eventually limited his attendance to examinations, citing a lack of resources to manage his condition. In response, his parents significantly reduced academic expectations, hoping to alleviate any potential stressors, but his symptoms persisted. Initial structured assessments and interviews did not reveal any overt psychological distress or identifiable external stressors. However, a deeper exploration using the "Children's Apperception Test (CAT)" uncovered recurring themes of abandonment and familial vulnerability in the father's absence. This suggested that his symptoms might serve a dual purpose—first, as an unconscious attempt to bring his father into closer physical proximity, and second, as a means of securing secondary gains, such as exemption from schoolwork and academic pressures.

With Master C, the therapist adopted a structured approach by sitting with him as he completed his school-related work while engaging him in conversations about his day, his friends, and anything that would interest him. However, whenever he began to hyperventilate, the therapist would calmly shift focus back to her own work instead of reinforcing the symptom with immediate attention. Over time, it was observed that during his interactions with the therapist, Master C became increasingly engaged in constructive activities such as completing classwork, painting along with the therapist, discussing his day, etc. As a result, both the intensity and frequency of his episodes significantly diminished. Alongside individual therapy, the father, who was in inpatient care with the child, was provided with psychoeducation on the importance of getting the child back to regular schooling and maintaining academic expectations independent of his symptom trajectory. He was guided to avoid inadvertently reinforcing the episodes with excessive attention and was specifically advised against immediately taking leave to visit the child whenever symptoms appeared to worsen, as this could unintentionally serve as a secondary gain. The unconscious nature of these gains was emphasized to reduce any tendencies toward blame or criticism. He was also encouraged to provide warmth and support contingently—recognizing and reinforcing positive behaviors such as engaging in schoolwork and hobbies, socializing with peers and openly communicating with family. This approach aimed to gradually reduce symptom-related primary and secondary gains.

To further enhance adaptive behavior, *activity scheduling* helps both the child and parents to be more goal directed in their approach. DD often leads to school refusal, academic decline, social isolation, and reduced extracurricular involvement. A therapist can aim to boost functionality by developing a structured timetable that includes a balance of mastery-oriented activities (such as studying and completing school tasks) and pleasurable activities (such as hobbies, socializing, and spending time with family). Breaking the syllabus into manageable chunks and scheduling regular breaks can help to alleviate academic pressure, while engaging in enjoyable activities promotes a sense of normalcy and control. A structured activity schedule, collaboratively designed with the child or adolescent can reinforce engagement in activities of daily life. This schedule should outline expected activities throughout the week, with specific reinforcements for successful completion. As the child becomes more engaged in this routine, stressors like parental expectations or pressures often diminish, thus activity scheduling have twofold benefit of not only maintaining adaptive behavior but also reduce risk factors associated with DD as mentioned above. It can be seen that activity scheduling was used in all the illustrated cases.

In addition, teaching *relaxation techniques* such as paced breathing, diaphragmatic breathing, and progressive muscle relaxation as well as *distraction techniques* such as counting backward, talking to a friend, listening to music, watching a movie or playing engaging games can help the child to manage overwhelming emotions. These methods reduce physiological arousal associated with stress and anxiety, allowing children and adolescents to better cope with emotional challenges.

Behavior therapy including *environmental manipulation* is highly effective for very young children or those with alexithymia who struggle to express their emotions. The therapeutic focus often shifts toward modifying the child's environment—through improved parenting practices, shared family activities such as meals, and engagement in extracurricular pursuits—to reinforce positive coping behaviors, rather than directly targeting the child's symptoms. These strategies help to create a supportive environment, fostering emotional growth and symptom improvement.

Cognitive Behavioral Therapy

Adolescents, with their developing cognitive capacities and ability of abstraction, can benefit from techniques such as cognitive restructuring and visualization to challenge biases and distortions related to stressors and their impact on well-being. This is especially true for adolescents from upper socioeconomic status who in our clinical practice have been observed to be highly creative and expressive.

Problem-solving therapy (PST) is a crucial cognitive behavioral therapy (CBT) intervention that helps children systematically to identify problems, evaluate potential solutions, select the most effective option, and implement it. This process can be practiced during therapy sessions using both hypothetical scenarios and real-life challenges, such as peer pressure, bullying or academic difficulties. By actively engaging in structured problem-solving, children develop essential skills to navigate stressors more effectively and reduce reliance on maladaptive coping strategies.

Family-based Interventions

It is essential to recognize cultural differences between India and Western nations, where the CBT was developed. While CBT traditionally limits family involvement to psychoeducation, this approach may not be suitable in India, where family is integral to child and adolescent's sense of self. Therefore, family involvement play an active role in managing dissociative symptoms.

Parents are trained in differential reinforcement and extinction techniques to maintain consistency in reinforcing adaptive behaviors. However, many hesitate to withhold attention during episodes due to safety concerns. To address this, psychoeducation helps them to understand how primary and secondary gains sustain dissociative behaviors. Parents are also guided on ensuring the child's safety while gradually reducing reinforcement of symptoms, fostering a sense of control in the child.

Family communication is also a key focus in therapy. Critical comments, passive-aggressive interactions, rigid rules, and unjustified punishments can significantly strain the parent–child relationship, exacerbating symptoms. Therapy should help parents to improve communication—not only with their children but also with each other—by setting clear expectations, expressing emotional support, and managing conflicts constructively. With adolescents, therapy emphasizes boundary-setting that respects their need for autonomy and parents can be encouraged to create spaces where the adolescent can openly express their concerns, talk about their day and share quality family time, while with younger children, parents are trained to model healthy emotional expression and regulation to reduce reliance on dissociation as a coping mechanism. The impact of parenting styles on the child's difficulties should be explored in depth.

If parental discord is present, it should be prioritized with discussions on its role in triggering or maintaining the child's symptoms. In *Case vignette 1*, individual sessions with each of the parents were required to address extramarital issues and to resolve couple conflict. Family sessions were also conducted to demonstrate the faulty communication patterns and to make the father understand the difference between parent-child interaction and parent-adult interaction.

Another key modification in the Indian context is the nature of core beliefs, which often take spiritual forms (e.g., "God is unhappy with me," and "God will not save me") or value-based forms (e.g., "I am not valuable to my family," "I am not honest or sincere" and "My relatives think I am bad"). Cognitive restructuring should therefore be adapted to reflect these cultural nuances. In *Case vignette 1*, the mother developed internal acceptance of her spouse's past behavior and became more optimistic, attributing this change to her strengthened faith in "God's decisions."

Enhancing Coping Skills

Dissociative disorder usually emerge as means to cope with everyday challenges that the child perceives to be stressful. Hence, teaching children and adolescents age-appropriate skills to manage common stressors such as academic demands, societal expectations, sibling rivalry, and parental criticism in an effort to build psychological resilience and reduce relapse. By equipping them with effective coping mechanisms, therapy aims to decrease reliance on dissociation as a primary means of regulating distressing emotional experiences. A key aspect of this process is teaching both problem-focused and emotion-focused coping, including their relevance, appropriate contexts for use and specific techniques involved. In *Case vignette 1*, after strong therapeutic alliance was formed and the patient had become verbose in sessions, cognitive restructuring was used to make the patient understand the link between stress/symptoms and coping style and ways of developing alternate ways for resolving the problem whereas in *Case vignette 4*, the patient had low creativity, and thus patient had to be given precise suggestions so as to enable her to adopt positive coping style.

Working with Underlying Conflicts

Given that chronic or severe traumatic experiences—such as sexual or physical abuse, neglect, violence, loss, and prolonged stress—significantly increase the risk of developing DD,[24,25] effective treatment requires a thorough assessment of these stressors to guide intervention. Children and adolescents often rely on avoidance-based coping mechanisms in response to emotionally intense situations which initiate the development of dissociative episodes. Therapists can utilize structured interventions such as picture books and storytelling to help children process traumatic experiences in a nonthreatening manner. These methods allow for gradual exposure while ensuring that the therapeutic environment remains safe and supportive for steady development of adaptive coping mechanisms. With young children, playing with dolls or coloring can be most effective in gradual articulation of distress, *for instance, colors can be incorporated to symbolize emotions such as blue color can be used to symbolize shame, red can be used to show anger or yellow to show tension and a narrative can be crafted using different colors.*

This method provides a structured yet gentle approach for the child to explore their internal experiences while mitigating emotional overwhelm and reducing the likelihood of avoidance through dissociative symptoms. However, any disclosure of sexual or physical abuse during sessions must be taken seriously and reported to the appropriate authorities in accordance with the POSCO Act (2012). It is equally important for the therapist to reflect on their own curiosity about the traumatic events, as excessive inquiry can sometimes hinder recovery. Trauma disclosure should only be encouraged when the therapist feels competent to handle the socioemotional consequences of such revelations. The therapist's primary goal in such a situation is to provide psychoeducation on the effects of trauma, ensure the child's safety, and build essential coping skills to manage the aftermath of such experiences. Incorporating trauma exposure through storytelling or creative arts can further enhance the child's sense of mastery.[26]

CASE VIGNETTE 4

Miss D, a 17-year-old female, presented with symptoms of regressive behavior, including thumb-sucking, speaking in a child-like manner, biting her mother, seeking constant reassurance, and frequently throwing temper tantrums when her demands were not met. Additionally, she experienced fainting spells that were abrupt in onset and continuous in course. Premorbidly, D was functionally well, studying in a boarding school with an average academic performance and no prior decline.

One week before her examinations, she lost consciousness at school and was hospitalized. Despite multiple episodes of loss of consciousness (LOC), her CT scan, MRI, and blood reports indicated normal physiological functioning. Upon referral to a psychiatrist and subsequent evaluation by a clinical psychologist, a diagnosis of "Functional Neurological Disorder" was made, given the absence of clear organic markers.

Detailed assessments provided insight related to how staying away from home and a perceived lack of parental response contributed to feelings of abandonment and insecurity. Her parents, preoccupied with caring for her ailing grandparents, had unknowingly neglected her emotional needs. We also gathered information relating to the patriarchal family structure where the father and brother held dominant roles, while D and her mother occupied subordinate positions. Her brother often assumed an authoritarian, pseudo-father role, which D resented, leading to a push-and-pull struggle for autonomy. By the time she met the therapist, she had been out of school for 3 months, disengaged from studies and sleeping excessively (13–15 hours a day).

Therapeutic intervention initially focused on building rapport and enhancing motivation. Given her love for cooking, therapy sessions involved discussions about recipes and her favorite dishes. Activity scheduling was introduced by encouraging her to cook for the therapist, facilitating a shift away from the sick role while fostering trust. Once the therapeutic alliance was established, structured engagement in mastery activities was prioritized. A timetable was designed to reintroduce an academic routine, incorporating 1–2 hours of daily study across different subjects along with pleasurable activities like cooking and dancing. D also expressed a desire to assist her mother with household chores, which further contributed to her sense of engagement and responsibility. This structured approach not only aided her transition back to routine but also alleviated parental anxiety regarding her academic stagnation and future prospects.

Family counseling was crucial in addressing reinforcement patterns. Her mother would usually end up reinforcing the dissociative symptom out of her concern for D's safety. She was educated on the importance of responding only to age-appropriate behaviors and to reduce secondary gains associated with the symptoms. Similarly, her brother was counseled to recognize how his controlling behavior exacerbated her distress. Being the youngest child in a sheltered environment, she developed core schemas such as "I need protection to be safe," "I cannot tolerate distress," and "I am weak." Moving to a new city for boarding school, coupled with reduced perceived family support heightened her vulnerability. The stress of preparing for her 12th-grade preboard examinations triggered these schemas, leading to distress, avoidance, and the emergence of symptoms as a coping mechanism to shield her from the fear of failure. Treatment also focused on helping her to recognize cognitive distortions in real-time and replace them with balanced, realistic thoughts.

As therapy progressed, D disclosed that she had been a victim of sexual cyber-harassment a year before symptom onset when her intimate image was shared on social media. This deeply traumatic event led to feelings of shame. Though her parents were initially upset, they supported her and filed a police case under Section 66E of the IT Act (Violation of Privacy). She revealed that performing well in examinations became her way of atoning for this incident, and when she struggled academically, overwhelming anxiety about failing and disappointing her parents triggered the initial episode.

Regression to childhood allowed her to view herself as an "innocent, gullible child" who is protected from the awareness of these instances. Her need for reassurance, wherein the mother would have repeated that "you are a good child" was situated in the guilt and shame associated with this incident. Therapeutic work centered on normalizing her emotional response to trauma and reassuring her that her experiences were valid. She was encouraged to express her feelings whenever overwhelmed and was advised to maintain a journal to document a narration of her emotions. Additionally, she was guided to write a self-compassionate letter, forgiving herself and acknowledging her strengths. These strategies were aimed to foster self-acceptance and emotional processing of the trauma in a gradual manner.

Supportive Psychotherapy Techniques

Even when underlying conflicts are present, if the intensity of intrapsychic conflict in children and adolescents is too great to explore due to their developing and often inefficient ego functioning, supportive psychotherapy (SP) should be recommended over insight-oriented dynamic therapy. The primary aim of treatment is to validate the child's experiences in order to strengthen self-esteem and promote the development of adaptive coping skills, rather than to explore unconscious conflicts or delve deeply into the inner psyche. In many cases, a child or adolescent may only be available for therapy for a short duration of time and, hence, an expedient therapy process such as this becomes essential in addressing the symptoms and reducing distress associated with it. As in any other form of psychotherapy, a strong therapeutic alliance and an appropriate disclosure become the basis of psychotherapy. Techniques such as acceptance, praise, reassurance, modeling, advising, guidance, suggestion, psychoeducating the client, focusing, and reinforcing strengths are used. For example, in *Case vignette 5*, the patient, due to limited ability, could not be initiated into active discussions, thus indirect suggestions and reassurance along with creating positive environment helped in recovery. **Figure 1** shows the trajectory of symptom resolution over time.

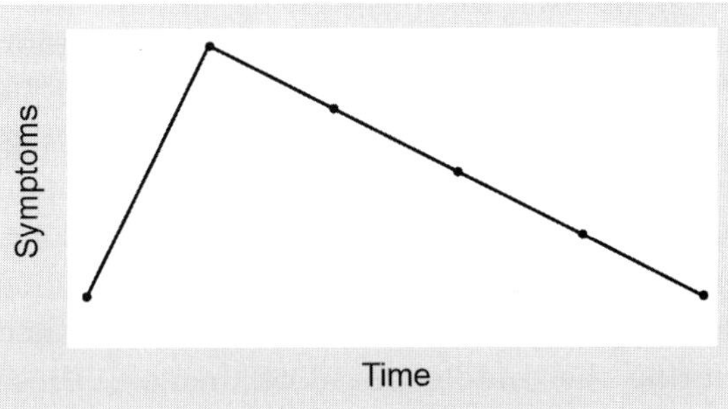

Fig. 1: The trajectory of symptom resolution may not be linear and may follow the following pattern.

Note: As the therapy proceeds, initially there may be worsening of symptoms, at which point new symptoms may arise or older symptoms may be at its highest intensity, in behavioral term "extinction burst" may be noticed. After this temporary increase in symptoms, there will be a gradual diminishing of pathological dissociation and improvement will be noticed across the symptoms. Novice therapist must be aware of this temporary increase in symptoms and skillfully navigate their own anxiety and parental concern about the effectiveness of therapy in reducing the symptoms of dissociation. Failure to do so may lead to premature termination of therapy, thereby hindering the child's progress.

To prevent dropout and maintain parental trust in the therapist's competence, it is essential to provide psychoeducation with the expected course of symptoms, in a clear and jargon-free manner. By fostering an understanding of the expected course of symptom progression, parents can be reassured so as to ensure that the treatment adherence is ensured.

Emotional Regulation

One of the important goals in therapy sessions is enhancing emotional awareness and regulation among children with DD. Children can be guided in understanding their emotions, recognizing their function, naming, and labeling them, and developing strategies to regulate them during moments of emotional vulnerability. With younger children, these skills can be taught using developmentally appropriate methods such as dolls, toys, storybooks, cartoons, painting, or role plays. These approaches provide a nonthreatening medium for expressing distress, reducing defensiveness, and enhancing the therapist's ability to teach effective emotion regulation techniques. Furthermore, children can be taught practical strategies to navigate distressing experiences and emotions through relaxation techniques. Methods such as paced breathing, progressive muscle relaxation, and grounding techniques can be introduced and integrated during the middle phase of therapy. These techniques help children to develop self-soothing abilities, enhance emotional regulation, and reduce physiological arousal associated with distress.

Mindfulness-based Stress Reduction Techniques

Mindfulness has been shown to reduce symptoms of dissociation and promote adaptive functioning in adolescents.[27] Mindfulness-based stress reduction (MBSR) is a structured and patient-centered program that uses mindfulness meditation to help children and adolescent to manage stress, learn adaptive emotional skills, and reduce internalizing problems.[28]

Interpersonal Skills Training

Since intrafamilial stressors are a common trigger for the onset of DD, therapy with adolescents should include interpersonal skills training. These interventions can help them to navigate conflicts that frequently arise with parents over autonomy, control, and independence in decision-making. Assertiveness training focuses on teaching adolescents how to express dissatisfaction or disagreement in a respectful and constructive manner, assert boundaries without resorting to anger or aggression, and develop perspective-taking skills to improve their responses to criticism.

Dealing with Nonresponsive Adolescent

Adolescents with low intelligence or of extremely introverted nature may not be forthcoming with their problems. In such cases, assessment using projective tests may help in identifying the conflicts besides helping in rapport formation. Supportive therapy using indirect suggestions may help in resolving dissociative symptoms as shown in *Case vignette 5*.

CASE VIGNETTE 5

A 17-year-old girl studying in 11th class, presented with selective mutism in the OPD. The family belonging to the lower middle class had been in contact with doctors (physician and mental health professionals) for the past 3 years. The past treatment history showed that she would start talking after every contact with a therapist but would relapse after a few months. Prior to the referral to the first author, she was being given electric shock (placebo) with the suggestion that her vocal chords opened with mild shock.

The patient had one elder sister who was not only doing well in studies but also shared several responsibilities with her mother. The father was an auto driver. A detailed clinical interview with family members and the patient did not yield any apparent stressor. After psychoeducation sessions with respect to psychogenic illness, the parents were asked to continue with sessions when the patient becomes verbose and the adherence with follow-up was reinforced by scheduling appointments as per their convenience.

However, the patient would only give focused specific responses to any queries. Since she was cooperative, "Draw a Person Test and TAT" was administered. The unstructured tests helped in unraveling the unspoken dilemmas that the patient was undergoing. The feeling of hopelessness, worthlessness, low self-esteem along with the criticism by the family came forth on the tests. The test performance also indicated a need for evaluation of intellectual ability which suggested a dull average level of intelligence.

Separate sessions with mother, father, and sister focused on improving communication patterns by identifying situations that precipitated negative interactions. Roles and responsibilities were redistributed that boosted confidence level in the patient. Since she was never verbose to share her thoughts, indirect suggestions through stories of hypothetical situations and people were narrated to provide her with options for adaptive coping and her future course. Her relapses gradually reduced and in 2 years' time, she recovered fully.

Termination Phase

Termination of therapy should be a gradual and structured process, and initiated once the patient demonstrates significant improvement in symptoms. This phase involves reviewing the techniques and strategies learned throughout therapy, reinforcing the progress made, and acknowledging the growth. When working with parents, it is essential to set realistic expectations regarding the possibility of symptom re-emergence during times of stress or crisis. They should be reassured that this does not necessarily indicate a relapse but rather a natural part of the healing process. Parents must be equipped to navigate such situations by helping the child to revisit coping skills, recognize their own strengths, and apply learned strategies to manage stressors. Additionally, reinforcing and rewarding the child's efforts—rather than just symptom reduction—encourages long-term improvement.

EFFECTIVENESS OF MANUALIZED TREATMENT

Goldstein's CODES study, LaFrance et al.'s CBT-informed psychotherapy (CBT-ip), and Sharpe's CBT-based guided self-help interventions have shown significant effect in the improvement in symptoms amelioration and enhanced overall well-being of the patients.[29-31] However, it has been noted that a strict adherence to manualized treatment approaches, which are often effective for other psychological disorders, may not neatly apply to DD. Qualitative analyses of therapists' experiences with DD highlight the limitations of manualized CBT protocols, which are not universally effective due to the considerable heterogeneity in symptom presentation and underlying factors among patients with DD. Therapists also emphasized that focusing on enhancing patients' overall well-being and their ability to manage the episodes, rather than solely aiming to reduce seizure frequency led to better control over seizures and reduced dysfunction associated with the conditions.[32,33] Similarly, research indicates that a 12-month follow-up of patients with dissociative convulsions treated with manualized CBT, standardized medical care, or combined treatment demonstrated comparable outcomes. All three approaches led to significant improvements in avoidance behaviors, symptom-related discomfort, and work-related functionality. However, none of the treatments showed a significant reduction in seizure frequency, highlighting the absence of a clear superiority of one approach over the others in addressing DD rather than an eclectic approach to treatment may lead to efficacious outcomes.

SUMMARY AND CONCLUSION

Dissociative disorders are relatively common among children and adolescents, yet their management presents significant challenges in the Indian context. Our understanding of the factors primarily emerges from the western literature as Indian research among children and adolescents is sparse and treatment approaches are often shaped by prevailing cultural and religious beliefs. Since treatment primarily relies on nonpharmacological interventions that often require prolonged engagement, adherence can be difficult. Regardless of their educational background or socioeconomic status, families often lack psychological awareness, leading to misconceptions about the disorder and its treatment. Effective management, therefore, necessitates culturally sensitive strategies to foster a strong therapeutic alliance. In India, where societal attitudes and stigma can hinder psychological interventions, developing indigenous approaches may be key to overcoming these barriers—potentially addressing a significant portion of the treatment challenge.

REFERENCES

1. Irpati AS, Avasthi A, Sharan P. Study of stress and vulnerability in patients with somatoform and dissociative disorders in a psychiatric clinic in North India. Psychiatry Clin Neurosci. 2006;60(5):570-4.
2. American Psychiatric Association. (2013). Diagnostic and statistical manual of mental disorders: DSM-5. [online] Available from https://psychiatryonline.org/doi/book/10.1176/appi.books.9780890425596 [Last accessed 19 November, 2025].
3. World Health Organization. Clinical descriptions and diagnostic requirements for ICD-11 mental, behavioural and neurodevelopmental disorders. Geneva: World Health Organization; 2024.
4. Chaturvedi SK, Desai G, Shaligram D. Dissociative disorders in a psychiatric institute in India—a selected review and patterns over a decade. Int J Soc Psychiatry. 2010;56(5):533-9.
5. Srinath S, Bharat S, Girimaji S, Seshadri S. Characteristics of a child inpatient population with hysteria in India. J Am Acad Child Adolesc Psychiatry. 1993;32(4):822-5.
6. Blanz B, Lehmkuhl G. Conversion symptoms in childhood and adolescence. Fortschr Neurol Psychiatr. 1986;54(11):356-63.
7. Mohamed R, Koparde V, Chate S, Patil N. Study of Clinical Profile and Short-term Outcome of Dissociative Disorder in Children and Adolescents—An Observational Study. J Indian Assoc Child Adolesc Mental Health. 2025;21(1):67-71.
8. Rana SK, Garg S, Mishra P, Kumar M, Pandey JM. Dissociative disorder in children and adolescents and their personality profile: a comparative study. Int J Res Med Sci. 2015;3(10):2639-42.
9. Agarwal V, Sitholey P, Srivastava C. Clinical practice guidelines for the management of dissociative disorders in children and adolescents. Indian J Psychiatry. 2019;61(Suppl 2):247-53.
10. Jayan P, Kashyap H, Thippeswamy H. Dissociative Disorders in India: Cultural Influence on Psychopathology and Treatment. Indian J Psychol Med. 2025;47(2):183-6.
11. Garg H, Sharan P, Kumaran SS, Bhargava R, Patra BN, Tripathi M. fMRI Analysis of Dissociative Convulsions: A Case-Controlled Study. Neurology India. 2023;71(3):476-86.
12. Reddy LS, Patil NM, Nayak RB, Chate SS, Ansari S. Psychological Dissection of Patients Having Dissociative Disorder: A Cross-sectional Study. Indian J Psychol Med. 2018;40(1):41-6.
13. Satyanarayana VA, Chandra PS, Sharma MK, Sowmya HR, Kandavel T. Three sides of a triangle: gender disadvantage, resilience and psychological distress in a sample of adolescent girls from India. Int J Cult Mental Health. 2016;9(4):364-72.
14. Emran A, Sharma V, Singh R, Jha M, Iqbal N. Lived Experiences of Women with Dissociative Disorder: An Interpretative Phenomenological Analysis. Indian J Psychol Med. 2021: 025371762110448.
15. Bhati N, Bhargava R, Sagar R, Chadda RK. Adolescent and psychotherapist views of psychosocial factors in Dissociative Neurological Symptom Disorder: A mixed-method study. Eur J Trauma Dissoc. 2025;9(1):100491.

16. Lynn SJ, Maxwell R, Merckelbach H, Lilienfeld SO, van Heugten-van der Kloet D, Miskovic V. Dissociation and its disorders: Competing models, future directions, and a way forward. Clin Psychol Rev. 2019;73:101755.
17. Malhotra S, Singh G, Mohan A. Somatoform and dissociative disorders in children and adolescents: A comparative study. Indian J Psychiatry. 2005;47(1):39.
18. Gentile JP, Dillon KS, Gillig PM. Psychotherapy and pharmacotherapy for patients with dissociative identity disorder. Innov Clin Neurosci. 2013;10(2):22-9.
19. Sutar R, Sahu S. Pharmacotherapy for dissociative disorders: A systematic review. Psychiatry Res. 2019;281:112529.
20. Woolard A, Boutrus M, Bullman I, Wickens N, Gouveia Belinelo PD, Solomon T, et al. Treatment for childhood and adolescent dissociation: A systematic review. Psychol Trauma. 2024;16 (Suppl 3):S483-S491.
21. Cronin E, Brand BL, Mattanah JF. The impact of the therapeutic alliance on treatment outcome in patients with dissociative disorders. Eur J Psychotraumatol. 2014;5(1):22676.
22. Neki JS. Psychiatry in south-East Asia. Br J Psychiatry. 1973;123(574):257-69.
23. De Sousa A. Ethical issues in child and adolescent psychotherapy: A clinical review. Indian J Med Ethics. 2010;7(3):157-61.
24. Putnam FW. Dissociative disorders in children: Behavioral profiles and problems. Child Abuse Neglect. 1993;17(1):39-45.
25. Nowak M, Szyszka M, Lewicka W. Dissociative disorders in children–literature review. Pediatria Polska-Polish J Paediatr. 2023;98(3): 223-8.
26. Cohen JA, Mannarino AP, Deblinger E. Treating trauma and traumatic grief in children and adolescents. New York: Guilford Publications; 2016.
27. Sharma T, Sinha VK, Sayeed N. Role of mindfulness in dissociative disorders among adolescents. Indian J Psychiatry. 2016;58(3):326-8.
28. Vohra S, Punja S, Sibinga E, Baydala L, Wikman E, Singhal A, et al. Mindfulness-based stress reduction for mental health in youth: A cluster randomized controlled trial. Child Adolesc Mental Health. 2019;24(1):29-35.
29. Goldstein LH, Mellers JD, Landau S, Stone J, Carson A, Medford N, et al. COgnitive behavioural therapy vs standardised medical care for adults with Dissociative non-Epileptic Seizures (CODES): a multicentre randomised controlled trial protocol. BMC Neurol. 2015;15:1-3.
30. LaFrance WC, Baird GL, Barry JJ, Blum AS, Webb AF, Keitner GI, et al. Multicenter pilot treatment trial for psychogenic nonepileptic seizures: a randomized clinical trial. JAMA Psychiatry. 2014;71(9):997-1005.
31. Sharpe M, Walker J, Williams C, Stone J, Cavanagh J, Murray G, et al. Guided self-help for functional (psychogenic) symptoms: a randomized controlled efficacy trial. Neurology. 2011;77(6):564-72.
32. Fritzsche K, Baumann K, Götz-Trabert K, Schulze-Bonhage A. Dissociative seizures: a challenge for neurologists and psychotherapists. Deutsches Ärzteblatt Int. 2013;110(15):263.
33. O'Connor PJ, Reuber M. 'It's both challenging and probably the most rewarding work'–A qualitative study of psychological therapy provider's experiences of working with people with dissociative seizures. Epilepsy Behav. 2021;122:108156.

CHAPTER 18 Trauma and Stressor-related Disorders

Satya Raj

INTRODUCTION

Trauma and stressor-related disorders is a chapter newly included in the *Diagnostic and Statistical Manual of Mental Disorders, 5th Edition* (DSM-5). This includes reactive attachment disorder (RAD), disinhibited social engagement disorder (DSED), post-traumatic stress disorder (PTSD), acute stress disorder, adjustment disorders, other specified trauma and stressor-related disorders, and unspecified trauma and related disorders. All the above-mentioned disorders share a common feature: exposure to a stressor or a traumatic event.[1] The unique feature of this class of disorders is that the etiology is included as a part of the diagnostic criteria. The common cause is exposure to traumatic events, abuse, or severe neglect during childhood.

EFFECTS OF TRAUMA ON THE DEVELOPING BRAIN

Early adversity has significant effects on the developing brain, this has been shown in multiple animal studies, but recently there has also been increasing evidence for the same in humans. It has also been shown that there are certain sensitive periods for the development of language and intelligence. Windsor et al.[2] had shown that children who were in institutional placements, when placed in foster families before 15 months of age were more likely to exhibit normal expressive and receptive language, compared to the children who were placed at a later age. Therefore, it can be stated that the absence of the needed input during a sensitive period, or excessive unwanted input, can lead to adverse outcomes in children and adolescents.[3]

Response to childhood adversity and trauma can become manifested by a wide range of behaviors that can be considered as adaptive behaviors to overcome the stressor and cope with it at that point in time, but when the behaviors persist even after the stressor or the inciting traumatic event is removed or when it no longer exists, they are said to be maladaptive behaviors that result in psychopathology.

ACUTE STRESS DISORDER

DSM-5 describes acute stress disorder, as the symptoms that are being experienced by an individual, immediately after a traumatic event and should last for at least 3 days, and the duration of such symptoms must not exceed 4 weeks. They can present with significant anxiety, heightened reactivity, and re-experiencing of the trauma. The symptoms must be noted in the following domains of intrusion in the form of flashbacks, or nightmares, negative mood, dissociative symptoms, avoidance like avoiding memories and reminders, and arousal symptoms like sleep disturbances, irritability, and hypervigilance. A diagnosis of acute stress disorder can be made if there are at least nine of these symptoms associated with significant distress or impairment. If the symptoms persist beyond 4 weeks, then the person must be reassessed, and PTSD must be considered.

POST-TRAUMATIC STRESS DISORDER

INTRODUCTION

Post-traumatic stress disorder in children and adolescents has been under-recognized by parents and even mental health professionals. There is a wide variation in the prevalence of post-traumatic stress disorder depending on the assessment measure, the severity of the trauma, the duration of exposure to the trauma, and the methodology used. Multiple studies have shown that the response to traumatic events and the symptom presentation in PTSD are dependent on many sociocultural factors.

DEFINITION

Post-traumatic stress disorder is characterized by a group of symptoms that occur following an exposure to a frightening incident or event that is overwhelming to the individual. The traumatic event may be directly experienced by the child, or may witness it occurring to others, or may even hear about its occurrence and then can have PTSD symptoms. Children may exhibit varied symptoms like hyperarousal, anxiety, and negative mood triggered by thoughts of the event, and may also have flashbacks or nightmares, and avoidance.

Post-traumatic stress disorder can occur after any life-threatening event like an accident, natural disaster, violence, abuse, physical, emotional, or sexual abuse, and neglect.

PREVALENCE

International studies: The Great Smoky Mountain study reported that in the community sample studied 68% of the children had experienced a traumatic event at least once, and 37.0% of them had exposure to more than one traumatic event. Only 0.5% of them met criteria for PTSD, and 13% of children developed post-traumatic symptoms.[4]

Indian studies: Kar N et al.,[5] in their study, showed that following a natural disaster, 30.6% of children had PTSD and 13.6% had subsyndromal PTSD, and they also opined that PTSD in the Indian context is a valid entity. John PB et al.,[6] in a study among Tsunami survivors, reported a prevalence of 70.7% for acute PTSD and 10.9% for delayed onset PTSD. They had also opined in their study that PTSD was more prevalent among girls, and the PTSD symptoms were more severe among adolescents exposed to loss of life or property.

Multiple studies[7,8] have shown that the prevalence of PTSD was higher in areas of conflict and war, like Kashmir, and that the lifetime experience of traumatic events was as high as 58.69%.

Mathew et al.,[9] in a study done in Kerala to assess PTSD following the floods, reported a prevalence of 34.9% of probable PTSD in adolescents. Bhaskaran et al.,[10] in a retrospective chart review done among children presenting with a history of sexual abuse at a tertiary care hospital in India, reported that 25% of them had stressor-related disorders like acute stress disorder and PTSD.

CLINICAL PRESENTATION

Katie McLaughlin et al.[11] reported that distressing intrusive thoughts, avoidance, hyperarousal, and heightened emotional reactivity are common symptoms in children with PTSD. Bad dreams and nightmares are also common in children, and this can result in sleep difficulties.

It was also highlighted that children with PTSD have an increase in negative emotions such as fear, anger, guilt, and shame, and they also have an overall reduction in positive emotions. Children with an abuse history also tend to develop negative views about themselves, others, and the world, and perceive this world as an unsafe place, due to the early traumatic experience. Children with PTSD have difficulty concentrating on their studies, and they also present with an academic decline. Children can also present with hypervigilance and separation anxiety symptoms.

It is also known that children can at times re-experience the trauma or relive the distressing event. The trauma reminders for the same can be internal triggers like thoughts or memories, and external triggers like a place or person.

COURSE

Most of the PTSD symptoms in children tend to gradually remit over time, however, Scheeringa et al.,[12] in their study showed that PTSD in preschool children does not remit quickly and seems to have a prolonged course.

NEUROBIOLOGY OF POST-TRAUMATIC STRESS DISORDER

Dysregulation of multiple neurotransmitter systems—serotonin, norepinephrine, dopamine, and gamma-aminobutyric acid (GABA) have been implicated in PTSD. The hypothalamo-pituitary adrenal axis is mainly involved in mediating the stress responses. Exposure to chronic or severe stress can result in elevated corticotropin-releasing hormone (CRH) levels for long periods of time and this results in sympathetic overactivity and hyperarousal in PTSD can be explained by the above mechanism.[13]

Heim et al.[14] suggested that children with PTSD had elevated levels of cortisol in the saliva, and they were also found to have abnormalities in brain electrical activity as noted on the EEG.

Multiple studies[15,16] have shown that PTSD can be explained by a learning model in which the main reason suggested is the failure to inhibit fear, and a weak extinction memory that fails to inhibit the original fear memory even in the presence of safety cues.

Studies[17-22] have implicated that multiple brain regions have been involved in PTSD. It has been shown that heightened amygdala activation, reduced activity in the ventromedial prefrontal cortex, and rostral anterior cingulate cortex in response to emotional or threatening cues, and elevated activity in the dorsal anterior cingulate cortex during fear conditioning, extinction learning recall are noted in PTSD. Reduced hippocampal volume has also been consistently observed among individuals with PTSD.[23]

DIAGNOSIS

Post-traumatic stress disorder in children manifests differently as compared to adults and, therefore, DSM-5-TR gives two sets of diagnostic criteria for PTSD, one for children under 6 years of age and another set of criteria for older children and adults. This is because children <6 years of age can have varied presentations following a traumatic event, compared to older children and adolescents.[24,25]

Box 1 shows the "DSM-5 Diagnostic Criteria for Post-traumatic Stress Disorder".

Box 2 shows that children less than 6 years of age have separate diagnostic criteria for PTSD.

RISK FACTORS

There are multiple factors, like the type of trauma, child and family factors that contribute to the PTSD presentation in children and adolescents. Trauma with a high degree of life threat, interpersonal violence or sexual abuse, and exposure to war and/or displacement are risk factors for PTSD. Female gender and comorbid mental illness are the individual risk factors for the development of PTSD. Poor family functioning, parental PTSD, and poor social support are the family-related risk factors.[26,27]

BOX 1: DSM-5 Diagnostic Criteria for post-traumatic stress disorder.

Note: The following criteria apply to adults, adolescents, and children older than 6 years.

A. Exposure to actual or threatened death, serious injury, or sexual violence in one (or more) of the following ways:
   1. Directly experiencing the traumatic event(s)
   2. Witnessing, in person, the event(s) as it occurred to others
   3. Learning that the traumatic event(s) occurred to a close family member or close friend. In cases of actual or threatened death of a family member or friend, the event(s) must have been violent or accidental
   4. Experiencing repeated or extreme exposure to aversive details of the traumatic event(s) (e.g., first responders collecting human remains; police officers repeatedly exposed to details of child abuse)

Note: Criterion A4 does not apply to exposure through electronic media, television, movies, or pictures, unless this exposure is work related

B. Presence of one (or more) of the following intrusion symptoms associated with the traumatic event(s), beginning after the traumatic event(s) occurred:
   1. Recurrent, involuntary, and intrusive distressing memories of the traumatic event(s). *Note:* In children older than 6 years, repetitive play may occur in which themes or aspects of the traumatic event(s) are expressed
   2. Recurrent distressing dreams in which the content and/or affect of the dream are related to the traumatic event(s). *Note:* In children, there may be frightening dreams without recognizable content
   3. Dissociative reactions (e.g., flashbacks) in which the individual feels or acts as if the traumatic event(s) were recurring. (Such reactions may occur on a continuum, with the most extreme expression being a complete loss of awareness of present surroundings.) *Note:* In children, trauma-specific re-enactment may occur in play
   4. Intense or prolonged psychological distress at exposure to internal or external cues that symbolize or resemble an aspect of the traumatic event(s).
   5. Marked physiological reactions to internal or external cues that symbolize or resemble an aspect of the traumatic event(s).

C. Persistent avoidance of stimuli associated with the traumatic event(s), beginning after the traumatic event(s) occurred, as evidenced by one or both of the following:
   1. Avoidance of or efforts to avoid distressing memories, thoughts, or feelings about or closely associated with the traumatic event(s).
   2. Avoidance of or efforts to avoid external reminders (people, places, conversations, activities, objects, and situations) that arouse distressing memories, thoughts, or feelings about or closely associated with the traumatic event(s).

D. Negative alterations in cognitions and mood associated with the traumatic event(s), beginning or worsening after the traumatic event(s) occurred, as evidenced by two (or more) of the following:
   1. Inability to remember an important aspect of the traumatic event(s) (typically due to dissociative amnesia, and not to other factors such as head injury, alcohol, or drugs).
   2. Persistent and exaggerated negative beliefs or expectations about oneself, others, or the world (e.g., "I am bad," "No one can be trusted," "The world is completely dangerous," "My whole nervous system is permanently ruined").
   3. Persistent, distorted cognitions about the cause or consequences of the traumatic event(s) that lead the individual to blame himself/herself or others.
   4. Persistent negative emotional state (e.g., fear, horror, anger, guilt, or shame)
   5. Markedly diminished interest or participation in significant activities.
   6. Feelings of detachment or estrangement from others.
   7. Persistent inability to experience positive emotions (e.g., inability to experience happiness, satisfaction, or loving feelings).

Contd...

Contd...

E. Marked alterations in arousal and reactivity associated with the traumatic event(s), beginning or worsening after the traumatic event(s) occurred, as evidenced by two (or more) of the following:
1. Irritable behavior and angry outbursts (with little or no provocation), typically expressed as verbal or physical aggression toward people or objects.
2. Reckless or self-destructive behavior
3. Hypervigilance
4. Exaggerated startle response
5. Problems with concentration
6. Sleep disturbance (e.g., difficulty falling or staying asleep or restless sleep)

F. Duration of the disturbance (Criteria B, C, D, and E) is >1 month.

G. The disturbance causes clinically significant distress or impairment in social, occupational, or other important areas of functioning.

H. The disturbance is not attributable to the physiological effects of a substance (e.g., medication and alcohol) or another medical condition.

Specify whether: With dissociative symptoms: The individual's symptoms meet the criteria for post-traumatic stress disorder, and in addition, in response to the stressor, the individual experiences persistent or recurrent symptoms of either of the following:
1. *Depersonalization:* Persistent or recurrent experiences of feeling detached from, and as if one were an outside observer of, one's mental processes or body (e.g., feeling as though one were in a dream; feeling a sense of unreality of self or body or of time moving slowly).
2. *Derealization:* Persistent or recurrent experiences of unreality of surroundings (e.g., the world around the individual is experienced as nreal, dreamlike, distant, or distorted). *Note:* To use this subtype, the dissociative symptoms must not be attributable to the physiological effects of a substance (e.g., blackouts and behavior during alcohol intoxication) or another medical condition (e.g., complex partial seizures). Specify whether: With delayed expression—if the full diagnostic criteria are not met until at least 6 months after the event (although the onset and expression of some symptoms may be immediate).

BOX 2: DSM-5-TR diagnostic criteria for post-traumatic stress disorder for children 6 years of age and younger.

Criterion A: Stressor

In children 6 years and younger, exposure to actual or threatened death, serious injury, or sexual violence in one (or more) of the following ways:
- Directly experiencing the traumatic event(s)
- Witnessing, in person, the event(s) as it occurred to others, especially primary caregivers. This does not include events witnessed only in electronic media, television, movies, or pictures.
- Learning that the traumatic event(s) occurred to a parent or caregiving figure.

Criterion B: Intrusion symptoms

Presence of one (or more) of the following intrusion symptoms associated with the traumatic event(s), beginning after the traumatic event(s) occurred as follows:
- Recurrent, involuntary, and intrusive distressing memories of the traumatic event(s)
- Recurrent distressing dreams in which the content and/or effect of the dream are related to the traumatic event(s)
- Dissociative reactions in which the child feels or acts as if the traumatic event(s) were recurring
- Intense or prolonged psychological distress on exposure to internal or external clues that symbolize or resemble an aspect of the traumatic event(s)
- Marked physiological reactions to reminders of the traumatic event(s)

Contd...

Contd...

Criterion C: Avoidance

One (or more) of the following symptoms, representing either persistent avoidance of stimuli associated with the traumatic event(s) or negative alterations in cognitions and mood associated with the traumatic event(s), must be present, beginning after the event(s) or worsening after the event(s).

- Persistent avoidance of stimuli
- Avoidance of or efforts to avoid activities, places, or physical reminders that arouse recollections of the traumatic event(s)
- Avoidance of or efforts to avoid people, conversations, or interpersonal situations that arouse recollections of the traumatic event(s)
- Negative Alterations in Cognitions
- Substantially increased frequency of negative emotional states
- Markedly diminished interest or participation in significant activities, including constriction of play
- Socially withdrawn behavior
- Persistent reduction in the expression of positive emotions

Criterion D: Alterations in arousal and reactivity

Alterations in arousal and reactivity associated with the traumatic event(s), beginning or worsening after the traumatic event(s) occurred, as evidenced by 2 (or more) of the following:

- Irritable behavior and angry outbursts (with little or no provocation) typically expressed as verbal or physical aggression toward people or objects (including extreme temper tantrums)
- Hypervigilance
- Exaggerated startle response
- Problems with concentration
- Sleep disturbance

Criterion E: Duration

Persistence of symptoms in Criterion A, B, C, and D for more than 1 month.

Criterion F: The disturbance causes significant functional impairment or distress in various areas of life, such as social or educational.

Criterion G: The disturbance is not attributable to substance use, medication, or another medical illness.

The subjective experience of traumatic event, cognitive and emotional responses to the trauma, peritraumatic fear, and social support are factors associated with an increased risk for PTSD in children.[28]

COMORBIDITY

Post-traumatic stress disorder in children has been associated with multiple comorbid conditions such as anxiety, depression, suicidal ideation, and somatic symptoms.[29] Some of them have externalizing disorders and substance abuse. Dissociative symptoms can also be seen commonly in children with PTSD.

ASSESSMENTS

A detailed clinical interview is needed for making a diagnosis of PTSD in children and adolescents and it must be done with utmost care and sensitivity, to prevent retraumatization. Creating a safe space for them is essential, and this would help children to discuss the trauma. Children may not be able to talk about their traumatic experiences during the very first interview and may take multiple sessions before they are able to open up and discuss about their trauma and distress.

There are a few objective assessments for PTSD in children and adolescents. The child PTSD symptom scale is a 20-item self-rated scale.

The Clinician-Administered PTSD Scale for Children and Adolescents (CAPS-CA5) is a 30-item structured interview that can be used to assess PTSD symptoms in children above 7 years of age.[30]

"Trauma Symptom Checklist for Children" can also be used to objectively assess PTSD in preschool children.[31-33]

MANAGEMENT

Trauma-focused psychotherapies must be used as the first line of management for PTSD in children and adolescents. Psychoanalytic, attachment, and cognitive-behavioral treatment models have been studied.[34-36] Psychological debriefing and EMDR have also been shown to be effective in treating PTSD.

Studies have shown that SSRIs may be beneficial in reducing child PTSD symptoms.[37] Other medications that have been tried are benzodiazepines, MAOA inhibitors. Medications are mainly used in children and adolescents only when there is comorbid anxiety or depression.

CONCLUSION

Post-traumatic stress disorder in children and adolescents is a valid diagnostic construct and is quite prevalent in this population. Evidence-based interventions and developmentally sensitive approaches are needed to effectively manage childhood PTSD.

Primary prevention strategies include creating safe environments for children, promoting positive parenting, and implementing trauma-informed practices in schools and the community. Identifying high-risk and vulnerable children, providing trauma-related psychoeducation, and working on their resilience will help decrease the risk of developing PTSD.[38]

Early diagnosis and management are needed for better recovery, reducing functional impairment, and improving long-term outcomes.

CASE VIGNETTE

A 13-year-old girl child, in grade 8, coming from a lower socioeconomic background, presented with a 3-month history of recurrent intrusive thoughts regarding a traumatic event, hyperarousal, and anxiety. The symptoms started following her being involved in a road traffic accident with her father 3 months back when they were travelling on a motorcycle.

She avoided going anywhere on the bike and started insisting that her father must also refrain from driving the bike. She reported having a startle response even when she heard a horn sound or screeching noise of the brakes; her sleep was disturbed, and she had bad dreams almost every night.

She was unable to focus on her studies when she was at school and kept worrying if her father had reached his office safely.

The birth and development history was uneventful. Nil significant past or family history.

Mental status examination—revealed intrusive traumatic thoughts, significant anxiety, hyperarousal, and avoidance.

DIAGNOSIS

Post-traumatic stress disorder.

MANAGEMENT

Psychotherapy is the mainstay of treatment. Establish rapport with the child, allow the child to ventilate, and provide emotional support. Considering the significant anxiety and hyperarousal symptoms, the child would benefit from relaxation exercises, Jacobson's progressive muscle relaxation. The child would benefit from trauma-focused CBT. The steps involved in trauma-focused CBT are *PRACTICE*—*P*sychoeducation, *R*elaxation techniques, *A*ffective modulation, *C*ognitive coping, *T*rauma narrative, *I*n vivo exposure, *C*onjoint *T*rauma narrative, and *E*nhancing safety. SSRIs can be given for managing the anxiety symptoms, if required.

Take Home Points

- Post-traumatic stress disorder in children and adolescents has been under-recognized by parents and even mental health professionals.
- Early adversity and traumatic experiences have a significant effect on the developing brain.
- Post-traumatic stress disorder in children manifests differently as compared to adults, and, therefore, DSM-5-TR gives separate diagnostic criteria for PTSD in children under 6 years of age.
- Detailed clinical interview is needed for making a diagnosis of PTSD in children and adolescents and it must be done with utmost care and sensitivity to prevent retraumatization.
- Evidence-based interventions and developmentally sensitive approaches are needed to effectively manage childhood PTSD.
- Creating safe environments for children and working on their resilience will help in decreasing the risk of developing PTSD.
- Early diagnosis and management are needed for better recovery, reducing functional impairment, and improving long-term outcomes.

GRIEF IN CHILDREN

INTRODUCTION

The death of a loved one is a significant loss to a child or adolescent, and they experience grief like any other adult. Grief in children and adolescents is an area that is mostly overlooked by professionals and society at large. Loss of a loved object like even a toy can result in distressing emotions in a child. The death of a family member, caregiver, or parent is a significant loss in the life of a child and results in grief in them.

DEFINITION OF GRIEF

William Worden defined grief as "an experience of loss due to the death of a loved one".[39] Later the concept was broadened to include other losses as well. Grief can be conceptualized as a natural response to loss. Grief affects emotional well-being and has an impact on the physiological, psychological, spiritual, social, cognitive, and behavioral functioning.[40] The death of a parent, sibling, or close relative is very distressing to the child, and this radically changes their view of the world.[41]

DEFINITION OF BEREAVEMENT

Bereavement is defined as a state following the loss of a loved object and constitutes grief and mourning processes associated with it.[42] The intensity and duration of the grieving process depend on multiple factors like the type of loss, relationship and attachment with the deceased person, circumstances leading to the loss, and personal factors like personality, and coping styles.

Multiple studies[43,44] have shown that childhood bereavement is associated with a range of mental health problems, such as depression and post-traumatic stress reactions. It can also result in substance use[45] and suicide-related behaviors.[46]

TYPES OF GRIEF

Grief can be broadly classified into two types, namely uncomplicated and complicated grief.

Uncomplicated Grief

Usually it occurs in everyone, following a loss, and is characterized by physical or bodily changes, changes in thought, emotion, and behavior, and it gradually resolves, and the child or adolescent can eventually accept the loss and move forward. There can be repeated thoughts about the deceased person, a sense of loss, helplessness, emotions such as anger and sadness, and biological changes in sleep and appetite.[40]

Complicated Grief

In complicated grief, children and adolescents have similar symptoms as in uncomplicated grief, but the intensity of symptoms can be more severe, or the duration can be more prolonged. In complicated grief, there is difficulty in integrating the loss, adapting to it, and moving forward. The children are unable to get back to their routine functioning. There are many types of complicated grief namely, chronic grief reaction, delayed grief reaction, exaggerated grief reaction, masked grief reaction, or distorted grief reaction.

Anticipatory Grief

It is the grief experienced by a person, days or months before losing someone. It is due to the distress of impending loss of a loved one. It is also referred to as preparatory grief.[47]

Disenfranchised Grief

Another type of grief that is a little more complicated is "Disenfranchised grief", which occurs when the loss cannot be openly acknowledged, or it cannot be socially supported in the grieving process or cannot be publicly mourned. It is seen in cases where there is a stigma associated with the type of death, e.g., death by suicide, or the relationship with the person who died is not a socially acceptable one, then this can disenfranchise the child as a griever and, hence, complicates the grieving process.[48]

Regrieving

It is when a childhood loss comes back to memory, and grief is re-experienced. Triggers or reminders of the deceased cause re-grief.

Recently, there has been increased recognition of grief and its importance, resulting in the inclusion of prolonged grief disorder (PGD) in the 11th edition of the International Classification of Diseases (ICD-11; WHO, 2018) and in Section II of the Fifth Diagnostic and Statistical Manual for Psychiatric Disorders text revision (DSM-5-TR; APA, 2020).[49]

Prolonged Grief Disorder (Box 3)

Studies have shown that symptoms of PGD are characterized by intense yearning, difficulties in accepting the loss, anger, and a sense that life is meaningless, and this is unique and makes it different from other presentations that can occur post-trauma or loss, as in PTSD and depression.[51,52] The way in which PGD symptoms present in different age groups may be very different depending on the age of the child and the developing cognitive capacity.[53]

BOX 3: Prolonged grief disorder (PGD) in the Fifth Diagnostic and Statistical Manual for Psychiatric Disorders Text Revision (DSM-5-TR).

PGD in the DSM-5-TR (APA, 2020) can be diagnosed in children:

A. After at least 6 months have passed since the death of someone close

B. The child experiences intense yearning or preoccupation regarding the deceased person.

C. Accompanied by at least three out of eight symptoms of identity disruption, disbelief about the death, avoidance (characterized by efforts to avoid reminders in children and adolescents), emotional pain related to the loss, difficulties in moving on with life, emotional numbness, a sense that life is meaningless, and intense loneliness, nearly every day or more often, for at least 1 month

D. Cause distress or functional impairment

E. Exceed cultural and contextual norms

F. Not better explained by another mental disorder or substance use[50]

CHILDHOOD GRIEF—THEORIES

There are multiple grief theories, and they have conceptualized grief in different ways. Understanding them helps in getting a holistic picture of the same.

- *Freud* describes "grief as the individual search for a lost attachment". The loss needs to be internalized, accepted, and processed, and only then can new attachments be formed.
- *Elisabeth Kübler-Ross,* in her book "On Death and Dying", described stages of grief, namely denial, anger, bargaining, depression, and acceptance.[54]
- *Bowlby* conceptualized grief from the perspective of the loss of an attachment figure. He described the phases of mourning as numbing, yearning-searching, disorganization, and reorganization.[55]
- *Multidimensional grief theory:* According to this theory, childhood grief reactions can be characterized by three dimensions, namely, separation distress, existential/Identity distress, and circumstance-related distress. This theory is based on the assumption that both maladjustment and positive adjustment can manifest in each domain, and sometimes both can co-occur.[56,57]
- *Relational developmental systems (RDS) metatheory:* It proposes that developmental processes are dynamic and transactional, and that adaptation is the result of reciprocal interactions between children, their families, and culture.[58] The theory suggests that grief reactions are informed by cognitive, socioemotional, and identity developmental processes and that the ways in which bereavement-related problems manifest change according to the developmental stages and transitions.[59]
- *Therese A Rando* et al. described *the six "R" Model,* which goes through three phases namely avoidance, confrontation, and accommodation. He described six tasks that happen sequentially, recognising the loss, reaction to the separation, recollection and re-experience, relinquishing old attachments, readjusting, and reinvesting.[60]
- *Stroebe and Schut dual process model of grief:* They described normal grieving as a dynamic regulatory process oscillating between the stress of loss-oriented and restoration-oriented domains. The griever confronts, and at times avoids the different tasks of grieving, and keeps oscillating between both states.[61]
- *Kenneth J Doka and Terry L Martin model:* They described that grieving is a complex process and unique to every individual. They also stated that there were two types of grievers, the intuitive type, and the instrumental type, where the pattern is affective, and cognitive respectively.[62]

DEVELOPMENTAL ASPECTS IN "UNDERSTANDING DEATH"

Children and adolescents understand death in different ways, and this depends on the age and developmental stage of the child. Multiple studies[63-65] have shown that the main concepts that are foundational to understanding death are: universality, finality, irreversibility, inevitability, and causality. By 5–7 years of age, children develop a fair understanding of the concept of death. Children, at times, may have repetitive questioning about the death of a loved one, this may be to get a better understanding of how and why it happened, and in such situations, it is best to answer the child rather than avoiding and explaining in simple terms helps.

Secondary Loss

When children lose a close relative, they grieve the loss of that person and all the memories associated with them. Change in their life situation, relocation to another place, loss of shared memories, and decreased sense of safety and trust, are all secondary losses.[66]

GRIEF TRIGGERS AND ANNIVERSARY REACTIONS

Sudden reminders of the deceased person can evoke very strong emotional responses in a grieving child; identifying the triggers and managing them is needed. Anniversary reaction happens in children grieving the loss of a loved one, birthdays, death anniversaries, and special days can trigger sad feelings and anxiety.

Adaptive grief reaction—the intensity and severity of grief reaction decreases over time, and the child is able to access positive memories of the deceased and they are able to find meaning in the life.[49]

The key factors that moderate the grief are:

1. Circumstances of death
2. Time since the loss
3. Relationship of the child to the deceased
4. Culture, race, and ethnicity
5. Caregiving contexts

Childhood Traumatic Grief

Cohen JA et al.[67] described childhood traumatic grief as a condition where the trauma symptoms are overwhelming and interfere with the natural grieving process. Re-experiencing the trauma through traumatic memories, distressing thoughts, avoidance, hyperarousal, emotional dysregulation, and learning difficulties are seen.

ASSESSING GRIEF IN CHILDREN AND ADOLESCENTS

Grief in children and adolescents can present in multiple ways. Common symptoms include low mood, feelings of emptiness, somatic complaints, anxiety symptoms, anger, guilt, social withdrawal, and sleep and appetite disturbances. Diagnosing complicated grief in children is an area of ongoing debate.

There are self-report questionnaires, clinician-administered scales, and structured interviews to assess grief. The following measures can be used to assess grief, namely, Adolescent Grief Inventory, Adolescent Grief Response Inventory, Grief Facilitation Inventory, Grief Process Scale, Hogan Inventory of Bereavement, Inventory of Youth Adaptation to Loss, Two-Track Model of Bereavement Questionnaire (TTBQ), and the UCLA Grief Inventory-Revised, etc.

Maladaptive grief reactions can also be assessed by the "Extended Grief Inventory, Grief Cognitions Questionnaire for Children, Grief Screening Scale, Intrusive Grief Thoughts Scale, Inventory of Complicated Grief Revised for Children, Inventory of Prolonged Grief for Adolescents Inventory of Prolonged Grief for Children, Persistent Complex Bereavement Disorder Checklist, Prolonged Grief Questionnaire for Adolescents, Prolonged Grief-13 Child, Texas Revised Inventory of Grief, and the Traumatic Dissociation and Grief Scale".[68]

However, most of these measures have been validated in Western populations and, therefore, need to be validated in the Indian context, as there are huge social and cultural differences in the expression of grief.

MOURNING

Mourning can be described as an outward expression of grief. William Worden et al.[69] described it is a process in which four tasks are involved, namely, (1) To accept the reality of the loss, (2) To process the pain of grief, (3) To adjust to a world without the deceased, and (4) To find an enduring connection with the deceased while embarking on a new life. Sandra Fox et al.[70] developed the "Good Grief Program Model", where similar tasks were described, such as understanding, grieving, commemoration, and going on.

TREATMENT

Children and adolescents are very resilient and, therefore, cope with the loss and work through the grief effectively. However, some of them may require grief therapy to come to terms with the loss. Multiple strategies can be used to work with grief, namely writing a letter to the deceased, drawing, role-playing, visual imagery, and cognitive strategies. Play and art can be used as a medium for therapy, as children can express their emotions through the same.

Trauma-focused CBT helps in working with children with traumatic grief. TF-CBT consists of the following steps: psychoeducation, relaxation strategies, affective modulation skills, cognitive coping, trauma narrative, processing of the traumatic event, and in vivo mastery of trauma reminders. Once the child is emotionally ready, then conjoint sessions are planned with the child and parent, and this helps the parent in validating the child's emotions and supporting them. Ensuring future safety and enhancing the developmental trajectory is an essential task of trauma-focused CBT.

CONCLUSION

Children and adolescents usually overcome distress and effectively work on the grief and soon adapt to the new situation. However, a few of them who experience complicated grief, and prolonged grief may need specific interventions, and this needs to be delivered in a timely manner for better outcomes.

Take Home Points

- Children and adolescents experience grief, just like adults, but the presentation is different.
- Grief can be either uncomplicated or complicated.
- Children understand death in different ways, and this depends on the age and developmental stage of the child.
- Grief in children and adolescents can present in multiple ways, and diagnosing the same in children is complex.
- Children and adolescents are very resilient and cope with the loss and work through the grief effectively.
- Strategies like writing a letter to the deceased, drawing, role-playing, visual imagery, play and cognitive strategies can be used to work with grief in children.
- Trauma focused CBT can be used in traumatic grief.

ATTACHMENT DISORDER

INTRODUCTION

John Bowlby described attachment as a "lasting psychological connectedness between human beings".[71] He was one of the first attachment theorists, who was interested in studying the anxiety and distress in children when they were separated from their primary caregivers and Mary Ainsworth later expanded on this work.

Attachment can be defined as a "deep and enduring emotional bond that connects one person to another across time and space".

The main construct of attachment theory is that when the primary caregiver is emotionally available and responsive to an infant's needs, the child develops a sense of security. This creates a secure base for the child, and he or she can explore the world.

ATTACHMENT DISORDER

Attachment disorder can be defined as abnormal or aberrant attachment behaviors due to trauma, neglect, or emotional deprivation. The two common clinical presentations are those of RAD, and DSED. It can be seen as two extremes of disturbed attachment where, in RAD, the child is very emotionally withdrawn and inhibited, and, in DSED, the child is indiscriminately social and disinhibited.

REACTIVE ATTACHMENT DISORDER

The DSM-5 classifies RAD as a trauma and stressor-related condition of early childhood that is caused due to social neglect or maltreatment.

The children with RAD are emotionally withdrawn, lack positive emotions, do not seek comfort from the primary caregiver when they are distressed, and they can also react with extreme violence or meltdowns even with minimal change in their routines and have erratic mood fluctuations. Failure to develop selective attachment relationships is a characteristic feature of children with RAD. Social neglect is the most important underlying cause for RAD, and the onset of symptoms is before 5 years of age.

Etiology

Severe social neglect of children in institutional care, overcrowded placements where the child did not receive nurturing care from the primary caregiver, or in families where parents have a mental illness and, therefore, are unable to emotionally relate to the child, all of the above scenarios can lead to social and emotional deprivation in children, and increase the risk of developing RAD. Gradually, these children turn inward and stop seeking comfort from the caregiver when distressed. Due to disruption in the emotional nurturing and responsive caregiving, these children have social, emotional, and cognitive delays as well as behavioral dysfunction.[72]

The neurobiological basis of RAD needs to be studied more, and there is no conclusive evidence to date. Few neuroimaging studies[73,74] have reported reductions in grey and white matter volumes in institutionalized children, however, this is not specific to RAD.

Prevalence

Pritchett R et al.,[75] in their study, reported a prevalence of RAD to be 1–2%. The prevalence of RAD comes from studies of children adopted out of institutional care or foster care homes. Even in this high-risk population group, the rate of attachment disorders is <10%, and RAD was less common compared to the DSED. The Bucharest Early Intervention Project highlighted that children who were in institutional care for longer periods had more stable symptoms.[76]

Symptoms of Reactive Attachment Disorder

The symptoms of RAD can be different and varied in every child. The most common symptoms include avoiding physical contact, limited eye contact, inability to experience positive emotions like joy and comfort in interactions with the primary caregiver and are also fearful and irritable on most occasions.

In addition to the above symptoms, Stinehart et al.[77] described a few symptoms like feeding difficulties, failure to gain weight, lack of empathy, and poor impulse control behaviors in children with RAD. The DSM criteria for RAD are as below **(Box 4)**.[24]

Assessment and Diagnosis

A comprehensive biopsychosocial history and structured observation of the child-caregiver interaction are essential. The "Disturbances of Attachment Interview" can also be used to obtain additional information.[78]

Comorbidity in Reactive Attachment Disorder

The comorbidity in RAD can be described in three age groups, namely, 0–3 years, 4–6 years, and 7–9 years. Developmental disorders of speech and language and ASD is common in 0–3 years of age. In the 4–6 years age group, behavioral and emotional disorders, attention-deficit hyperactivity disorder, anxiety disorder,

BOX 4: Fifth Diagnostic and Statistical Manual for Psychiatric Disorders (DSM-5) criteria—Reactive Attachment Disorder.

- The patient demonstrates a chronic pattern of being emotionally withdrawn and inhibited, which is demonstrated by rarely seeking or responsive to comfort when distressed
- There is evidence of a chronic social and/or emotional perturbation, responsiveness to others, negative effect, unfounded or inexplicable episodes of irritability, fearfulness, or sadness—or out of proportion reactions to normative stress.
- The patient presents with a history of extremely insufficient care, entailing of one of the following: deprivation or social neglect of basic emotional needs for stimulation, comfort, and affection by caring caregivers; the constant flux of caregivers, resulting in a destabilized home environment; growing up in an unusual setting which limits the ability to form selective attachments.
- The child cannot also meet the diagnostic criteria for autism spectrum disorder as the two diagnoses (autism spectrum disorder and reactive attachment disorder) are mutually exclusive.
- The behavioral perturbation should manifest prior to the age of 5 years of age.
- The child must have a developmental age of at least 9 months in order to qualify for the diagnosis.

affective disorder, enuresis, and encopresis were common comorbid conditions. Children aged 7–9 years had comorbid conduct disorder, reaction to severe stress, adjustment disorder, and tic disorder.[79]

Differential Diagnosis

Autism spectrum disorder, intellectual disabilities, and depressive disorders should be considered as differential diagnoses of RAD.[78]

Treatment

Children with RAD when placed in nurturing caregiving environments show steady improvement in symptoms. Child-parent psychotherapy, circle of security, attachment and biobehavioral catch-up are interventions that improve the emotional communication between the child and the caregiver and help in the development of secure attachment between parents and young children who have experienced adversity.[80-82]

DISINHIBITED SOCIAL ENGAGEMENT DISORDER

Disinhibited social engagement disorder is an attachment disorder, in which children are socially disinhibited, overly familiar with stranger adults, do not check if the caregiver is present when venturing out, and have history of early childhood adversities and difficulty in forming selective stable attachments with caregivers. They are impulsive and violate verbal and physical boundaries. Some theories suggest that this indiscriminate social behavior is an adaptive mechanism in the context of significant emotional deprivation.[83] They seek contact as they did not receive nurturing care from their caregivers.

Etiology

Multiple factors have been implicated in the causation of DSED, namely, genetic factors, biological factors, cognitive factors, attachment status, and degree and length of deprivation.[84]

Soares et al. had implicated that children with socially indiscriminate behaviors can have specific polymorphisms within the Williams syndrome critical region. There are individual differences noted in the responsiveness to changes in the caregiving environment, and this has been associated with the functional polymorphisms in the serotonin transporter gene and brain-derived neurotrophic factor.[85]

Stunting of growth, cognitive delay, and indiscriminate social behavior—all can be seen to arise in children who come from impoverished backgrounds, but a causal relationship with DSED cannot be established.

Prevalence

The epidemiology of DSED has not been studied extensively. The Bucharest Early Intervention Project reported that the signs of DSED remained moderately stable between the ages of 30 and 54 months among children with a history of institutional rearing. Stability of the symptoms was higher in children who were continuously in institutionalized care.[86]

Symptoms of Disinhibited Social Engagement Disorder

The symptoms that are commonly seen in children with DSED include, wandering away from the caregiver, no anxiety in leaving the parent and willing to go with strangers, lack the inhibition or fear on meeting strangers, being overfamiliar with strangers, increased levels of hyperactivity, impulsivity and poor motor skills, and social functioning **(Box 5)**.

Assessment and Diagnosis

Detailed history and structured interview regarding the attachment patterns are essential. Observation of the child-caregiver dyadic interactions is very useful in analyzing attachment patterns.

"Attachment Formation Rating Scale and Disinhibited Social Behavior Observational Measure.[87] "Waiting Room Observation (WRO)" is a quick and easy observational scale.[88]

Differential Diagnosis

Attention-deficit/hyperactivity disorder is a common differential diagnosis, that needs to be ruled out.

Treatment

Sensitive, responsive caregiving and nurturance can decrease the symptoms of DSED and promote the development of stable and secure attachments.[3] Emphasising social boundaries and ensuring safety are essential.

Evidence-based interventions that promote attachment can be effectively used in children with DSED. Child-parent psychotherapy, Attachment and Biobehavioral Catch-up, Video-feedback Intervention to Promote Positive Parenting and Sensitive Discipline, and Circle of

BOX 5: Fifth Diagnostic and Statistical Manual for Psychiatric Disorders (DSM-5) criteria—Disinhibited Social Engagement Disorder.

A. A pattern of behavior in which a child actively approaches and interacts with unfamiliar adults and exhibits at least two of the following:
   1. Reduced or absent reticence in approaching and interacting with unfamiliar adults. Overly familiar verbal or physical behavior (that is not consistent with culturally sanctioned and with age-appropriate social boundaries)
   2. Diminished or absent checking back with adult caregiver after venturing away, even in unfamiliar settings. Willingness to go off with an unfamiliar adult with minimal or no hesitation

B. The behaviors in Criterion A are not limited to impulsivity (as in attention-deficit/hyperactivity disorder) but include socially disinhibited behavior

C. The child has experienced a pattern of extremes of insufficient care as evidenced by at least one of the following:
   - Social neglect or deprivation in the form of persistent lack of having basic emotional needs for comfort, stimulation, and affection met by caregiving adults
   - Repeated changes of primary caregivers that limit opportunities to form stable attachments (e.g., frequent changes in foster care). Rearing in unusual settings that severely limits opportunities to form selective attachments (e.g., institutions with high child-to-caregiver ratios)

D. The care in Criterion C is presumed to be responsible for the disturbed behavior in Criterion A (e.g., the disturbances in Criterion A began following the pathogenic care in Criterion C)

E. The child has a developmental age of at least 9 months (APA, 2013a)

Security can be used, but it must be noted that none of these approaches has clear guidelines for the treatment of DSED.

FUTURE DIRECTIONS

The classification of attachment disorders has been based on the phenotypic presentation, course, and response to treatment. However there needs to be further studies looking into the differential risk factors involved in developing one disorder over the other. A deeper understanding of the trajectories of the RAD and DSED can help in assessing long-term outcomes, and help in framing preventive programs, and early interventions.

Take Home Points

- DSM-5 classifies attachment disorder as a trauma and stressor-related condition of early childhood that is caused due to social neglect or maltreatment.
- Reactive attachment disorder and disinhibited social engagement disorder are common presentations.
- In RAD, the child is very emotionally withdrawn and inhibited, and, in DSED, the child is indiscriminately social and disinhibited.
- Early identification and intervention are key to better prognosis.
- Safe environment and nurturing and responsive caregiving are of paramount importance.
- Evidence-based interventions that promote attachment can be effectively used in children with attachment disorders, such as child-parent psychotherapy, attachment and biobehavioral catch-up, video-feedback intervention, and circle of security.

ADJUSTMENT DISORDER IN CHILDREN

INTRODUCTION

Adjustment disorder is an unhealthy or maladaptive emotional or behavioral response to a stressful event or change in a person's life. The reaction occurs within 3 months of the stressful event. Change of place, death of a close relative, parent or sibling, chronic illness in a family member, parental separation, or bullying, can serve as a trigger. Adjustment disorders are listed in the category of trauma and stress-related disorders, in the DSM-5.

Adjustment disorder can be seen in children following a stressor or a significant life event, and presents with symptoms of depression, anxiety, or conduct symptoms, causing significant impairment in functioning.

EPIDEMIOLOGY

Adjustment disorder is said to be common in children and adolescents, but the prevalence rates are varied, depending on the setting, criteria, and measures used for the diagnosis.

In a study done by Maercker et al.,[89] 0.9% of the adolescents were found to have adjustment disorder. Bird et al.,[90] in their study, reported a prevalence of 4.2% in the Puerto Rican children. Higher incidence rates have been reported in clinic settings and emergency department presentations. Mulligan A et al.,[91] in their study, reported that 30% of the adolescents presenting to the emergency department have a diagnosis of adjustment disorder.

Children with chronic medical illness had higher incidence rates of adjustment disorder. LeBlanc LA et al.,[92] in their study, showed that the rates of adjustment disorder varied from 36 to 60% in children and adolescents with chronic medical illnesses like diabetes.

ETIOLOGY

The presence of a stressor is required to make a diagnosis of adjustment disorder, but the stressor

BOX 6: Fifth Diagnostic and Statistical Manual for Psychiatric Disorders (DSM-5)—diagnostic criteria for Adjustment Disorder.

A. The development of emotional or behavioral symptoms in response to an identifiable stressor(s) occurring within 3 months of the onset of the stressor(s)

B. These symptoms or behaviors are clinically significant, as evidenced by one or both of the following:
1. Marked distress that is out of proportion to the severity or intensity of the stressor, taking into account the external context and the cultural factors that might influence symptom severity and presentation.
2. Significant impairment in social, occupational, or other important areas of functioning

C. The stress-related disturbance does not meet the criteria for another mental disorder and is not merely an exacerbation of a pre-existing mental disorder.

D. The symptoms do not represent normal bereavement.

E. Once the stressor or its consequences have terminated the symptoms do not persist for more than an additional 6 months.

Adjustment disorder can have varied presentations, hence has six subtypes, namely:

(1) With depressed mood, (2) With anxiety, (3) With mixed anxiety and depressed mood, (4) With disturbance of conduct, (5) With mixed disturbance of emotions and conduct, and (6) Unspecified category.

can be any difficult situation or life event. When the stress is over and above what the child can manage, when it overwhelms the child's coping mechanism, then it results in emotional and behavioral disturbance. It must be understood that not all children having stressors develop, this is due to the individual and environmental factors that mediate the impact of stress on the individual. Some stressors are manageable, can be tolerated and overcome with the individual coping and the care and support from a responsive adult.[93]

The individual factors that affect response to stress include the temperament of the child, cognitive ability, coping, and problem-solving skills. Responsive parenting, a favorable family environment, and good social support are protective against adverse stress responses.[94,95]

The common stressors include stressors at home, at school, with peers, and stressors in the larger community. Bullying at school, change of school, academic difficulties, problems with teachers, and relationship issues are common stressors. Problems in the primary support group, parental separation or divorce, and illness or death of a parent or caregiver can lead to adjustment-related problems in children and adolescents. Chronic medical illness in the child or adolescent can also adversely affect them and lead to adjustment disorders **(Box 6)**.[24]

ADJUSTMENT DISORDER: DSM-5 VERSUS ICD-11

The ICD-11 criteria for adjustment disorder bring a greater specificity to the symptom requirements, indicating a preoccupation with the stressor, excessive worry, recurrent distressing thoughts, or rumination about the stressor. The symptom onset is within 1 month of the stressor, and functional impairment is also present. The subtypes of adjustment disorder have been eliminated.[96]

CLINICAL PRESENTATION OF ADJUSTMENT DISORDER

Children and adolescents can present with varied symptoms following a stressor. Symptoms can include sadness, anxiety, irritability, social withdrawal, difficulty in concentrating, changes in sleep and appetite, and academic or behavioral issues. This follows a significant stressor, and there is functional impairment as well.

Adjustment Disorders—Controversies

Adjustment disorder is diagnosed when there are subthreshold depressive, anxiety, or other emotional symptoms, in the context of a clear stressor. However, it cannot be diagnosed when the depressive symptoms are severe enough to qualify for a depressive disorder. This makes it difficult to rationalize as the symptom severity and the functioning can be equally affected in both conditions.[97]

Pelkonen M et al.,[98] in their study, reported that 25% of adolescents with a diagnosis of adjustment disorder engage in suicidal behavior. Moreover, up to one-third of the young people who die by suicide have a diagnosis of adjustment disorder.[99] Therefore, calling it a mild disorder may not be correct as it has a significant effect on the behavior.

Adjustment disorder is said to occur in the context of a stressor, but all reactions of distress following a stressful event cannot be labeled as adjustment disorder, as there is a risk of medicalizing even normal reactions to stress. Therefore, understanding the culture, and personal attributes to cope with stress, is essential in making a diagnosis of adjustment disorder.[100]

Assessments

A detailed history focusing on the symptoms, stressors, and the temporal correlation is essential. History regarding the child's temperament, coping and problem-solving skills, and resilience will help in addressing the stressors with appropriate supportive interventions. Relationship with parents, family, and social support also needs to be assessed. This will help in the diagnostic formulation and making a clear treatment plan.

Differential Diagnosis

The most common differential diagnoses for adjustment disorder are mood disorder, anxiety disorder, disruptive behavior disorder like oppositional defiant disorder, conduct disorder, or post-traumatic stress disorder.

Treatment

The main goal of treatment in adjustment disorder is to decrease emotional and behavioral disturbance and improve psychosocial functioning. Psychotherapy is the mainstay of treatment. We need to work with the child on providing simple strategies for stress management, enhancing their coping skills, building problem-solving skills, and fostering resilience.

Depressive and anxiety symptoms can be addressed with cognitive behavior therapy. The core components of which are, psychoeducation, behavioral activation, cognitive restructuring, and problem-solving.[95] Mindfulness-based therapies have been shown to be effective in adults with adjustment disorder, however, need to be researched in children and adolescents.[101]

Parents play a pivotal role in management; psychoeducating them about the stressor and its impact, can help to empower them to work with their child on improving coping skills and promoting recovery.[102]

Addressing the stressor and identifying the precipitating and perpetuating factors and removing them may help in symptom reduction and functional recovery as well.

Pharmacological interventions do not have a well-established evidence base in the treatment of adjustment disorders. SSRI's and benzodiazepines have been used to manage anxiety and depressive symptoms in adjustment disorders, and have been clinically helpful in symptom reduction, but overall impairment and functioning needs to be addressed with nonpharmacological strategies.

SUMMARY AND CONCLUSION

Adjustment disorder is relatively common in children and adolescents, and early identification and management are needed. Empowering primary care physicians and pediatricians to identify and intervene early will decrease the burden of the problem.

Take Home Points

- Adjustment disorder is an unhealthy or maladaptive emotional or behavioral response to a stressful event or change in a person's life. The reaction occurs within 3 months of the stressful event.
- Adjustment disorder is said to be common in children and adolescents.
- Individual and environmental factors mediate the impact of stress on the child.
- Children can present with sadness, anxiety, irritability, social withdrawal, difficulty concentrating, changes in sleep and appetite, and academic or behavioral issues.
- Significant functional impairment is seen.
- Identifying the stressor, decreasing the stress, and working on resilience and functional recovery is essential.

REFERENCES

1. Stein DJ, Craske MA, Friedman MJ, Phillips KA. Anxiety disorders, obsessive-compulsive and related disorders, trauma- and stressor-related disorders, and dissociative disorders in DSM-5. Am J Psychiatry. 2014;171(6):611-3.
2. Windsor J, Benigno JP, Wing CA, Carroll PJ, Koga SF, Nelson CA 3rd, et al. Effect of foster care on young children's language learning. Child Dev. 2011;82:1040-6.
3. Thakur A, Creedon J, Zeanah CH. Trauma- and Stressor-Related Disorders Among Children and Adolescents. Focus (Am Psychiatr Publ). 2016;14(1):34-45.
4. Copeland WE, Keeler G, Angold A, Costello EJ. Traumatic events and posttraumatic stress in childhood. Arch Gen Psychiatry. 2007;64:577-84.
5. Kar N, Mohapatra PK, Nayak KC, Pattanaik P, Swain SP, Kar HC. Post-traumatic stress disorder in children and adolescents one year after a super-cyclone in Orissa, India: exploring cross-cultural validity and vulnerability factors. BMC Psychiatry. 2007;7:8.
6. John PB, Russell S, Russell PS. The prevalence of posttraumatic stress disorder among children and adolescents affected by tsunami disaster in Tamil Nadu. Disaster Manag Response. 2007; 5(1):3-7.
7. de Jong K, Kam SV, Ford N, Lokuge K, Fromm S, van Galen R, et al. Conflict in the Indian Kashmir Valley II: Psychosocial impact. Confl Health. 2008;2:11.
8. Margoob MA, Firdosi MM, Banal R, Khan AY, Malik YA, Ahmad SA, et al. Community prevalence of trauma in south asia—experience from Kashmir. JK-Practitioner. 2006;13(suppl 1):s14-7.
9. Mathew G, Varghese AD, Sabu AM, Joseph A. Screening for post-traumatic stress disorder among adolescents following floods—a comparative study from private and public schools in Kerala, India. BMC Pediatr. 2021; 21:462.
10. Sowmya BT, Seshadri SP, Srinath S, Girimaji S, Sagar JV. Clinical characteristics of children presenting with history of sexual abuse to a tertiary care centre in India. Asian J Psychiatry. 2016;19:44-9.
11. McLaughlin K, Brent DA, Friedman M. Post-traumatic stress disorder in children and adolescents: Epidemiology, clinical features, assessment, and diagnosis. UpToDate. 2025.
12. Scheeringa MS, Zeanah CH, Myers L, Putnam FW. Predictive validity in a prospective follow-up of PTSD in preschool children. J Am Acad Child Adolesc Psychiatry. 2005;44:899-906.
13. Charney DS, Deutch AY, Krystal JH, Southwick SM, Davis M. Psychobiologic mechanisms of posttraumatic stress disorder. Arch Gen Psychiatry. 1993;50:295-305.
14. Heim C, Nemeroff CB. Neurobiology of post-traumatic stress disorder. CNS Spectr. 2009; 14(1 Suppl 1):13-24.
15. Jovanovic T, Norrholm SD. Neural mechanisms of impaired fear inhibition in posttraumatic stress disorder. Front Behav Neurosci. 2011;5:44.
16. Milad MR, Quirk GJ. Fear extinction as a model for translational neuroscience: ten years of progress. Annu Rev Psychol. 2012;63:129.
17. Rauch SL, Shin LM, Phelps EA. Neurocircuitry models of posttraumatic stress disorder and extinction: human neuroimaging research—past, present, and future. Biol Psychiatry. 2006;60:376.

18. Pitman RK, Rasmusson AM, Koenen KC, Shin LM, Orr SP, Gilbertson MW, et al. Biological studies of post-traumatic stress disorder. Nat Rev Neurosci. 2012;13:769-87.
19. Etkin A, Wager TD. Functional neuroimaging of anxiety: a meta-analysis of emotional processing in PTSD, social anxiety disorder, and specific phobia. Am J Psychiatry. 2007;164:1476.
20. Shin LM, Wright CI, Cannistraro PA, Wedig MM, McMullin K, Martis B, et al. A functional magnetic resonance imaging study of amygdala and medial prefrontal cortex responses to overtly presented fearful faces in posttraumatic stress disorder. Arch Gen Psychiatry. 2005;62:273-81.
21. Rauch SL, Whalen PJ, Shin LM, McInerney SC, Macklin ML, Lasko NB, et al. Exaggerated amygdala response to masked facial stimuli in posttraumatic stress disorder: a functional MRI study. Biol Psychiatry. 2000;47:769-76.
22. Shin LM, Whalen PJ, Pitman RK, Bush G, Macklin ML, Lasko NB, et al. An fMRI study of anterior cingulate function in posttraumatic stress disorder. Biol Psychiatry. 2001;50:932.
23. Kitayama N, Vaccarino V, Kutner M, Weiss P, Bremner JD. Magnetic resonance imaging (MRI) measurement of hippocampal volume in posttraumatic stress disorder: a meta-analysis. J Affect Disord. 2005;88:79-86.
24. American Psychiatric Association. Diagnostic and statistical manual of mental disorders, 5th edition. Arlington, VA: American Psychiatric Association; 2013.
25. De Young AC, Scheeringa MS. PTSD in children 6 years and younger. In: Stoddard FJ Jr, Benedek DM, Milad MR, Ursano RJ (Eds). Trauma- and stressor-related disorders. Oxford: Oxford University Press; 2018. pp. 85-102.
26. McLaughlin KA, Koenen KC, Hill ED, Petukhova M, Sampson NA, Zaslavsky AM, et al. Trauma exposure and posttraumatic stress disorder in a national sample of adolescents. J Am Acad Child Adolesc Psychiatry. 2013;52:815-30.e14.
27. Lewis SJ, Arseneault L, Caspi A, Fisher HL, Matthews T, Moffitt TE, et al. The epidemiology of trauma and post-traumatic stress disorder in a representative cohort of young people in England and Wales. Lancet Psychiatry. 2019;6: 247-56.
28. Trickey D, Siddaway AP, Meiser-Stedman R, Serpell L, Field AP. A meta-analysis of risk factors for post-traumatic stress disorder in children and adolescents. Clin Psychol Rev. 2012;32:122-38.
29. Brady KT, Killeen TK, Brewerton T, Lucerini S. Comorbidity of psychiatric disorders and posttraumatic stress disorder. J Clin Psychiatry. 2000;61(7):22-32.
30. Nader, K., Kriegler, K. A., Blake, D. D., Pynoos, R. S., Newman, E., & Weathers, F. W. (1996). Clinician-Administered PTSD Scale For Children and Adolescents (CAPS-CA) [Database record]. APA PsycTests. 1996.
31. Levendosky A, Huth-Bocks A, Semel M, Shapiro D. Trauma symptoms in preschool-age children exposed to domestic violence. J Interpers Violence. 2002;17(2):150-64.
32. Dehon C, Scheeringa M. Screening for preschool posttraumatic stress disorder with the Child Behavior Checklist. J Pediatr Psychol. 2005;31(4):431-5.
33. Briere J. Trauma Symptom Checklist for Children (TSCC). Odessa, FL: Psychological Assessment Resources; 1996.
34. Cohen JA. Practice Parameter for the Assessment and Treatment of Children and Adolescents With Posttraumatic Stress Disorder. J Am Acad Child Adolesc Psychiatry. 2010;49(4):414-30.
35. Cohen JA, Deblinger E, Mannarino AP, Steer R. A multisite, randomized controlled trial for children with sexual abuse-related PTSD symptoms. J Am Acad Child Adolesc Psychiatry. 2004;43(4):393-402.
36. Lieberman AF, Van Horn P, Ippen CG. Toward evidence-based treatment: Child Parent Psychotherapy with preschoolers exposed to marital violence. J Am Acad Child Adolesc Psychiatry. 2005;44(12):1241-8.
37. Margoob MA, Ali Z, Andrade C. Efficacy of ECT in chronic, severe, antidepressant- and CBT-refractory PTSD: an open, prospective study. Brain Stimul. 2010;3(1):28-35.
38. Torrico TJ, Mikes BA. Posttraumatic Stress Disorder in Children. In: StatPearls [Internet]. Treasure Island (FL): StatPearls Publishing; 2024.
39. Bonanno GA, Kaltman S. The varieties of grief experience. Clin Psychol Rev. 2001;21(5):705-34.

40. Sanghvi P. Grief in children and adolescents: a review. Indian J Mental Health. 2020;7(1):6.
41. Weaver D. Parental mortality and outcomes among minor and adult children. Popul Rev. 2019;58:2.
42. Nader K, Salloum A. Complicated grief reactions in children and adolescents. J Child Adolesc Trauma. 2011;4(3):233-57.
43. Cerel J, Fristad MA, Verducci J, Weller RA, Weller EB. Childhood bereavement: Psychopathology in the 2 years postparental death. J Am Acad Child Adolesc Psychiatry. 2006;45(6):681-90.
44. Keyes KM, Pratt C, Galea S, McLaughlin KA, Koenen KC, Shear MK. The burden of loss: Unexpected death of a loved one and psychiatric disorders across the life course in a national study. Am J Psychiatry. 2014;171(8):864-71.
45. Kaplow JB, Saunders J, Angold A, Costello EJ. Psychiatric symptoms in bereaved versus non-bereaved youth and young adults: A longitudinal epidemiological study. J Am Acad Child Adolesc Psychiatry. 2010;49(11):1145-54.
46. Hill RM, Kaplow JB, Oosterhoff B, Layne CM. Understanding grief reactions, thwarted belongingness, and suicide ideation in bereaved adolescents: Toward a unifying theory. J Clin Psychol. 2019;75(4):780-93.
47. Venkatesan S. Loss, grief, bereavement, mourning in children. Int J Recent Sci Res. 2022;13[03(B)]:619-24.
48. Doka KJ. Disenfranchised grief. Bereavement Care. 1999;18(3):37-9.
49. Alvis L, Zhang N, Sandler IN, Kaplow JB. Developmental Manifestations of Grief in Children and Adolescents: Caregivers as Key Grief Facilitators. J Child Adolesc Trauma. 2023;16:447-57.
50. Prigerson HG, Boelen PA, Xu J, Smith KV, Maciejewski PK. Validation of the new DSM-5-TR criteria for prolonged grief disorder and the PG-13-Revised (PG-13-R) scale. World Psychiatry. 2021;20(1):96-106.
51. Dillen L, Fontaine JRJ, Verhofstadt-Denève L. Confirming the distinctiveness of complicated grief from depression and anxiety among adolescents. Death Studies. 2009;33(5):437-61.
52. Spuij M, Reitz E, Prinzie P, Stikkelbroek Y, de Roos C, Boelen PA. Distinctiveness of symptoms of prolonged grief, depression, and post-traumatic stress in bereaved children and adolescents. Eur Child Adolesc Psychiatry. 2012;21(12):673-9.
53. Kentor RA, Kaplow JB. Supporting children and adolescents following parental bereavement: Guidance for healthcare professionals. Lancet Child Adolesc Health. 2020;4(12):889-98.
54. Kübler-Ross E, Kessler D. On grief and grieving: Finding the meaning of grief through the five stages of loss. New York: Simon & Schuster; 2005.
55. Tyrrell P, Harberger S, Siddiqui W. Kubler-Ross Stages of Dying and Subsequent Models of Grief. In: StatPearls [Internet]. Treasure Island (FL): StatPearls Publishing; 2025.
56. Kaplow JB, Layne CM. Sudden loss and psychiatric disorders across the life course: Toward a developmental lifespan theory of bereavement-related risk and resilience. Am J Psychiatry. 2014;171(8):807-10.
57. Layne CM, Kaplow JB, Oosterhoff B, Hill RM, Pynoos RS. The interplay between posttraumatic stress and grief reactions in traumatically bereaved adolescents: When trauma, bereavement, and adolescence converge. Adolesc Psychiatry. 2017;7(4):266-85.
58. Lerner RM, Brindis CD, Batanova M, Blum RW. Adolescent health development: A relational developmental systems perspective. In: Halfon N, Forrest CB, Lerner RM (Eds). Handbook of Life Course Health Development. Cham (CH): Springer; 2018. pp. 109-21.
59. Kaplow JB, Layne CM, Pynoos RS, Cohen J, Lieberman A. DSM-V diagnostic criteria for bereavement-related disorders in children and adolescents: Developmental considerations. Psychiatry. 2012;75(3):242-65.
60. Solomon RM. (2024). 'The "R" Processes of Mourning', EMDR Therapy Treatment for Grief and Mourning: Transforming the Connection to the Deceased Loved One (Oxford, 2024; online edition, Oxford Academic, 21 Mar. 2024). [online] Available from https://doi.org/10.1093/oso/9780198881360.003.0010. [Last accessed 20 November, 2025].
61. Stroebe M, Schut H. The dual process model of coping with bereavement: rationale and description. Death Studies. 1999;23(3):197-224.

62. Doka KJ, Martin TL. Grieving Beyond Gender, Understanding the Ways Men and Women Mourn, Revised Edition. London, United Kingdom: Routledge; 2024.
63. Emswiler M, Emswiler J. Guiding Your Child Through Grief. New York, NY: Bantam Books; 2000.
64. Panagiotaki G, Nobes G, Ashraf A, Aubby H. British and Pakistani children's understanding of death: cultural and developmental influences. Br J Dev Psychol. 2015;33(1):31-44.
65. Schonfeld DJ. Talking with children about death. J Pediatr Health Care. 1993;7(6):269-74.
66. Schonfeld DJ, Demaria T. AAP Committee on psychosocial aspects of child and family health, disaster preparedness advisory council. Supporting the Grieving Child and Family. Pediatrics. 2016;138(3):e20162147.
67. Cohen JA, Mannarino AP. Supporting children with traumatic grief: What educators need to know. School Psychol Int. 2011;32(2):117-31.
68. Zhang T, Krysinska K, Alisic E, Andriessen K. Grief Instruments in Children and Adolescents: A Systematic Review. Omega (Westport). 2025;91(4):2183-225.
69. Worden JW. Grief counselling and grief therapy: A handbook for the mental health practitioner. New York City: Springer Publishing Company; 2018.
70. Fox GC, Reid GE, Salmon A, Mckillop-Duffy P, Doyle C. Criteria for traumatic grief and PTSD. Br J Psychiatry. 1999;174(6):560-6.
71. Bowlby J. Attachment and Loss: Vol. 1. Loss. New York: Basic Books. 1969.
72. Spratt EG, Friedenberg SL, Swenson CC, Larosa A, De Bellis MD, Macias MM, et al. The Effects of Early Neglect on Cognitive, Language, and Behavioral Functioning in Childhood. Psychology (Irvine). 2012;3(2):175-82
73. Sheridan MA, Fox NA, Zeanah CH, McLaughlin KA, Nelson CA 3rd. Variation in neural development as a result of exposure to institutionalization early in childhood. Proc Natl Acad Sci USA. 2012;109:12927-32.
74. Bick J, Zhu T, Stamoulis C, Fox NA, Zeanah C, Nelson CA. Effect of early institutionalization and foster care on long-term white matter development: a randomized clinical trial. JAMA Pediatr. 2015;169:211-9.
75. Pritchett R, Pritchett J, Marshall E, Davidson C, Minnis H. Reactive attachment disorder in the general population: a hidden ESSENCE disorder. Sci World J. 2013;2013:818157.
76. Smyke AT, Zeanah CH, Gleason MM, Drury SS, Fox NA, Nelson CA, et al. A randomized controlled trial comparing foster care and institutional care for children with signs of reactive attachment disorder. Am J Psychiatry. 2012;169:508-14.
77. Stinehart M, Scott DA, Barfield HG. Reactive attachment disorder in adopted and foster care children: implications for mental health professionals. Fam J. 2012;20(4):335-60.
78. Zeanah CH, Smyke AT. Attachment disorders and severe deprivation. In: Rutter M, Bishop D, Pine D (Eds). Rutter's Child and Adolescent Psychiatry, 6th edition. London: Blackwell Publishing; 2018.
79. Hong M, Moon DS, Chang H, Lee SY, Cho SW, Lee KS, et al. Incidence and Comorbidity of Reactive Attachment Disorder: Based on National Health Insurance Claims Data, 2010-2012 in Korea. Psychiatry Investig. 2018;15(2):118-23.
80. Berlin LJ, Zeanah CH, Lieberman AF. Prevention and intervention programs for supporting early attachment security. In: Cassidy J, Shaver PR (Eds). Handbook of Attachment, 3rd edition. New York: Guilford Press; 2018.
81. Powell B, Cooper G, Hoffman K, Marvin B, Zeanah J. The Circle of Security Intervention: Enhancing Attachment in Early Parent-Child Relationships. New York: Guilford Press; 2013.
82. Ellis EE, Yilanli M, Saadabadi A. Reactive Attachment Disorder. [Updated 2023 May 1]. In: StatPearls [Internet]. Treasure Island (FL): StatPearls Publishing; 2024.
83. Chisholm K. A three-year follow-up of attachment and indiscriminate friendliness in children adopted from Romanian orphanages. Development and Psychopathology. 1998;10:607-23.
84. Zeanah CH, Gleason MM. Annual Research Review: attachment disorders in early childhood—clinical presentation, causes, correlates, and treatment. J Child Psychol Psychiatry. 2015;56:207-22.

84. Soares I, Belsky J, Mesquita AR, Osório A, Sampaio A. Why do only some institutionalized children become indiscriminately friendly? Insights from the study of Williams Syndrome. Child Dev Perspect. 2013;7:1-6.
85. Drury SS, Gleason MM, Theall KP, Smyke AT, Nelson CA, Fox NA, et al. Genetic sensitivity to the caregiving context: the influence of 5httlpr and BDNF val66met on indiscriminate social behavior. Physiol Behav. 2012;106:728-35.
86. Gleason MM, Fox NA, Drury S, Smyke A, Egger HL, Nelson CA 3rd, et al. Validity of evidence-derived criteria for reactive attachment disorder: indiscriminately social/disinhibited and emotionally withdrawn/inhibited types. J Am Acad Child Adolesc Psychiatry. 2011;50:216-31.
87. Bruce J, Tarullo AR, Gunnar MR. Disinhibited social behaviour among internationally adopted children. Develop Psychopathol. 2009;21:157-71.
88. McLaughlin A, Espie C, Minnis H. Development of a Brief Waiting Room Observation for Behaviours Typical of Reactive Attachment Disorder. Child Adolesc Ment Health. 2010;15(2):73-9.
89. Maercker A, Forstmeier S, Pielmaier L, Spangenberg L, Brähler E, Glaesmer H. Adjustment disorders: prevalence in a representative nationwide survey in Germany. Soc Psychiatry Psychiatr Epidemiol 2012;47:1745-52.
90. Bird HR, Gould MS, Yager T, Staghezza B, Canino G. Risk factors for maladjustment in Puerto Rican children. J Am Acad Child Adolesc Psychiatry. 1989;28:847-50.
91. Mulligan A. Adjustment disorders in child and adolescent psychiatry. In: Casey P (Ed). Adjustment Disorder: From Controversy to Clinical Practice. Oxford: Oxford Academic Press: 2018.
92. LeBlanc LA, Goldsmith T, Patel DR. Behavioral aspects of chronic illness in children and adolescents. Pediatr Clin North Am. 2003;50: 859-78.
93. Shonkoff JP, Garner AS; Committee on Psychosocial Aspects of Child and Family Health; Committee on Early Childhood, Adoption, and Dependent Care; Section on Developmental and Behavioral Pediatrics. The lifelong effects of early childhood adversity and toxic stress. Pediatrics. 2012;129:e232-46.
94. Newcorn JH, Strain J. Adjustment disorder in children and adolescents. J Am Acad Child Adolesc Psychiatry. 1992;31:318-26.
95. Alvarado GL. Adjustment disorder in the pediatric population. Pediatr Med. 2022;5:19.
96. International Classification of Diseases, Eleventh Revision (ICD-11), World Health Organization (WHO) 2019
97. Casey P, Maracy M, Kelly BD, Lehtinen V, Ayuso-Mateos JL, Dalgard OS, et al. Can adjustment disorder and depressive episode be distinguished? Results from ODIN. J Affect Disord. 2006;92:291-7.
98. Pelkonen M, Marttunen M, Henriksson M, Lönnqvist J. Suicidality in adjustment disorder, clinical characteristics of adolescent outpatients. Eur Child Adolesc Psychiatry. 2005;14:174-80.
99. Lönnqvist JK, Henriksson MM, Isometsä ET, Marttunen MJ, Heikkinen ME, Aro HM, et al. Mental disorders and suicide prevention. Psychiatry Clin Neurosci. 1995;49:S111-6.
100. Casey P, Bailey S. Adjustment disorders: the state of the art. World Psychiatry. 2011;10:11-8.
101. O'Donnell ML, Metcalf O, Watson L, Phelps A, Varker T. A systematic review of psychological and pharmacological treatments for adjustment disorder in adults: Review of treatments for adjustment disorder. J Trauma Stress. 2018;31:321-31.
102. Shaw RJ, DeMaso DR. Clinical manual of pediatric psychosomatic medicine: Mental health consultation with physically ill children and adolescents. Washington, DC: American Psychiatric Publishing; 2007.

CHAPTER 19

Deliberate Self-Harm and Suicide

Pratap Sharan, Nishtha Chawla, Sarthak Kukreja

INTRODUCTION

Suicide has been known to occur since antiquity. The meaning, perspectives, modes, and motives for suicide vary across nations, religions, and cultures, e.g., from being considered acceptable (e.g., *"Sati"* or *"Samadhi"* or *"Kamikaze"* or "Medically assisted suicide") to being considered unacceptable or even punishable at different times in different societies.[1]

Suicide and self-harm are major public health concerns across the globe with suicide being one of the leading causes of death among adolescents. A characteristic of suicides in India sets it apart from the age-specific rates in the majority of other nations—the first peak of suicide rates in India occurs among those aged 15–24.[2] Further, unlike the West, psychosocial factors play a major role in contributing to suicides in India compared to psychiatric illnesses, which could possibly be due to significantly higher psychosocial stressors for the vulnerable population such as young women and minorities.

Deliberate self-harm (DSH) is another phenomenon closely resembling suicide but is often associated with little or no intent to die and comes under the umbrella of maladaptive coping mechanisms to underlying distress. While DSH and suicide share the common ground of emotional distress and psychological pain, DSH is typically a nonfatal act intended to manage overwhelming emotions, whereas suicide involves the intent to end one's life.

In this chapter, we discuss definitions, epidemiological patterns and risk factors, and assessment and management of these conditions (suicide and DSH), with a focus on children and adolescents in the Indian context.

DEFINITION

Different terms have been used to understand suicide and self-harm.[3] *Suicidality* is a broad term which often encompasses thoughts or behaviors (actions as well as omissions) of a person aimed toward ending her/his own life. *Suicidal behaviors* entail a spectrum ranging from suicidal ideations, planning of suicide, attempting suicide, and suicide itself.[4] *Suicide* is the act carried out by an individual intentionally to end his/her life. *Suicide attempt* is a nonfatal act or preparation on the part of an individual with the intent of killing himself/herself. An attempt could be interrupted (by external forces) or aborted (by self).

The terms *parasuicide, DSH, and nonsuicidal self-injury (NSSI)* are often used interchangeably in literature. DSH has been defined as "intentional self-poisoning or self-injury irrespective of the type of motive or the extent of suicidal intent".[5] DSH is an important predictor of completed suicide.[6] NSSI simply refers to injury inflicted on self without the intent of suicide.[7] Parasuicide is a "nonsuicidal (i.e., without the intent of killing oneself) behavior which is not habitual and can be potentially life-threatening."[3]

Two terms refer to suicide risk, viz., suicidal *intent* and *lethality* of suicide attempt. While intent is subjective expectation that an act of self-harm is likely to cause death, lethality is an objective assessment of possibility of a self-harming behavior or method to potentially cause death. It is important to understand that lethality may not always correlate with the individual's expectation of how dangerous (likely to cause death) the attempt was.[8]

EPIDEMIOLOGY

Suicide contributes to 6% of all-cause mortality among youth globally. A global school-based survey estimates suicidal ideations to be present in 16% and 12% of adolescent females and males, respectively, with figures for suicidal plans reaching nearly 8% and 6%, respectively. Almost 75% of youth suicide occurs in low- and middle-income countries (LMIC).[4] The two most common modes of suicide and self-harm among youth in LMIC are poisoning followed by hanging.[9,10]

Literature suggests that NSSI can begin as early as 11 years of age and reach adult level by 16 years of age.[11] Lifetime prevalence rates among adolescents range from 17.2 to 22.9%, indicating an increase over time. 12-month prevalence rates are around 18%. Prevalence is higher in clinical settings, reaching up to 60–82% in inpatient samples excluding adolescents with psychosis or intellectual disabilities. Among children under age 12, lifetime prevalence is 6.2% in community samples and 37.4% in clinical samples.[11]

Up to 30% of teenagers with DSH report having had prior incidents, many of which went untreated. In the ensuing year, at least 10% of people with DSH relapse, with relapses most likely to occur in the first 2 or 3 months. Following DSH, the probability of suicide ranges from 0.24 to 4.30%.[12]

As per burden of diseases estimates, global suicide prevalence is nearly 11.1 per 100,000 population.[13] The suicide rates in India are much higher—17·9 per 100,000.[14] The risk of dying by suicide before the age of 15 years was estimated at 1.3% in a nationally representative sample from India.[15] A verbal autopsy study from southern India at the turn of the century showed that suicide accounted for death in nearly a quarter of young men and around 50–75% of young women, which was alarmingly higher than global figures.[16]

Adolescent females' high suicide death rates have drawn attention, as suicides now rank higher worldwide than maternal mortality. This high suicide rate has been linked to gender role differences and gender-based discriminatory factors, such as early marriage; and a higher risk of depression in females.[16]

Compared to adult suicidality, youth suicidality is more frequently impulsive, linked to externalizing traits (aggression, substance abuse, etc.), greatly influenced by peers and the media (copycat suicide), temporally related to life stressors (family, relationship, academic conflicts, etc.), and more reliant on the availability of suicide methods.[4,15]

ETIOLOGY AND RISK FACTORS

It is necessary to study and identify risk factors to predict and prevent suicide and self-harm.[17] It is particularly important for children and adolescents since young age of onset is associated with higher burden and morbidity over the life course.[6]

Suicide is a complex phenomenon with a variety of risk factors and biopsychosocial determinants. Besides factors such as gender, suicide risk is determined by other important but understudied social factors, such as culture and politics.[9] These are believed to be the reasons behind differences in suicide rates among youth between LMIC and high-income countries.

Some common characteristics discovered by psychological autopsy among adolescents who died by suicide were broken homes (parental separation, divorce, or death), family history of psychiatric disorder or suicidal behavior, personal history of psychiatric disorder or behavioral disturbance, history of substance misuse, and prior history of self-harm.[12] On the other hand, youth who present with DSH or NSSI express different cognitions ranging from wanting to die and escape from unbearable pain to an act to change the behavior of others, to show desperation to others, to take revenge or make the other person feel guilty, or to escape from a situation, or gain relief of tension and seeking help. Thus, the primary purpose of NSSI is understood to be emotional regulation, including relief from overwhelming feelings, self-punishment, or communicating distress.[12]

Hink et al. (2022) classify risk factors for adolescent suicide into three broad categories, viz., (i) individual factors (male, psychiatric or substance use disorders, past suicidal ideations/ attempts, impulsivity, etc.), (ii) interpersonal/ family factors (bullying, neglect, adoption, parental mental illness/separation, etc.), and (iii) community factors (social isolation, economic distress, firearm laws, etc.).[18] Regional data may vary. For example, being female poses a higher risk of suicide among adolescents in India due to various cultural factors including oppression of females.[18] Other risk factors for youth suicide highlighted in different studies include bullying, poor social support, having family problems, substance use, assault (physical/sexual), love affairs, failure in examinations, etc.[4,9] **Table 1** summarizes risk factors and determinants identified in LMIC, particularly in India.[18]

A study conducted on middle and high school children in urban areas of Chandigarh found that around 6% of students reported having suicidal ideations and 0.4% reported having made an attempt.[19] Academic decline was a significant association with suicidal thoughts compared to those with no such thoughts. Relationships with parents and peers also had a significant impact on psychological health. Other factors which may play a significant role in adolescent suicide and self-harm include influence of social media.

Nearly 21% of COVID-19 related suicide deaths occurred in youth.[20] In a multicentric study from Spain, mental health consultations in pediatric emergency from March 2019 to March 2020 and March 2020 to March 2021 were analyzed. The results showed a 122% increase in the diagnosis of "nonaccidental drug intoxication" and 56% increase in "suicide/suicide attempt/ suicidal ideation." A prospective analysis on 281 youth with suicide attempts showed that the modal patient was female (90%) and 15-year-old. While 35% did not have a prior psychiatric diagnosis, 58% had engaged in suicide behavior in the past.[21]

Sociodemographic and clinical risk factors identified till date, cumulatively account for weak prediction of suicide in clinical situations. The most well-known risk factor for suicidal conduct is the presence of mental illnesses, particularly depression, and prior suicide attempts, while other circumstances also play a role (family, personal, or social).[18] Most risk factors interact with each other and may have additive effects when present together (demonstrated in **Case Vignette 1**).

Nonsuicidal Self-injury

Various psychological, social, and biological influences contribute to the development of NSSI. Emotion dysregulation is a key factor, as many individuals engage in NSSI to manage overwhelming emotions. Meta-analyses have found that greater difficulties in emotional regulation are strongly associated with an increased likelihood of NSSI across different populations.[22] The risk is particularly high in individuals who struggle to access effective emotion regulation strategies. Individuals with emotional disorders, especially depression and

TABLE 1: Biopsychosocial determinants of suicide in adolescents.[9,18]

Biological	*Psychological*	*Socio-environmental*
• Late adolescence (14–18 years) • Female gender • *Neurobiological correlates:* – *Structural abnormalities:* Hippocampal and dorsolateral prefrontal cortex (DLPFC) abnormality – *Functional abnormalities:* Abnormally increased connectivity with the cerebellum and left lingual gyrus, and decreased connectivity with the right posterior cingulate cortex and the right precuneus • *Neurochemical abnormalities:* – Higher binding to 5HT2A receptors in the postmortem brains (with prominent involvement of the PFC and hippocampus) – Increased proinflammatory markers such as interleukin-1b, tumor necrosis factor-alpha (in PFC of a deceased teenager), and serum CRP (among the suicide attempters compared to the controls) in youth with suicidal behaviors – Decreased brain-derived neurotropic factor (BDNF) in PFC • Genetics and epigenetics • *Familial factors:* Parental psychopathology, suicidal behavior, and impulsivity (in addition to genetic predisposition) • Psychiatric illness and substance use	• *Affective processes:* – Negative valence like low self-esteem, worthlessness, and neuroticism – Lack of positive valence anhedonia recurrent suicidality – Blunted reward responsivity and reward learning deficit – Difficulty identifying emotions • *Cognitive-conative processes:* – Impulsivity-aggression trait – Selective-information-processing and related biases (attentional and memory related) – Suppression and rumination increase risk, while distraction and problem-solving are protective • *Social processes:* – Thwarted belongingness among the females and perceived burdensomeness among the males (interpersonal theory of suicide) – Social communication and response processing are critical to interpersonal relationships	• *Childhood maltreatment/abuse:* Physical, sexual, or emotional • *Bullying/peer victimization:* Social exclusion, verbal or physical assault, or peer coercion • *Peer influence:* Peer suicide may lead to complicated grief, social participation, modeling, and assortative relationships • *Media influence:* Sensationalizing suicide by media, especially celebrity suicide, with the determinants being the duration of reporting, elaboration of means of suicide, and live discussion on suicide • *Drifting:* Getting disconnected from one's support system (family, work, and school). Migration, sociopolitical changes, involvement in substance use, and illegal activities • *Family constellation:* Disrupted family, poor parent-child relationships, and parental loss/separation • Minorities/ethnicities and caste-based discrimination • Availability of lethal means • Accessibility and availability of mental health resources • Perceived stigma

anxiety, are more prone to NSSI, with associations also observed with panic disorder and PTSD, though not always statistically significant.[23]

Research indicates that early-life adversity, including childhood maltreatment, parental separation, and attachment disruptions, contributes to NSSI risk.[24] Recent findings suggest a modest but significant association between childhood sexual abuse and NSSI; its impact may be mediated by factors such as dissociation,

CASE VIGNETTE 1

A 16-year-old female presented to the emergency department accompanied by her mother, reporting a paracetamol overdose. The patient ingested 10 tablets of paracetamol two nights prior, went to sleep, and experienced no immediate adverse effects. The overdose was discovered the following morning when the patient's mother found an empty medication strip by her bedside. Upon confrontation, the patient admitted to the ingestion.

She had a 3- to 4-month history of low mood, along with difficulty concentrating on studies, perceived decline in academic performance, and fear of failing upcoming board examinations (scheduled for next month). There was avoidance of peer interaction at school, and increased reprimands from teachers due to declining academic attendance. Sleep disturbances and decreased appetite, accompanied by reported weight loss over the past few months, were corroborated by the mother.

The patient reports that the decision to overdose was precipitated by receiving the examination schedule earlier that week. She expressed a belief that ending her life was preferable to facing perceived humiliation due to anticipated academic failure and thought that consuming a strip of paracetamol would be sufficient to die. She, however, reported regrets about her behavior (self-harm) to her mother later and agreed to take psychiatric help.

Discussion:

The ingestion of 10 paracetamol tablets, while not objectively lethal, represents a suicide attempt with high perceived lethality and intent to die, precipitated by acute academic stress, specifically the receipt of her examination schedule. The patient's belief that ending her life was preferable to facing perceived academic humiliation underscores the severity of her distress and the potential for future self-harm.

The 3- to 4-month history of low mood, impaired concentration, social withdrawal, sleep disturbances, and decreased appetite strongly suggests a depressive episode.

Risk factors for future attempts in her case include self-harm behavior, depression, significant academic stress, social isolation, and nondisclosure about the attempt. Protective factors are parental support, subsequent presentation to the emergency department, and the patient's readiness to take psychiatric treatment.

self-blame, and alexithymia.[25] Similarly, adolescents with adverse childhood experiences (ACEs) face heightened risk, particularly when employing maladaptive coping mechanisms.[26] However, not all individuals engaging in NSSI have experienced trauma or have a diagnosed mental health condition.

Bullying, whether as a victim or perpetrator, has also been identified as a significant risk factor for NSSI, especially among younger adolescents.[27] Strong parental support can mitigate this risk. Compared to peer support, parental support and connection appear to be more protective against NSSI.[28] In contrast, parental criticism increases the risk, particularly when adolescents internalize negative parental feedback.[29]

Other psychological risk factors include self-criticism and low self-esteem, both of which are associated with a greater likelihood of NSSI.[30] Studies suggest that individuals with a history of NSSI who exhibit high self-criticism endure pain longer and may even experience mood improvements during painful experiences.[31]

Traits associated with borderline personality disorder (BPD) are often linked to NSSI, though research indicates that NSSI occurs across various psychiatric conditions.[31] Although impulsiveness is commonly associated with NSSI, findings are mixed. While individuals who engage in NSSI often perceive themselves as impulsive—especially in response to distressing emotions—objective measures of impulsivity do not consistently differentiate between those who self-injure and those who do not.[32] Some evidence suggests that shifts in emotional states preceding NSSI are detectable hours in advance, rather than occurring suddenly before the act. Self-efficacy—the belief that one can resist self-injurious urges—mediates the relationship between impulsivity and NSSI.[33]

One needs to understand the immediate triggers which could lead to self-harm or suicide attempt, namely conflicts with parents/siblings/peers, problems at school/college/work, difficulties in romantic relationships, physical ill health, depression or low self-esteem, bullying, sexual problems, alcohol and drug abuse, family members/friends becoming aware of their self-harm. While these may be the immediate triggers, there are certain lifetime risk factors which predispose the individual to a higher risk of harming self than other, viz., history of self-harm in the past (most significant risk factor), disturbances in personality, psychiatric illnesses, particularly depression, alcohol or drug abuse, psychosocial issues including disturbed family relationships, history of alcohol dependence in the family, social isolation, and academic difficulties.[12]

DIAGNOSIS AND ASSESSMENT

Suicide and self-harm are classified as a potentially life-threatening psychiatric emergency (class I) as per Rosenn urgency classification.[34,35] While NSSI may not have suicidal intent, it may also accidentally lead to death. They may present in emergency or out-patient settings. The first thing to do for a child/adolescent is to ensure his/her safety. A formal risk assessment must be carried out and documented. The basic principles of risk assessment include triaging the patient, curtailing risks associated with the condition, looking for medical etiology (if any), and stabilizing the crisis through psychological interventions or pharmacotherapy, or both.[36]

Clinical Approach

The basic approach for assessing children/adolescents with suicidal risk is the same as in adults, which includes the reasons for presentation, detailed history of presenting illness, past, medical, family, and developmental history, and a detailed mental status examination including assessment of judgment and insight. Important clinical considerations while examining children/adolescents include:[36] empathetic approach, interviewing the parents and child together and then separately as well, collecting corroborative information from other available collateral sources, interacting as per the child's age and cognitive development (very young children interact better with play, drawing, story-telling), understanding the child's concept of death and suicide, giving them adequate space and time if they take more time to engage, and avoiding confrontation. Children/adolescents may not be cognitively positioned to articulate their thoughts or verbalize their symptoms. Behavior is often a significant indicator of suicidality and comorbid diagnosis. Involvement of parents/legal guardians is necessary in assessing and managing children/adolescents with imminent suicidality.

The clinician should not be hesitant in asking direct questions about suicide in children/adolescents, just like in adults. Skillfully asking questions related to suicide/self-harm has in fact been shown to improve rapport with the youth; by showing them one's concern and supporting their autonomy by showing a willingness to talk about a sensitive topic. Beginning the conversation with consent/assent, and normalizing thoughts and behaviors related to suicide may be helpful in building rapport and lowering the child's/adolescent's defenses. However, it is not uncommon for the youth to express unwillingness to talk about self-harm, in which case respecting their choice and gently exploring into their reason for hesitation in this regard may be pursued. An open and empathetic dialog may often lead to increasing their willingness to talk. However, continued refusal may need to be balanced with safety as risk assessment is necessary rather than optional. In such cases, explaining the professional responsibility for assessing risk and ensuring the minor's safety, and need for assessment or admission must be conveyed.[37]

Another important information that should be conveyed by clinicians to the child/adolescent is the limits of confidentiality. They should be informed prior to risk assessment about the need to breach confidentiality to ensure their safety. While it is likely that the child/adolescent may not open up fully after knowing this, it must still be conveyed a priori to avoid breaking their trust or making them feel betrayed. It might be helpful to assure them that only the "necessary" information, which is required to keep them safe, will be conveyed to the legal guardian.

After seeking permission and informing about limits of confidentiality, clinicians may interview the minor and their legal guardian together as well as separately, as both may be more comfortable revealing certain information on a one-to-one interview. Any discrepancy in reporting should be clarified individually, and wherever discrepancies remain, it is better to err on the side of caution rather than disregarding that information. The most significant evidence-based risk factor remains past history or suicide/NSSI. Based on current thoughts, plans, preparatory actions, and attempts, the risk may be graded into low, moderate, and high-risk categories, and the management may ensue accordingly. A case of suicide attempt with low intent and low lethality is demonstrated in **Case Vignette 2**.

CASE VIGNETTE 2

A 17-year-old girl presented to the emergency department accompanied by her aunt. She reportedly ingested a small amount of a diluted corrosive solution following a heated argument with family members. She had poured approximately one cap of a household cleaning solution in a glass of water and had started drinking it when her aunt stopped her.

Both her parents died in a road traffic accident 5 years ago, and since then she had been staying with her uncle and aunt. She reported a history of strained relationships and frequent conflicts with them. When they did not comply with her demand to acknowledge her perceived mistreatment on their part, she impulsively ingested the cleaning solution in her aunt's presence, who stopped her from drinking more of it. She described an immediate burning sensation in her throat, followed by ghabrahat, prompting her family to bring her to the emergency department. She reported having threatened similar actions in the past during arguments but had never actually consumed anything.

When asked if she had wished she were dead, she stated, "Yes, I suppose so, but I mainly wanted them to understand how upset I was." When asked if she still harbored thoughts of killing herself, she stated, "No, I don't want to die." She denied having planned it. She also stated, "I didn't really think about the consequences."

Discussion:

This 17-year-old girl presented following the ingestion of a small amount of diluted corrosive solution. The patient's actions were driven by a desire to convey her distress and elicit acknowledgment of perceived mistreatment from her family, rather than a well-thought-out plan to end her life. Her statements, denying any current wish to be dead, along with the impulsive nature of the act, suggest low suicidal intent.

While the ingestion of a corrosive substance carries potential lethality, the dilution and small quantity ingested indicate low actual lethality. However, the behavior itself, alongside the reported history of similar threats, suggests a need for further assessment and intervention. The patient's emotional dysregulation and the dysfunctional family dynamics are crucial factors to consider.

Risk factors include impulsivity, a history of using threats of self-harm, and the presence of ongoing conflict within the family. Protective factors include her denial of clear suicidal intent and promptly seeking medical attention.

Management should focus on safety planning, addressing the underlying emotional distress, and improving coping mechanisms. It is important to educate the patient about the potential dangers of her actions and to develop strategies for managing conflict and expressing her emotions in a healthier manner. Family therapy may be beneficial to address dysfunctional relationship patterns.

As clinicians, it is important for us to understand that impulsive DSH may turn out to be fatal, even though the intent among the individual may be low. Ensuring safety and timely intervention becomes important in such individuals.

Assessment of suicidal and self-harm behaviors requires skillful evaluation of what is said and done. Regarding suicidal intent, one should not always just go by what is said or denied but be vigilant for behaviors indicating intent. Some behaviors indicative of high intent include conducting the act in isolation, timing the act in a way when intervention is unlikely (being alone at home when parents are away), taking precautions to avoid discovery, making preparations, expressing such thoughts beforehand to other people, writing a suicide note, not alerting others during or after the act.[12] One should gather collateral information before labeling an adolescent as low-risk (demonstrated in **Case Vignette 3**).

CASE VIGNETTE 3

A 19-year-old male, student, son of a police constable, presented to the psychiatry outpatient clinic following an interrupted suicide attempt. He was intercepted by a neighbor near his home while holding a loaded service revolver, poised to place it against his temple. The patient reports a several-month history of progressive, persistent and pervasive low mood. He describes persistent fatigue, loss of interest in previously pleasurable activities, including recent family festivities, sleep difficulties, decreased appetite, and the family members reporting that his clothes have recently become loose. He would also complain of impaired concentration, impacting his performance at school. He also reported worries related to the financial strain due to impending retirement of his father, which he felt might impact his career choices.

He reports experiencing recurrent suicidal ideation for several weeks, with persistent thoughts of ending his life. Initially, he explored various methods of suicide but lacked a definitive plan. He subsequently decided to use a firearm and picked up his father's service revolver, while the latter was asleep. He planned to carry out the suicide attempt at a deserted park near his home at 5:00 AM, when all family members would be asleep. However, when he went out that morning to execute his plan, he was interrupted by his neighbor, who discovered him accidentally and then alerted his family.

The patient was taken to a psychiatrist the same day to whom, patient did not disclose many details initially. He expressed annoyance for not planning his attempt better and refused to have detailed conversation since he believed the doctor could not reduce his suffering. His father reported history of completed suicide in mother when the patient was 2 years old. The patient was being brought up by his grandparents and father and resides in a joint family with his elder sibling, cousins, and uncle. The family relations are cordial.

Discussion:

This 19-year-old boy presents with a clinical picture suggestive of a major depressive episode. The progression from passive suicidal ideation to a concrete plan involving a firearm, coupled with his intent to carry it out, signifies high suicidal intent and potential lethality (firearm). Despite the interrupted attempt, the risk remains significant, emphasizing the critical need for thorough assessment and prompt intervention.

Risk factors include the interrupted suicide attempt with a lethal method, detailed suicide plan with intent, severe depressive symptoms, family history of suicide, and access to firearms. Conversely, protective factors such as family support and acceptance of a mental health referral are important in management.

Hospitalization is essential to ensure patient safety, facilitate detailed assessment, and initiate pharmacological and nonpharmacological interventions. Critical to the management is the immediate removal of access to firearms and safety planning to mitigate future risks.

Assessment Instruments

Some commonly used instruments, which may help in a more objective assessment of self-harm behaviors are described here:

- *Columbia suicide severity rating scale:*[38] It is a reliable tool that has been validated for adolescents, and available in public domain.
- *Self-injurious thoughts and behaviors interview:*[39] It is a 72-item Likert-type scale assessing suicidal behaviors and NSSI separately. It is a reliable and valid tool for adolescents, and available in public domain.
- *Short-term assessment of risk and treatability-adolescent version (START-AV):*[40] It evaluates a young person's risk of experiencing different negative outcomes (such as violence, victimization, or NSSI between the ages of 12 and 18. It consists of 24 items divided into three clusters: (1) Response to interventions, (2) relationships and environment, and (3) individual adolescent.
- *Risk-rescue rating scale (RRRS):*[41] This scale has 5 items each on risk and rescuability of the suicide attempt. Each item is scored on a Likert-type scale. Composite score is calculated based on the risk and rescue scores. It is a reliable, valid, quick-to-administer tool, and available in public domain.

- *Scale for assessment of lethality of suicide attempt (SALSA):*[42] It has two components; The first component has four items indicating seriousness of the attempt and its likely consequences and the second component is the global impression of lethality. Studies suggest that lethality scores of SALSA differentiate known groups with different lethality, e.g., deceased and survived, and attempters with different levels of medical intervention: in-patient only, intensive care, ventilator support. It is a reliable, valid, quick-to-administer tool, and available in public domain.
- *Ask suicide-screening questions (ASQ):*[43] It is a brief validated tool for use among both youth and adults. Additional materials to help with suicide risk screening implementation are available in the ASQ Toolkit, a free resource for use in various medical settings (emergency, inpatient, and outpatient/primary care). The material for youth versions takes into account developmental considerations. *The ASQ is a set of four screening questions that takes 20 seconds to administer.* In a NIMH study, a "yes" response to one or more of the four questions identified 97% of youth (aged 10–21 years) at risk for suicide.[43]

Legal Implications

One must be aware of the legal implications of managing minor patients with psychiatric illness, as per the provisions of the Mental Healthcare Act (MHCA) 2017 and Protection of Children from Sexual Offences Act (POCSO) 2012.

The MHCA mandates that decisions with respect to treatment of a minor must be taken into consultation with a nominated representative. The procedure for admitting a minor as per MHCA comes under Section 87, which also prescribes that minor be admitted in a separate setting than adults, with separate washrooms, and must have a nominated representative always staying with them. Section 94 deals with emergency treatment. Certain procedures such as electroconvulsive therapy cannot be given to minors as per provisions in Section 95 of MHCA unless approved by mental health review board (MHRB).

While it is important to ensure confidentiality, e.g., use of psychoactive substances, it is important to do mandatorily report certain sexual encounters under POCSO (even a consensual sexual encounter may be subsumed under POCSO for a minor).

MANAGEMENT AND PREVENTION

Both psychosocial and pharmacological measures may be needed while managing adolescents or children with suicidal or self-harming behavior.

Psychosocial Measures

Management begins with ensuring safety of the child/adolescent. Different safety planning approaches have been studied in context of suicide and self-harm. Safety planning intervention (SPI) is a tactic which was initially developed for application in adults like a cognitive therapy for suicide prevention.[44] It was later adapted to a cognitive behavioral therapy (CBT) for suicide prevention for adolescents.[45] It is seen that suicidal crises are typically time-limited, consisting of a period of suicidal desire and urges followed by a decline in the desire to attempt suicide. This is the principle behind SPI. By stopping someone from acting on strong suicide thoughts and cravings, we can give the suicidal crisis time to pass. The six steps in the SPI are given in **Box 1**. It is important to explain the essence of SPI to the children/adolescents and their parents for it to be work.

The strongest evidence for suicide prevention exists for behavior change, skill-enhancement, and strengthening of interpersonal bonds in

BOX 1: Six steps of suicide prevention intervention.[37]

1. Generating a list of personal warning signs that immediately precede suicidal crisis, indicating the need to initiate safety plan
2. Generating a list of internal coping strategies to distract themselves from suicidal crisis/thoughts (immediate crisis management strategy until long-term emotion regulation strategies can be developed and employed)
3. Generating a list of people (who have positive and stable relations with the child/adolescent; could be peers/adults) or social settings (online/offline) which can act as distractors
4. Generating a list of people (preferably adults with positive and stable relationships) to ask for help. The safety plan may be discussed with a few of the listed adults
5. Generating a list of professional resources including treating clinicians, nearby emergencies, etc.
6. Collaboration between youth, caregivers, clinicians, and other resource persons who can help make the environment safe and restrict/limit access to lethal means

adolescents. A combination of individual and family therapy usually works better than alone. For example, integrated cognitive behavioral therapy (I-CBT), and attachment-based family therapy (ABFT), an interpersonal approach to individual and family therapy and parent skill training to amplify love, empathy, enhance affective attunement, and enhance the quality of attachment bonds between the adolescents and their parents have shown persistent positive results compared to control arm (also received active intervention).[46]

Individual therapies aiming to improve the youth's psychological and interpersonal skills have also shown promising results for both suicide and DSH. For instance, dialectic behavior therapy-adolescent (DBT-A), which involves basic components of DBT (mindfulness, emotional regulation, distress tolerance, and interpersonal skill training) and family therapy has shown positive results on long-term follow-up.[47] Similarly, interpersonal therapy (IPT) for youth in school settings (IPT-A-IN) (therapy adapted for adolescents, and addressing the interpersonal and social precipitants of suicide) for depressed youth with the risk of suicide has shown efficacy over counseling as usual; however, long-term efficacy data are lacking for IPT-A-IN.[48]

Brief intervention during crisis/postcrisis: Postdischarge period from the emergency department (ED) and acute care setting is critical for the suicide reattempt. Crisis management interventions (multiple-component post-ED interventions and SAFETY Program) that involve safety planning for decreasing suicidal behavior in youth have got empirical support. Crisis management involves psychoeducation of youth and their parents, safety planning, linkage, and ensuring compliance with the follow-up care.[49,50] Such interventions have been found to have high acceptability and utility as a coping strategy during suicide-related crises.[51,52]

Pharmacological Measures

The underlying psychiatric symptoms need to be treated. Common comorbidities associated with self-harming behavior include depression, anxiety, adjustment disorder, personality disorder, attention-deficit/hyperactivity disorder, and psychotic disorders. Since depression is a common association of suicidal behavior, anti-depressant medications, particularly selective serotonin reuptake inhibitors (SSRIs) have a role in reducing suicidal behavior. However, treating clinicians should be cautious against SSRI-induced akathisia in the initial phase, which may contribute to higher suicidal risk. Tricyclic antidepressants are generally avoided due to narrow therapeutic index to ensure safety in cases of intentional overdose.[9]

Among the mood stabilizers, lithium has shown positive results in youth with suicidality. Lithium has shown improvement in impulsivity, disruptive behavior, and personality disorders.

The role of valproate and carbamazepine is not much investigated in youth. Second-generation antipsychotics, particularly clozapine, also have evidence in reducing suicidality in schizophrenia. Other second-generation antipsychotics such as aripiprazole, risperidone, and olanzapine also have protective effects, provided they are uptitrated gradually and cautiously.[9]

An age-old biological therapy that has anti-suicidal property is electroconvulsive therapy. Some other newer agents such as ketamine have shown promising results; however, more evidence on effectiveness and safety is required in the youth.[9]

Nonsuicidal Self-injury

Nonsuicidal self-injury mainly involves skin lesions (e.g., cutting, self-biting; self-tattooing; burning or freezing the skin; self-hitting). Swallowing sharp or nonedible objects and nonsuicidal self-poisoning also occurs.

Individuals, who engage in self-injury often use it as a (dysfunctional) coping method for:[3,53]

- Regulation of emotions (anxiety, anger, frustration, and sadness)
- Control of thoughts or memories (distraction from problems and stopping suicidal thoughts)
- Regulation interpersonal relationship (secure care and attention and influence others), and/or
- Self-punishment

Most NSSIs in adolescents resolve spontaneously by the time they become young adults. Self-harm was more likely to persist in females, and it is associated with depression and anxiety, antisocial behavior, high risk alcohol use, cannabis use, and cigarette smoking.[3]

Assessment

Every child or adolescent who has self-harmed should be assessed for risk of repetition and suicide risk. Parents and other important caregivers should be included in the assessment.

The assessment should consider:[3]

- Methods and frequency of current and past self-harm
- Current and past suicidal intent
- Depressive symptoms and psychiatric illnesses and their relationship to self-harm
- Contextual and specific factors preceding self-harm (e.g., unpleasant affective states and relational stressors)
- Coping strategies that the person has used to limit or avert self-harm or to contain the impact of contextual factors preceding episodes of self-harm
- Significant relationships that may either be supportive or represent a threat
- Immediate and longer-term risks

Management

Patients severely harming themselves may need the same close supervision as patients with high or moderate suicide risk.

Treatment goals may include:

- Preventing escalation of self-harm and reducing harm arising from self-harm
- Reducing or stopping self-harm and other risk-related behavior
- Improving associated mental health condition and socio-occupational functioning

Immediate management efforts should include: (i) Ensuring safety and close monitoring, e.g., providing first aid, medical evaluation, and treatment (e.g., injection tetanus toxoid); and (ii) providing emotional support in an empathetic and nonjudgemental manner.[53]

A risk management plan should be developed covering strategies to deal with the risks identified (psychological, pharmacological, social, and relational). This plan should include self-management strategies and ways of accessing services and receiving support during a crisis when self-management strategies fail.[3]

Further management involves building a psychotherapeutic relationship to provide validation of the adolescent's emotional state and psychoeducation to both parents and the adolescent (including medical consequences). The adolescent is helped to understand the connection of the behavior with distressing experiences (unhelpful coping with stressful situation), helped to take a firm view regarding avoiding future self-injury; and gradually develop more functional coping strategies.[53]

Despite encouraging results from pilot studies, empirical evidence for the efficacy of psychosocial interventions in the treatment of self-injuring behavior in adolescents is limited. There is also no evidence supporting the use of medication to reduce self-harm, although medication may be indicated to treat comorbid disorders.[53]

SUICIDE PREVENTION STRATEGIES IN INDIA

Globally various ways of reducing and preventing suicide have been studied. Some evidence-based methods identified in literature include: (i) Restricting access to lethal means, especially with regard to control of analgesics; (ii) identifying and restricting hot-spots for suicide by jumping; (iii) school-based awareness programs and educating youths on depression and suicidal behavior; (iv) training primary care physicians in depression recognition and treatment; (v) effective treatment of depression and active outreach to psychiatric patients after discharge or a suicidal crisis; (vi) cognitivebehavioral therapy and dialectical behavior therapy; (vii) certain pharmacotherapy agents such as antidepressants, clozapine, lithium, and ketamine.[54,55] Evidence on effectiveness of education of gatekeepers about youth suicidal behavior is lacking due to paucity of randomized trials.

WHO recommends four key interventions which may be useful in prevention, viz., (i) restricting access to means of suicide, (ii) ensuring responsible reporting of suicide by the media, (iii) helping the youth to develop coping strategies to cope with day-to-day stressors of life, and (iv) early identification and management of those with high risk for suicide. The WHO strategy for suicide prevention is called LIVE LIFE. LIVE stands for leadership, interventions, vision, and evaluation, and LIFE stands for less means of suicide, interact with media, form the youth, and early identification.[56]

The Ministry of Health and Family Welfare introduced the national suicide prevention strategies (NSPS) in 2022.[57] The strategy aims to reduce deaths due to suicide by 10% by the year 2030. The NSPS hopes to accomplish this goal by implementing efficient monitoring systems (by 2025), offering suicide prevention services through the District Mental Health Programme in every district (by 2027), and incorporating a mental health curriculum into every educational institution (by 2030). NSPS delineates REDS path which stands for reinforcing leadership, partnership, and institutional capacity in India, enhancing the capacity of health services, developing community resilience, and societal support to reduce stigma around suicide, strengthening surveillance and evidence generation.

The National Mental Health Programme of India incorporates certain in-built activities for prevention of suicide. It has led to development of various resources, e.g., facilitator's manual on life skill education, stress management and suicide prevention, manuals of mental health for various medical/mental health professionals such as medical officers, psychiatry social workers, and psychologists. Under the District Mental Health Programme (DMHP), targeted intervention techniques have been defined for catering to needs of vulnerable individuals or adverse life situations such as poverty, unemployment, depression, and alcohol/drug use. Suicide prevention is also an important element in various other national programs targeted toward youth such as Nasha Mukt Bharat, Rashtriya Bal Swasthya Karyakram, and Rashtriya Kishore Swasthya Karyakram.

RECOMMENDATIONS AND FUTURE DIRECTIONS

From a public health perspective, suicide prevention should focus first on health promotion, which may partly be done with the help of public awareness campaigns, incorporating awareness programs in schools, building resilience, and strength. Three levels of prevention include: (i) Universal (all adolescents, e.g., curriculum changes), (ii) selective (adolescents identified as at-risk), and (iii) indicated (those exhibiting suicidal ideations and behavior).[6] Two interventions, which promise positive results but have limited evidence in support include: (i) Gatekeeper training, which could be people in community with face-to-face contact with individuals at-risk, e.g., school teachers and (ii) peer-based intervention, who can acts as a bridge between the distressed peer and the gatekeeper.[6]

Research also indicates that in India, suicide prevention can be achieved through the use of lay counseling (SHAPE: School Health Promotion and Empowerment Programme).[58] In India and other LMIC nations, school-based screening surveys have been conducted for mental illnesses and teenage suicidality. These kinds of programs ought to be expanded to include colleges and workplaces. Putting together community-level camps with the help of NGOs and civic society can also be beneficial, particularly for young people who are homeless, in observation and childcare facilities, or who have dropped out of school or college.[59]

Suicide management and prevention require a multimodal and multisectoral approach. To stop suicidal thoughts and actions, primary, inpatient, and mental healthcare services for the pediatric population should be improved. To prevent child and teen suicide, it is essential that school personnel have specialized training, and pediatricians and nurses receive training in child and adolescent psychiatry. Pediatricians must also receive training on how to respond to inquiries regarding suicide and develop the ability to conduct interviews with a compassionate and encouraging demeanor, as they may often be the first contact for children and adolescents presenting with self-harm.

Utilization of digital and technological means in research on behavior and thoughts related to suicide and self-harm may enhance our understanding of the phenomenon, leading to a better real-time prediction and eventually prevention.[60]

At national level, national suicide prevention strategies need to be planned and executed utilizing the available resources in the best possible manner. The regular evaluation and modifications in the strategy must be made as per the outcomes assessed and updates available from on-going research. Since the current NCRB data is unreliable in estimating the problem, the nation should create a strong national and regional suicide reporting system. Incorporating local demands into the development of interventions and resource allocation would also benefit from this. Further, youth-friendly policies that protect their rights to health, education, employment, and freedom from discrimination in society can lower stress levels and enhance the quality of life for young people, particularly those from underrepresented and minority groups. This has the potential to reduce the risk factors for suicide.

SUMMARY AND CONCLUSION

Suicide is a complex phenomenon with various biopsychosocial determinants. Rates of suicide and self-harm behavior among children and adolescents are concerning with majority burden being borne by LMIC including India. Any individual with history of self-harm, irrespective of the intent, should be assessed with priority with details on risk assessment. Various pharmacological and nonpharmacological measures have moderate evidence in reducing suicidal behavior. Efforts have been made at global and national level to prevent youth suicide. With the launch of national suicide prevention strategy of India in 2022, we aim and hope to achieve a significant reduction in the suicide rates in India.

REFERENCES

1. Radhakrishnan R, Andrade C. Suicide: An Indian perspective. Indian J Psychiatry. 2012; 54(4):304-19.
2. Mythri SV, Ebenezer JA. Suicide in India: Distinct Epidemiological Patterns and Implications. Indian J Psychol Med. 2016;38(6):493-8.
3. Jans T, Vloet TD, Taneli Y, Warnke A. Suicide and self-harming behaviour. In: Rey JM (Ed). IACAPAP e-Textbook of Child and Adolescent Mental Health. Geneva: International Association for Child and Adolescent Psychiatry and Allied Professions; 2018.
4. McKinnon B, Gariépy G, Sentenac M, Elgar FJ. Adolescent suicidal behaviours in 32 low- and middle-income countries. Bull World Health Organ. 2016;94(5):340-50F.
5. Hawton K, Saunders KE, O'Connor RC. Self-harm and suicide in adolescents. Lancet. 2012; 379(9834):2373-82.
6. Patra BN, Sen MS, Sagar R, Bhargava R. Deliberate self-harm in adolescents: A review of literature. Ind Psychiatry J. 2023;32(1):9-14.
7. Nock MK. Understanding Nonsuicidal Self-Injury: Origins, Assessment, and Treatment. American Psychological Association; 2009.
8. Boland R, Verduin M, Ruiz P (Eds). Kaplan & Sadocks's Synopsis of Psychiatry, 12th edition. Wolters Kluver; 2022.
9. Gupta S, Basera D. Youth Suicide in India: A Critical Review and Implication for the National Suicide Prevention Policy. OMEGA - J Death Dying. 2023;88(1):245-73.
10. National Crime Records Bureau (NCRB). Accidental Deaths and Suicide in India. Ministry of Home Affairs, Government of India; 2022.
11. Jung KY, Kim T, Hwang SY, Lee TR, Yoon H, Shin TG, et al. Deliberate Self-harm among Young People Begins to Increase at the Very Early Age: A Nationwide Study. J Korean Med Sci. 2018; 33(30):e191.
12. Hawton K, James A. Suicide and deliberate self-harm in young people. BMJ. 2005;330(7496): 891-4.
13. Naghavi M. Global, regional, and national burden of suicide mortality 1990 to 2016: systematic analysis for the Global Burden of Disease Study 2016. BMJ. 2019;364:l94.
14. Dandona R, Kumar GA, Dhaliwal R, Naghavi M, Vos T, Shukla DK, et al. Gender differentials and state variations in suicide deaths in India: the Global Burden of Disease Study 1990–2016. Lancet Public Health. 2018;3(10):e478-89.
15. Patel V, Ramasundarahettige C, Vijayakumar L, Thakur JS, Gajalakshmi V, Gururaj G, et al. Suicide mortality in India: a nationally representative survey. Lancet. 2012;379(9834):2343-51.
16. Aaron R, Joseph A, Abraham S, Muliyil J, George K, Prasad J, et al. Suicides in young people in rural southern India. Lancet Lond Engl. 2004;363(9415):1117-8.
17. Franklin JC, Ribeiro JD, Fox KR, Bentley KH, Kleiman EM, Huang X, et al. Risk factors for suicidal thoughts and behaviors: A meta-analysis of 50 years of research. Psychol Bull. 2017;143(2):187-232.
18. Hink AB, Killings X, Bhatt A, Ridings LE, Andrews AL. Adolescent suicide—Understanding unique risks and opportunities for trauma centers to recognize, intervene, and prevent a leading cause of death. Curr Trauma Rep. 2022;8(2):41-53.
19. Arun P, Chavan B. Stress and suicidal ideas in adolescent students in Chandigarh. Indian J Med Sci. 2009;63(7):281.
20. Dsouza DD, Quadros S, Hyderabadwala ZJ, Mamun MA. Aggregated COVID-19 suicide incidences in India: Fear of COVID-19 infection is the prominent causative factor. Psychiatry Res. 2020;290:113145.

21. Vázquez López P, Armero Pedreira P, Martínez-Sánchez L, García Cruz JM, Bonetde Luna C, Notario Herrero F, et al. Self-injury and suicidal behavior in children and youth population: Learning from the pandemic. An Pediatr Engl Ed. 2023;98(3):204-12.
22. Wolff JC, Thompson E, Thomas SA, Nesi J, Bettis AH, Ransford B, et al. Emotion dysregulation and non-suicidal self-injury: A systematic review and meta-analysis. Eur Psychiatry. 2019;59:25-36.
23. Bentley KH, Cassiello-Robbins CF, Vittorio L, Sauer-Zavala S, Barlow DH. The association between nonsuicidal self-injury and the emotional disorders: A meta-analytic review. Clin Psychol Rev. 2015;37:72-88.
24. Gratz KL. Risk factors for and functions of deliberate self-harm: An empirical and conceptual review. Clin Psychol Sci Pract. 2003;10(2):192-205.
25. Liu RT, Scopelliti KM, Pittman SK, Zamora AS. Childhood maltreatment and non-suicidal self-injury: A systematic review and meta-analysis. Lancet Psychiatry. 2018;5(1):51-64.
26. Wan Y, Chen R, Wang S, Clifford A, Zhang S, Orton S, et al. Associations of coping styles with nonsuicidal self-injury in adolescents: Do they vary with gender and adverse childhood experiences? Child Abuse Neglect. 2020;104:104470.
27. Claes L, Luyckx K, Baetens I, Van de Ven M, Witteman C. Bullying and victimization, depressive mood, and non-suicidal self-injury in adolescents: The moderating role of parental support. J Child Fam Stud. 2015;24:3363-71.
28. Taliaferro LA, Jang ST, Westers NJ, Muehlenkamp JJ, Whitlock JL, McMorris BJ. Associations between connections to parents and friends and non-suicidal self-injury among adolescents: The mediating role of developmental assets. Clin Child Psychol Psychiatry. 2020;25(2):359-71.
29. Wedig MM, Nock MK. Parental expressed emotion and adolescent self-injury. J Am Acad Child Adolesc Psychiatry. 2007;46(9):1171-8.
30. Zelkowitz RL, Cole DA. Self-criticism as a transdiagnostic process in nonsuicidal self-injury and disordered eating: Systematic review and meta-analysis. Suicide Life Threat Behav. 2019; 49(1):310-27.
31. Fox KR, Toole KE, Franklin JC, Hooley JM. Why does nonsuicidal self-injury improve mood? A preliminary test of three hypotheses. Clin Psychol Sci. 2017;5(1):111-21.
32. Hamza CA, Willoughby T, Heffer T. Impulsivity and nonsuicidal self-injury: A review and meta-analysis. Clin Psychol Rev. 2015;38:13-24.
33. Hasking P, Whitlock J, Voon D, Rose A. A cognitive-emotional model of NSSI: Using emotion regulation and cognitive processes to explain why people self-injure. Cogn Emot. 2017;31(8):1543-56.
34. Pon N, Asan B, Anandan S, Toledo A. Special Considerations in Pediatric Psychiatric Populations. Emerg Med Clin North Am. 2015; 33(4):811-24.
35. Edelsohn GA, Braitman LE, Rabinovich H, Sheves P, Melendez A. Predictors of urgency in a pediatric psychiatric emergency service. J Am Acad Child Adolesc Psychiatry. 2003;42(10): 1197-202.
36. Deep R, Bhargava R. Psychiatric emergencies. In: Gupta P, Bagga A, Ramji S (Eds). Principles of Pediatric and Neonatal Emergencies, 4th edition. New Delhi: Jaypee Brothers Medical Publisher; 2020. pp. 553-64.
37. Pettit JW, Buitron V, Green KL. Assessment and Management of Suicide Risk in Children and Adolescents. Cogn Behav Pract. 2018;25(4):460-72.
38. Posner K, Brown GK, Stanley B, Brent DA, Yershova KV, Oquendo MA, et al. The Columbia–Suicide Severity Rating Scale: Initial Validity and Internal Consistency Findings from Three Multisite Studies with Adolescents and Adults. Am J Psychiatry. 2011;168(12):1266-77.
39. Nock MK, Holmberg EB, Photos VI, Michel BD. Self-Injurious Thoughts and Behaviors Interview: Development, reliability, and validity in an adolescent sample. Psychol Assess. 2007;19(3):309-17.
40. Viljoen J, Nicholls T, Cruise K, Desmarais S, Webster C. Short-term assessment of risk and treatability: Adolescent version (START: AV)–User guide. Ment Health Law Policy Inst. 2014.
41. Weisman AD, Worden JW. Risk-rescue rating in suicide assessment. Arch Gen Psychiatry. 1972;26(6):553-60.
42. Kar N, Arun M, Mohanty MK, Bastia BK. Scale for assessment of lethality of suicide attempt. Indian J Psychiatry. 2014;56(4):337-43.

43. Brown GK, Ten Have T, Henriques GR, Xie SX, Hollander JE, Beck AT. Cognitive therapy for the prevention of suicide attempts: a randomized controlled trial. JAMA. 2005;294(5):563-70.
44. Aguinaldo LD, Sullivant S, Lanzillo EC, Ross A, He J-P, Bradley-Ewing A, et al. Validation of the ask suicide-screening questions (ASQ) with youth in outpatient specialty and primary care clinics. Gen Hosp Psychiatry. 2021;68:52-8.
45. Stanley B, Brown G, Brent DA, Wells K, Poling K, Curry J, et al. Cognitive-behavioral therapy for suicide prevention (CBT-SP): treatment model, feasibility, and acceptability. J Am Acad Child Adolesc Psychiatry. 2009;48(10):1005-13.
46. Diamond GS, Wintersteen MB, Brown GK, Diamond GM, Gallop R, Shelef K, et al. Attachment-based family therapy for adolescents with suicidal ideation: A randomized controlled trial. J Am Acad Child Adolesc Psychiatry. 2010;49(2):122-31.
47. Miller AL, Rathus JH, Linehan MM, Wetzler S, Leigh E. Dialectical behavior therapy adapted for suicidal adolescents. J Psychiatr Pract. 1997; 3(2):78.
48. Tang TC, Jou SH, Ko CH, Huang SY, Yen CF. Randomized study of school-based intensive interpersonal psychotherapy for depressed adolescents with suicidal risk and parasuicide behaviors. Psychiatr Clin Neurosci. 2009;63(4): 463-70.
49. Asarnow JR, Hughes JL, Babeva KN, Sugar CA. Cognitive-behavioral family treatment for suicide attempt prevention: a randomized controlled trial. J Am Acad Child Adolesc Psychiatry. 2017;56(6):506-14.
50. Asarnow JR, Porta G, Spirito A, Emslie G, Clarke G, Wagner KD, et al. Suicide attempts and nonsuicidal self-injury in the treatment of resistant depression in adolescents: findings from the TORDIA study. Focus. 2012;10(3):380-8.
51. Kennard BD, Biernesser C, Wolfe KL, Foxwell AA, Craddock Lee SJ, Rial KV, et al. Developing a brief suicide prevention intervention and mobile phone application: a qualitative report. J Technol Hum Serv. 2015;33(4):345-57.
52. Stanley B, Brown GK. Safety planning intervention: a brief intervention to mitigate suicide risk. Cognit Behav Pract. 2012;19(2):256-64.
53. Shetty VB, Kiragasur RM. Self-injury and suicidal behaviour in adolescents. In: Kiragasur RM, Kommu JV, Kumar CN, Shetty VB, Parthasarathy R, Math SB (Eds). Child and Adolescent Mental Health: A Manual for Medical officers. Bengaluru: National Institute of Mental Health and Neuro Sciences; 2020.
54. Mann JJ, Michel CA, Auerbach RP. Improving Suicide Prevention Through Evidence-Based Strategies: A Systematic Review. Am J Psychiatry. 2021;178(7):611-24.
55. Zalsman G, Hawton K, Wasserman D, van Heeringen K, Arensman E, Sarchiapone M, et al. Suicide prevention strategies revisited: 10-year systematic review. Lancet Psychiatry. 2016;3(7):646-59.
56. National Suicide Prevention Strategies: Progress, Examples and Indicators, 2018th edition. World Health Organization; 2018.
57. National Suicide Prevention Strategy. Ministry of Health and Family Welfare, Government of India; 2022.
58. Rajaraman D, Travasso S, Chatterjee A, Bhat B, Andrew G, Parab S, et al. The acceptability, feasibility and impact of a lay health counsellor delivered health promoting schools programme in India: a case study evaluation. BMC Health Serv Res. 2012;12(1):127.
59. Gupta S, Sagar R. Juvenile Justice System, Juvenile Mental Health, and the Role of MHPs: Challenges and Opportunities. Indian J Psychol Med. 2020;42(3):304-10.
60. Allen NB, Nelson BW, Brent D, Auerbach RP. Short-term prediction of suicidal thoughts and behaviors in adolescents: Can recent developments in technology and computational science provide a breakthrough? J Affect Disord. 2019; 250:163-9.

CHAPTER 20

Eating and Feeding Disorders

Pratap Sharan, Akanksha Shukla

INTRODUCTION

In this chapter on eating and feeding disorders, we will be focusing on anorexia nervosa, bulimia nervosa, binge eating disorder, avoidant/restrictive food intake disorder (ARFID), pica, rumination disorder, and psychogenic vomiting. Eating disorders usually occur in adolescence or early adulthood, while feeding disorders are more common in childhood. They share similar psychopathology involving a persistent disturbance of eating or eating-related behaviors that produce a change in the consumption or absorption of food, causing a significant impact on physical and psychological health. They retain a good prognosis in childhood and adolescence; however, their prognosis worsens if they persist in adulthood. Early diagnosis and management of cases in children and adolescents are essential.

The first medical description of an anorexic illness was published in 1689 by Richard Morton. In 1873, Sir William Gull gave the term "anorexia nervosa," and at the same time, Ernest Charles Lasegue published case reports of "anorexie hysterique." Hilde Bruch gave the earliest modern description of anorexia nervosa and described three pathognomonic issues: "disturbance in body image of delusional proportions"; "disturbance in the accuracy of perception or cognitive interpretation of stimuli arising in the body"; and "paralyzing sense of ineffectiveness." She emphasized the crucial role of weight correction as the initial component of treatment, with a focus on individual therapy. In 1978, Salvador Minuchin included families in therapy in his work. The final two decades of the 20th century saw a dramatic increase in public awareness of eating disorders and a concomitant rise in their incidence in various parts of the world. This was followed by increased professional interest, new and refined treatment concepts and methods and the development of various treatment programs in multiple settings. Expanded research into the disciplines of neurobiology, cognitive neuroscience, genetics, and psychopharmacology has produced promising results that have contributed to our understanding of eating disorders and their treatment.[1]

NOSOLOGY

The Diagnostic and Statistical Manual, published by the American Psychiatric Association, in its third edition (DSM-III) in 1980, first introduced a section on eating disorders. It included anorexia nervosa (which had appeared under other sections in DSM-I and DSM-II) and bulimia (a new entry).[1] The DSM-IV and the International Classification of Diseases—10th edition (of the World Health Organization, ICD-10) brought in minor modifications. The chapter on Feeding and Eating Disorders in DSM-V included several changes to better represent these conditions across the lifespan. Major changes were the recognition of binge eating disorder, and the inclusion of pica, rumination, and ARFID. DSM-IV listed these under the section on Disorders Usually First Diagnosed during Infancy, Childhood, or Adolescence, which has been removed from DSM-5. Significant revisions to the diagnostic criteria for anorexia nervosa and bulimia nervosa include the exclusion of criteria on amenorrhea from anorexia nervosa, and reduction of binge frequency threshold to once per week. DSM-V also specifies criteria for partial remission, full remission, and severity. It utilizes sex and developmental norms, and physical health and body mass index data to contextualize the interpretation of diagnostic criteria.[2]

The ICD-11 also combines feeding and eating disorders in one section and parallels the developments of DSM-5.[3] It is not clear whether psychogenic vomiting is a mental disorder and thus has been removed from ICD-11 as a diagnostic entity. Now, cases of psychogenic vomiting would be diagnosed as an unspecified eating disorder, a cultural variant of rumination disorder or cyclical vomiting (not a mental disorder).[4]

EPIDEMIOLOGY

The pooled lifetime prevalence rate of any eating disorder was 1.69% in a recent meta-analysis. The lifetime prevalence rates were the lowest for anorexia nervosa (0.16%), followed by bulimia nervosa (0.63%) and binge eating disorder (1.53%).[5]

Adolescent and young adult populations are at an increased risk, with the age of onset for anorexia nervosa being earlier than bulimia nervosa or binge eating disorder. A two-normal components model (early and late onset) best fitted the observed distribution of onset of anorexia nervosa [mean age at onset: 18 years; early onset: mean 16.2 years (75%); late onset: mean 23.6 years (21%)] and bulimia nervosa [mean age at onset: 18.2 years, early onset: mean 16.7 years (83%); late onset: mean 25.3 years (17%)].[6] Binge eating disorder is found to have a later mean age at onset of 23.3 years.[7]

The prevalence rate of anorexia nervosa in India is estimated at 22.3/100,000 with a male: female ratio of 1:3.7.[8] The rates are much lower than those reported globally, which could reflect cultural or methodological issues. Higher rates have also been reported in some studies, e.g., a study conducted in Gujarat reported prevalence rates of 25.2%, 0.6%, and 0.2%, respectively, for suspected eating disorders, other specified feeding or eating disorders, and bulimia nervosa on screening.[9] Multiple clinical studies in India have highlighted adolescents as the most susceptible age group for developing eating disorder symptoms. A file review involving 43 cases of anorexia nervosa revealed a mean age at presentation of 13.4 years, with an average age of onset at 12.4 years.[10] A 10-year (2002–2012) study from a Children and Adolescent Psychiatry hospital in Bengaluru reported a prevalence rate of ED as 0.063%, of which 75% were diagnosed with anorexia nervosa.[11]

A recent systematic review found the prevalence of ARFID to range from 32% to 64% in specialist feeding clinics, 5–22.5% in specialized eating disorder services, 0.3% to 15.5% in nonclinical samples and 2.02 per 100,000 patients in children and adolescents in a national surveillance. Studies conducted in eating disorders services found that patients with ARFID are generally younger at presentation: The mean age in ARFID ranged from 11.1 to 14.6 years.[12] The epidemiological characteristics of ARFID in children are unclear, and there is a lack of validated screening tools in India and internationally.

Pica is common in India. In a robust epidemiological study conducted in Bengaluru, it was the second most common behavioral disorder among children aged 0–3 years (more common in rural than urban areas).[13] In a recent study of children 4–18 years of age attending a psychiatric clinic, 5.6% had a feeding and eating disorder, of which most (5.4%) had pica.[14]

Psychogenic vomiting is commonly reported in clinical populations. A retrospective chart review of a pediatric population found that the 6-year period prevalence of eating disorder was 1.25%, with psychogenic vomiting (85.4%) being the most common.[15]

The lifetime prevalence rates of eating disorders were higher in females (2.58%) than in males (0.74%). Anorexia nervosa, bulimia nervosa, and binge eating disorder had a female-to-male ratio of 15.5, 3.2, and 2.1, respectively.[5] Similarly, Indian survey data consistently demonstrate a significant female predominance among individuals with eating disorders.[16] Psychogenic vomiting is also more common in females, with a female: male ratio of 2:1.5.[15] ARFID is equally prevalent in males and females, but when associated with ASD, it is more common in males.[2]

ETIOLOGY

Animal Models

The starvation-induced hyperactivity model shows that among rodents with access to a running wheel, kept on a restricted feeding schedule, a proportion (predominantly females) chose to exercise instead of eating, even to the point of starvation and death.[17] In another animal model of anorexia, around 40% of adolescent female mice with the *BDNF-Val66Met* gene variant, exposed to social isolation stress and caloric restriction, showed severe self-imposed dietary restriction, sometimes to the point of death, showing the interaction of genetic and environmental factors.[18]

Binge eating behaviors have been explained from an addiction-based model. It suggests that the salience of food rewards is heightened in those with a genetic predisposition, especially following dietary restrictions and in the paucity of other sources of rewards (e.g., in stress and competition). The intermittent consumption of palatable foods with high glycemic index, impulsivity traits, and purging behaviors causes wide fluctuations in blood glucose levels, altering dopamine firing levels, leading to neuroadaptation and a habitual pattern. Thus, the drive to eat is no longer in response to hunger but to food cues.[19]

Human Studies

Eating disorders are associated with complex genetic factors. Twin studies have confirmed the heritability of anorexia nervosa, with estimates ranging from 0.28 to 0.74. Positive polygenic correlations with obsessive compulsive disorder (OCD), neuroticism, educational attainment, and activity have been observed in anorexia nervosa. Research is still limited on the genetics of binge spectrum disorders, which have slightly lower levels of heritability (0·35–0·45) and positive genetic correlations with alcohol problems and obesity.[20]

Social neuroscience theories have shown that brain activations and variations (e.g., in frontal lobe regions) in responding to social cues, such as physical self-perception and social evaluations, were distinct in people with eating disorders, and on recovery, when compared to controls.[21] Altered functional connectivity in networks/areas (such as corticolimbic circuit and insula) has been linked to domains of anorexia nervosa, such as impaired cognitive control and body image disturbances. Seed-based resting state functional magnetic resonance imaging (fMRI) studies showed alterations in the functional connectivity between dorsal anterior cingulate cortex (ACC) and the precuneus, thalamus-frontal circuits and in the right inferior frontal gyrus. These are associated with cognitive control processes and rumination on weight and body shape. In patients with bulimia nervosa and binge eating disorder, hypoactivity in the frontostriatal circuits, abnormal responses to different stimuli in the insula, amygdala, middle frontal gyrus, and occipital cortex and increased regional cerebral blood flow (rCBF) on single-photon emission computed tomography (SPECT) in relation to disorder-related stimuli have been observed.[22]

Studies have indicated that the reinforcing value of food is reduced in anorexia nervosa, while it is increased from the properties of food that are associated with binge eating in bulimia nervosa. The dopamine reward pathway has been linked to anorexia, bulimia, and pica, similar to addiction.[23,24] Altered executive functioning has also been implicated in the inability to control food intake in eating disorders.[21] Current data suggest that control systems—broadly focused on cortico-striato-thalamo-cortical pathways—are affected in bulimia nervosa and may reflect altered neurodevelopment. Examination of maladaptive behavior in anorexia nervosa has indicated that there are differences in neural mechanisms of decision-making about food.[23] A three-dimensional model for ARFID has been proposed wherein neurobiological abnormalities in homeostatic appetite, sensory perception and negative valence systems underpin the three primary ARFID presentations of lack of interest in eating, sensory sensitivity and fear of aversive consequences, respectively.[25]

Studies on the metabolic underpinnings of eating disorders have found that insulin sensitivity is increased in anorexia nervosa and decreased in bulimia nervosa and binge eating disorders.[26] Atypical intestinal microbial composition has also been implicated—archeon methanobrevibacter smithii being higher in the fecal microbiota of participants with anorexia nervosa.[27] Micronutrient deficiencies have been associated with pica, such as iron (strongest evidence), calcium, zinc, and vitamin B complex.[28] Cannabis use may precipitate cyclical vomiting.[29]

A history of childhood adversities is linked with bulimia spectrum disorders.[30] Neglect, lack of stimulation, stressful life situations, relationship difficulties with parents, and temperamental anxiety is also seen in children with rumination disorder.[2]

Five major psychological theories have been hypothesized to explain the development of eating disorders:

1. Self-esteem theory, which says that low self-esteem maintains the exacerbated body shape concerns, resulting in disturbed eating behavior.
2. Interpersonal theory explains how social factors affect eating patterns; interpersonal problems lead to dysfunctional eating, as a maladaptive stress response.
3. Emotional regulation theory talks about emotional stress reactivity. Those with anorexia try to enhance their sense of emotional and self-regulation through extremely restrictive dieting, while in bulimia nervosa, they try to numb negative emotions through binge eating and compensatory behaviors.
4. Transdiagnostic theory proposes common psychological themes underlying the various eating disorders, with the core cognitive concern being excessively influenced by weight and body shape.
5. The theory of mind, from a developmental psychology perspective, addresses the rigidity and impairment in taking others' perspectives, with difficulty in proper emotion recognition and realistic understanding displayed in sufferers of disordered eating.[21]

The various factors involved in eating disorders have been summarized in **Table 1**.[30]

CLINICAL FEATURES

Anorexia Nervosa

Anorexia nervosa is characterized by:

- Significantly low body weight in the context of age, developmental trajectory, sex, and physical health, which is taken as BMI for age below the 5th percentile for children and adolescents (for adults, BMI of <18.5 kg/m^2).

TABLE 1: Etiology of eating disorders.

	Restrictive-type eating disorders	*Bulimic spectrum eating disorders*
Biological factors	Genetic vulnerability, perinatal stressors	Asians
	Females >> Males (10:1)	Females > Males (3:1)
	Mid puberty	Late puberty
	Metabolic vulnerability	
	Behavioral susceptible to appetite dysregulation	
Psychological factors	Reduced theory of mind	Childhood adversity
	Obsessive-compulsive or autistic spectrum traits	ADHD traits (inattention and impulsivity)
	Sensitive to social ranking and threat	Problems in social cognition with emotional avoidance
	High reward delay ability, high control over drives, and cognitive rigidity	Low reward delay ability
	Body image disturbance	
	Alexithymia	
Psychosocial factors	Middle-to-high socioeconomic status and high parental education	Fat shaming by peers, family, and authority figures
	Bullying	
	Exposure to trauma	
	Social isolation	
	Western culture and idealization of thinness	
Behavioral factors	Overcontrol of weight and eating	Weight control behaviors
	Excess concern with body mass index	
	Avoidance coping	

Sometimes, underweight may present in children as failure to gain expected weight. Rapid weight loss within 6 months of >20% of total body weight may also be considered for diagnosis if other criteria are met. A specifier for dangerously low body weight has been described in ICD-11 as BMI <14 kg/m^2 or BMI-for-age of <0.3 percentile, which represents patients at a high risk for medical complications and mortality.

- A persistent pattern of restrictive eating to establish or maintain the low weight.
- Intense fear of gaining weight, which is not alleviated by weight loss. Weight gain is considered a failure of self-control. Children with anorexia may not recognize or acknowledge this fear. Thus, information from collateral sources such as parents, physical examination, and laboratory findings or unexplained persistent behaviors to remain thin, is helpful.
- *Preoccupation with weight or shape:* A sense of having more weight overall or on specific body parts; usually accompanied by excessive weighing, measuring, and looking in the mirror. Insight is usually poor. Thus, patients are usually brought by family members, while those who come on their own usually present

with somatic or psychological sequelae of starvation.[2,3]

Anorexia nervosa is often associated with serious and life-threatening medical complications; these include:[30]

- *Cardiovascular:* Hypotension, bradycardia, prolonged QT, arrhythmias, and cardiomyopathy
- *Dermatological:* Dry, scaly skin and brittle hair (hair loss), lanugo
- *Endocrine and metabolic:* Hypoglycemia, hypokalemia, hyponatremia, hypothermia, altered thyroid function, hypercortisolemia, amenorrhea, delay in puberty, arrested growth, and osteoporosis
- *Gastrointestinal:* Prolonged gastrointestinal transit (delayed gastric emptying, altered antral motility, gastric atrophy, and decreased intestinal mobility), constipation, transaminitis, and liver failure
- *Hematologic:* Anemia, leukopenia, and thrombocytopenia
- *Neurological:* Peripheral neuropathy, loss of brain volume, ventricular enlargement, sulcal widening, cerebral atrophy (pseudoatrophy—correction occurs with weight gain)
- *Oral:* Dental caries
- *Skeletal:* Osteopenia
- *Renal:* Renal calculi and acute kidney injury (from dehydration and purging)
- *Reproductive:* Amenorrhea, infertility, and low birthweight infant.

The severity and consequences of somatic sequelae depend on the age of the patient, duration of illness, intensity of purging, extent and rate of weight loss, and current weight. Children in general suffer from more medical comorbidities due to a smaller fat mass.[31]

Bulimia Nervosa

Bulimia nervosa is characterized by:

- *Recurrent episodes of binge eating:* Defined as eating an amount of food that is definitely more than what most people would eat in a discrete period (usually <2 hours), usually lasting till the person feels uncomfortably full. These episodes are associated with a sense of lack of control, in the form of being unable to control eating or stopping once started. In contrast, some patients may completely abandon efforts to control. These episodes are commonly triggered by negative effects, interpersonal relationship issues, negative perceptions about the body, boredom, and dietary restrictions. A sense of shame often accompanies these binges. Hence, binges usually occur in secrecy. The binge episode temporarily improves the triggering symptoms but leads to negative self-evaluation and dysphoria, thus creating a vicious cycle. The type of food also differs in binges, usually involving foods that one would otherwise avoid.
- *Recurrent inappropriate compensatory behaviors to avert weight gain:* Most commonly, this is done by self-induced vomiting—using fingers or instruments to induce the gag reflex at will or using emetics. Vomiting reduces the fear of weight gain and also the abdominal discomfort from overeating. It can also be done through other purging behaviors like the use of laxatives, diuretics, enemas, thyroid hormone, skipping insulin in diabetes, fasting, and excessive exercise.
- Excessive preoccupation with body weight/shape and self-evaluation that is unduly influenced by it.
- The episodes of binge eating and inappropriate compensatory behaviors occur at least once a week for 1 month (3 months as per DSM-5).[2,3]

Medical complications occur due to the effects of starvation (similar to anorexia nervosa) or purging:[30]

- *Cardiovascular:* Arrhythmias, cardiac failure (can cause sudden death)

- *Endocrine and metabolic:* Electrolyte disturbances [K^+, Na^+, Cl^-, metabolic acidosis (due to laxatives) or alkalosis (due to vomiting)]
- *Gastrointestinal:* Constipation or steatorrhea, gastric or duodenal ulcers, pancreatitis, esophageal or gastric erosions, or perforation
- *Hematological:* Leukopenia or lymphocytosis
- *Oral:* Dental erosion
- *Renal:* Acute renal injury.

Binge Eating Disorder

Recurrent episodes of binge eating: Similar to those seen in bulimia nervosa, associated with distress and occurring at least once a week for 3 months (DSM-5). These episodes of binge eating should not regularly be associated with compensatory behaviors. This is often seen in overweight and obese individuals.[2,3]

Avoidant/Restrictive Food Intake Disorder

It is characterized by a feeding disturbance, leading to a persistent failure in meeting the appropriate nutritional or energy needs. The intake of an insufficient variety or quantity of food needed to meet adequate nutritional or energy requirements. This must not be due to the unavailability of food or preoccupation with body weight and image. This results in clinically significant nutritional deficiencies, significant weight loss, dependence on oral nutritional supplements, or tube feeding, or otherwise negatively affects the physical health of the individual. This may present as a lack of interest in eating, avoidance of food based on its sensory characteristics of food, or concerns about the aversive consequences of eating.[2,3]

The differentiating features of eating disorders are summarized in **Table 2** and case scenarios discussed as shown in **Box 1**.

Pica

Pica is characterized by regular eating of nonnutritive, nonfood substances for at least 1 month. It must be persistent or severe enough to warrant clinical attention and developmentally and socioculturally inappropriate. It is usually diagnosed after the age of 2 years. Typically ingested substances are chalk, soil, hair, paper, cloth, soap, string, talcum powder, wool, gum, metal, paint, pebbles, ice, starch, ash, coal, etc.[2,3]

The phenomenology of pica was described on the compulsive-impulsive spectrum. Those on the compulsive end of the spectrum had other OCD symptoms and those on the impulsive end described the nonnutritive food eating reminiscent of an impulse control disorder.[24,32] The psychopathology of pica has also been compared to that of addictions with intense cravings, failures in treatment, and relapses.[33] Pica has also been explored from a cultural perspective: Geophagy is seen as an expression

TABLE 2: Differences between eating disorders.

		Binge eating	*Purging*	*Body image issues*	*Weight*
Anorexia nervosa	Restricting type	–	–	+	Low and stable
	Binge eating/purging type	+	+	+	Low and fluctuating
Bulimia nervosa		+	+	+	Normal and overweight/obese
Binge eating disorder		+	–	+	Overweight/obese
Avoidant/restrictive food intake disorder		–	–	–	Low

BOX 1: Cases of avoidant/restrictive food intake disorder (ARFID).

A case with onset in childhood

Master R, a 9-year-old boy, presented to the psychiatry outpatient department with history of delayed language milestones, difficulty in interacting with children of his age and preference for solitary play. The mother and child had difficulty establishing a breastfeeding routine and the child was top fed with formula milk from the age of 1 month and later shifted to semi-solid baby food. When the parents tried introducing solid foods, he would become irritable and was mostly continued on semi-solid food. He was shown to various pediatricians, but no organic abnormality was found. He became even more selective, rejecting many semi-solid food items and would take only 1 meal per day of dal and rice mashed together. At the time of presentation, his weight was at the 12th percentile. A diagnosis of autism spectrum disorder and avoidant/restrictive food intake disorder (ARFID) was made. After a dietician consultation, a high-calorie formula feed was introduced as a short-term measure. He was started on low-dose olanzapine. Behavioral intervention was applied to introduce other types of foods.

A case with onset in adolescence

Ms YB is a 17-year-old girl student with a 4-year history of multiple physical symptoms, including nausea, abdominal pain, and loose stools, worsening with meals. She consulted multiple gastroenterologists and underwent investigations, which were normal. She was compliant with the treatments but would also self-medicate with antacids and home remedies. As symptoms worsened with meals, she started altering her diet—initially excluding spices and oil; then certain pulses, vegetables, and fruits, based on the advice of Ayurveda practitioners. Later she started restricting the quantity of food and took only one meal per day. She started losing weight, felt weak, and was unable to maintain her routine and studies. Despite medical advice, she persisted with this dietary pattern.

At presentation, she was admitted because of extremely low weight (BMI 14.6), and a detailed evaluation was done. She reported a normal appetite and hunger pangs but would not increase the quantity of food because of the concern about her abdominal symptoms. She acknowledged the decrease in her weight and wished to regain it, provided her abdominal symptoms were ameliorated.

A diagnosis of ARFID was made based on her progressive restriction of food quantity and types due to fears of adverse consequences of eating and the absence of body weight and image concerns. She responded to behavioral management and was able to maintain her weight (BMI = 18.2) and diet in the normal range while continuing treatment. Her concern about abdominal complaints persisted, although at a reduced intensity.

of soil play, e.g., an observational study from western Uttar Pradesh suggested that mud eating may be culturally sanctioned and reported examples of all members of certain families eating mud. Geophagia, seen in tropical climates, is also hypothesized to protect from food-borne pathogens since clay has adsorptive properties. Pica may be associated with electrolyte and metabolic imbalances, heavy metal poisoning (lead and mercury), parasitic infections, intestinal obstruction, and perforation.[28] A case description is given in **Box 2**.

Rumination Disorder

Rumination disorder is characterized by repeated regurgitation of food, which may be chewed or swallowed again, or spit out. It must occur

BOX 2: Case of pica.

Ms A, a 6-year-old girl, was referred to the psychiatry OPD from the pediatrics department in view of unexplained pain abdomen. There was no history of fever, vomiting, and no signs of intestinal obstruction. She was found to have been ingesting mud for the past 3 years. Initially the frequency of mud ingestion was once a week, but it gradually increased to multiple times every day. At times, she would scrape off plaster from the wall and consume it. Blood investigations showed microcytic hypochromic anemia, low serum iron, and transferring-binding, suggestive of iron deficiency. No specific stressors or antecedent events could be found. A diagnosis of pica was made. She was started on iron supplements, and deworming was done. Behavioral therapy with differential reinforcement was started. The behavior gradually reduced over the next 3 months and stopped completely after 6 months.

several times a week for several weeks, after the developmental age of 2 years. It is not explained by an underlying medical condition that causes nausea/vomiting (e.g., pyloric stenosis) or regurgitation (e.g., esophageal strictures or neuromuscular disorders affecting the esophagus). Infants may take specific positions and grin while doing this and later appear irritable and hungry between episodes. Adolescents typically try to hide it by eating alone, covering their mouth or coughing. Sometimes, rumination may be subtle; however, in clinically salient cases, it is obvious and can cause marked dysfunction in everyday life. These children may be underweight (or fail to gain weight) and malnourished. Some cases of psychogenic vomiting may be a cultural variant of rumination disorder as per ICD-11.[2,3] Signs of rumination disorder include a persistent smell of stomach acid and dental decay due to enamel erosion. The act of rumination can have a self-soothing or self-stimulating function and increase under stress or anxiety.[34] A case is discussed in **Box 3**.

BOX 3: Case of rumination disorder.

MS is a 16-year-old boy, referred from gastroenterology because of "persistent vomiting" after each meal for 2 years for which medical-surgical causes could not be found. He reported a sense of fullness in his abdomen after meals but no nausea. The "vomiting" was preceded by no or minimal retching and the patient explained it as "a filling up of the mouth by food." He never induced "vomiting." He used to contract his abdominal muscles to facilitate "vomiting" earlier, but it had become automatic later. He reduced food intake by 75% to avoid vomiting. He had lost 11 kg (27%) of weight and had a BMI of 15. He had significant social and educational dysfunction. He did not consider himself overweight, denied any binge eating, conscious motivation to diet, and the use of laxatives or diuretics. He agreed that an effort to increase his weight was justified.

As per ICD-11, MS would not meet the diagnostic requirement for a typical case of rumination disorder. Although the food came up without retching, it was not rechewed/reswallowed or spat out, nor was it held in the mouth or go up and down the gullet. Instead, it comes up and is expelled in one movement similar to vomiting. In the culture-related features, ICD-11 clarifies that certain cases of "psychogenic vomiting" in South Asia may be cultural variants of rumination disorder characterized by repeated regurgitation of food along with emptying of the mouth (not rechewing or reswallowing). When compared to psychogenic vomiting, rumination disorder is diagnosed even when the regurgitation is effortless (automatic) but at least in the early stages of the disorder it appears to be volitional (e.g., by contracting abdominal muscles).

Psychogenic Vomiting

The term psychogenic vomiting is used when vomiting is the result of an emotional upset or of an underlying psychic disturbance, only after no organic pathology is found.[35]

The Rome-III diagnostic criteria are used to differentiate between three separate syndromes:

1. *Chronic idiopathic nausea:* Bothersome nausea, not usually associated with vomiting, not explained by endoscopy or metabolic disease, occurring at least several times per week
2. *Functional vomiting:* One or more episodes of vomiting per week, without any other psychiatric disorder, self-induced vomiting, chronic cannabinoid use, abnormalities of the central nervous system, or metabolic diseases. This is relatively rare and needs to be differentiated from rumination disorder.
3. *Cyclic vomiting syndrome:* Stereotypical episodes of vomiting regarding onset (acute) and duration (<1 week), with three or more discrete episodes in the previous year, in the absence of nausea and vomiting between episodes. Its supportive criteria are a history or family history of migraine headaches. Cannabis use may be associated as a precipitating factor or as self-medication to relieve the nausea.

All the above must last for the past 3 months, with the onset of symptoms at least 6 months before diagnosis.[36]

Psychogenic vomiting is not classified as a mental disorder in ICD-11.

COURSE AND PROGNOSIS

Eating disorders cause high morbidity and mortality. Among adolescents with a 12-month history of anorexia nervosa, bulimia nervosa, and binge eating disorder, 24.2%, 10.7%, and 8.7%, respectively, reported severe impairment, especially in social domains. Eating disorders, especially anorexia nervosa, have high mortality rates, with standardized mortality ratios of 5.86, 1.93, and 1.92 for anorexia nervosa, bulimia nervosa, and eating disorder not otherwise specified (EDNOS), respectively.[37]

The 6-year recovery rates were similar for anorexia nervosa, bulimia nervosa, and binge eating disorder (52.3%, 52.2%, and 63.8%, respectively). Relapse rates for those in remission were 26.0%, 17.7%, and 11.4%, respectively, among patients with anorexia nervosa, bulimia nervosa, and binge eating disorder. Crossover was also seen among eating disorders: 23.4% from anorexia nervosa to bulimia nervosa; 8.4% from bulimia nervosa to anorexia nervosa; 7.1% from binge eating disorder to bulimia nervosa; 8.4% from bulimia nervosa to binge eating disorder, respectively. The crossover between anorexia nervosa and binge eating disorder was virtually absent. Good outcomes were seen in those with lower concerns related to weight/shape and lower subjective binge eating episodes. In contrast, substance abuse and more subjective binge eating were associated with poorer outcomes.[38]

Little is known about the longitudinal course and outcome of ARFID. A study of 15–40 year-old ARFID patients in Japan reported that individuals with ARFID were less likely to die (0% vs. 15%), more likely to recover (51.9% vs. 35.5%), had more improvement in terms of eating behaviors (restrictive eating, binge eating, and purging behaviors), psychological state (excessive concern over weight and shape), and psychosocial state (emancipation from nuclear family, personal contacts, and social adjustment) than the AN group. There was no significant group difference in the physical state scores (body mass index score and menstrual pattern).[39]

Pica usually remits spontaneously in most cases.[28] Rumination disorder in infancy usually remits spontaneously. However, it can be life-threatening in some cases and can also take an episodic or continuous course.[2]

COMORBIDITY

Psychiatric Comorbidity

Psychiatric comorbidities are common and must be evaluated in all patients with eating disorders. They are a predictor of poor long-term outcomes.

In patients with anorexia nervosa, the lifetime prevalence of psychiatric comorbidity ranges from 45 to 97% and includes:

- Mood disorders are seen in up to 60% of adolescents with AN, with depressive symptoms more common in the binge/purge type than the restrictive type. Several studies have found an association between weight loss/starvation and depression. Emaciated patients complain of depressed mood, emotional emptiness, social withdrawal, anhedonia, loss of libido, and low self-esteem. Depressive states that result from starvation are often alleviated by nutritional rehabilitation and need to be differentiated from independent mood disorders.
- Anxiety disorders are seen in about 25% of patients with AN. The most common presentations are specific phobias, separation anxiety disorders, and social phobias.
- OCD must be differentiated from eating disorder-related obsessions and compulsions.
- Substance abuse is seen more commonly with the binge/purge subtype than with the restrictive subtype. Mostly, it includes amphetamine, cocaine, and nicotine.

- *Neurodevelopmental disorders:* Autism spectrum disorders are associated with anorexia nervosa.
- *Personality disorders:* Cluster C personality disorders (obsessive compulsive and avoidant) are seen in anorexia nervosa.
- Suicidal ideations are seen in half the patients and attempts in 3–7%, leading to 1 in 5 mortalities seen in anorexia. It is more prevalent in those with the binge/purge subtype, comorbid depression, and longer duration of illness.

Overall, comorbidities are lower in adolescents than in adults.

Comorbidities seen in patients with bulimia nervosa include:

- Mood disorders with a prevalence similar to that of anorexia nervosa
- *Anxiety disorders:* Commonly specific phobias, post-traumatic stress disorder (PTSD), and social phobias
- OCD with a prevalence lower or similar to that of anorexia nervosa
- Substance abuse is highest in bulimic patients with purging behaviors
- *Neurodevelopmental disorders:* Attention-deficit/hyperactivity disorder (ADHD) was associated with bulimia.
- *Personality disorder:* Impulsivity and borderline personality disorders, along with cluster C personality disorders, are seen in bulimia nervosa.
- *Suicidality:* Seen in half the patients with bulimia nervosa and attempts in one-third.

Studies on the comorbidities associated with binge-eating disorders are scarce. These include mood disorders, anxiety disorders, substance abuse disorders, ADHD, and personality disorders (cluster-C and cluster-B).[31]

Young people with ARFID often present with a comorbid psychiatric disorder, with anxiety disorders, especially generalized anxiety disorder, being very common. Between 8.2 and 54.7% of patients with ARFID have autism spectrum disorder, and 21–28% of children with autism spectrum disorder have an increased risk of ARFID.[12]

Feeding problems are common among children with autism and intellectual disability. Pica has also been associated with comorbid psychiatric disorders, especially autism spectrum disorder and intellectual disability.[24] There are also a few reports associating pica with OCD.[32] Rumination disorder may also be associated with intellectual disability and other neurodevelopmental disorders as a form of self-soothing or self-stimulating behaviours.[2] Cannabis use disorder may be present with cyclical vomiting syndrome.[29]

Medical Comorbidity

Eating disorders are associated with various medical comorbidities that can mask symptoms of the disorder, such as:

- *Diabetes:* Patients with insulin-dependent diabetes use insulin omission to lose weight. This causes poor glycemic control and can increase mortality for both diabetes and anorexia.
- Gastrointestinal conditions, epilepsy, cystic fibrosis, and cancer may predispose body-image-conscious youth to neglect treatments that can increase weight.
- Obesity is seen in patients with bulimia nervosa and binge eating disorder.[40]

ASSESSMENT

It is useful to gather information from multiple sources (family members and friends) because patients may be guarded about their symptoms. Indirect evidence of purging behaviors and dietary restrictions should also be considered. Directly observing a family meal at home may provide valuable insights. Menstrual history and input-output charting (daily food and liquid intake, purging behaviors) must also be obtained. Psychiatric comorbidities must be looked for in all patients.

The physical examination and investigations should include:

- Weight monitoring (the height and weight of the child should be plotted on standardized growth charts to see the percentile and trajectory of weight gain or loss)
- Physical assessment (heart rate, blood pressure, and body temperature)
- Oral examination (for caries)
- Complete blood count (for anemia and leukopenia)
- *Serum electrolytes:* Sodium, potassium, calcium, chloride, magnesium, and phosphate
- *Kidney function tests:* Creatinine and urea
- *Liver function tests:* Serum proteins, liver enzymes, amylase, and lipase
- *Blood glucose levels:* Low in starvation and high in uncontrolled diabetes
- Thyroid function tests
- *Electrocardiogram:* For cardiac status and severe electrolyte abnormalities
- Electroencephalography, magnetic resonance imaging, and computed tomography (in case of atypical eating disorder, e.g., in boys, children, or those with seizures)
- Bone density scans (for osteopenia)
- Urine pregnancy test (in patients with amenorrhea, vomiting, and weight fluctuations)
- Determination of iron, ferritin, zinc, and lead levels in patients with pica
- Obstruction series, plain abdominal radiographs, CT, and endoscopy may be necessary in case of obstruction in pica patients to find the etiology—parasites or bezoars.[24]
- Esophageal manometry (to rule out medical causes in rumination disorder)[34]
- Urinary drug screen (for cannabis use), upper GI endoscopy, X-ray abdomen, CT enterography, gastric emptying tests, tests to rule out Addison's disease, and mitochondrial diseases—in cases of cyclical vomiting
- Esophageal pH testing, upper GI endoscopy for structural abnormalities, and gastric scintigraphy to rule out gastroparesis—in cases of chronic idiopathic nausea.[29]

Scales

The SCOFF questionnaire by Morgan et al. is a validated, brief screening tool. It has five questions, out of which a yes in two or more indicates a likely case of anorexia nervosa or bulimia nervosa. The questions are as follows:

1. Do you make yourself *S*ick because you feel uncomfortably full?
2. Do you worry you have lost *C*ontrol over how much you eat?
3. Have you recently lost more than *O*ne stone (6 kg) in weight over a 3-month period?
4. Do you believe yourself to be *F*at when others say you are thin?
5. Would you say that *F*ood dominates your life?[41]

The Eating Disorder Assessment for DSM-5 (EDA-5) is a clinician-rated, semi-structured interview that can be used for confirming the diagnosis in the adolescent population. It also has a youth version available for children aged 8–14.[42] The Child Eating Disorder Examination Questionnaire (ChEDE-Q) has been adapted to a culturally appropriate, English language version for assessing disordered eating among urban Indian adolescents.[43] The Eating Disorder-15 for Youth (ED-15-Y) scale may be used to briefly assess eating disorder psychopathology in youth (8–18 years). It is sensitive to change very early in treatment and thus can be used to measure treatment outcomes.[44] The Pica, ARFID, and Rumination Disorder Interview (PARDI) has been developed to assess the presence and severity of these diagnoses for evaluation and treatment planning in clinical and research settings.[45]

MANAGEMENT

Eating disorders require prompt and often intensive management. The treatment setting can be outpatient or inpatient. Outpatient treatment offers the advantage of better continuity of school, daily activities, and interaction with family and peers. Indications for inpatient treatment are:

- Symptoms such as suicidality, aggression, and severity of illness (<75% median BMI for age and sex, >10% weight loss in 6 months or 20% in 1 year)
- *Medical instability:* Need for monitoring, intravenous fluids, or nasogastric feeding (bradycardia, postural hypotension, hypoglycemia, hypothermia, hyponatremia/hypokalemia/hypophosphatemia/hypomagnesemia).
- *Severe complications:* QTc prolongations, ECG abnormalities, seizures, syncope, cardiac failure, pancreatitis, arrested growth, and development
- *Comorbidity affecting management:* Medical or psychiatric
- Severe psychosocial stressors and poor social support
- Inability to decrease dietary restrictions and purging behavior without monitoring
- Poor motivation and compliance with treatment, failure of outpatient treatment.[46]

Anorexia Nervosa

Weight Restoration and Nutritional Rehabilitation

Weight restoration is a crucial part of recovery. Individualized weight targets need to be set, which can be based on premorbid height, weight, BMI percentiles, and current pubertal stage or the weight at which reproductive physiology normalizes (e.g., restoration of normal menstruation and ovulation or testicular function). Menses typically resume at approximately 90–95% of median BMI. Dieticians can make specific meal plans and include calorie-dense liquids in between meals. Nasogastric tube feeding may be necessary for short periods in some cases while transitioning to oral feeding.[46] Earlier, high-caloric diets were avoided initially for fear of refeeding syndrome. However, recent studies do not show any difference between the two regimens (even with very low BMI). Rather than total caloric intake, lower BMI at admission may predict hypophosphatemia.[47] Care should be taken with refeeding smaller children who may experience faster dehydration and deterioration.

Psychological Interventions

Psychological treatments are considered essential for the management of eating disorders. The APA recommends eating disorder-focused family-based treatment (FBT) for adolescents with an involved caregiver.[46] A wide range of manualized psychotherapeutic treatments exist for anorexia nervosa, which are described here.[48]

Family-based treatment (well established): It involves both patients and their families. It consists of hour-long sessions in 3 phases—phase 1 focuses on absolving parents from the burden of causing the disorder and appreciating the positive aspects of their parenting styles. The family is encouraged to find the best way to help restore the child's weight on their own. This phase lasts 3–5 months with weekly sessions. In phase 2, sessions are conducted every 2–3 weeks, where parents are encouraged to shift control of eating and weight back to the adolescent. In phase 3, monthly sessions focus on building a healthy relationship between the parents and the adolescent, and issues about normal adolescent development are addressed. Shorter courses of 10 sessions over 6 months may be used for those with intact families and without obsessive-compulsive features.[49]

Maudsley family therapy (MFT) (well established): It considers the family as a valuable resource to be mobilized to help the adolescent, rather than placing blame on them and acknowledges the effect of the disorder on the entire family. MFT also consists of three phases. The first is focused on the approach to family meals, in which parents decide their attitude toward eating, which can be either initial control over all eating habits or considering that the eating is none of their business. The second phase starts when there is steady weight gain and tries to maintain it with minimum tension. It addresses family issues from the perspective of how it affects their task of helping the child. In the third phase, the responsibility for the weight is transferred back to the patient. A return to normalcy and healthy parent-child relationships are built.[50]

Family system therapy (FST; probably efficacious): It focuses on how patterns develop in a family to diffuse anxiety. Its goal is to assist family members in reducing blaming and reactivity and taking more responsibility for themselves through greater levels of differentiation.[51]

Adolescent-focused therapy (AFT; probably efficacious): It is an individual-based therapy that helps patients identify and define their emotions and tolerate these affective states instead of numbing themselves through starvation.[52]

Cognitive behavioral treatment (enhanced; CBT-E) (experimental): It is considered a transdiagnostic personalized psychological treatment. It is divided into four stages: Problem identification and behavior modification; progress monitoring and formulation of treatment plan; addressing perpetuating factors; maintenance of progress; and dealing with setbacks.[53]

Pharmacotherapy

There is limited evidence of pharmacological treatments, with most of the studies on pharmacological treatments conducted on adults. Medications should be used with caution due to their effect of prolonging the QTc interval. Low-dose olanzapine may be used to increase the tolerance of weight gain and decrease ruminations in patients with anorexia nervosa.[54] There is mixed evidence when it comes to the role of selective serotonin reuptake inhibitors (SSRIs) in treatment. Initial reports that fluoxetine might reduce relapse in weight-recovered anorexic patients failed to be replicated in later studies.[40] Oral hormone replacement therapy has at times been used to improve bone mineral density in patients with amenorrhea, but this must be weighed against the risks of early epiphyseal fusion and false reassurance of weight normalcy when more weight gain is required. It can be considered for older adolescents (bone age ≥15 years; BMD Z score <–2). Supplementation with oral vitamin D and calcium can be done in those with deficiency, weighing against the risk of renal stones and cardiovascular calcification at high doses.

The duration of treatment varies with the treatment approach and for individual patients, but treatment is usually continued even after weight restoration to prevent relapse of symptoms.[46]

Bulimia Nervosa and Binge Eating Disorder

Treatment with family-based psychotherapy or individual disorder-focused cognitive behavioral therapy is indicated for patients with bulimia nervosa.[46] Interpersonal therapy is a brief treatment focusing on the social and interpersonal context in which the disorder began and is maintained. It is a strongly supported evidence-based treatment of bulimia nervosa and binge eating disorder.[55]

In terms of pharmacotherapy, antidepressants may be considered.[46] SSRIs (up to 60 mg of fluoxetine) are also indicated, especially if there is minimal response to psychotherapy.[54] Bupropion (due to the risk of seizures) and drugs prolonging QTc should be avoided, especially in those with purging behaviors (laxative use and self-induced vomiting).

Avoidant/Restrictive Food Intake Disorder

Children with ARFID with inadequate oral intake need support in the form of intensive behavioral interventions, oral nutritional formula supplementation, and tube feeding delivered in day care or inpatient settings. Tube feeding is at times considered earlier in treatment for ARFID (compared to anorexia), prior to less invasive interventions. However, its benefits must be weighed against the risk of iatrogenic effects (e.g., reduced expectation for solid food consumption and reinforcement of sick role) and difficulty in weaning off the tube.

Nonpharmacological strategies, especially behavioral interventions, have been most widely studied for ARFID, which include systematic desensitization or operant conditioning paradigms to increase the quantity and variety of food consumed.[25] However, there is controversy regarding behavioral interventions—Satter's influential Feeding Dynamics Model suggests that parents should never apply pressure to encourage children with ARFID to increase or expand their dietary intake.[56] Family-based therapy has also been used in the management of ARFID.[25] A new form of cognitive-behavioral therapy for ARFID (CBT-AR) has been developed, which teaches skills for approaching novel foods in a stepwise fashion, interoceptive and in vivo exposure for addressing phobic responses to traumatic experiences such as vomiting or choking and involves parental support.[57]

Pharmacotherapy has been used for the management of ARFID but always as an adjunct to psychotherapy. Though cyproheptadine, olanzapine, and mirtazapine have been used for their appetite-stimulating properties, more research is needed on their efficacy.[58,59]

Pica

There is no specific treatment for pica. Treatment should focus on identifying and correcting the underlying physical and psychological causes. Behavioral interventions, cognitive behavioral therapy, and appropriate management of the environment can be done.[28,34] Addressing nutritional deficiencies (iron, calcium, zinc, and vitamin B complex), especially iron supplementation, has been shown to be effective. Deworming may be useful in some cases.[60] SSRIs have been shown to be effective in case reports. Those with comorbid OCD may respond to higher doses of SSRIs, with gradual improvement in OC symptoms, while those with impulsive pica require more caution with pharmacotherapy.[32] The use of olanzapine has mixed evidence, with case reports of it both causing and treating pica.[24,61]

Rumination Disorder

Current treatment recommendations include behavioral approaches, such as habit reversal training, as well as cognitive-behavioral approaches for older children able to access this form of therapy. There is limited evidence for pharmacologic treatment, and this modality is not generally recommended as a first-line intervention.[34]

Psychogenic Vomiting

Acute episodes of vomiting may require intravenous fluids and antiemetics. There are no treatment guidelines for the treatment of psychogenic vomiting in children and adolescents. Usually, its management requires a tailor-made approach that combines various strategies.

Nonpharmacological approaches include supportive psychotherapy, behavioral therapy, cognitive and social skills training, self-monitoring with suppression of the urge to vomit, autogenic training, and integrating systems theory and attachment theory.

The pharmacological treatment discussed below has usually been studied on adults and should be used with caution in children.

In case of cyclical vomiting, triptans (in those with a history of migraine) for acute attacks and low-dose tricyclic antidepressants for prophylaxis can be used. Limited evidence is currently available for the use of β-blockers like propranolol, antiepileptics like levetiracetam and zonisamide, ketorolac, and prochlorperazine. Cyclical vomiting associated with cannabis use may be resolved on abstinence from cannabis.

There is a lack of evidence for the treatment of functional vomiting. Antidepressants such as tricyclic antidepressants (TCAs) and escitalopram have been found to be useful in some cases.

Chronic idiopathic nausea may be treated using prokinetics like domperidone, anticholinergics like prochlorperazine, and promethazine and 5HT3 antagonists like ondansetron. TCAs may also be used in refractory cases.[29,62]

Newer Treatments

Newer therapies developed for the management of eating disorders (discussed in this section) have mostly been studied on adults.

Cognitive remediation therapy has been tried in anorexia nervosa to target cognitive inflexibility; however, few controlled trials have been conducted and data on efficacy are not consistent.[63] Exposure and Response Prevention for Anorexia Nervosa (AN-EXRP) is a new therapy that targets eating-related fear and anxiety to improve maladaptive eating behaviours.[64] Virtual reality is now being used for assessing and managing patients with eating disorders. This helps decrease patients' negative emotional responses to virtual food or body image stimuli.[65]

Topiramate is also a promising new agent for binge eating disorder and obesity.[66] Meta-analysis of data pooled from three RCTs favor lisdexamfetamine over placebo for binge eating disorder. However, it is currently unavailable in India, and its side effects and high attrition rates need to be weighed against its positive effects.[67]

Neuromodulation techniques have been tried in adults with anorexia nervosa, such as deep brain stimulation (involving the splenium of the corpus callosum and the nucleus accumbens) and noninvasive brain stimulation techniques; however, further studies are needed to see the long-term effects of the treatment.[68,69]

PREVENTION

Awareness about eating disorders is essential among children, parents, and teachers. A review found common themes among successful eating disorder prevention programs to be:[70]

- Based on a cognitive or behavioral approach
- Target risk factors
- Include discussions on media literacy, sociocultural pressures, healthy eating, nutrition, and body acceptance/body satisfaction
- In younger ages, include boys and girls together, while in older ages, target women alone
- Group based
- Have multiple sessions
- Have interactive sessions.

SUMMARY AND CONCLUSION

Eating disorders have a lifetime prevalence of about 1.7% in global populations. They are more common among adolescent and young adult females. The rates in India may be lower, with less typical presentations and ARFID, pica, and psychogenic vomiting being common.

They have a complex biopsychosocial etiology. Medical complications are common in patients with feeding and eating disorders and can lead to mortality. Psychiatric comorbidities are present in majority of patients with eating disorders and need to be evaluated. Various tools such as the SCOFF questionnaire and Child Eating Disorder Examination Questionnaire may be used for assessment. Management includes weight restoration and nutritional rehabilitation. Psychotherapy is considered essential for management, while limited evidence exists for pharmacotherapy.

REFERENCES

1. Marks A. The evolution of our understanding and treatment of eating disorders over the past 50 years. J Clin Psychol. 2019;75(8):1380-91.
2. American Psychiatric Association. Diagnostic and Statistical Manual of Mental Disorders. Fifth Edition. American Psychiatric Association; 2013.
3. World Health Organization. International Classification of Diseases, 11th Revision. World Health Organization; 2019.
4. Sharan P, Hans G. Cultural Issues Related to ICD-11 Mental, Behavioural and Neurodevelopmental Disorders. Consort Psychiatr. 2021;2(2):7-15.
5. Qian J, Wu Y, Liu F, Zhu Y, Jin H, Zhang H, et al. An update on the prevalence of eating disorders in the general population: a systematic review and meta-analysis. Eat Weight Disord. 2022;27(2):415-28.
6. Volpe U, Tortorella A, Manchia M, Monteleone AM, Albert U, Monteleone P. Eating disorders: What age at onset? Psychiatry Res. 2016;238:225-7.
7. Kessler RC, Berglund PA, Chiu WT, Deitz AC, Hudson JI, Shahly V, et al. The prevalence and correlates of binge eating disorder in the World Health Organization World Mental Health Surveys. Biol Psychiatry. 2013;73(9):904-14.
8. Mohandoss AA. A Study of Burden of Anorexia Nervosa in India - 2016. J Ment Health Hum Behav. 2018;23(1):25.
9. Raval CM, Bhatt RB, Tiwari DS, Panchal BN. Prevalence and characteristics of eating disorders among college students of a nonmetro city of Gujarat. Ind Psychiatry J. 2022;31(1):74-80.
10. Prasad KE, Rajan RJ, Basker MM, Mammen PM, Reshmi YS. Clinical Profile of Adolescent Onset Anorexia Nervosa at a Tertiary Care Center. Indian Pediatr. 2021;58(8):726-8.
11. Jacob P, Sadananda S, Sagar J, Srinath S, Seshadri S. A study of eating disorders in children and adolescents from a tertiary care centre in India. Arch Ment Health. 2016;17(1-2):1-5.
12. Sanchez-Cerezo J, Nagularaj L, Gledhill J, Nicholls D. What do we know about the epidemiology of avoidant/restrictive food intake disorder in children and adolescents? A systematic review of the literature. Eur Eat Disord Rev. 2023;31(2):226-46.
13. Srinath S, Girimaji SC, Gururaj G, Seshadri S, Subbakrishna DK, Bhola P, et al. Epidemiological study of child & adolescent psychiatric disorders in urban & rural areas of Bangalore, India. Indian J Med Res. 2005;122(1):67-79.
14. Sahu S, Menon P, Kumar S, Saldanha D. Sociodemographic Profile of Psychiatric Disorders among Children in a Tertiary Care Hospital in Western India. Int J Contemporary Med Res. 2020;7(9).
15. Mammen P, Russell S, Russell P. Prevalence of eating disorders and psychiatric co-morbidity among children and adolescents. Indian Pediatr. 2007;44(5):357.
16. Vaidyanathan S, Menon V. Research on feeding and eating disorders in India: A narrative review. Indian J Psychiatry. 2024;66(1):9-25.
17. Guttierrez E. A rat in the labyrinth of anorexia nervosa: contributions of the activity-based anorexia rodent model to the understanding of anorexia nervosa. Int J Eat Disord. 2013;46(4):289-301.
18. Madra M, Zeltser LM. BDNF-Val66Met variant and adolescent stress interact to promote susceptibility to anorexic behavior in mice. Transl Psychiatry. 2016;6(4):e776.
19. Treasure J, Leslie M, Chami R, Fernández-Aranda F. Are trans diagnostic models of eating disorders fit for purpose? A consideration of the evidence for food addiction. Eur Eat Disord Rev J Eat Disord Assoc. 2018;26(2):83-91.
20. Bulik CM, Flatt R, Abbaspour A, Carroll I. Reconceptualizing anorexia nervosa. Psychiatry Clin Neurosci. 2019;73(9):518-25.

21. Zanella E, Lee E. Integrative review on psychological and social risk and prevention factors of eating disorders including anorexia nervosa and bulimia nervosa: seven major theories. Heliyon. 2022;8(11).
22. Donnelly B, Touyz S, Hay P, Burton A, Russell J, Caterson I. Neuroimaging in bulimia nervosa and binge eating disorder: a systematic review. J Eat Disord. 2018;6:3.
23. Steinglass JE, Berner LA, Attia E. Cognitive Neuroscience of Eating Disorders. Psychiatr Clin North Am. 2019;42(1):75-91.
24. Schnitzler E. The Neurology and Psychopathology of Pica. Curr Neurol Neurosci Rep. 2022;22(8): 531-6.
25. Thomas JJ, Lawson EA, Micali N, Misra M, Deckersbach T, Eddy KT. Avoidant/Restrictive Food Intake Disorder: A Three-Dimensional Model of Neurobiology with Implications for Etiology and Treatment. Curr Psychiatry Rep. 2017;19(8):54.
26. Ilyas A, Hübel C, Stahl D, Stadler M, Ismail K, Breen G, et al. The metabolic underpinning of eating disorders: A systematic review and meta-analysis of insulin sensitivity. Mol Cell Endocrinol. 2019;497:110307.
27. Schwensen HF, Kan C, Treasure J, Høiby N, Sjögren M. A systematic review of studies on the faecal microbiota in anorexia nervosa: future research may need to include microbiota from the small intestine. Eat Weight Disord. 2018;23(4): 399-418.
28. Bhatia M, Kaur J. Pica as a Culture Bound Syndrome. Delhi Psychiatry J. 2014;17(1).
29. Talley NJ. Functional nausea and vomiting. Aust Fam Phys. 2007;36(9):694-7.
30. Treasure J, Duarte TA, Schmidt U. Eating disorders. Lancet Lond Engl. 2020;395(10227):899-911.
31. Herpertz-Dahlmann B. Adolescent eating disorders: update on definitions, symptomatology, epidemiology, and comorbidity. Child Adolesc Psychiatr Clin N Am. 2015;24(1):177-96.
32. Stein DJ, Bouwer C, Van Heerden B. Pica and the obsessive-compulsive spectrum disorders. Afr Med J. 1996;86(12 Suppl):1586-8, 1591-2.
33. Young SL. Craving Earth: Understanding Pica—the Urge to Eat Clay, Starch, Ice, and Chalk. Columbia University Press; 2011:240.
34. Bryant-Waugh R. Feeding and Eating Disorders in Children. Psychiatr Clin North Am. 2019;42(1):157-67.
35. Leibovich MA. Psychogenic Vomiting: Psychotherapeutic Considerations. Psychother Psychosom. 2010;22(2-6):263-8.
36. Drossman D, Corazziari E, Delvaux M, Spiller R, Talley N, Thompson WG, et al. Rome III: The Functional Gastrointestinal Disorders, 3rd edition. Degnon Associates; 2006.
37. Arcelus J, Mitchell AJ, Wales J, Nielsen S. Mortality rates in patients with anorexia nervosa and other eating disorders. A meta-analysis of 36 studies. Arch Gen Psychiatry. 2011;68(7):724-31.
38. Castellini G, Lo Sauro C, Mannucci E, Ravaldi C, Rotella CM, Faravelli C, et al. Diagnostic crossover and outcome predictors in eating disorders according to DSM-IV and DSM-V proposed criteria: a 6-year follow-up study. Psychosom Med. 2011;73(3):270-9.
39. Nakai Y, Nin K, Noma S, Hamagaki S, Takagi R, Teramukai S, et al. Clinical presentation and outcome of avoidant/restrictive food intake disorder in a Japanese sample. Eat Behav. 2017;24:49-53.
40. Hay P, Morris J. Eating disorders. In: Textbook of Child and Adolescent Mental Health. IACAPAP; 2016.
41. Morgan JF, Reid F, Lacey JH. The SCOFF questionnaire: assessment of a new screening tool for eating disorders. BMJ. 1999;319(7223): 1467-8.
42. Sysko R, Glasofer DR, Hildebrandt T, Klimek P, Mitchell JE, Berg KC, et al. The eating disorder assessment for DSM-5 (EDA-5): Development and validation of a structured interview for feeding and eating disorders. Int J Eat Disord. 2015;48(5):452-63.
43. Ahuja L, Diedrichs P, Garbett K, Chaudhry A, Hasan F, Uglik-Marucha N, et al. Adaptation and Validation of the Child Eating Disorder Examination Questionnaire (ChEDE-Q) for Use in English among Adolescents in Urban India. Nutrients. 2023;15(17):3836.
44. Accurso EC, Waller G. A brief session-by-session measure of eating disorder psychopathology for children and adolescents: Development and psychometric properties of the Eating

Disorder-15 for Youth (ED-15-Y). Int J Eat Disord. 2021;54(4):569-77.
45. Bryant-Waugh R, Micali N, Cooke L, Lawson EA, Eddy KT, Thomas JJ. Development of the Pica, ARFID, and Rumination Disorder Interview, a multi-informant, semi-structured interview of feeding disorders across the lifespan: A pilot study for ages 10–22. Int J Eat Disord. 2019;52(4): 378-87.
46. Crone C, Fochtmann LJ, Attia E, Boland R, Escobar J, Fornari V, et al. The American Psychiatric Association Practice Guideline for the Treatment of Patients With Eating Disorders. Am J Psychiatry. 2023;180(2):167-71.
47. Mosuka EM, Murugan A, Thakral A, Ngomo MC, Budhiraja S, St Victor R. Clinical Outcomes of Refeeding Syndrome: A Systematic Review of High vs. Low-Calorie Diets for the Treatment of Anorexia Nervosa and Related Eating Disorders in Children and Adolescents. Cureus. 2023; 15(5):e39313.
48. Zipfel S, Giel KE, Bulik CM, Hay P, Schmidt U. Anorexia nervosa: aetiology, assessment, and treatment. Lancet Psychiatry. 2015;2(12): 1099-111.
49. Lock J, Grange DL. Treatment Manual for Anorexia Nervosa, Second Edition: A Family-Based Approach. Guilford Press; 2012.
50. Russell GFM. An Evaluation of Family Therapy in Anorexia Nervosa and Bulimia Nervosa. Arch Gen Psychiatry. 1987;44(12):1047.
51. Brown J. Bowen Family Systems Theory and Practice: Illustration and Critique. Aust N Z J Fam Ther. 1999;20(2):94-103.
52. Lock J, Le Grange D, Agras WS, Moye A, Bryson SW, Jo B. Randomized clinical trial comparing family-based treatment with adolescent-focused individual therapy for adolescents with anorexia nervosa. Arch Gen Psychiatry. 2010;67(10): 1025-32.
53. Fairburn C. Cognitive Behavior Therapy and Eating Disorders. Guilford Press; 2008.
54. Couturier J, Lock J. A review of medication use for children and adolescents with eating disorders. J Can Acad Child Adolesc Psychiatry. 2007;16(4):173.
55. Karam AM, Fitzsimmons-Craft EE, Tanofsky-Kraff M, Wilfley DE. Interpersonal Psychotherapy and the Treatment of Eating Disorders. Psychiatr Clin North Am. 2019;42(2):205-18.
56. Satter E. Feeding dynamics: Helping children to eat well. J Pediatr Health Care. 1995;9(4): 178-84.
57. Thomas JJ, Eddy KT. Cognitive-Behavioral Therapy for Avoidant/Restrictive Food Intake Disorder: Children, Adolescents, and Adults. Cambridge University Press; 2018.
58. Thomas JJ, Brigham KS, Sally ST, Hazen EP, Eddy KT. Case 18-2017: An 11-Year-Old Girl with Difficulty Eating after a Choking Incident. N Engl J Med. 2017;376(24):2377-86.
59. Brewerton TD, D'Agostino M. Adjunctive Use of Olanzapine in the Treatment of Avoidant Restrictive Food Intake Disorder in Children and Adolescents in an Eating Disorders Program. J Child Adolesc Psychopharmacol. 2017;27(10): 920-2.
60. Advani S, Kochhar G, Chachra S, Dhawan P. Eating everything except food (PICA): A rare case report and review. J Int Soc Prev Community Dent. 2014;4(1):1.
61. Lerner AJ. Treatment of pica behavior with olanzapine. CNS Spectr. 2008;13(1):19.
62. Koparde V, Ramesh V, Ninan PA, Poornima N, Girimaji SC. Treatment of chronic psychogenic vomiting in an adolescent - successful use of multiple therapeutic strategies. J Indian Assoc Child Adolesc Ment Health. 2019;15(3): 83-9.
63. Kim EJ, Bahk YC, Oh H, Lee WH, Lee JS, Choi KH. Current Status of Cognitive Remediation for Psychiatric Disorders: A Review. Front Psychiatry. 2018;9:461.
64. Steinglass JE, Albano AM, Simpson HB, Wang Y, Zou J, Attia E, et al. Confronting fear using exposure and response prevention for anorexia nervosa: A randomized controlled pilot study. Int J Eat Disord. 2014;47(2):174-80.
65. Clus D, Larsen ME, Lemey C, Berrouiguet S. The Use of Virtual Reality in Patients with Eating Disorders: Systematic Review. J Med Internet Res. 2018;20(4):e157.
66. Nourredine M, Jurek L, Angerville B, Longuet Y, de Ternay J, Derveaux A, et al. Use of Topiramate in the Spectrum of Addictive and Eating Disorders: A Systematic Review Comparing Treatment

Schemes, Efficacy, and Safety Features. CNS Drugs. 2021;35(2):177-213.

67. Fornaro M, Solmi M, Perna G, De Berardis D, Veronese N, Orsolini L, et al. Lisdexamfetamine in the treatment of moderate-to-severe binge eating disorder in adults: systematic review and exploratory meta-analysis of publicly available placebo-controlled, randomized clinical trials. Neuropsychiatr Dis Treat. 2016;25:1827-36.
68. Hsu TI, Nguyen A, Gupta N, Godbole N, Perisetla N, Hatter MJ, et al. Effectiveness of Deep Brain Stimulation in Treatment of Anorexia Nervosa and Obesity: A Systematic Review. World Neurosurg. 2022;168:179-89.
69. Lee DJ, Elias GJB, Lozano AM. Neuromodulation for the treatment of eating disorders and obesity. Ther Adv Psychopharmacol. 2018;8(2): 73-92.
70. Ciao A, Loth K, Neumark-Sztainer D. Preventing eating disorder pathology: common and unique features of successful eating disorders prevention programs. Curr Psychiatry Rep. 2014;16:1-3.

CHAPTER 21

Childhood Trauma, Child Sexual Abuse, and Family Violence

Eesha Sharma, Shekhar Seshadri

INTRODUCTION

What is Childhood Trauma?

Operationalizing Trauma in Terms of Adverse Childhood Experiences

The Diagnostic and Statistical Manual of Mental Disorders, Fifth Edition (DSM-5) defines trauma as actual or threatened death, serious injury, or sexual violence that is either directly experienced, witnessed, or learnt as having happened to someone close to an individual.[1] It also talks about *re-traumatization* through repeated or extreme exposure to details of a traumatic event. This operationalization is included to ensure reliability in the elicitation of trauma history and communication across liaising care services. However, research has shown that children's development and well-being are impacted by a much broader gamut of events encompassed under *adverse childhood experiences* (ACEs).[2] These could happen at the individual (physical/emotional/sexual abuse or neglect), family (violence, mental illness, parental separation or loss, incarceration), or community (collective violence) level and are known to increase risk for all types of noncommunicable disorders, including mental illnesses. From a developmental psychopathology perspective,[3] they comprise significant exposures that interact with a child's developmental characteristics to influence further development and well-being. These observations have strong clinical concordance, wherein a multiplicity of adverse exposures is seen to exacerbate developmental challenges and trigger and maintain mental morbidity. Therefore, in this chapter as we discuss about trauma, violence, and child sexual abuse (CSA) in the context of child and adolescent psychiatry, we will be taking the broader trauma conceptualization that ACEs entail rather than the reliable but narrow definition that DSM-5 offers. Throughout the chapter, unless otherwise specified, the term "child" will cover ages 0–17 years.

From an ACE's perspective, trauma includes stressors that overwhelm a child's ability to cope. Such stressors may be single and apparent, for example, in the case of a 15-year-old girl who presented with low mood and intrusive recollections after sexual abuse by her neighbor. However, in most instances, stressors are multiple and have long-term developmental and mental health impact, such as in the case of a 10-year-old autistic boy, who presented with obsessive–compulsive symptoms, in the background of significant family violence and parental discord. For the 15-year-old girl the traumatic event may well be *causal* in her psychiatric morbidity, whereas for the 10-year-old boy, the adversities play a key *pathoplastic* role, that is, they are developmentally nonconducive and could contribute to maintenance of the obsessive–compulsive symptoms.

In the clinic, history of trauma may be readily reported or suspected when children present with disorders like post-traumatic stress disorder (PTSD), dissociation, or attachment disorders. However, trauma and adversity may also be frequently, incidentally, discovered when children have other psychiatric disorders, like anxiety, mood disorder, eating disorders, and oppositional defiance, or have symptoms, like self-harm, suicidality, aggression, and school refusal. It is implied that the clinician must keep a high index of suspicion for trauma and adversity.

Concept of Complex Trauma

Adversities are not uncommon in life. Epidemiological studies have shown that majority of young people have faced at least one adversity during childhood.[4] Not every child who faces an adversity is impacted by it. Adversities are more likely to impact children when their care and protection systems are inadequate. The concept of *complex trauma* perhaps arises from this. Complex trauma is defined as a situation when a child has experienced repeated or multiple traumas and has disrupted attachment relationships.[5] Clinical presentations can be quite variable, from mood and anxiety to dissociation or even PTSD. The occurrence of repeated or multiple traumas signifies high threat, while the disrupted attachments signify high deprivation. High threat and deprivation are understandably nonconducive to children's development and well-being.

Complex trauma—a case illustration: Z, a 14-year-old girl, brought by her parents, was reported to be steadily declining from being a star student in school, over the past 2 years. She also had instances of absences from home, despite the recent COVID-19-related lockdowns. Parents reported that Z had been a "compliant" child with no problems at school or home. Z, however, reported that she had always been terrified of her father who would often use physically punitive methods, especially for academic performance, increasingly so in the past 2 years. The father was perceived as "strict" and punitive by mother too the child, and her younger sibling. Around 2 years ago, Z had been in an intimate relationship with a school classmate for a few months. The relationship abruptly ended for unclear reasons. Z said she had been emotionally invested in this boy, and she felt, for the first time, that she could "talk" to someone. Z was devastated after the breakup. She tried to hide her distress from her family and friends for a few months. She tried to focus on her studies but found it hard. Gradually, she found herself getting into sexual encounters with classmates and even strangers on two occasions. She described these as "flings" and did not feel there was anything "wrong". She noted that at times, she found it difficult to recall the sequence of events of these "flings". Parents' response to learning about her breakup and subsequent "flings" was to ask her to "forget" and "forgive" like they were doing and to return to focusing on her studies. Z expressed that she wanted help to be able to handle her father's anger better, to be able to study, and to get back with her boyfriend. In therapy sessions, Z appeared eager to get help but found it difficult to follow through on any discussions.

Z's history illustrates how relational and emotional adversities occurred in the background of her difficult attachment relationships with her parents. Academic difficulties and upsets in romantic relationships are not uncommon in teenagers. However, they can become triggers for mental morbidity when there is inadequate support from attachment relationships that could help buffer the negative impact.

CHILD SEXUAL ABUSE

The World Health Organization (WHO) defines CSA as a child's involvement in sexual activity for which the child is not developmentally ready, that the child is not capable of fully comprehending, and to which the child is incapable of giving informed consent.[6] Developmental readiness—in terms of physical, cognitive, emotional, and sexual maturity—evolves over childhood, especially adolescence. Sexual expression and explorations are normative among adolescents; however, if any of them arise in the context of coercion, by a person of the same or older age, it is abusive. According to international and national estimates, CSA is more common than was previously thought. Nearly 8% boys and 18% girls report CSA.[6] As we discuss later in the chapter, CSA can have complex dynamics determining the long-term developmental and mental health impact. Age at onset of the abuse, duration of the abuse, severity of violence, identity of the perpetrator, grooming, location of the abuse, and form of abuse (e.g., contact vs. noncontact) play a role in the impact of CSA.

IMPACT OF CHILDHOOD TRAUMA—FROM NEUROBIOLOGY TO THE CLINIC

Neurobiological Impact of Childhood Trauma

The impact of trauma has been well researched.[7] Studies have looked at structural and functional brain integrity, in addition to the cognitive, emotional, and behavioral impact it can have on mental health and illness. Neurobiologically, developmental impediment is seen in several areas of the brain including the frontal lobes, corpus callosum, right cerebral hemisphere, and hippocampus. In addition, certain brain regions seem to become hyperactivated, including the center of fear-based learning in the amygdala and the cortisol pathways. These changes have been reported in the context of various studies on trauma exposures, including neglect, disrupted attachment, physical and sexual abuse. Neuroimaging findings in these brain regions are manifest as thinner cortices, lower regional volumes, and lower functional activation. Neurochemical findings include an exaggerated release of stress hormones including cortisol and norepinephrine.

What do the above brain structural and functional changes mean in terms of observable behaviors? These include difficulties in emotional regulation, integration of experiences, stress modulation, executive functioning, social interaction, and attachment behaviors. All these manifested difficulties are commonly seen in the clinic when assessing children with trauma-related disturbances. Whereas emotional regulation, coping, executive functioning, and social skills can be impaired in various disorders even without trauma history, it is perhaps the difficulty in integration of experiences and attachment behaviors that is more specifically impacted by trauma.

Researchers have spoken about a *right hemispheric versus left hemispheric dysfunction*. The terms right hemisphere and left hemisphere are used in a functional sense, rather than an anatomical sense. While the *left hemisphere* refers to the language and linear processing skills, the *right hemisphere* refers to nonverbal and emotionally focused skills. Trauma can disrupt the integration of experiences and laying down of autobiographical memories resulting in psychopathological breakdown. Trauma experiences are emotionally overwhelming and the resulting, excessive functional right brain activation is inadequately accompanied by the functional left brain's ability to process and integrate it. This is one of the purported mechanisms for symptoms seen in PTSD, like flashbacks and intrusive memories, as well as in dissociative disorders. In both these presentations, therapists often help the patient to "work through" their experiences while supporting and managing the accompanying overwhelming emotions.

The neurobiological impact of trauma is spread over different brain regions and networks and determined by the age at onset and chronicity of trauma; and concomitant developmental and environmental risks. According to the *dynamic systems theory*, the more rapidly moving a dynamic system is, the more influence any perturbation will have.[8] The brain is a rapidly changing system in childhood. Therefore, the neurobiological impact of childhood trauma is more pronounced the younger a child is, and especially when there are repeated or chronic exposures. Adverse experiences early in life especially impact the emerging regulatory systems in an individual. It is important to remember that the nature of trauma and the determinants of the neurobiological impact of trauma result in substantial heterogeneity, evident in clinical presentations too.

Developmental and Behavioral Impact of Childhood Trauma

The impact of trauma on development and behavior is summarized in **Table 1**. It depicts the interdependent influence on different aspects of individual functioning. Bronfenbrenner's socioecological model places a child at the center of multiple layers of the environment, the most proximate being the layer of caregivers or parents. Ideally, parents and caregivers, through their consistent presence in the child's life and a secure attachment relationship, should be able to buffer possible impacts of childhood trauma. However, when the caregivers around a child are either abusive themselves, or unable to protect a child from trauma and abuse, children develop significant attachment difficulties. They relate to the adults around them as not caregivers or protectors whom they can turn to in distress but as selfish and dangerous. They may be hyperalert, and anxious around them, and find it difficult to develop working models for trusting relationships. Children also carry the models from these troubled relationships to other relationships they form that also tend to be conflicted and multilayered.

Similarly, children also tend to have significant challenges in their social skills, emerging self-concept, and world view. The unpredictability, and uncontrollability of trauma, with little room for reflective skill nurturing can result in chronic low self-worth and self-confidence. The world around them may be seen as unsafe and selfishly motivated. These social, self, and world view disturbances can trigger feelings of helplessness, inappropriate social behaviors, and adjustment difficulties in multiple social spaces. An interesting behavioral pattern seen in children who have been abused is a *reverse engagement* wherein the child takes the lead in establishing rapport with the clinician. This presents as a cheerful demeanor, appeasing behaviors, and easy agreements on tasks. Frontal lobe involvement in the neurobiology of trauma manifests as learning difficulties, affective dysregulation, and poor behavioral control. What manifests as clinical disorders are various combinations of the disturbances outlined in **Table 1**.

Specific symptoms in children, like dissociation, academic difficulties, and socially inappropriate behaviors, may originate from the neurobiological and developmental impact of adverse experiences and trauma.

This is especially important to bear in mind when the impact of trauma can be misconstrued as oppositional and conduct disorders. **Box 1** lists several behaviors that may seem disruptive and indicative of a conduct disorder, but these may have emerged from patterns of engagement determined by trauma and adverse adult–child relationships.

Finkelhor's Traumagenic Dynamics Model of Child Sexual Abuse

David Finkelhor's traumagenic dynamics model of CSA explains the multiple dynamics that play

TABLE 1: Impact of trauma on children's self and social worlds.

	Domain	*Impact*	*Clinical evaluation*
Interdependent	Attachment	• Difficulty relating to adults/authority figures • Seek out security/nurturance (vulnerability) • Difficulties with empathy, trust	Conflicted, multilayered relationships
	Biology	• Physical growth low for age • Delayed puberty • Chronic injuries/somatic complaints • NDDs—attention, sensory processing, language, learning	
	Affect regulation	• *Have little or no emotion:* Apathy • *Have little or no emotional awareness:* Alexithymia • *Have little or no emotional control:* Dysregulation	• Dissociative symptoms • Outbursts
	Behavioral control	• Anger outbursts • Regression • Manipulation	
	Cognition	Impaired learning ability	• Poor academic performance • "Gaps" in memory/ forgetfulness
	Self-concept	• Low self-worth • Low self-confidence	• Feelings of helplessness • Sexualized behavior • Reverse engagement
	World view	• Unpredictable and unsafe • Selfishly motivated	Adjustment difficulties in multiple social spaces
	Social development	Poor social skills—perception, cue-processing, and expression	• Attention-seeking behaviors • Sexualized behaviors • Antisocial behaviors

(NDDs: neurodevelopmental disorders)

out in a child's mind when he or she is sexually abused.[9] These dynamics determine the manifest thinking and behavioral patterns, as described in **Table 2**.

Traumatic sexualization refers to the inappropriate circumstances under which a child's sexuality is shaped in a developmentally inappropriate and interpersonally dysfunctional way. For instance, abusers tend to use rewards in exchange for sexual experiences and may also perpetuate misconceptions about gender and sexuality. Children may adopt similar tendencies in their behavioral repertoire such that their sexual identities and behaviors may be developmentally and interpersonally dysfunctional. The dynamics of *betrayal* that is perceived immediately or in the future inculcates a sense of mistrust and unsafety in their relationships with caregivers, and this will also play out in their future intimate relationships. *Stigmatization* may emerge from behaviors and words of the abuser or may emerge spontaneously in the child's self-reflections which can significantly threaten the developing selfhood. As the child faces betrayal and stigmatization, they may feel *powerless* given their age, limited sense of agency, and without any consistent support from

BOX 1: Conduct-like disturbances arising from adverse childhood experiences and adverse adult–child relationships.

- *Defiance:* Because social order (wanting to listen to authority) needs trust, loyalty, and engagement
- *Manipulation:* Because being direct and honest is dangerous
- *Splitting:* Because relationships are built in whatever way feels safest, varying across people, places, and time
- *Lying:* Because truth can be dangerous
- *Stealing:* Because that is what adults do to get things done
- *Aggression:* Because that is what adults do to get things done
- *Attention-seeking:* Because there is not enough!!
- *Dependency:* Because there is nothing wrong in it... we are an interdependent species!!
- *Age-inappropriate behavior:* Because of lack of skills!!

those around them, to do something about the situation.

Signs of Trauma over Childhood from Preschoolers to Adolescents

Trauma affects cognitive ability, affective experience and regulation, and behavioral control. The manifestations of disturbances in cognition, affect, and behavior vary over childhood, as is true for psychiatric disorders in general. We will focus on two rather extreme ends of the childhood age span, i.e., preschoolers and adolescents. Manifestations in the ages in between can be extrapolated from these descriptions.

Preschoolers are observant of their environments, and they can share their experiences and feelings with basic use of language. However, the

TABLE 2: Finkelhor's traumagenic dynamics model of child sexual abuse.

Traumatic sexualization	Conditions under which a child's sexuality is shaped in a developmentally inappropriate and interpersonally dysfunctional way: • Use of (rewarded) sexual behaviors to manipulate others • Fetishized body parts • Misconceptions about sexual behavior and morality • Traumatized sexuality	Impacts on • Capabilities • Self-concepts • World view
Betrayal	• Concurrent with abuse or belatedly realized • Determined by degree and nature of erstwhile trust and relationship • By offender and nonoffending family members • In realizing the limitations of their own parents' power to protect them	
Stigmatization	Negative messages about self—evilness, worthlessness, shamefulness, guilt • Stated directly or through furtiveness and pressures for secrecy • Reinforced by comments at disclosure—"spoiled" (girls), "queer" (boys) • From the fact of having been abused—"Why me?"	
Powerlessness	*Invasion:* Against child's will, wishes, sense of efficacy • Physical, psychological, and social space invaded *Threat:* Of injury and annihilation • Experience of violence, coercion, threat to body and life *Powerlessness is exacerbated:* • When child tries to fight back and fails • When child has to face the "adult world" following disclosure	

complexity of a traumatic experience and their lack of a template through which to understand what happened to or around them makes verbal sharing challenging. Instead, there can be a range of observable nonverbal changes and behaviors. Some of these are indicative of emotional distress in general, not necessarily specific to traumatic exposures. These include clinginess, difficulty in sleeping, and moodiness. Changes that are perhaps more commonly observed in children who have been abused or traumatized include recreating the traumatic event in play, physical complaints (may be located to the area of injury or abuse), over- or under-reactivity to the environment, as well as increased worry about safety of self and others (indicative of heightened threat perception), worries about recurrence of the traumatic event, new-onset fears, and statements and questions about death and dying or questions related to the nature of the trauma or abuse.

At the other end of the childhood age span, adolescents' experience of trauma involves an almost adult-like processing of the facts of the trauma. However, given their socioemotional immaturity they may find it challenging to regulate themselves affectively and behaviorally. They may be worried about safety, recurrence of trauma, and consequences of trauma. They may have uncomfortable feelings of seeking revenge. They may find it hard to trust others and have significant difficulty in dealing with authority or criticism. There may be mixed mood and conduct-like disturbances arising out of the emotional turmoil—irritability and aggression, school absenteeism, decline in academic performance, reduced concentration, high impulsivity and risk-taking, and substance use. They may experience PTSD-like symptoms with trauma re-experiencing and may have thoughts about death and dying.

At any age in childhood, the prominent dimensions of disturbances might include mood disturbance, trauma re-experiencing, anxiety and heightened threat perception, impulsivity and risk-taking, and decline in occupational and developmental functioning. Sometimes, the clinical manifestations in children may be largely characterized by somatic complaints and dissociation. Here, the expected sense of unpredictability and threat underlying the dimensions described previously is seemingly blocked out, and the internalized distress manifests somatically or as dissociated experiences. The blocking is understood to emerge from the previously described difficulties with integrating experiences. Besides the common somatic complaints that the child may "tell" about, and the conversion symptoms, dissociation may sometimes be also playing a role in observed regressive behaviors, gaps in learning and memory, and varying demeanor in different situations. In all of these, the troublesome (trauma-related) experiences are poorly integrated with the conscious self. The affect-laden experiences then find a way out through somatic or dissociative presentations.

Diagnostic Categories under Trauma-related Disorders

From a clinical and research perspective, it is important to be well versed with the categorical taxonomies of trauma and stress-related disorders. These are described in **Table 3**.

CLINICAL APPROACH TO CHILDHOOD TRAUMA

Trauma-informed Clinical Practice

Clinicians working with children understand that ACEs are commonly elicited from children presenting with mental health problems. The elicitation may at times take a few meetings and rapport establishment with the child and family. Clinicians need to take a trauma-informed

TABLE 3: Trauma and stress-related disorders in DSM-5.

Disorder	*Trauma/Stressor*	*Diagnostic requirements*	*Clinical characteristics*
Reactive engagement disorder	Social neglect (absence of adequate caregiving) during childhood, e.g., foster care	• Developmental age ≥9 months • Presentation <5 years	• Internalizing and depressive symptoms • Lack of comfort-seeking • Low emotional responsiveness
Disinhibited social engagement disorder		Developmental age ≥9 months	• Disinhibition and externalizing behavior • Low social referencing • "Superficial" relationships
Post-traumatic stress disorder	Actual/ threatened death/injury/sexual violence	• Symptoms at least >1 month • Any age >1 year • Onset usually within 3 months	• Intrusion • Negative mood • Dissociation • Avoidance • Arousal • Depersonalization/ derealization
Acute stress disorder		• Onset immediately after trauma • Duration at least 3 days • Usually, resolution in 1 month	
Adjustment disorders	Any identifiable stressor, of any severity	• Onset within 3 months • Termination within 6 months of stressor removal	Combination of trauma and symptom cluster differ from acute stress/PTSD

approach as a general practice rule, given the commonality of trauma and adverse experiences.[10] Trauma-informed clinical practice essentially involves the following:

- *Realizing* the widespread impact of trauma and understanding the potential pathways for recovery
- *Recognizing* signs and symptoms of trauma
- *Responding* by incorporating knowledge about trauma into policies, procedures, and practices
- Actively *resisting* re-traumatization

The *responding* part of the trauma-informed clinical practice is where a trauma-informed care (TIC) model comes in. It involves:

- Facilitating *resources and routines* that promote normalized activities, and a sense of agency and control
- *Responding* in words and behaviors, which are validating and supportive, from clinical team, family, school, and peers
- *Provision of choices* in routines, treatment options, and scheduling appointments, which again convey a sense of control
- *Support* through spending healing time, jointly managing cues that trigger distress, and liaising with school and other spaces that the child occupies.

Eliciting Trauma History

Eliciting the child's account of trauma requires specific skill building. Beyond orientation to developmentally appropriate engagement skills, the clinician needs to establish the child's capacity to establish accuracy and the ability to narrate experiences **(Box 2)**.[11] Young children may have immature language skills, display developmentally normative imaginary play, interact with fantasy figures, and may also be prone to complying with all instructions of adults, depending upon their caregiving environment. These may interfere with eliciting their account of trauma, and therefore,

BOX 2: Developmental considerations in eliciting a child's account of trauma.

Capacities to establish accuracy:
- Differentiate truth from lies
- Say "I don't understand"
- Tell when a person "is not right"

Ability to narrate experiences:
- Understand questions
- Memory of experiences
- Narration

the clinician must first be able to establish these skills before making further enquiries about traumatic experiences. This would also be applicable to children with neurodevelopmental disorders where developmental age may be lower than their chronological age.

Once these capacities and abilities are established, the clinician must proceed with largely open-ended questions to elicit an unbiased account from the child. The use of close-ended questions is not entirely ruled out; however, they need to be judiciously used in the context of established rapport with the child and for purposes of clarification of already narrated experiences. The reader is referred to clinical practice guidelines on CSA, published in 2016, for a more detailed understanding of skills and processes in eliciting trauma history from children.

Neurosequential Model of Therapeutics

Bruce Perry has spoken about *core elements of positive, developmental, educational, and therapeutic experiences.* These are characterized by activities that are respectful (in keeping with the child's family culture), relational (safe), relevant (developmentally matched), repetitive (patterned), rewarding (pleasurable), and rhythmic (resonant with neural patterns). These same elements underlie the neurosequential model of therapeutics.[12] This is a developmentally sensitive and neurobiologically informed approach to best meet the child's needs. It facilitates the assessment of a child in terms of putative dysfunction at different levels of brain structure and functioning. Depending upon the apparent dysfunction, responsive interventions can be planned. **Figure 1** illustrates manifestations of brain dysfunction at different levels and suitable interventions for the same. This model specifically lays emphasis on the role of patterned, repetitive somatosensory activities based on music, movement, yoga, and even drumming and therapeutic massage. In states of high physiological arousal, these interventions can be an important regulation aid. At high arousal, children may not be amenable to self-regulate and participate in more cognitive or emotionally focused discussions.

Attachment Informed Phase-oriented Therapy

Pierre Janet and Judith Herman described a phase-oriented therapy for individuals suffering from trauma-related disorders.[13] The larger goal of this approach is recovery from trauma and childhood adversities. However, it prioritizes child development that may have been missed by several children with complex trauma histories. The treatment is divided into three phases, sequential but not always linear, with possibility of revisiting an earlier phase based on the ongoing mental health circumstances. The three phases are *safety and stabilization*, *processing of trauma memories*, and *reconnection and integration*, as shown in **Figure 2**.

The tasks in the phase of *safety and stabilization* include strengthening of attachment, affective and behavioral regulation, and daily coping skills with a normalization of activities. This is considered the key phase in therapy and may last for variable duration of times for different individuals. Sometimes, especially in children

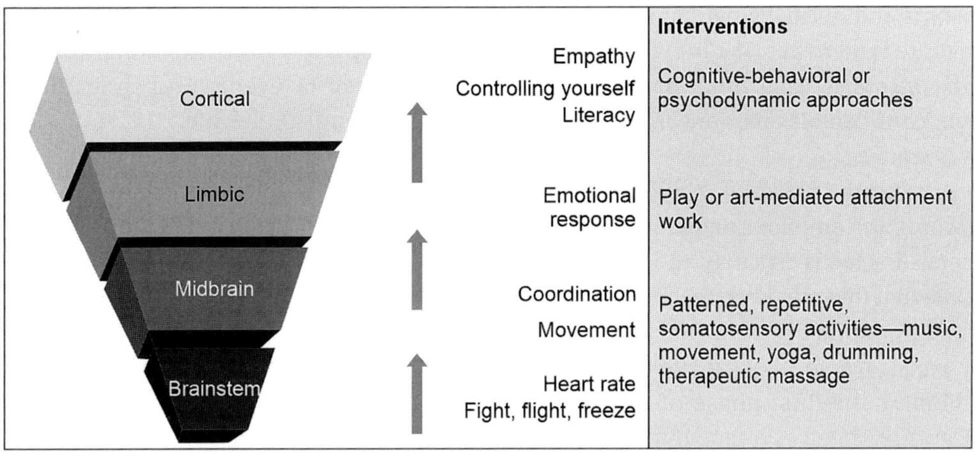

Fig. 1: Neurosequential model of therapeutics—a neurobiologically informed intervention approach to childhood trauma.

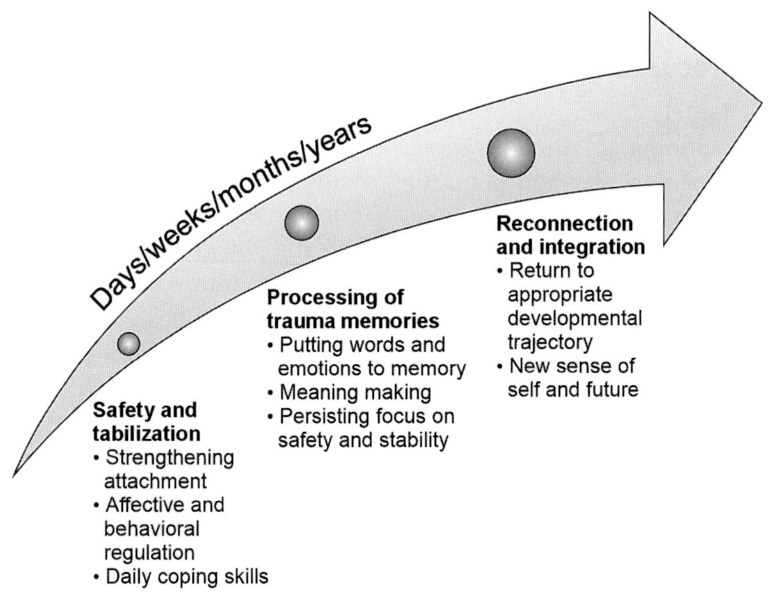

Fig. 2: Attachment-informed phase-oriented therapy.

and emotionally vulnerable persons, it may last for months to years. Janet and Herman allude to the role of *window of tolerance* propounded by Daniel J Siegel[14] that the clinician or therapist must be able to assess for the individual in therapy. The window of tolerance defines the range of emotion that a person can optimally tolerate without becoming overwhelmed. If the experience goes beyond this window, it may result in an undesirable re-traumatization. Therefore, a lot of time is spent in engaging the individual in an emotionally safe space while stabilizing relationships and normalizing daily activities. As evident, there is no rush to get into the *processing of trauma memories* that must be approached only when considerable emotional and functional stability is reached.

The *processing of trauma memories* involves putting words and emotions to memory, however, with a persisting focus on safety and stabilization. At any time that the individual feels overwhelmed or there is possibility of re-traumatization, the therapy can traverse back to the stabilization phase. Finally, the final phase of *reconnection and integration* involves a return to appropriate developmental trajectory with a new sense of self and future. The individual looks at restoring a balance of self-identity, aspirations, desires, relationships, and social networks.

Specific Trauma-focused Interventions

This chapter has largely taken a conceptual approach to understanding childhood trauma, from broader ACEs' perspective, and planning interventions that prioritize safety, development, and functionality. When children are ready for it, specific trauma-focused work can be undertaken. In fact, these trauma-focused interventions can be alternatives for the *processing of trauma memories* phase in attachment-informed phase-oriented therapy. The scope of this chapter does not allow for a detailed discussion of these techniques. For the sake of completion, we list some of these techniques below. It is important to note that these techniques have been successfully used in children and, like other psychotherapy approaches for children, often involve a parent or caregiver in the treatment.

- *Fractionated abreaction,*[15] described by Rick Kluft and Catherine Fine, processes each memory slowly and in small amounts, stopping frequently to ground, regulate, and allow the child to connect emotionally. The therapist serves as an empathic witness, soothing and coregulating. The final goal is to develop a *co-created meaning,* i.e., a coherent narrative of events and their place in the child's and family's life.
- *Trauma-focused cognitive behavior therapy (Tf-CBT)*[16,17] takes a cognitive-behavioral approach to modifying distorted or unhelpful thinking and negative cognitive and behavioral reactions, including fear and guilt. The parent's involvement in therapy focuses on coaching in stress management, communication, and parenting skills.
- *Eye movement desensitization and reprocessing (EMDR),*[18] a technique described by Francine Shapiro, involves focusing on traumatic memories, as in exposure therapy, while engaging in side-to-side eye movements or other forms of bilateral stimulation.

SUMMARY AND CONCLUSION

Childhood adversity or all kinds is not uncommon. While some adversities may be physically and immediately graver than others, all adversities have the potential to disrupt child development and create future vulnerabilities for a range of mental health issues. For all professionals working with children, it is important to hone a trauma-informed approach. Manifestations of adverse experiences can vary with the age of the child, trauma-related and child-related determinants, and the neurobiological impact they would have had. Child mental health professionals need to hone their skills in several specific areas like eliciting children's account of the trauma, TIC, and safety- and stabilization-focused interventions for child survivors of trauma. Readers are encouraged to refer to the reference list at the end of the chapter for further nuanced understanding.

REFERENCES

1. American Psychiatric Association. Diagnostic and Statistical Manual of Mental Disorders:

DSM-5, 5th edition. American Psychiatric Association; 2013.
2. World Health Organization. (2020). Adverse childhood experiences international questionnaire (ACE-IQ). [online]. Available from https://www.who.int/publications/m/item/adverse-childhood-experiences-international-questionnaire-(ace-iq) [Last accessed 19 November, 2025].
3. Cicchetti D, Cannon TD. Neurodevelopmental processes in the ontogenesis and epigenesis of psychopathology. Dev Psychopathol. 1999; 11(3):375-93.
4. Zhang Y, Vaidya N, Iyengar U, Sharma E, Holla B, Ahuja CK, et al. The Consortium on Vulnerability to Externalizing Disorders and Addictions (c-VEDA): an accelerated longitudinal cohort of children and adolescents in India. Mol Psychiatry. 2020;25(8):1618-30.
5. McLaughlin KA, Sheridan MA. Beyond Cumulative Risk. Curr Direct Psychol Sci. 2016;25: 239-45.
6. World Health Organization. (2024). Lifetime prevalence of child sexual abuse (%). [online]. Available from. https://www.who.int/data/gho/data/indicators/indicator-details/GHO/lifetime-prevalence-of-child-sexual-abuse-(-) [Last accessed 19 November, 2025].
7. Gomez-Perales N. Attachment-focused trauma treatment for children and adolescents: Phase-oriented strategies for addressing complex trauma disorders, 1st edition. London: Routledge; 2015.
8. Thelen E, Smith LB. Dynamic systems theories. In Lerner RM, Damon W (Eds). Handbook of Child Psychology: Theoretical Models of Human Development, 6th edition. New York: Wiley; 2006. pp. 258-312.
9. Finkelhor D. The trauma of child sexual abuse: Two models. J Interpers Viol. 1987;2(4):348-66.
10. Pynoos RS, Fairbank JA, Steinberg AM, Amaya-Jackson L, Gerrity E, Mount ML. The National Child Traumatic Stress Network: Collaborating to improve the standard of care. Prof Psychol Res Pract. 2008;39(4):389-95.
11. Seshadri S, Ramaswamy S. Clinical Practice Guidelines for Child Sexual Abuse. Indian J Psychiatry. 2019;61(Suppl 2):317-32.
12. Perry B, Hambrick E. The Neurosequential Model of Therapeutics. J Strengths-Based Intervent. 2008;17:38-43.
13. Herman JL. Trauma and Recovery. United States: Basic Books; 1997.
14. Siegel DJ. The Developing Mind. New York: Guilford; 1999.
15. Kluft RP. Treating the traumatic memories of patients with dissociative identity disorder. Am J Psychiatry. 1996;153(7 Suppl):103-10.
16. Deblinger E, Cohen J, Mannarino A. Child and Parent Trauma-Focused Cognitive Behavioral Therapy Treatment Manual. Pittsburgh, PA: Allegheny General Hospital Center for Traumatic Stress in Children and Adolescents; 2003.
17. Cohen JA, Mannarino AP, Deblinger E. Treating Trauma and Traumatic Grief in Children and Adolescents. New York: Guilford; 2006.
18. Shapiro F. The role of eye movement desensitization and reprocessing (EMDR) therapy in medicine: addressing the psychological and physical symptoms stemming from adverse life experiences. Perm J. 2014;18(1):71-7.

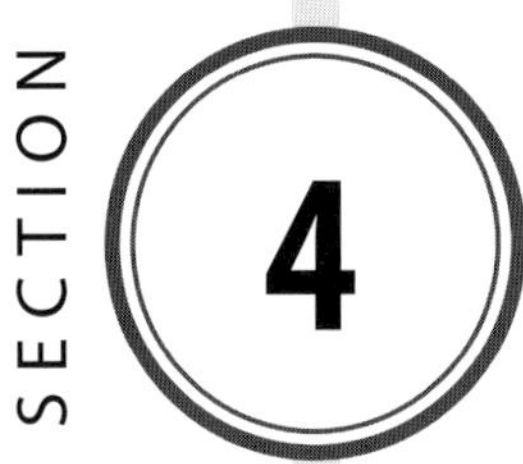

SECTION 4 Management and Aftercare

CHAPTER 22

Management of Child and Adolescent Mental Illnesses: An Overview

Savita Malhotra

INTRODUCTION

Treatment of childhood psychiatric disorders comprises not just the treatment of problems with which the child is brought but also to ensure that the child will have an opportunity for optimal growth and development in future as much as possible. Thus, the management has to be holistic including promotive, preventive, curative, and rehabilitative components. This would require intervention in multiple settings in most cases, like the clinic, home, school, community, or other healthcare facilities.

In child psychiatry, the treatment of current disorder contributes to prevention of other disorders in future, and therefore an element of prevention is always there. For example, treating attention-deficit/hyperactivity disorder (ADHD) early can minimize the occurrence of substance-use disorder or conduct disorders in future. On the other hand, primary prevention may require strategies for universal intervention for the whole population in a given locality or community. Nutritional supplementation or life skills training programs for the whole school can be examples of universal intervention. The other is selective intervention where children at higher risk for mental health problems are targeted, e.g., children with physical illness or those who live in deprivation or in institutions or in war zones or those with any disability constituting specific risk groups. Indicated prevention targets those children who present with subclinical symptoms, as in the prodromal phase of psychosis or subthreshold depression. Any treatment done for the present disorder, i.e., secondary prevention, must incorporate advice for prevention of the same or other disorders in future (primary prevention) and for reduction of disability, i.e., tertiary prevention. All levels of intervention are needed for every child from time to time. There is a need for timely recognition and early management of specific vulnerabilities to reduce the burden of future morbidity.

There are a few guiding principles in the management of childhood psychiatric disorders:[1,2]

- *Integration of mental health care in general health*: Mental health issues generally coexist with physical ill health and are better addressed together. All pediatric settings must have child psychiatric services available. It will lead to early recognition and better handling of mental health issues. It will also help to remove stigma.
- There should be intersectoral coordination and access to other social, psychological, remedial, educational, and occupational interventions. Child and adolescent psychiatric (CAP) disorders require interdisciplinary team and services comprising medications, psychotherapies, family therapy, speech therapy, occupational therapy, and special education. So it is a teamwork between psychiatrists, clinical psychologists, speech therapists, occupational therapists, remedial teachers, and social workers.

- Child's mental health is closely linked to parental, societal, school, and community level ecosystem in which the child lives. So the intervention plans must include the entire ecosystem of the child. Intervention extends much beyond the clinics and the psychiatrist has to liaise with the teachers in school, child protection teams, parents, families, and whoever else is relevant in the life of the child.
- There is a need to adopt a lifecycle approach where the entire life experience of the child from in utero to postnatal phase should be incorporated in planning intervention. Interventions must also aim to reduce the risk for mental disorder and promote resilience and effective coping.
- Effort should be made to address the known or hypothesized etiological factors of the disorders that the child is brought with. Etiological factors contributing to the occurrence of psychiatric disorders in children generally arise from multiple sources such as biological, physical or organic, psychological, and social. These should all be incorporated in the treatment plan.

Thus, the treatment is multimodal and requires multidisciplinary inputs. Ideally, the treatments in child psychiatry are carried out by a multidisciplinary team of professionals, i.e., psychiatrists, pediatricians, psychologists, social workers, and teachers. Other members of the team required are those who have specialized expertise in fields like speech therapy, art therapy, occupational therapy, remedial education, and the like. However, reality is far from the ideal. In India, there is an overall shortage of manpower. Very few psychiatrists are involved in the care of children, and there is still a fewer number of other mental health professionals to the extent that the treatment models practiced or advocated as ideal become inapplicable. Therefore, there is a great need to adapt the management approaches advocated in the West and create our own models of care for the Indian situation.

In India, we have to depend a great deal on the resource that is available in plenty, i.e., parents and families and to some extent teachers. They are, although, not trained mental health professionals, but they are, by and large, exceptionally valuable, motivated, and dependable individuals who must become not only our allies in treatment but also co-therapists. Most of the treatment, therefore, is carried through the parents, teachers, and other significant adults in the child's life.

In addition to lack of qualified professionals, there is also lack of sensitivity and awareness to identify psychological problems or to bring them to a service facility among population. In the absence of a psychiatric facility or due to lack of knowledge about it, most of the problems present to a general healthcare facility. It is often the general physician or the pediatrician who is the first point of contact and who, depending upon his/her own knowledge, sensitivity, and experience, also determines the need for psychiatric referral. In clinic populations, therefore, we see mostly children with neuropsychiatric or psychosomatic problems. In schools or at the community level, a wide range of emotional, behavioral, and learning problems exist which may never reach a health facility. Infrequently, parents or family members directly or on advice from schoolteachers bring the child over to a psychiatry clinic.

In India, specialized child psychiatric services including in-patient care are available only in a few large metropolitan cities, that too varying in levels of expertise and care. Mental health care for children at the primary and secondary levels is almost unavailable. Most CAP services are provided in general psychiatry facilities without availability of child psychiatrists or other supporting professionals. Due to the absence of child psychiatry units or qualified child psychiatrists in most of the institutions running

MD psychiatry courses, general psychiatrists have negligible or no training in child psychiatry during their postgraduation.

Most of the treatment is and has to be done in the outpatients setting or at the community level. In-patient treatment is available in very few places in the country.

There are no standard treatment packages. General practice guidelines are available to deal with most of the commonly occurring problems and disorders, but these are mostly derived from western guidelines and lack Indian perspectives. There is a need for considerable adaptation, and fine-tuning is needed in treatment approaches to make them suitable to Indian sociocultural situations. Broadly, the treatment is palliative, promotive, and preventive and not always curative.

For a comprehensive management plan, it is helpful to make multiaxial diagnosis as per Diagnostic and Statistical Manual of Mental Disorders, 5th Edition (DSM-5). Axis I covers the clinical disorder for which treatment is needed. Axis II addresses the presence of personality disorders and intellectual developmental disorders or delays which may be the problem by itself or may constitute a factor of biological vulnerability that needs to be kept in mind while dealing with axis I disorders. Axis III refers to general medical conditions, as it is equally important to pay attention to the physical status of the child and deal with any associated physical disorder. Psychosocial and environmental problems are coded on axis IV. In most cases, there is some disorder of psychosocial situation (axis IV) which may or may not be causally related to the clinical disorder but needs intervention. Axis V is global assessment of functioning. Assessment procedure and diagnosis, particularly if done on a multiaxial framework, facilitate formulation of a comprehensive management plan.

The objectives of the management of psychiatric disorders in children generally include:[3,4]

- Removal or minimization of symptoms
- Enhancement of adjustment, coping, and resilience
- Reduction of impairment or handicap
- Promotion of optimum growth and development

Depending upon the nature of the problems, several strategies of management can be used. Usually, combinations of more than one treatment method are required, targeting the specific objectives of management, given above and applicable in a given case. Specific management in each case has to be prepared keeping in mind the nature of problems, the unique characteristics of the particular child, the general background of the family, and specific psychosocial and environmental factors that are relevant.

General level of functioning and psychosocial disability, as coded on axis VI, measures and monitors the course and indicates rehabilitative needs.

After the diagnostic workup, a problem-oriented analysis of the case provides the broad framework within which the case should be managed. Problems can be broadly categorized as predominantly:

- Problems of emotions causing personal distress and suffering, e.g., anxiety, depression, somatic symptoms, fears, tension, dissociation, poor coping, etc.
- Problems of behavior and conduct causing disruption in family and social life, e.g., overactivity, impatience, intolerance, defiance, challenging behavior, obstinacy, demandingness, aggressiveness, anger as seen in ADHD, conduct disorder, oppositional defiant disorder, delinquency, or antisocial personality
- Problems of learning or lower scholastic performance, as in specific learning difficulties, borderline intelligence

- Problems of development manifesting as arrested, delayed, and/or deviant development as in mental retardation; poor eye contact or poor social cognition as in pervasive or specific developmental disorders, growth retardation, etc.
- Abnormal/odd behavior; severe disturbance of thought, affect, or behavior as in psychosis, mania stupor, aggressiveness, excitement; obsessions, compulsions, suicidality
- Other problems, e.g., drug abuse, trauma, sexual, or physical abuse

These are transdiagnostic groupings, arbitrarily identified, to help in making a simpler mental framework and for ease of comprehension. It is helpful to conceptualize each case along the above-mentioned guidelines in planning management. Given below is a method for conceptualizing, analyzing, and planning treatment and gives a very broad outline of treatment approaches. A clinician must first decide on what is needed for the patient and then make a specific plan on how to go about it.

PREDOMINANT PROBLEMS OF EMOTIONS

Problems of emotions are generally managed by encouraging the child to express and describe, in detail, the symptom, the emotional component associated with the symptoms, the psychosocial factors or the setting within which the problem is experienced, the events and factors that trigger or aggravate the symptoms, and also those which relieve it. All these aspects are explored for a comprehensive assessment, but this exploration has a significant therapeutic value. This gives the child a chance not only to express and ventilate but also to focus attention on various situations and events that are closely linked to the symptoms, suggesting casual connections and thereby facilitating insight. A similar exercise undertaken with parents also serves a similar purpose and helps them to understand the symptom in the context of events. This comprises psychoeducation and also is a form of supportive psychotherapy.

The next step involves making efforts to deal with specific issues in the psychosocial situation, the environment or the handling of the child, in the direction of making these suit or match the legitimate needs, desires, and capabilities of the child. Here, there is the maximum role of parent advice, guidance, and counseling and these are used extensively. In most cases, the problems are often solved at this level of intervention itself.

In certain cases, where there is severe pathology in the family setting or in the social environment such as parental mental illness, alcoholism, abuse, parental discord, a systematic family therapy and treatment of parents themselves or environmental manipulation needs to be carried out.

Sometimes, the symptoms in the child are severe to the extent that it is difficult to engage the child in psychological therapy or the symptoms do not respond to the above measures of psychological exploration, education, parent advice, guidance, and supportive psychotherapy. Medication is then used as an adjunct to psychosocial management. Depending upon the nature of symptoms and basic diagnosis, antidepressants can be used which act as both anxiolytics and antidepressants. In certain instances where symptoms are deeply rooted in psychopathology or are unaffected by changes in the environment or psychosocial situation, a specific symptom-oriented approach to management, i.e., behavior therapy, is instituted. Symptoms such as obsessional thoughts, rituals or repetitive behavior, tics, habit symptoms, and certain dissociative symptoms are effectively managed with behavior therapy as the primary mode of treatment. The technique of behavior therapy that is to be used is chosen after a careful behavioral analysis. It is usually a combination of therapeutic techniques that is most effective and is invariably used in the management of emotional disorders. In very young children and those who have limited repertoire of speech, play therapy is used instead of verbal psychotherapy. Details of psychotherapy, behavior therapy, or play therapy in children are discussed in other relevant chapters.

Before embarking on these formal and specific types of psychotherapies, it is important to establish a therapeutic relationship. Generally, during the initial interview sessions when most of exploration into history is done, it is possible to establish a good therapeutic relationship between the child and his family and the psychiatrist.

To foster a positive therapeutic relationship, it is important that:

- Relationship is based on faith and trust the patient has in the psychiatrist
- Genuineness and concern shown by the psychiatrist is paramount
- Patient has confidence in the ability of the psychiatrist to help
- Nonjudgmental attitude and an attitude of acceptance for the patient and the family despite all their difficulties and shortcomings is exceedingly necessary.

Sometimes, there is a need for an active effort on the part of the therapist to establish a therapeutic relationship. In the absence of this relationship, any psychotherapy has little chance to succeed.

Parents have to be dealt with using the same psychotherapeutic principles as above. While pointing out their shortcoming or at their contribution to problems, there is a need for observing a great deal of sensitivity and skill in order to avoid indication of blame. Parents have to be treated as partners in therapy who though are equally interested in the child's welfare but could be working at counter purposes out of ignorance, misconception, their own compulsions of personality, and so on. There is a need for a step-by-step correction of these attitudes imparting education, modification of their behavior, and training for a more healthy and adaptive functioning. Parental advice and counseling have both therapeutic and preventive value.

PREDOMINANT PROBLEMS OF BEHAVIOR AND CONDUCT

Disorders that manifest with predominant symptoms (obstinacy, temper tantrums, defiance, aggressiveness, impulsiveness, stealing, lying, truancy, cruelty, and the like) of behavior and conduct require handling in multiple domains. Mild-to-moderate intensity of such symptoms can be managed with psychosocial measures alone, whereas severe forms of disruptive behavior disorders may need medication as well. ADHD is best managed with stimulant drugs, i.e., methylphenidate, atomoxetine, or pemoline. In case of nonavailability or of contraindication to the use of these drugs, there are alternatives available, i.e., imipramine, buspirone, clonidine, guanfacine, or even small doses of antipsychotics (haloperidol or chlorpromazine). Medication can bring about improvement in gross symptoms so that the other psychosocial and educational inputs in therapy can take effect.

Since these symptoms indicate the presence of disinhibition and dyscontrol, effort is made to structure and control the environment and alter handling methods for the child. Parents are advised to be firm and consistent, set firm limits to behavior, and make a structured routine for the child. Use of operant conditioning principles to modify behavior in the form of reward for good behavior and withdrawal of reward or punishment for bad behavior are effective strategies. The entire family must enter into therapy in this situation so that the whole environment can be structured and controlled. The essential message to the child is that he cannot get away with what he does and that there are other ways to achieve the desired goal, i.e., by behaving well or by complying with parents or teachers, etc. Parents are advised not to lose patience or get frustrated at the bad behavior of the child. The child is engaged in planning of the contingency contract where the behavior and its consequent rewards or punishments are clearly specified and agreed upon. The parents are advised to enforce this under supervision. Many a times, parents do not want or are unable to carry through the above advice. But there are no shortcuts, and parental/family's engagement is absolutely necessary.

When these symptoms occur in the setting of an underlying biological or organic brain disorder, as, for example, in association with birth trauma, perinatal difficulties, epilepsy, postencephalitic sequelae, and mental retardation, then medication has a greater role in management. If these symptoms are seen in the setting of a pathological environment like highly restrictive or punitive parents, extreme poverty and deprivation, membership of a delinquent peer group, etc., then the predominant thrust of management is psychosocial and behavioral. Every effort is made to organize the environment in such a way that at least the basic biological (food, clothes, house) and minimum essential psychological (care, love, education, play, security) needs of the child are met. Overall management here requires a high degree of involvement and supervision by adults in whose care the child lives. These adults do well by undergoing specific training by mental health professionals.

PREDOMINANT PROBLEMS OF LEARNING

Problems of learning and scholastic underachievement are among the most common problems that the urban, middle-class parents are concerned with. These are managed depending upon the underlying casual factors. Very often, the child has low average or borderline intelligence and he/she is unable to cope with the pressure of studies. In such a situation, parents are educated and counselled to bring down their demand and expectations to match with the child's ability. Sometimes, the problem is seen due to poor teaching techniques or facilities in school and poor interest and motivation in teachers. Parents are advised to either change school or arrange extra coaching to help the child. There are some children who have poor motivation to study. Many of such children come from either very rich or very poor backgrounds for whom education may have low value. There is a new trend in the urban middle class who although places a very high value on education but is getting increasingly attracted by the wave of consumerism and hedonism as a symbol of modernization and westernization. Children from these homes are caught in a conflict and are easily swayed by the dominant influence of adopted luxurious lifestyle and social media. These children lose interest in studies and have serious problems of adjustment and relationships with parents. These problems are often seen with older children and adolescents. Management here requires family therapy in addition to individual psychotherapy for the child. Effort is made to reduce the gap between the expectations and attitudes of parents and the child. Children do well with cognitive or rational psychotherapy where they are made to see the fallacy in their own thinking and logic.

Education and learning, which is the major casualty in the conflict-ridden situation, is brought back to its place of priority. Use of assertiveness training and prestige suggestion to enhance self-esteem and self-efficacy is beneficial. For these problems, most of the therapeutic work is done with the child and the parents mainly provide support.

Another significant but ill-understood and unrecognized cause of learning difficulties in the child is the group of conditions diagnosed as specific developmental disorders of scholastic skills. In these conditions, there is a specific difficulty in learning arithmetic, spellings, reading, or writing in the child who has adequate intellectual potential to learn these skills. Schoolteachers as well as parents generally complain about the child as being "careless" or "unmotivated" rather than being incapable. Since specific learning disorder (SLD) is a definite pathology based on the biological maturational processes of the brain, these children require special or remedial education.

These children require specialized methods of teaching involving multisensory inputs and slow and systematic approach. Unfortunately, this is the area where facilities and expertise are seriously lacking in India. Even in good child psychiatry centers, not to talk of school, this facility is not available. It requires specially trained teachers who are only a handful for a vast country like India. As of now, these children remain underachievers to the great frustration and anguish of parents. The best that can be done under the prevailing circumstances is to advise parents and the child to make more effort in the direction that helps the child learn best; e.g., if the child can learn better by listening or discussion rather than by silent reading, then he should learn by reading aloud or by listening to someone. Cooperation and involvement of teachers is essential. The problem must be discussed with the teachers, and strategies to help the child should be planned together. Counseling to the child and the parents helps in preventing the secondary morbidity.

PREDOMINANT PROBLEMS OF DEVELOPMENT

Delayed or arrested development manifesting as mental subnormality is one of the most common presenting problems in the clinic samples. Depending upon the degree of mental retardation and also whether it is primary or secondary, parents need to be counseled accordingly. They are given education about the nature of problems, its course and outcome, probable cause, and possible intervention. They are encouraged and advised to accept the intellectual level the child has and the capabilities associated with it and to make the best of what the child has. There is no point lamenting on what the child cannot do. The child should be helped to realize his/her full potential. Parents go through several psychological reactions themselves like guilt, anger, and depression which needs to be worked through. Specific training to the child directly or through parents for teaching life and social skills is highly useful. Depending upon other associated problems like speech difficulty, behavior problems, etc., targeted management is instituted.

Pervasive developmental disorders (PDDs) are more severe disorders involving not only simple delay but also deviance in the development of speech and language, social communication, and certain types of behavioral problems. These are again managed by parental advice, guidance, counseling, and parent training for handling of the child and for facilitating communication and language functions. Specific treatment for associated problems like speech therapy for speech problems, behavior therapy for behavioral problems, remedial education for learning difficulties, and occupational therapy for motor or social skills is necessary. As the management of PDDs is very intensive and the progress is very slow, it is highly taxing, often frustrating for the parents as well as for the therapist.

Another not-so-uncommon problem is that of suboptimal physical growth and development, i.e., nonorganic failure to thrive. As this problem is seen in families with poor education, low socioeconomic status, and child neglect or abuse, the management involves family therapy and education. Parents, particularly the mother, need to understand the child's nutritional needs as well as psychological needs. Children living in abnormal situations such as in foster homes or other institutions or with foster/step parents are often victims of these problems. They need to be put in alternative care if possible. Unfortunately, in India, as we do not have many options for alternative care, we have to work with the same caretakers who are responsible for neglect. Effort is made to make them our allies in treatment as much as possible.

SUMMARY AND CONCLUSION

To summarize and conclude, treatment in child psychiatry is approached not merely from the perspective of symptomatic relief, but from holistic concern aimed at managing etiological contributors in the entire ecosystem of the child and fostering optimum growth and development as much as possible.

Alongside symptomatic relief, targeted intervention at the contributing etiological factors is essential for comprehensive management. Transdiagnostic emergency conditions like trauma, physical abuse, sexual abuse, suicidality, or substance use require complex management strategies, including inpatient care, and are discussed in respective chapters. Detailed treatment for specific psychiatric disorders is given in the respective chapters.

REFERENCES

1. Malhotra S. Child mental health in India: Needs and priorities. In Malhotra S, Malhotra A, Varma VK (Eds). Child Mental Health in India. Noida: Macmillan.
2. Malhotra S. Challenges for providing mental health services for children and adolescents in India. In: Gerald J, Ferrari YP (Eds). Designing Mental Health Services and Systems for Children and Adolescents: A Shrewd Investment. New York: Brunner Mazel.
3. World Health Organization. (2005). Mental health policy, plans and programme. Geneva: World Health Organization.
4. Malhotra S. Clinical Assessment and Management of Childhood Psychiatric Disorders, 3rd edition. New Delhi: CBS Publishers; 2025.

Psychological Therapies for Emotional and Behavioral Disorders-I (Psychotherapies, Counseling, Psychoeducation, Play, and Art Therapies)

Uma Hirisave, Uttara Chari

INTRODUCTION

Psychological intervention is often the first-line treatment for emotional/behavioral issues in children and adolescents (henceforth referred to as "young persons"). This comprises individual psychotherapy, family therapy, parenting interventions, and school/community-centric interventions. The focus of this chapter will be on individual psychotherapy. While counseling is often used synonymously with psychotherapy, both of them differ in focus, intensity, goals, and approach in working with a young person. In this chapter, counseling will be addressed under the rubric of psychoeducation.

What is meant by psychological intervention?

Psychological interventions engage the "psyche", i.e., persons (self and/or other) in bringing about a change in the current situation in the young person's life. Specifically, psychotherapy is defined as:

"The treatment, by psychological means, of problems of an emotional nature in which a trained person deliberately establishes a professional relationship with the patient, with the object: (1) Of removing, modifying, or retarding existing symptoms; (2) of mediating disturbed patterns of behavior; and (3) of promoting positive personality growth and development".[1]

All three objectives hold relevance for young persons with emotional and behavioral issues. Often, behavioral issues have emotional underpinnings. Subjective distress is often mitigated when there is symptomatic improvement. Improving self and relationships with others is engaged as the therapeutic process progresses.

PSYCHOLOGICAL INTERVENTION IN CHILD AND ADOLESCENT MENTAL HEALTH

Children and adolescents are dynamic, actively engaging with the world around them, for their development. The ecological systems theory proposes that young persons are enveloped in systems that include other persons such as parents, teachers, peers, community members, government policy makers, and so forth.[2] Each of these systems interacts with each other producing a synergistic effect on the young person's life. Thus, it is expected that any psychological intervention in the child and adolescent's mental health involves as many systems as feasible, hence the scope of parenting interventions, family therapy, and school/community-based interventions. This makes it distinct from interventions for adults, where the focus is often primarily on the individual.

Psychological interventions vary on dimensions of how structured they are, the lead taken by the therapist in delivering them, and the generic focus of the intervention. Generally, psychotherapeutic approaches, such as those of psychodynamic, narrative, play, and art, are less structured and more child directed, with greater emphasis on enhancing intra- and interpersonal functioning. Behavioral and cognitive behavioral therapies (CBT) are often more structured and clinician directed, focusing on symptomatic improvement.

EMOTIONAL AND BEHAVIORAL DISORDERS IN CHILDREN AND ADOLESCENTS

The current conceptualization of emotional and behavioral disorders in young persons stems from the prior classification of externalizing and internalizing problems. A disorder is useful merely for purposes of research and clinician understanding. For a given child/adolescent, they experience "problems" which need mitigation. **Box 1** lists some of these problems. As stated earlier, behavioral issues may also rise out of negative emotional states (e.g., nail biting, thumb sucking).

BOX 1: Internalizing and externalizing problems in children and adolescents.

Internalizing problems:
- Low interest
- Shyness
- Fear/anxiety
- Sadness/crying
- Increased sensitivity to criticism
- Nail biting/thumb sucking
- Jealousy
- Bed wetting/soiling clothes
- Somatic complaints
- Decreased self confidence

Externalizing problems:
- Overactivity/restlessness
- Impulsivity
- Disturbing other children
- Destructive
- Lying/stealing
- Demanding/stubborn behavior
- Aggression/temper tantrums
- Bullying

SPECIFIC PSYCHOLOGICAL INTERVENTIONS FOR CHILDREN ADOLESCENTS

Interventions are developmentally indexed, bearing in mind the cognitive capacities of the child/adolescents as per their age. **Figure 1** roughly suggests relevant interventions, appropriate to developmental stages.

- *Psychoeducation:* The focus is to educate on probable causes and management of mental health issues. It is based on the premise that knowledge enhances motivation and agency to get better. Every individual will have their own understanding of their problems. However, the purpose here is to give a more scientific and empirically based knowledge.
- *Supportive psychotherapy:* It is an approach that has an explicit focus on strengths and seeks to enhance them, rather than on problematic areas in self-functioning. The premise is that the young person already has all the resources within him/her to be better.

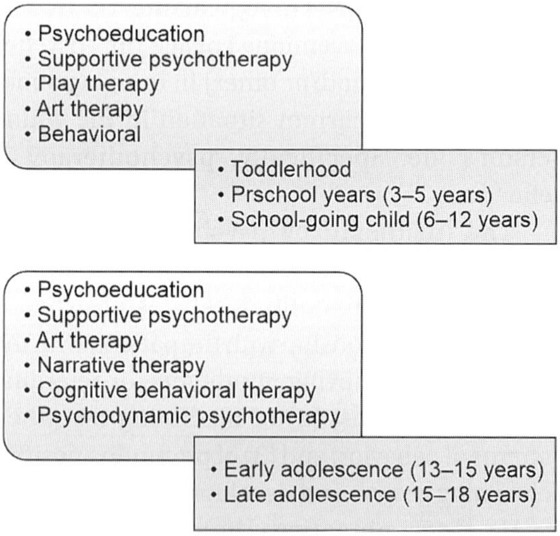

- Psychoeducation
- Supportive psychotherapy
- Play therapy
- Art therapy
- Behavioral

- Toddlerhood
- Prschool years (3–5 years)
- School-going child (6–12 years)

- Psychoeducation
- Supportive psychotherapy
- Art therapy
- Narrative therapy
- Cognitive behavioral therapy
- Psychodynamic psychotherapy

- Early adolescence (13–15 years)
- Late adolescence (15–18 years)

Fig. 1: Developmentally appropriate psychotherapeutic approaches.

The therapist catalyzes these resources into action by being supportive.

- *Play therapy:* Based on the premise that play is a child's spontaneous medium of communication, this therapeutic approach utilizes toys and other play materials to facilitate self-expression. Emotional difficulties and distressing thoughts are "played out" in sessions, and resolution is achieved.
- *Art therapy:* This approach uses art materials and art-based activities (drawing/coloring) to engage the young person to express, discuss, and resolve concerns. Art is symbolic and offers a medium of expression and a less-threatening means to communicate and resolve emotional concerns.
- *Narrative therapy:* This is a therapeutic approach, wherein one's life is construed as a story, with the young person being the narrator. This facilitates having a third person perspective on one's experiences, thereby promoting construction of a healthier narrative regarding oneself and his/her life.
- *CBT:* A very popular approach due to a structured therapeutic process, CBT focuses on changing maladaptive thought and behavior patterns. This is done via having an objective, reality-based approach to one's thoughts and challenging them/putting them to test through behavioral experiments.
- *Behavior therapy:* Using principles of learning, this therapeutic approach focuses on changing overt behaviors. The approach seeks to either teach new adaptive behaviors and/or replace maladaptive behaviors, using functional analysis of behaviors and reinforcement strategies.
- *Psychodynamic psychotherapy:* Here, the focus is on making aware of impulses, thoughts, and feelings that are away from the conscious awareness of the young person. The premise of this therapeutic approach is that these facets in the young person's unconscious drive their attitude and behaviors toward self and others. Bringing these into conscious awareness facilitates a more psychologically healthy life.

Empirical Evidence

A quick online search will reveal multiple articles on psychotherapy with young persons, spanning from specific to generic therapies, across mental health conditions. However, two consistent findings will emerge: (1) All therapeutic approaches are beneficial in bringing about a facilitative change in mental health for young persons and (2) data from randomized controlled trials are not directly replicable in the clinical setting.

The superiority of one therapeutic approach over another has been researched as early as in the 1930s in Saul Rosenzweig's "Dodo bird verdict" that all psychotherapies were equally effective. Subsequent research has corroborated the same, with common factors across psychotherapies accounting for their benefit.[3] The contextual model proposes three pathways for the effect of common factors, i.e., (1) relationship between therapist and client, (2) client expectations on disorder and treatment, created by therapist explanations, and (3) client carrying out health-promoting actions.[4] There are fewer effectiveness studies in child and adolescent psychotherapy than efficacy studies.[5] This is unfortunate as young persons in the clinic do not present with the stringent and sanctified backgrounds demanded in research. Thus clinically, it would seem prudent to adhere to a common factors approach, given the ubiquitous benefit of all psychotherapies. It is pertinent to state that the foundational therapeutic approach of the common factors approach is client-centered psychotherapy,[6] which is often used in working with young persons.

PSYCHOTHERAPEUTIC PRACTICE WITH CHILDREN AND ADOLESCENTS WITH EMOTIONAL CONCERNS

Clinical psychotherapeutic work with young persons rests on a bedrock of common factors. It is pertinent to understand these, prior to delving into specific psychotherapies.

Relationship between Therapist and Client

Conceptualized as "*therapeutic alliance*", this is indexed on a collaborative relationship between therapist and young person, the emotional bond between them, and an agreement on treatment goals and tasks.[7] It is the responsibility of the therapist to ensure a therapeutic alliance; of course, the young person's motivation and attitude toward therapy do influence. In this regard, establishing a therapeutic alliance with adolescents is often a challenge.[7]

Few clinical pointers for establishing therapeutic alliance are as follows:

- As much as possible, in the first session, speak to the young person first, rather than the adult who has brought him/her. Even if parents insist on being seen first, emphasize that you would like to speak to the young person first, assuring the parents that their perspective will be heard subsequently. This is especially pertinent for adolescents.
- However, it is important that the young person is comfortable with being spoken to alone. So, ensure to get the young person's consent for this in the presence of the parents. If the young person declines, follow through on whatever he/she finds comfortable.
- As much as possible, have the young person in the room, when parents express their concerns. Again, the consent of the young person is necessary for this.
- Assure confidentiality to the young person (with parents being present), explicitly stating that any expression of harm to self or others will have to be informed to parents.
- Inquire into the young person's understanding/perspective on what contributed to their consultation with a mental health professional. If they express that they do not have a problem, validate that and communicate your understanding of being brought forcibly.
- Speak to the young person about their interests and hobbies and anything that they would like to talk about. Slowly build into discussing issues and problems, at the pace and priority perceived by the young person.
- Establish your role as a therapist and the scope of your work.
- Speak to them in a neutral tone of voice, appearing friendly and nonthreatening.
- Assure that you will be available for them, for anything that they would like to talk about.
- If you would like to take notes, seek permission from the young person for the same.

Client Expectations

Expectations of young persons vary, depending on their socioeconomic background, awareness of mental health issues and treatments, age, education, and cognitive capacities. It is natural for children to be apprehensive about visiting a "doctor" and for adolescents to be skeptical/cynical. It is on the therapist to correct any misconceptions and establish accurate expectations for the young person. Few clinical pointers for the same are as follows:

- Inquire into the young person's knowledge and experience with mental health professionals. Listen to what they say, without interruption, even if grossly misinformed.
- Empathize with any unpleasant experiences they may have had with mental health professionals in the past. Also, express hope that experiences may vary across professionals.

- Emphasize that you would like to get to know him/her better and understand and work along with them to help them. Add that you are not here to judge, to take sides as to who is right, but to help.
- Assert that your primary interest is their well-being. Elicit their motivation to seek professional help, specifically from you.
- Educate on how the therapeutic process progresses—what will be done within sessions, any take-home tasks, therapeutic approach, number and frequency of meeting, termination, etc. It is important that this is done, keeping in mind the age of the child. For younger children, only the most pertinent details in a simple language are adequate.
- Ensure that the young person has had an adequate understanding, by asking for feedback and questions. His/her expectations may need to be periodically corrected over the course of therapy, as evident.

Health-promoting Actions

- These refer to tasks that are done by the young person, either within or outside sessions. These are tasks that are conjointly decided by the therapist and young person.
- At the outset, it is important that the young person feels accepted as they are, as a person's strengths and weaknesses. This "unconditional positive regard" is communicated to the young person by the therapist in their manner of speech and actions.
- The understanding that the young person *has a problem and is not the problem* needs to be established. Only then are therapeutic tasks acceptable.
- Discuss these problems, communicating your understanding in a curious rather than judgmental manner. This implies that your understanding is put forward more as a hypothesis rather than fact. For younger children, this may be achieved by stating this as a situation with others and checking if it applies for the child.
- Seek permission to suggest and do certain tasks. You may have to present it as an enjoyable and interesting task for younger children and as an experiment for adolescents.
- Offer simple tasks that are acceptable and doable by the young person. Discuss possible impediments in carrying out the task and probable solutions. Communicate confidence in the young person's ability to do the task.
- If the young person fails to do the task as discussed, do not criticize or judge. Elicit reasons for being unable to do the task. Reframe it as a difficulty in doing the task, rather than the young person's failure. Revisit the tasks and discuss alternatives.

SPECIFIC THERAPEUTIC APPROACHES

Counseling

While psychotherapy aims to make changes in the young person's "*psyche*", i.e., thought, emotional, and behavioral patterns, counseling is more situation-specific, offering specific guidance on resolving circumscribed issues. As such, counseling is more behavioral in its approach, offering specific strategies to manage issues.

Box 2 offers examples of certain specific techniques for common internalizing and externalizing problems. Again, the focus is on individual-level interventions. It goes without saying that parents and teachers must be included in the intervention, depending on the problem. Only then is counseling comprehensive.

Psychoeducation

Psychoeducation is rarely a standalone intervention in clinical care. It is usually utilized as a precursor to the standard intervention,

BOX 2: Techniques for specific emotional and behavioral problems.

Internalizing problems

Shy/socially anxious:
- Specific social skill tasks such as greeting, initiating conversations, asking to join play, sharing, engaging in a conversation, participating in a class activity, speaking to teachers, etc.
- Behavioral exposure toward practicing social skills
- Reinforce efforts to practice social skills

Bed-wetting:
- Schedule toileting time
- Waking child up at night to use toilet
- Minimizing liquid intake for 2 hours before sleep

Externalizing problems

Overactive/restless:
- Break down tasks into smaller chunks
- Work on enhancing sitting time, by starting short duration tasks—focus on task engagement, rather than completion
- Reinforce efforts made—fade out reinforcement gradually by moving from continuous to periodic

Aggression/temper tantrum:
- Ignore this behavior—facilitate time out
- Examine and make aware feelings underlying aggressive behavior
- Teach adaptive ways of expressing distress
- Practice differential reinforcement, wherein adaptive behavior is reinformed and maladaptive behavior is penalized

toward enhancing knowledge on the probable causes of distress, etiology of the mental health issues, available avenues for management, prescribed management protocol, and roles of clinician/therapist, young person, and caregivers. It is pertinent to note that psychoeducation must necessarily include caregivers. The World Health Organization's Mental Health Gap Action Programme (mhGAP) offers some inputs on psychoeducation for young persons with emotional and behavioral disorders.[8] In India, the Psychological Vaccine for Immunization against Mental Health Problems (PsychoVac) was attempted with low-resource community settings in Karnataka.[9] This program, which is didactic in its approach, educated parents to promote psychological development and mental well-being for preschool children and was found feasible and effective.[9]

Supportive Psychotherapy

This therapeutic approach, inspired from the psychodynamic psychotherapy, currently falls closer to the client-centered approach. Therapy seeks to promote symptomatic relief, through tapping into the existing internal resources of the young person, while providing a supportive therapeutic atmosphere.[10] There is no active focus on personality vulnerabilities and any maladaptive behaviors.[10] Supportive psychotherapy is often utilized as an initial therapeutic approach with a young person, toward building therapeutic alliance and enhancing emotional capabilities. Following this, more in-depth approaches such as psychodynamic psychotherapy or CBT may be utilized to facilitate personality change. Techniques of supportive psychotherapy may be noted in other approaches. However, supportive psychotherapy has relevance as a standalone therapeutic approach, with its own assessment and intervention methods.[11]

Play Therapy

Play therapy, as is generally practiced, is nondirective.[12] This implies that the child leads the play session, within the structured parameters of a given time and frequency of sessions. Whilst novel and typical toys are provided to the child, there are rules on their appropriate use, without breaking them. So, the purpose is for the child to express their fantasies, fears, thoughts, and other feelings within the playroom, using the play materials provided. These play materials may be adapted to the context of the child and the problem. **Figures 2 and 3** show the play materials that were utilized in play therapy, for children

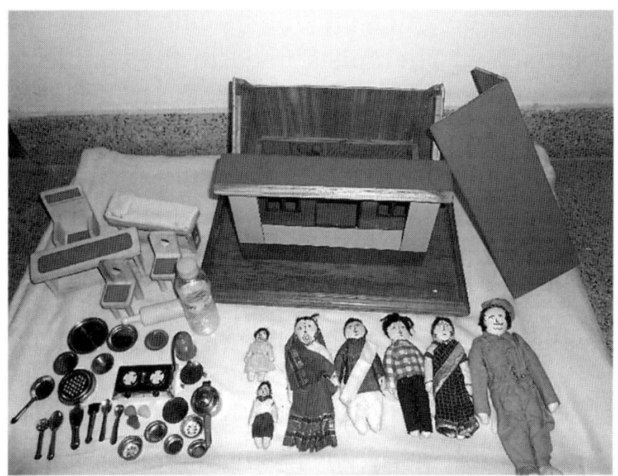

Fig. 2: Novel and typical toys.

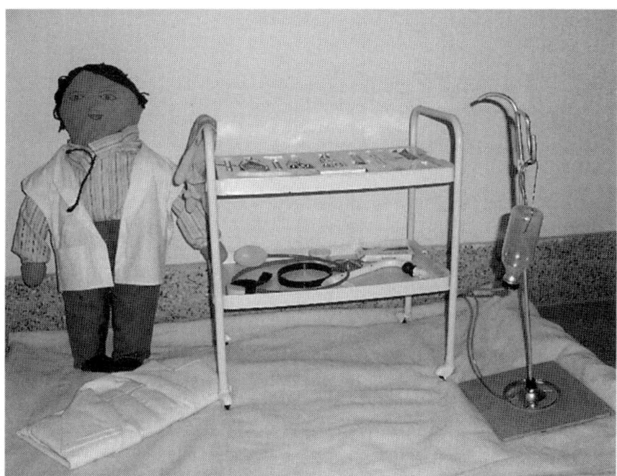

Fig. 3: Medical toys.

undergoing treatment for cancer.[13] It is beyond the scope of this chapter to give individual case illustrations for each therapeutic approach. Interested readers are referred to Chari et al.[14] for a case report of play therapy with one such child diagnosed with cancer and to Reddy and Hirisave[15] for a case report on play therapy with a child with probable emotional disorder.

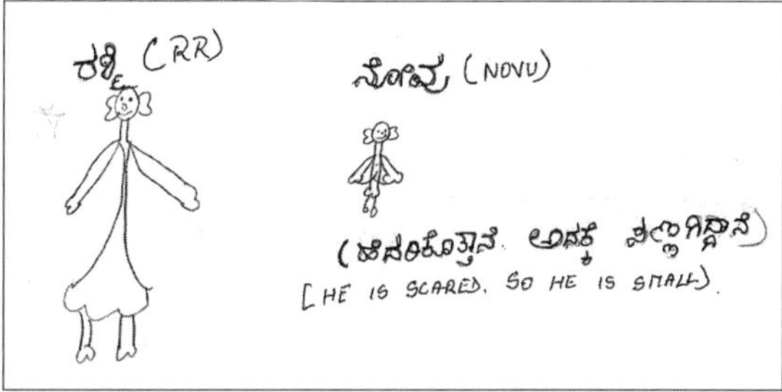

Fig. 4: Conceptualizing fear and its impact.

Art Therapy

As mentioned earlier, art materials are utilized to facilitate expression of emotional distress and resolution. The premise is that visual image-making is an important aspect of the natural learning process for young persons. In the presence of the art therapist, they can get in touch with feelings that are difficult to express verbally, thereby contributing to self-discovery and self-efficacy, paving the way for problem-solving.[16] Art therapists may interpret artwork from any angle, such as the use of color, content of the art, story of the art work, and theoretical basis. For an understanding of the mechanism of change in art therapy, please refer to Bosgraaf et al.[16] Hanes[17] presents a case report of art therapy with an adolescent girl.

Narrative Therapy

Narrative approaches lend themselves readily for use with young persons in India. Stories are an intrinsic aspect of Indian culture, and often children are raised on mythological stories, family stories, and stories of daily life. In narrative therapy, the young person is encouraged to construct their life story as it has happened thus far. This facilitates the young person to externalize their problems, witness them as an observer, and construct a new narrative of themselves and their experiences. In this process, art and other activities may be utilized; illustrated in **Figures 4 and 5**. Narrative therapy is gaining popularity in its use with young persons in the country, due to its flexibility in its approach. This case report

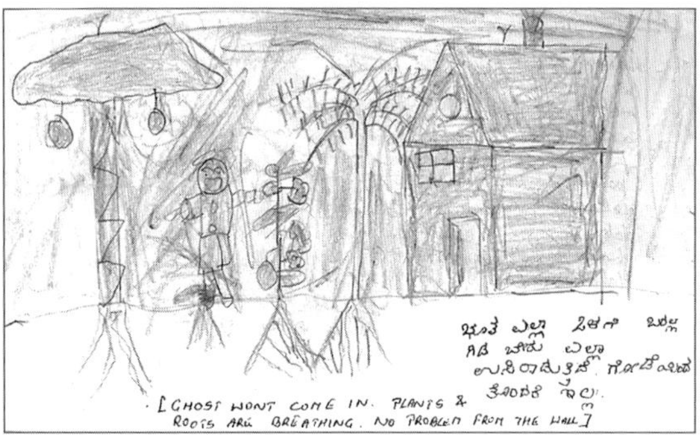

Fig. 5: Overcoming fear.

documents the application of narrative therapy with a young adolescent.[18]

Psychodynamic Psychotherapy

This therapeutic approach works on the premise that overt mental health concerns are reflections of deeper (unconscious) unresolved psychic conflicts. Child and adolescent psychotherapists inadvertently have a psychodynamic approach, when they consider relational and attachment patterns, and early childhood experiences. However, the practice of structured psychodynamic psychotherapy with young persons is not as common, given that many years of training is required to become a psychodynamic psychotherapist and limited empirical literature. Nonetheless, there is evidence to suggest that psychodynamic psychotherapy is especially beneficial in internalizing issues such as depression and anxiety, emerging personality issues, and trauma.[19] However, it may find benefit even for overt behavioral issues such as self-harm, as documented in this case report.[20]

CASE ILLUSTRATIONS

While psychotherapies are practiced in their purist forms, in clinical practice, often an eclectic approach is adopted. This is a necessity, rather than a lacuna. Children/adolescents and families cannot be expected to strictly adhere to the criteria to be amenable for specific therapeutic approaches. Therapists need to be flexible to accommodate to the varied therapeutic needs of the young persons. The following cases demonstrate the use of therapeutic approaches and techniques on two young persons—one each with an externalizing and internalizing problem. Names and some contextual details have been changed to ensure anonymity.

Internalizing Problem[21]

Background: Alwyn was an 8-year-old male child, from upper middle socioeconomic status. He presented with episodes during sleep, which lasted for around 10 minutes, wherein he would wake up and appeared to be searching for something. He seemed frightened and ran around the house. He spoke in an unusual manner and the parents would not be able to decipher the language. During these episodes, he did not comprehend or respond to others. After about 10 minutes, the child would be forcibly taken to the toilet by his mother, where he would urinate and then return to his bed and fall asleep. The child had no recollection of this episode the next morning. These episodes occurred once/twice per week, over the last 5 years. All medical tests were insignificant. However, he had a history of adenoid gland inflammation, speech delay, and recent academic decline. His parents reported that he did not like going to school or completing his schoolwork in the last 2 years. He was also particularly sensitive to loud sounds and suffered from frequent headaches. Allwyn was diagnosed with night terrors.

Allwyn was the older of two siblings. His intellectual functioning was clinically found to be average. Temperamentally, he was reported as slow to warm but was friendly with schoolmates and cousins.

Assessment on projective tests was carried out to understand unconscious processes and elicit information about anxieties, which Allwyn may be unaware of. Subjective distress regarding difficulties with sleep was noted on the Children's Apperception Test. On the Raven's Controlled Projection Test, Allwyn expressed dreams to be frightening and that the protagonist dreams of a snake eating everyone. Additionally, aggression toward mother and younger figures was elicited. The father figure remained largely absent from stories. On the draw-a-person test, Allwyn expressed female figures as being weaker and less happy. Conflict with his sister was noted.

Psychotherapy: A total of 18 sessions were carried out, on an out-patient basis, combining supportive, art, and play therapies. Initial sessions used common therapeutic factors of creating and accepting and validating therapeutic atmosphere for the child, toward establishing therapeutic alliance. Within the supportive framework, specific parental guidance on improving their child's sleep quality was given. Allwyn was also taught relaxation using imagery and breathing exercises, to be practiced before bedtime. The frequency of the sleep episodes decreased.

Mid-therapy, art therapy was introduced, and themes in Allwyn's artwork were explored. These included family, holiday, school, and ideas of safety and fear. During this time, the child recalled having a dream of a dinosaur attacking him and he drew this in the session. The theme of fire emerged repeatedly in the child's drawings as well as in his accounts of imagination. He would report/draw that he was running away from a large fire and would describe falling buildings and people running to save them. Artwork on both dinosaurs and fire was reframed, toward making Allwyn more empowered in such situations. Thus, they were made less fearful. Family drawings revealed conflict and aggressive impulses toward the younger sister. This conflict was also verbalized by Allwyn, wherein he expressed that he loved her but preferred not to play with her, as he was a "big boy".

Simultaneous sessions with parents toward clarifying history revealed likely repressed trauma regarding his circumcision experience and suppressed fears of his father being in the midst of a terror attack and anxieties about being replaced with birth of sibling.

In artwork, phallic symbols, possibly reflecting repressed memories, emerged, such as in dinosaurs with missing finger in drawings. Also, discussions on the father's presence during a terrorist attack were marked by Allwyn relating this to emotional valence. Unlike psychotherapy with adults, the underlying interpretations of anxieties and symptoms are not actively pursued in therapy session discussions with children. Thus, play therapy was introduced as a means for Allwyn to resolve any underlying intrapsychic conflicts in a nonthreatening manner.

Utilizing a child-directed approach, Allwyn was initially hesitant to explore the playroom. Subsequently, however, he became comfortable. He liked the sandpit and filling buckets with sand. He made clay sculptures and sought the therapist's approval for the same. With dolls, he was aggressive, with elders being harsh with children in disciplining. He engaged in puppet-play, seeking the therapist to also join. The story revolved around a boy who was loved and happy at home and at school. Allwyn reported to enjoy the playroom the most.

Toward the last few sessions, Allwyn was given the freedom to choose whatever activity he preferred in therapy. He chose to draw and talk to the therapist. Over the course of psychotherapy, Allwyn was better able to verbalize his feelings. The frequency of night terror episodes decreased to once in a month. He was happier at home and felt less scared, although not fully sure of what he was sacred of. He was also keener to complete his schoolwork. Parents also reported better adjustment with his sister. Psychotherapy was terminated. Gains were maintained during follow-up.

Impression: In this case illustration, the initial supportive approach facilitated the way for more deeper art and play therapies. Supportive psychotherapy also facilitated initial symptom relief. The pertinence of adhering to the common factors is evident. While psychodynamic material emerged over the course of therapy, this was not actively discussed, given the child-directed framework. It is pertinent to progress at the pace as determined by the child. Parents were informants for clinical history, as is usually the case with young persons. The case demonstrates the necessity to periodically check with history with parents, over the duration of psychotherapy with the child.

Externalizing Problem[22]

Background: Suhas was a 7-year-old child from a lower socioeconomic background, in rural India. He presented with complaints of being physically aggressive, having anger outburst, and using foul language, in the last 2.5 months. Temperamentally, he was described to be difficult.

Suhas had witnessed his mother being murdered by his father, who subsequently ran away, leaving Suhas alone with the body of his mother for many hours. Following this, for about 2 weeks, he was physically unwell and withdrawn, after which he started displaying the reported complaints. The father was arrested, and Suhas was in the care of his maternal grandmother and great-grandmother. He was diagnosed with adjustment disorder–mixed, with disturbance in emotions and conduct, admitted in the inpatient child and adolescent psychiatry wards.

Psychotherapy: Psychotherapy was carried out over a period of 3 months of admission. A combination of play, art, and narrative therapies was adopted. Given his young age, nondirective play therapy was initiated at the outset. These sessions facilitated to provide a safe space for Suhas to explore and express. Autonomy was encouraged via the freedom to choose any of the toys and play as per his desire, in the background of unconditional acceptance from the therapist. Initially sullen and minimally communicative, Suhas spontaneously used dolls and re-enacted scenes of his father beating him, within a week of play sessions.

Subsequently, a narrative therapy approach, utilizing art and music as expressive mediums, was incorporated. Suhas was encouraged to narrate stories, making use of drawings while doing so. Initial stories were nihilistic, such as in the context of animals falling into a well, and ruminative, such as in drawings of his home with his mother's belongings. However, with subsequent narrations, stories became more hopeful and current/future-oriented. Constructed narratives and drawings did not feature any of his mother's belongings; instead, they depicted those of grandmothers'. Simultaneously, he was also taught a song conveying faith and hope, with the help of his grandmother. This helped further strengthen their relationship, while the song also became a means for Suhas to soothe himself when distressed.

Toward learning some adaptive social behaviors, Suhas was engaged in group play sessions. Rules were firmly stated and implemented, ensuring an equal opportunity for all children to play. While initially Suhas was impulsive, demanding, and demonstrated difficulty in sharing, subsequently he was able to await his turn and demonstrated enhanced frustration tolerance and prosocial behaviors.

A breakthrough was achieved 1 month into therapy, when Suhas had an emotional breakdown, crying for his mother. This was cathartic, as this was the first time that he directly expressed grief on his mother's death, instead of acting out. This episode was discussed by the therapist with him, reflecting and validating his feelings and addressing the pain of losing his mother. Suhas was able to verbally engage in this session and reconstruct the loss and its meaning, and integrate it into his life story. It appeared that Suhas had internalized and accepted the finality and irreversibility of death and was on the path to seeking a future for himself without his mother's presence.

Inpatient psychotherapy was terminated gradually, by engaging in dialogue regarding plans for himself at the village. It appeared that he was adequately secure in his relationship with the therapist, to process separation without undue distress. This was pertinent, especially in the background of the abrupt loss of his mother.

Gains made during inpatient stay such as improvement in mood, reduced aggression, improved verbalizing of emotional distress, and managing peer relationships were maintained even at outpatient follow-ups. However, his traits of reported difficult temperament, such as stubbornness, persisted.

Impressions: The basic principles (common factors) facilitated to building a strong therapeutic relationship with Suhas. The sequentially timed and appropriate use of play and narrative therapies with art/music encouraged expression and cathartic processes. The structures of group play inculcated adaptive social behaviors. Psychotherapy helped beyond symptomatic relief. Temperamental changes require more long-term therapies and were not immediately warranted. Developmental trajectories often mediate changes in temperament, and Suhas will be followed up for the same.

SUMMARY AND CONCLUSION

Psychological interventions are often the first-line treatment for emotional/behavioral disorders in children and adolescents. Psychotherapy in clinical practice with young persons deals with emotional problems and behavioral issues, not disorders. These interventions vary in their intensity and focus of treatment, based on underlying theoretical assumptions. The purpose of this chapter was to give an overview of commonly used supportive-expressive therapeutic approaches for emotional and behavioral issues in children and adolescents.

Any psychotherapeutic approach needs to based on universal factors that are facilitative of therapy. These include the therapeutic alliance, client expectations, and health-promoting behaviors carried out by the young person. As such, there is evidence to suggest that all psychotherapeutic approaches are effective, if there is a good fit between the type of problem and approach, and therapist's competence. Practice of any therapeutic approach mandates adequate training. It is hoped that the descriptions with references to case reports give the reader a basic understanding of these approaches. This chapter has focused only on working individually with the child/adolescents. Parenting and family interventions and CBTs are described in subsequent chapters.

REFERENCES

1. Sethi BB, Chaturvedi PK. Psychotherapy for the developing world. In: Pichot P, Berner P, Wolf R, Thau K (Eds). Psychiatry the State of the Art. Boston, MA.: Springer; 1985.
2. Darling N. Ecological systems theory: The person in the center of the circles. Res Hum Dev. 2007;4(3-4): 203-17.
3. Laska KM, Gurman AS, Wampold BE. Expanding the lens of evidence-based practice in psychotherapy: A common factors perspective. Psychother. 2014;51(4):467-81.
4. Wampold BE. How important are the common factors in psychotherapy? An update. World Psychiatry. 2015;14(3):270-7.
5. Weisz JR, Jensen AL. Child and adolescent psychotherapy in research and practice contexts: Review of the evidence and suggestions for improving the field. Eur Child Adolesc Psychiatry. 2001;10(Suppl 1):12-8.

6. Rogers CR. The necessary and sufficient conditions of therapeutic personality change. J Consult Psychol. 1957;21(2):95-103.
7. Stubbe DE. The therapeutic alliance: The fundamental element of psychotherapy. Focus (Am Psychiatr Publ). 2018;16(4):402-3.
8. World Health Organization. (2016). mhGAP Intervention Guide-Version 2.0, 2016. [online] Available from https://www.who.int/publications/i/item/9789241549790 [Last accessed 19 November, 2025].
9. Hirisave U. A pilot study for promotion of psychological development and mental health in early childhood using PsychoVac program. Bengaluru: National Institute of Mental Health and Neuro Sciences.
10. Winston A, Pinsker H, McCullough L. A review of supportive psychotherapy. Hosp Community Psych. 1986;37(11):1105-14.
11. Grover S, Avasthi A, Jagiwala M. Clinical Practice Guidelines for Practice of Supportive Psychotherapy. Indian J Psychiatry. 2020;62(Suppl 2):S173-82.
12. Axline VM. Play Therapy. New York: Ballantine Books; 1974.
13. Chari U. Childhood leukaemia: An exploratory study of a hospital-based psychological intervention. PhD thesis, National Institute of Mental Health and Neuro Sciences, Bengaluru, India; 2013.
14. Chari U, Hirisave U, Appaji L. Exploring Play Therapy in Pediatric Oncology: A Preliminary Endeavour. Indian J Pediatr. 2013;80:303-8.
15. Reddy RP, Hirisave U. Child's play: Therapist's narrative. Indian J Psychol Med. 2014;36(2):204-7.
16. Bosgraaf L, Spreen M, Pattiselanno K, Hooren S. Art therapy for psychosocial problems in children and adolescents: A systematic narrative review on art therapeutic means and forms of expression, therapist behavior, and supposed mechanisms of change. Front Psychol. 2020;11:584685.
17. Hanes MJ. Catharsis in art therapy: A case study of a sexually abused adolescent. Am J Art Ther. 2000;38:70-4.
18. Vishwanatha K, Hirisave U. Using narrative approaches with a young girl in India. Int J Narrat Ther Comm Work. 2009;2:41-7.
19. Midgley N, Mortimer R, Cirasola A, Batra P, Kennedy E. The evidence-base for psychodynamic psychotherapy with children and adolescents: A narrative synthesis. Front Psychol. 2021;12:662671.
20. Thompson C, Mazet P, Cohen D. Treatment of a Suicide Attempt through Psychodynamic Therapy in a 17-Year-Old Boy with Depression: A Case Study. Isr J Psychiatry Relat Sci. 2005;42(2): 282-5.
21. Ahluwalia H, Hirisave U. The terrors of the night: Creative psychotherapeutic approach in a case of a child with parasomnia. J Indian Assoc Child Adolesc Ment Health. 2018;14(1):80-92.
22. Rupa M, Hirisave U, Srinath S. Psychological intervention for a child exposed to murder. Indian J Pediatr. 2013;81(5):509-10.

CHAPTER 24

Psychological Therapies for Emotional and Behavioral Disorders-II (Cognitive Behavioral Therapy, Behavioral Therapy, and Related Therapies)

Pragya Sharma, Prerna Sharma

INTRODUCTION

20% of adolescents may experience a mental health problem in any given year.[1] Around 50% of mental health problems are established by age of 14 years and 75% by the age of 24 years.[2] 10% of children and young people (aged 5–16 years) have a clinically diagnosable mental problem,[3] yet 70% of children and adolescents who experience mental health problems have not had appropriate interventions at a sufficiently early age.[4] According to a 2014 study, the prevalence of mental health disorders in children and adolescents in India is 6.46% in community-based studies and 23.33% in school-based studies.[5] A 2016 National Mental Health Survey of India (NMHS) reported a 7.3% prevalence of psychological morbidity among adolescents aged 13–17 years.[6]

In view of the above facts, early intervention is crucial for addressing mental health issues in children and adolescents for several reasons. Early intervention for childhood mental health issues is essential to optimize long-term outcomes. It mitigates developmental disruption, prevents chronicity, enhances coping mechanisms, improves treatment efficacy, and disrupts negative cycles, fostering a healthier trajectory for emotional well-being. In addressing mental health concerns in children and adolescents, evidence-based interventions like cognitive behavioral therapy (CBT) and behavioral therapies have emerged as powerful tools. These approaches target the link between thoughts, emotions, and behaviors, equipping young people with practical strategies for managing challenges.

A one-size-fits-all approach just will not work when it comes to CBT and behavioral therapy for children and adolescents. Adapting these techniques across age groups is crucial. It may be because of several reasons such as cognitive development—children's thinking abilities progress significantly throughout childhood and adolescence. Younger children may struggle with abstract concepts, while teenagers can handle more complex cognitive restructuring techniques. Tailoring the approach ensures the child can understand and apply the strategies effectively. Therapists need to adapt communication styles and activities to keep young people engaged and motivated throughout the therapy process. Each age group faces unique challenges according to the developmental stage of the child. Young children might struggle with emotional regulation, while adolescents grapple with self-esteem, peer pressure, and identity development. Adapting techniques allows therapists to directly address the specific concerns relevant to each stage. Lastly, parents play a vital role in supporting their child's mental health journey. Adapting therapy techniques can help to equip parents with age-appropriate strategies to reinforce what their child learns in therapy, fostering a more consistent and supportive environment. By adapting CBT and behavioral techniques, therapists can ensure the interventions resonate with the child's = developmental stage, maximizing the effectiveness of the treatment and empowering young people with the tools they need to thrive.

IMPORTANCE OF STRONG THERAPEUTIC ALLIANCE

Building trust and rapport with the children and their family is fundamental in child and adolescent therapy. It builds psychological safety; a strong relationship creates a safe space for children and adolescents to express themselves openly and honestly, even about difficult thoughts and emotions. It increases engagement; when young people feel understood and respected, they are more likely to actively participate in therapy and be receptive to interventions. Strong therapeutic alliance fosters collaboration between the therapist, child/adolescent, and family. This is crucial for developing and implementing treatment plans that everyone feels invested in. Building trust also motivates young people to continue therapy and adhere to treatment recommendations. This is especially important for long-term success. Involving families in the therapeutic process and building rapport with them allows therapists to provide guidance for supporting the child's mental health at home. The therapist's relationship with the child independently affects intervention outcomes. Direct communication with the child, acknowledging the child's understanding about the situation, and building even a simplistic but shared understanding plays a huge role in the effectiveness of interventions.

Strategies for Building Rapport

Warm, empathetic, and nonjudgmental demeanor: Therapists should create a welcoming environment where children and adolescents feel comfortable and respected.

Age-appropriate communication: Using language and activities tailored to the child's developmental level fosters understanding and engagement.

Active listening: Therapists should demonstrate genuine interest in the child's experiences and perspectives.

Building trust with families: Therapists should collaborate with families and caregivers to understand their concerns and perspectives, fostering a sense of partnership.

By prioritizing a strong therapeutic relationship, therapists can create a foundation for successful treatment and empower children and adolescents to thrive.

COGNITIVE BEHAVIORAL THERAPY PRINCIPLES

Cognitive Behavioral Model

Cognitive behavioral therapy posits that our thoughts, feelings, and behaviors are interconnected as shown in **Figure 1.**[7] The way people perceive a situation predicts their reaction to it, rather than the situation itself.

Consider an adolescent was called to her office by the school principal. Adolescent 1 thinks, "Oh, it must be about the great stage performance I gave yesterday and the principal wants to praise me." She is jubilant and walks into the principal's office, smiling and excited. On the other hand, adolescent 2 thinks, "Oh no, what wrong did I

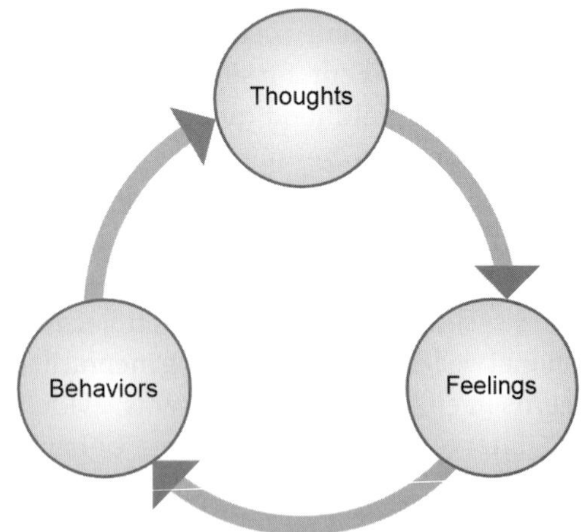

Fig. 1: Cognitive behavioral model.[8]

do now? I am sure the principal wants to scold me." She is nervous and jittery as she walks into the principal's office. The situation remained the same for both adolescents but what they thought determined their feelings and behaviors in the situation.

Cognitive behavioral therapy model recognizes that altering one component can influence the others. In the above example, changing the way the adolescent thought would change her feelings and behaviors.

Identifying and Challenging Negative Automatic Thoughts

Negative automatic thoughts (NATs) are often unconscious, fleeting thoughts that occur involuntarily in response to daily events. In order to have balanced feelings and engage in adaptive behaviors, it is crucial to learn to identify and challenge the validity of these NATs and work on replacing them with alternate perspectives.

Developing Adaptive Coping Mechanisms

The focus of CBT is on cultivating adaptive coping mechanisms to deal with stressful situations, resulting in better psychological well-being. These may include problem-solving, emotion regulation, and seeking social support. By practicing these skills, children and adolescents become better equipped to manage life's challenges effectively.

KEY TECHNIQUES

Cognitive Restructuring

This technique involves identifying and rectifying maladaptive cognitive patterns shown in **Figure 2 and Table 1**.[9] The unhelpful thought patterns are identified like catastrophizing or black-and-white thinking. These are then challenged by finding evidence, taking into account different viewpoints, and reframing them in a more realistic manner.

Behavioral Activation

Often, dysfunctional thoughts lead to negative mood states like depression and anxiety which then cause people to withdraw from once-enjoyable activities, thereby starting a vicious cycle of bad emotions. Children who receive behavioral activation are more likely to participate in enjoyable and fulfilling activities that make them feel happy and fulfilled, which improves their motivation and mood.[10]

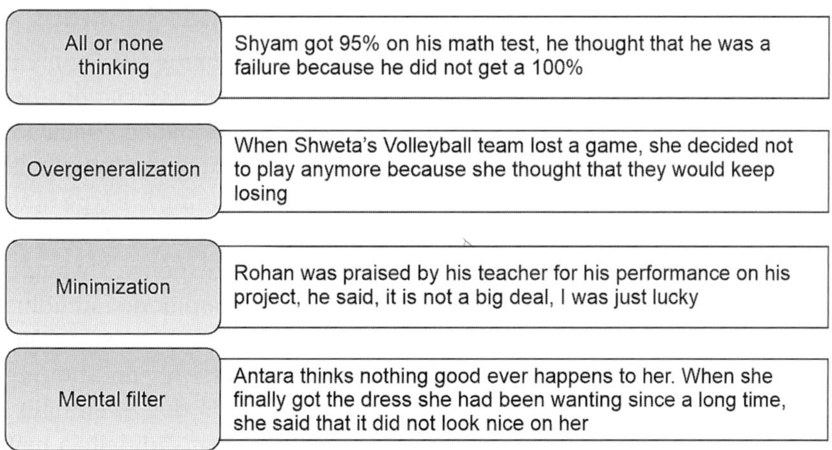

Fig. 2: Cognitive distortions.

TABLE 1: Few examples of cognitive distortions and cognitive restructuring.

Cognitive distortion	*Evidence against*	*Alternate thought*	*Reframed thought*
Catastrophizing "If I mess up this presentation, I will fail this grade."	"I have made mistakes before and did not fail a grade. My teacher has given me positive feedback in the past."	"If I mess up, I can explain myself and learn from the experience. My performance is not solely dependent on one presentation."	"It is normal to be nervous, but I have prepared well. Even if it does not go perfectly, it will not be the end of the world."
All or None Thinking "I'm a total failure."	"I have completed many successful projects in the past. One mistake does not define my overall performance."	"I made a mistake, but I have also done many things right. I can learn from this and improve."	"Everyone makes mistakes. This does not mean I am a failure; it means I am a human. I can use this experience to grow."

Exposure Therapy

Adolescents with anxiety-based disorders, such as phobias and obsessive-compulsive disorder (OCD), can learn to face their anxieties in a safe setting by gradually being exposed to feared stimuli or situations.[11]

Relaxation Techniques

Relaxation techniques such as deep breathing, progressive muscle relaxation, and mindfulness meditation offer children and adolescents a means to manage their stress-related behaviors effectively, giving them more control in anxiety-provoking situations.[12]

Social Skills Training

Social skills training focuses on communication-based training, assertiveness training, and imparting conflict resolution skills.[13] Role-playing exercises and real-life scenarios help children and adolescents to become more competent in social interactions.

By incorporating these practical techniques into the treatment approach, children and adolescents can be empowered to navigate the stress-provoking situations they frequently encounter.

BEHAVIORAL THERAPY APPROACHES

Behavioral approaches in psychotherapy are grounded in several key learning theories that explain how behaviors are acquired, maintained, and modified. Behaviorism assumes that all learning occurs through interactions with the environment and that environment shapes behavior. Behavioral approaches directly target problematic behaviors a child or adolescent exhibits. These therapies rely on established principles of learning, such as reinforcement and punishment, to shape desired behaviors.

Theoretical Underpinnings

Classical conditioning (Pavlov): This theory proposes that learned associations between stimuli can trigger emotional and behavioral responses. Discovered by Russian physiologist Ivan Pavlov, classical conditioning is a type of unconscious or automatic learning. This learning process creates a conditioned response through associations between an unconditioned stimulus and a neutral stimulus. Fear and aversive responses are typical examples of classical conditioning, e.g., a child who is bitten by a dog, eventually starts fearing all dogs, here dog is initially a neutral stimulus, biting is an unconditioned stimulus, fear is an unconditioned response. Now the child starts fearing all dogs and even at the sight of any dog he becomes fearful. Here, dog becomes a conditioned stimulus and fear a conditioned response. In simple terms, classical conditioning involves placing a neutral stimulus before a naturally occurring reflex. Taking a step further, if the child generalizes the fear response and gets fearful in presence of all animals then this phenomenon is called generalization in behavioral analysis. One may trace this phenomenon in agoraphobia, OCD, social anxiety disorder where the subject generalizes the response to more and more situations (stimuli) in the environment.

Operant conditioning (Skinner): This theory focuses on how the consequences of a behavior influence its future occurrence. Behavioral therapy techniques like positive reinforcement and extinction rely on operant conditioning principles to strengthen desired behaviors and weaken unwanted ones. It plays a powerful role in everyday learning. Operant conditioning is a method of learning that employs rewards and punishments for behavior. Through operant conditioning, an association is made between a behavior and a consequence (whether negative or positive) for that behavior.[14]

Operant conditioning was first described by behaviorist BF Skinner.[14] As a behaviorist, Skinner was more interested in how the consequences of people's actions influenced their behavior. Operant conditioning relies on a fairly simple premise: Actions that are followed by reinforcement will be strengthened and more likely to occur again in the future. If a person sings at a party and everybody enjoys, he is probably more likely to sing again in the future. Conversely, actions that result in punishment or undesirable consequences will be weakened and less likely to occur again in the future. If the person sings the same song again in another party, but nobody seems to enjoy this time, the person will be less likely to repeat the song again in the future.

There are four types of operant conditioning that can be utilized to change behavior: (1) Positive reinforcement (an increase in the probability of behavior due to an increase in the contingent event), e.g., a teacher praising kinds in class for good handwriting found this reinforcement resulted in more kids wanting to improve the handwriting, (2) negative reinforcement (it is an increase in the probability of behavior due to decrease in the contingent event), e.g., a child learns deep breathing to offset examination anxiety with a decrease in stress being a negative reinforcer, (3) positive punishment (a decrease in the probability of behavior due to an increase in the contingent event), e.g., if a child tells his math teacher he is having trouble keeping up with the class he is then given extra remedial work, then the extra work may act as a punisher resulting in a decrease in asking for help, and (4) negative punishment (decrease in the probability of behavior due to a decrease in the contingent event). This corresponds to a decrease in something desirable following some behavior, e.g., if a child throws a tantrum, then it may be stopped by cutting short screen time or taking away his favorite toy.

Social learning theory (Bandura): This theory emphasizes the role of observation and imitation in learning. Behavioral therapy techniques like modeling and social skills training leverage social learning principles to equip children and adolescents with new behaviors by observing and practicing them.

Techniques in Classical Conditioning

Flooding: This process involves exposing people to fear-invoking objects or situations intensely and rapidly. It is often used to treat phobias. During the process, the child is prevented from escaping or avoiding the situation. It is nongradual approach for producing extinction. It involves bombarding the child with anxiety producing stimuli and keeping the child in anxiety situation without escape. This approach is not very popular currently and the clinician/therapist should be careful to use flooding age appropriately since it can retraumatize the child who is not able to understand the rationale behind this technique especially in cases of high severity of anxiety. However, humans are continually confronted with situations that elicit some anxiety and if children are taught to normalize tolerating and confronting some amount of anxiety then this can be beneficial, e.g., making a presentation in front of class, talking about feelings to parents, and standing up to a bully.

Systematic desensitization: In this technique, people make a list of fears and then learn to relax while concentrating on these fears. Starting with the least fear-inducing item and working their way to the most fear-inducing item, people systematically confront these fears under the guidance of a therapist. Systematic desensitization is often used to treat phobias and other anxiety disorders.[15] This is based on the principle of counter conditioning which is eliciting a response incompatible with the undesired response such as some forms of relaxation may be to the anxiety provoking situations.

TECHNIQUES IN OPERANT CONDITIONING

Extinction: Another way to produce behavior change is to stop reinforcing behavior in order to eliminate the response. Time-outs are example of the extinction process. During a time-out, a person is removed from a situation that provides reinforcement. By taking away what the person found rewarding, unwanted behavior is eventually extinguished. A mother who stops giving attention during a tantrum of the child will likely to fade out sooner.

Token economies: This strategy relies on reinforcement to modify behavior. Parents and teachers often use token economies, allowing kids to earn tokens for engaging in preferred behaviors and lose tokens for undesirable behaviors. These tokens can then be traded for rewards such as candy, toys, or extra time playing with a favorite toy.[16]

ASSESSMENT AND CASE FORMULATION IN PSYCHOTHERAPY

Behavior analysis helps us to understand three vital aspects: (1) how behavior works, (2) how behavior is affected by the environment, and (3) how learning takes place. For the understanding of these aspects, it is equally vital to conduct a comprehensive child/adolescent mental health assessment in collaboration with parents/caregivers in order to develop a collaborative treatment plan with specific and measurable goals.[17]

Assessment

Following points must be covered in comprehensive clinical assessment **(Table 2)** for a case formulation which will aid in therapeutic management.

CASE CONCEPTUALIZATION

Case conceptualization is one of the core features of psychotherapy including CBT, and has been described as the "heart of evidence-based practice".[11] Conceptualization synthesizes the client's presenting problems, directs an intervention strategy, and provides a roadmap to guide treatment **(Fig. 3)**. Various factors are combined to understand a client's presenting problems. In preliminary stages, the clinician can attempt to best understand the current problems of the client with the help of 4P model and bio-psycho-social to conceptualize the case.[18] This can inform the clinician to synthesize the problems, later the case can be formulated with respect to the disorder and particular model

TABLE 2: Comprehensive clinical assessment.

Key points	*Description and method*
Information gathering from multiple sources	Multidisciplinary team (parents, psychiatric social worker, pediatrician, school counselor, teachers, and significant others)
Creating a child-centric environment—reduced anxiety, enhance cooperation, positive association for follow-up visits	Visual appeal in clinical space, playful activities, and drawing materials
Family functioning/parent and child interaction	Assess child's functioning within family and community context
Developmental/Cognitive functioning	Prenatal history, milestones, disruptions, other pertinent details, meeting developmental milestones, any delays (IQ and disability) is noted
School	Age-appropriate information (preschool, childcare, and school) is recorded via grade, behavior, achievement, attendance/ absence. Any expressive and receptive language problems or history of learning difficulties or impairment is noted
Self-care	Age-appropriate daily activities are recorded, including assistive technology, communication needs, self-preservation. History and current status of self-care skills (toileting, grooming, etc.)
Social support and functioning	Social skills, relationships, parental obligations, and family medical/psychiatric history. Difficulties in social skills, peer relationships, appropriate play, communication is noted. Community supports, connections, and sense of belonging
Caregiver resources and needs	*Record:* Family stress, housing, finances, organization, and community/social involvement
Trauma history	Record current status and history of family/household violence, abuse, neglect, and exploitation (history/current)
Child's strengths and abilities	Personal qualities (adaptability, persistence, curiosity, etc.), strengths in daily living, family, relationships, leisure/ recreational skills, and community resources available
Additional assessments	Medical/physical health summary, mental status examination (MSE), risk assessment, cultural and religious considerations, and sexuality and gender identity

(CBT, psychodynamic, etc.) detailing the process by which problems are developed and formed.

ANXIETY DISORDERS

Anxiety disorders that may begin in childhood include generalized anxiety disorder, social anxiety disorder, and separation anxiety disorder (collectively known as the "child anxiety triad"). Other prevalent anxiety disorders are OCD, panic disorder, agoraphobia, and specific phobia. Children and adolescents with anxiety disorders often experience significant functional impairment in educational, social, and familial domains, which lead to continued impairment in adulthood.[19]

Cognitive behavioral therapy has strong theoretical foundations on the principles

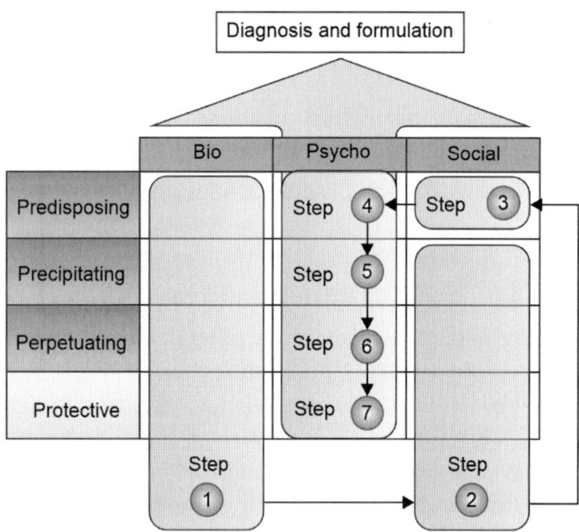

Fig. 3: Case conceptualization.

discussed previously. CBT model of anxiety is based on three constructs consisting of physiological, cognitive, and behavioral. Both cognitive factors (such as worry, obsessions, and dysfunctional beliefs) and behavioral factors (such as classical conditioning, operant conditioning, observational learning, or modeling) precipitate and maintain childhood anxiety.[20]

Cognitive behavioral therapy aims to change the beliefs or behaviors at the root of the anxiety, helping to ease symptoms. In order to understand how CBT works, it helps to understand how anxiety works. Once the fears are acquired through learning resulting in anxiety children learn to avoid the situations which maintain the fear. This is an instinctive response since this makes them feel better. This may bring temporary relief from anxiety and thus negatively reinforced. But as the child keeps avoiding their fears, the fears only grow more powerful. CBT helps kids to stop avoiding their fears. The goal in CBT is, essentially, to unlearn avoidant behavior. Most of the CBT-based treatment for anxiety disorders commonly share the process of exposure therapy; however, there are some additional points to consider such as in case of social anxiety disorder children must be encouraged to attend school as far as possible. Absence serves only to make them even more reluctant to attend school. In case of separation anxiety disorder behavioral therapy is practiced that systematically enforces regular separations. The goodbye scenes must be kept as brief as possible, and the mother (who is the primary attachment figure) should be coached to react to protestations calmly and firmly. Assisting the child in forming an attachment to one of the adults in the preschool or school may be helpful. Successfully treated children are prone to relapses after holidays and breaks from school. Because of these relapses, parents are often advised to plan regular separations during these periods to help the child remain accustomed to being away from the parents.

Core treatment component of CBT commonly shared for all anxiety disorders is discussed below:

Exposure Therapy

The basic premise is that children are exposed to the things that trigger their anxiety in structured and incremental steps and in a safe setting. As they get used to each trigger, the anxiety fades, and they are ready to take on another trigger. This is called exposure and response prevention.[21] Exposure therapy is very different from traditional talk therapy. It does not intent to explore the roots of the anxiety, in hopes of changing their behavior. In exposure therapy, we try to change the behavior to get rid of the fear. The child and the therapist will work together to come up with a list of the child's anxiety triggers. Then they will rank the fears on a scale of 1–10. Next, the child is exposed to their fear in its mildest possible form. The therapist supports the child until their anxiety fades. As their anxiety lessens, children feel more in control.

How does exposure therapy work?

The first step is identifying triggers. The clinician and the child collaboratively develop an exposure hierarchy, a series of incremental challenges or feared situations in order of the child-perceived difficulty. Instead of thinking in black and white terms—I *cannot* touch a cat or I *cannot* cross the road—kids are asked to consider degrees of difficulty. Clinician may ask the child who has fear of contamination—"On a scale of 1–10, how difficult would it be to touch the table top with one finger? To touch and sit on the chair?" By rating these different fears, kids come to see that some are less extreme, and more manageable, than they had thought.

The first exposure chosen should be one that the clinician expects the child can reasonably handle so that the child can experience mastery. Mastery can be enhanced by practicing the same exposure several times to test whether the feared outcome occurs and by showing children that they can tolerate the distress that they previously perceived as unbearable. Clinicians expose the child to the trigger in its mildest possible form, and support them until the anxiety subsides. Once clinicians worked through some exposures and child is feeling more confident, he may be assigned homework to practice what was done in the sessions. The idea is to really master their exposures before moving up the ladder. And, parents are taught to help kids progress by encouraging them to tolerate anxious feelings, rather than jumping in to protect them from their anxiety. Clinicians can monitor child reported SUDS throughout exposures. This technique is called habituation-based learning in exposure therapy. Until the child reports 50% reduction in SUDS from baseline the habituation may not have occurred. Treatment for mild-to-moderate levels of severity usually takes 8–12 sessions. Note that clinicians may use various creative ways to expose and move up and down the fear hierarchy as suited in the session. The choice of homework and mount of homework should also be given wisely suited to the capacity of the child. It must be ensured that child is practicing and generalizing the learning to other situations before the therapy is terminated.

Clinical Case Presentation

Reema is 12 years old and has fear of cats. She acquired this fear when she visited neighbor's house and their pet cat jumped on her and scratched her hand. She started avoiding visiting their house and even started to feel fearful from any furry object. She would feel *"ghabrahat"* at the thought of cats, a pinching sensation on her arms and hyperventilate when someone mentioned about visiting the neighbor's house. After a comprehensive evaluation, initial assessment of symptoms, functional impairment, and family accommodation the therapy was initiated. Reema was hesitant to speak to Dr Ajay and so most of the first session was focused on building rapport, therapeutic alliance by discussing her hobbies and some play activities. Reema and her parents were also provided with psychoeducation, which included an explanation of the development and maintenance of anxiety symptoms and the impacts of avoidance and reassurance seeking. Further, Dr Ajay discussed the CBT treatment model using developmentally appropriate language. A motivational reward mechanism was introduced, in which Reema earned tokens for attending sessions regularly, completing out-of-session homework, and practicing some exercises at home. The rewards in exchange of tokens were jointly decided with parents and Reema. Dr Ajay decided to collaboratively make a list of things she fears from the least fearing to most fearing on a 0–10 SUDS rating scale **(Table 3)**.

Dr Ajay also introduced a thought log in which Reema tracked the triggers, thoughts, and behaviors associated with her anxiety symptoms. She was taught how to identify anxious thoughts and replace them with more realistic alternative thoughts. For example, *"I can never touch a cat"*

TABLE 3: Exposure examples with rating.

Exposure exercise	*0–10 rating*
Petting a cat	10
Visiting the neighbor alone	9
Visiting the neighbor with someone	9
Wearing a furry jacket	8
Touching a stuff toy	8
Seeing a picture of a cat in the session	6
Talking about a cat with Dr Ajay	5
Watching a cat on TV	4
Seeing a cat from a distance	4
Passing by neighbor's house in car	3

to "I cannot touch a cat yet, but the feeling may change in future."

Most of the treatment sessions involved the following format: (1) Review exposure homework from the previous week, (2) discuss the thought log from the previous week (for situations in which Reema struggled to develop more realistic counter thoughts, the therapist used collaborative brainstorming to help to generate alternative thoughts), and (3) complete an in-session exposure exercise. During exposures, Reema experienced mastery little by little and tried to view fearful thoughts from a distance. Throughout treatment, Dr Ajay encouraged Reema's mother to coach her during the in-session exposure exercises to help to prepare them for exposure practice at home. The therapist also talked with her parents about the importance of not accommodating at home (e.g., not visiting neighbor's house, not keeping furry blankets at home, or bring soft toys at home for their younger child). Reema's parents had hard time not accommodating her requests related to anxiety provoking events. Psychoeducation related to maintenance of anxiety symptoms was reviewed, and Dr Ajay discussed how these accommodations can help to reduce Reema's anxiety and distress in the short term but often lead to more problems in the long term. He also reviewed Reema's progress in treatment, which was partially associated with her parents decreasing their reassurance and accommodations in different situations. As treatment progressed, her anxiety symptoms gradually decreased, and she avoided fewer situations in neighborhood and home. This led to less functional impairment in school, social, and familial domains. At the end of treatment, Reema was able to go about neighborhood and was okay with stray cats around the park. Reema faced her feared situations that she had previously avoided, and she discovered that her feared outcomes such as heavy breathing, sensations in body did not occur during the exposure exercises. Toward the end of treatment, sessions were spaced 2–3 weeks apart, and relapse prevention was discussed with Reema and her parents. Dr Ajay reviewed the techniques Reema learned in treatment and helped to prepare her for future events when anxiety symptoms occur.

MOOD DISORDERS

Diagnosing and treating mood problems in children and adolescents, especially depression, can be quite difficult.[22] It is critical to recognize the distinct ways that these illnesses present in young people and adjust interventions appropriately.

Depression

In contrast to adult depression, childhood and teenage depression frequently presents as irritation, social disengagement, scholastic deterioration, or somatic problems like headaches.[23] For pediatric depression, cognitive behavioral therapy, or CBT, has been proven to be beneficial.[24]

Cognitive Behavioral Therapy

Cognitive behavioral therapy involves using the previously stated methods. The child can benefit from cognitive restructuring by identifying and challenging maladaptive thoughts that are causing low mood. Their mood is elevated when they engage in meaningful and pleasurable activities as a result of behavioral activation. Interpersonal conflicts are addressed by teaching the child social, communication, and assertiveness skills.

Teaching the child social, communication, and assertiveness skills addresses interpersonal conflicts. In addition to these tactics, teaching the youngster to see early relapse warning signs is crucial to prevent a depressive or anxiety episode.

Effective treatment also includes working together with parents or other carers to address any environmental variables that may be contributing to the child's anxiety or depression as well as to reinforce therapeutic approaches at home. **Box 1** depicts a case scenario for CBT in depression in children

DISORDERS OF DISRUPTIVE BEHAVIOR

Behavioral disorders that cause disruption, such as attention-deficit/hyperactivity disorder (ADHD), oppositional defiant disorder (ODD), or conduct disorder (CD), are frequently identified mental health issues in children and teenagers.[25] As a stand-alone intervention or in combination with other modalities like medication or family therapy, CBT can assist in managing various problems.[26]

Attention-deficit/Hyperactivity Disorder

Enhancing executive functioning, impulse control, and organizational skills are the main goals of CBT for ADHD. Psychoeducation is beneficial for the child to understand their ADHD symptoms and how it affects their behavior and relationships.[27]

Implementing techniques like behavior modification, time management skills, and structured routines helps to improve self-regulation and reduces impulsivity.[28] Through social skills training, children can improve their social relationships by learning how to solve problems and take other perspectives. **Box 2** discusses a case scenario.

Oppositional Defiant Disorder/ Conduct Disorder

Cognitive behavioral therapy attempts to address maladaptive thought patterns and behavioral patterns that contribute to defiance and hostility for oppositional and conduct-related behaviors. With the use of anger management training, children can learn to identify what makes them angry and how to use coping mechanisms to control their feelings.[29] Training in conflict resolution skills aids in the development of positive strategies for resolving disputes with siblings, classmates, and authoritative figures.[30] A key component of the treatment plan is working closely with parents to establish consistent discipline techniques and reward positive behaviors at home in order to guarantee therapeutic improvements in real-life settings.

HOMEWORK AND PROGRESS MONITORING

A key component of CBT is giving homework assignments so that kids and teenagers can practice and reinforce the skills they acquire in treatment.[31] Assignments for homework could be recording one's thoughts, practicing relaxation methods, or doing studies on behavior to try out novel coping mechanisms.

In order to guarantee that therapeutic interventions continue after therapy sessions, cooperation with parents or other carers is essential. Parents can receive guidance on implementing behavioral methods at home and providing a supportive atmosphere that promotes their child's success by being involved in the treatment process.

BOX 1: Treatment plan for depression in an adolescent.

Ananya, a 15-year-old girl, has been diagnosed with depression. She was exhibiting symptoms of persistent sadness, loss of interest in activities she once enjoyed, fatigue, difficulty in concentrating, and feelings of worthlessness.

Cognitive Behavioral Therapy Treatment Plan

Psychoeducation and Building Rapport

- Educate Ananya and her parents about depression, its symptoms, and the cognitive-behavioral model
- Establish a trusting relationship with Ananya to ensure she feels safe and supported

Identifying and Monitoring Thoughts

Introduce a thought diary to help Ananya to identify and record her automatic negative thoughts

- *Situation:* Scored lower than expected on a science test
- *Thought:* "I am stupid and will never succeed"
- *Emotion:* Sadness and hopelessness

Challenging Cognitive Distortions

Cognitive restructuring: Teach Ananya to challenge and reframe her negative thoughts

- *Example:*
  - *Thought:* "I am stupid and will never succeed"
  - *Evidence for:* "I did not do well on this test"
  - *Evidence Against:* "I've done well on other tests before. This was just one test"

Behavioral Activation

- Encourage Ananya to engage in activities she used to enjoy to combat withdrawal and inactivity
- Start with small and manageable activities and gradually increase their complexity
- *Example activities:* Drawing, playing badminton, and spending time with friends

Developing Problem-solving Skills

- *Teach Ananya structured problem-solving skills to manage stressors effectively:*
  - Define the problem
  - Brainstorm possible solutions
  - Evaluate pros and cons of each solution
  - Choose the best solution
  - Implement the solution
  - Review the outcome

Relapse Prevention

- Equip Ananya with strategies to handle potential future depressive episodes
- Develop a plan for maintaining progress, including continued use of thought diaries and coping strategies
- Summarize progress and celebrate successes

It is crucial to regularly monitor progress in order to assess the success of interventions and make any required modifications to the treatment plan. This entails continuous evaluation of the patient's symptoms, functioning, and adherence to therapy, enabling therapists to customize interventions based on the patient's symptoms.

ETHICAL CONSIDERATIONS AND LIMITATIONS

Confidentiality and Informed Consent

Involving parents/caregivers while respecting the child/adolescent's autonomy.

Confidentiality allows them to disclose sensitive information freely, fostering trust, and

BOX 2: Case discussion.

Ajay, a 10-year-old boy diagnosed with ADHD, struggles with impulsivity, disorganization, and maintaining friendships at school. During the session, Ajay learns about ADHD and its effects on his behavior and relationships through psychoeducation. He understands his impulsiveness and understands why he sometimes has trouble concentrating or waiting his turn in conversations.

Ajay and his therapist use behavior modification techniques to reduce his impulsivity and disorganization. They set achievable goals, such as completing homework without distraction or following an independent morning routine. Ajay tracks his progress on a chart and earns rewards for reaching his goals, such as extra screen time or a special family outing.

Additionally, Ajay is learning time management skills that help him to stay on task. He breaks larger tasks into smaller, more manageable steps, and uses timers to focus on short periods of time. Ajay also creates a visual schedule for his daily routines, including set times for chores, homework, and free time.

To improve his social skills and build stronger friendships, Ajay participates in social skills exercises during therapy. He practices active listening, taking turns and solving problems in social situations. Through role-playing and real-life scenarios, Ajay gains the confidence to initiate conversations and resolve conflicts with his peers.

Over time, as Ajay consistently practiced these techniques both in therapy sessions and at home, his ability to regulate his behavior, manage his time effectively, and navigate social relationships improved. He is managing his ADHD symptoms and is more confident in his abilities to succeed both academically and socially.

effective treatment. However, therapists explain limitations beforehand, such as imminent harm or suspected abuse. Information sharing can be managed through a "therapeutic triangle" where confidentiality boundaries are clear for child, parents, and therapist.

Informed consent involves parental permission, but also the child's assent. Therapists explain therapy in age-appropriate terms and address concerns. This collaborative approach empowers children and builds trust. While parents remain informed about broader treatment goals, the child's privacy is respected.

Challenges include assessing a child understands confidentiality and navigating parental concerns. Therapists must be sensitive to family dynamics and ensure the child feels safe to express themselves openly.

Limitations of Cognitive Behavioral Therapy and Behavioral Therapies

Cognitive behavioral therapy relies heavily on a client's ability to identify and challenge negative thought patterns. Younger children may struggle with this due to their ongoing cognitive development. They might have difficulty expressing their emotions verbally or grasping abstract concepts like cognitive distortions. CBT and some behavioral therapies often require active participation and homework completion. Younger children might lack the focus or motivation to fully engage in these activities, requiring adaptations or incorporating parents/caregivers for support. CBT and behavioral therapies primarily address the thoughts and behaviors associated with a problem. However, complex emotional or environmental factors contributing to the child's struggles might not be fully addressed. Children might find it difficult to grasp abstract concepts and have limited emotional vocabulary hindering the identification of cognitive distortions. Exposing very young children to anxiety-provoking situations might be developmentally inappropriate or even retraumatizing. Children might not have developed enough coping skills to manage the anxiety successfully during exposure.

SUMMARY AND CONCLUSION

To summarize, CBT and behavioral therapies are excellent resources for addressing the complex mental health needs of children and adolescents. These approaches enable young people to comprehend and effectively regulate their thoughts, emotions, and behaviors by emphasizing practical interventions that are customized to each person's specific experiences and circumstances. The following is a summary of the main advantages of behavioral treatments and CBT for the mental health of children and adolescents:

Empowerment and skill-building: CBT gives kids and teenagers useful tools to deal with obstacles in life. Adolescents can take charge of their mental health by learning how to recognize and confront harmful thought patterns, manage their emotions, and change unhelpful behaviors.

Holistic approach: Behavioral therapies address the interconnectedness of mental health issues by adopting a holistic perspective. CBT provides all-encompassing treatment that targets the underlying causes of mental health issues rather than just treating symptoms by focusing on these many elements.

Collaboration and support: CBT places a strong emphasis on working together to create a supportive therapy environment between the therapist, the child, and family members. Therapists can encourage the continuous application of therapeutic procedures at home and strengthen the child's network of support by including parents or carers in the treatment process.

Evidence-based practice: CBT and behavioral therapies are grounded in empirical research and have demonstrated efficacy in treating a wide range of mental health conditions in children and adolescents, including anxiety disorders, depression, ADHD, and disruptive behavior disorders. Therapists can guarantee the provision of morally good interventions that are both effective and efficient by following evidence-based methods.

Importance of ongoing research and development: Even with the great advancements in the field of child and adolescent mental health, more study and development are still required. Sustained research funding is essential for expanding our knowledge of the fundamental causes of mental health issues in youth and discovering novel therapeutic modalities.

Digital and transdiagnostic interventions: Transdiagnostic techniques have the potential to improve treatment results and address comorbidity in children and adolescents by focusing on shared underlying processes that are shared by various mental health illnesses.[32]

Transdiagnostic therapies provide a more effective and economical way to provide individualized treatment by concentrating on shared causes such as cognitive biases, emotion dysregulation, and behavioral patterns.

Furthermore, incorporating digital technology into mental health interventions can improve their cost-effectiveness, scalability, and accessibility.[33] Digital platforms can overcome access constraints such as stigma and geographic distance by offering psychoeducation, self-help resources, symptom tracking tools, and even therapy interventions remotely.

Cognitive behavioral therapy and behavioral therapies offer tailored interventions empowering children and adolescents to navigate mental health challenges effectively. Grounded in evidence-based practices, these approaches foster collaboration, resilience, and holistic well-being. Embracing innovation and ongoing research holds the promise of further enhancing accessibility and efficacy in youth mental health interventions.

In conclusion, CBT is a structured and goal-oriented therapy focusing on the relationship between thoughts, emotions, and behaviors and modifying dysfunctional thinking leads to changes in emotions and behaviors. CBT techniques should be tailored to the child's or adolescent's developmental stage, using play-based methods for younger children and abstract cognitive strategies for adolescents. Key CBT techniques include cognitive restructuring, exposure therapy, behavioral activation, and problem-solving skills training, each implemented through age-appropriate methods. It is an important to engage parents in the therapeutic process to reinforce skills and strategies at home, ensuring consistency and support for the child's progress as is regular assessment and tracking of progress to adjust therapeutic strategies as needed, ensuring the therapy remains effective and responsive to the child's development.

REFERENCES

1. WHO. (2003). Caring for children and adolescents with mental disorders: Setting WHO directions. Geneva: World Health Organization. [online] Available from http://www.who.int/mental_health/media/en/785.pdf [Last accessed November, 2025].
2. Kessler RC, Berglund P, Demler O, Jin R, Merikangas KR, Walters EE. Lifetime prevalence and age-of-onset distributions of DSM-IV disorders in the National Comorbidity Survey Replication. Arch Gen Psychiatry. 2005;62(6): 593-602.
3. McGinnity Á, Meltzer H, Ford T, Goodman R. Mental health of children and young people in Great Britain, 2004. Basingstoke: Palgrave Macmillan; 2005.
4. Reitemeier B. The Good Childhood: An inquiry by the Children's Society. In: Childhood, Well-Being and a Therapeutic Ethos. 1st edition. Routledge; 2009:14.
5. Malhotra S, Patra BN. Prevalence of child and adolescent psychiatric disorders in India: a systematic review and meta-analysis. Child Adolesc Psychiatry Ment Health. 2014;8:1-9. (Erratum: Child Adolesc Psychiatry Ment Health. 2014;8:22)
6. Gautham MS, Gururaj G, Varghese M, Benegal V, Rao GN, Kokane A, et al. The National Mental Health Survey of India (2016): Prevalence, socio-demographic correlates and treatment gap of mental morbidity. Int J Soc Psychiatry. 2020;66(4):361-72.
7. Hollon SD, Beck AT. Cognitive and cognitive-behavioral therapies. In: Lambert MJ (Ed). Bergin and Garfield's Handbook of Psychotherapy and Behavior Change, 6th edition. New Jersey: John Wiley & Sons, Inc.; 2013. pp. 393-442.
8. Dobson KS. The science of CBT: toward a metacognitive model of change. Behav Ther. 2013;44(2):224-7.
9. Clark DA. Cognitive restructuring. In: Hofmann SG (Ed). The Wiley Handbook of Cognitive Behavioral Therapy. New Jersey: Wiley-Blackwell; 2013. pp. 1-22.
10. Martin F, Oliver T. Behavioral activation for children and adolescents: a systematic review of progress and promise. Eur Child Adolesc Psychiatry. 2019;28:427-41.
11. Bilek E, Tomlinson RC, Whiteman AS, Johnson TD, Benedict C, Phan KL, et al. Exposure-focused CBT outperforms relaxation-based control in an RCT of treatment for child and adolescent anxiety. J Clin Child Adolesc Psychology. 2022;51(4):410-8.
12. Hamdani SU, Zafar SW, Suleman N, Waqas A, Rahman A. Effectiveness of relaxation techniques 'as an active ingredient of psychological interventions' to reduce distress, anxiety and depression in adolescents: a systematic review and meta-analysis. Int J Ment Health Syst. 2022;16(1):31.
13. Elliott SN, Busse RT. Social skills assessment and intervention with children and adolescents: Guidelines for assessment and training procedures. School Psychol Int. 1991;12(1-2):63-83.
14. Wolpe J, Plaud JJ. Pavlov's contributions to behavior therapy: The obvious and the not so obvious. Am Psychol. 1997;52(9):966.
15. Hofmann SG. Cognitive processes during fear acquisition and extinction in animals and humans: Implications for exposure therapy of anxiety disorders. Clin Psychol Rev. 2008;28(2): 199-210.

16. Staddon JE, Cerutti DT. Operant conditioning. Ann Rev Psychol. 2003;54(1):115-44.
17. Srinath S, Jacob P, Sharma E, Gautam A. Clinical practice guidelines for assessment of children and adolescents. Indian J Psychiatry. 2019;61(Suppl 2):158-75.
18. Bieling PJ, Kuyken W. Is cognitive case formulation science or science fiction? Clin Psychol Sci Pract. 2003;10(1):52.
19. Weerasekera P. Formulation: A multiperspective model. Canad J Psychiatry. 1993;38(5):351-8.
20. Copeland WE, Angold A, Shanahan L, Costello EJ. Longitudinal patterns of anxiety from childhood to adulthood: the Great Smoky Mountains Study. J Am Acad Child Adolesc Psychiatry. 2014;53(1):21-33.
21. Stiede JT, Trent ES, Viana AG, Guzick AG, Storch EA, Hershfield J. Cognitive behavioral therapy for children and adolescents with anxiety disorders. Child Adolesc Psych Clin. 2023;32(3):543-58.
22. Hazell P. Depression in children and adolescents. BMJ Clin Evid. 2011;2011:1008.
23. Turk J, Graham P, Verhulst FC. Child and adolescent psychiatry: a developmental approach. Oxford: OUP Oxford; 2007.
24. Klein JB, Jacobs RH, Reinecke MA. Cognitive-behavioral therapy for adolescent depression: a meta-analytic investigation of changes in effect-size estimates. J Am Acad Child Adolesc Psychiatry. 2007;46(11):1403-13.
25. Turgay A. Aggression and disruptive behavior disorders in children and adolescents. Expert Rev Neurother. 2004;4(4):623-32.
26. Riise EN, Wergeland GJ, Njardvik U, Öst LG. Cognitive behavior therapy for externalizing disorders in children and adolescents in routine clinical care: A systematic review and meta-analysis. Clin Psychol Rev. 2021;83:101954.
27. Montoya A, Colom F, Ferrin M. Is psychoeducation for parents and teachers of children and adolescents with ADHD efficacious? A systematic literature review. Eur Psychiatry. 2011;26(3):166-75.
28. Nakashima M, Inada N, Tanigawa Y, Yamashita M, Maeda E, Kouguchi M, et al. Efficacy of group cognitive behavior therapy targeting time management for adults with attention deficit/hyperactivity disorder in Japan: a randomized control pilot trial. J Atten Disord. 2022;26(3):377-90.
29. Taher M, Aghae H, Hossein Khanzadeh AA. Effectiveness of Anger Management and Parenting Training on Inhibiting the Response of Students with Oppositional Defiant Disorder. J Except Children. 2022;22(4):117-30.
30. Lochman JE, Powell NP, Boxmeyer CL, Jimenez-Camargo L. Cognitive-behavioral therapy for externalizing disorders in children and adolescents. Child Adolesc Psychiatric Clin. 2011; 20(2):305-18.
31. Friedberg RD, McClure JM, Garcia JH. Cognitive therapy techniques for children and adolescents: Tools for enhancing practice. New York: Guilford Press; 2009.
32. Dalgleish T, Black M, Johnston D, Bevan A. Transdiagnostic approaches to mental health problems: Current status and future directions. J Consult Clin Psychol. 2020;88(3):179.
33. Lattie EG, Stiles-Shields C, Graham AK. An overview of and recommendations for more accessible digital mental health services. Nat Rev Psychol. 2022;1(2):87-100.

Psychological Therapies for Emotional and Behavioral Disorders-III (Family Therapy)

S Lokesh, Savithri Suresh, Veena A Satyanarayana

INTRODUCTION

A multifaceted approach is crucial while addressing mental health concerns experienced by children and adolescents. As they grow, children make sense of themselves and the world through interactions with their family members. They depend on their parents and caregivers for nurturance and protection. Family ties and relationships are highly valued in a collectivistic society like India. Indian families often have complex intergenerational structures and dynamics that influence the mental health of its different members. Family dynamics like communication styles, conflict-resolution strategies, etc., play an important role in developing psychological strengths and vulnerabilities in children. Family factors can predispose children and adolescents to develop emotional and behavioral disorders. Stressors within the family context may act as precipitating events that trigger or exacerbate symptoms. Some factors may perpetuate certain patterns or behaviors that impact their mental health and maintain the illness **(Table 1)**.

ROLE OF FAMILY THERAPY

While mental health professionals working with childhood and adolescent disorders consider the importance of family factors in the child's mental health, family members are usually underutilized in treatment.[7] Family therapy has an important role to play in the treatment of mental health disorders in children and adolescents. Family therapy often takes a systemic perspective, recognizing that an individual's mental health is influenced by various factors, including family dynamics, social environment, and cultural context. Addressing these factors can create lasting changes that promote resilience and well-being in children and adolescents. Families also serve as a child's first contact with the community and, hence, have a role to play in providing a protective and supportive environment for children and adolescents navigating mental health issues.[8] Family therapy may also be able to address the stress and burnout that caregivers and family members may experience when dealing with children with emotional and behavioral disorders.

Research[9-12] has also shown that involving family members in therapy leads to improved treatment outcomes for children and adolescents with mental disorders. Family therapy not only addresses the individual's symptoms but also strengthens familial bonds, improves coping mechanisms, and fosters a supportive environment conducive to long-term recovery.

Indicators for Family Therapy

Walrond-Skinner[13] describes how family therapy can be utilized as standalone as well as differential treatment where other treatments are given along with family therapy. There are certain indicators for family therapy. However, these are pointers, not fixed rules, as the overall picture of the clients may change based on the problems presented.

TABLE 1: Factors associated with the development and persistence of emotional and behavioral disorders.

	Adolescent factors	*Parental factors*
Predisposing factors	• Difficult temperament • Insecure attachment style • Gender identity-related issues[1] • Comorbid neurodevelopmental conditions (SLDs, ADHD comorbid)	• Parent(s) own attachment style • Parental mental health issues such as depression, substance misuse, personality disorders[2,3] • Unstable family environment • Maladaptive parenting style[4] • Maladaptive reinforcement strategies • Low socioeconomic background
Precipitating factors	• Child abuse • Developmental changes • Change in social environment (e.g., change in school) • Loss of peer relationship • New member(s) in the family • Loss of significant family member(s) • Substance abuse	• Increased parental conflict[5,6] • Domestic violence • Loss of employment • Separation or divorce • Difficulty adjusting to life cycle transitions
Perpetuating factors	• Maladaptive internal working models • Difficulties in communication • Attribution bias • Cognitive distortions • Dysfunctional coping strategies (e.g., avoidance)	• Parental psychological issues • Inconsistent parental discipline • Overinvolvement from the parent(s) • Disengaged and neglecting the child • Poor communication with the child • Reinforcing problem behavior • Dysfunctional attributional style • Lack of understanding about the condition
Protective factors	• Average intelligence • No previous history of emotional or behavioral problems • High self-efficacy • Adaptive coping strategies • Adhering to intervention	• Secure parent–child attachment • Authoritative parenting • Reinforcing adaptive behavior • Adaptive coping strategies • Parental internal locus of control • Healthy social support systems

(ADHD: attention-deficit/hyperactivity disorder; SLD: specific learning disability)

- Symptoms expressed appear to be a product of underlying dysfunctional family relationships.
- Conflicts and communication issues between family members which threaten the emotional environment of the family.
- Providing help to make changes in the relationship will be crucial to reduce the distress than individual family members.
- Families with an adolescent trying to separate from one's family or helping the children to achieve differentiation from family members.
- Family members whose roles are not defined leading to poor functioning individuals in the family.

Contraindications for Family Therapy

Research about contraindications for family therapy is found to be scarce. It should be recognized that contraindications may be a reflection of the therapist's training and competence to treat certain types of families. Hence, these conditions should be carefully evaluated before beginning therapy, as various forms of family therapy can be utilized to address these contraindications. Some of the contraindications given are as follows:[14]

- Nonavailability of one or more family members
- Lack of motivation among family members.
- Family violence, aggression or incest that could threaten the safety of the family member(s).
- Acute psychiatric distress in one or more family members which makes it challenging to engage in family therapy
- Family emotional equilibrium is poorly sustained; attempting to change may lead to severe disorganization in the family.

Principles of Family Therapy

Family therapy understands psychiatric symptoms as influenced by bidirectional interactions between individual factors and the interpersonal family environment.[15] It usually involves a comprehensive assessment of the family across different life cycle stages and generations to identify potential strengths and vulnerability factors. Therapy involves analyzing the interaction and dynamics of all family members, identifying dysfunctional interactional patterns, and working toward improving overall family health.

The conceptualization of problems and therapy processes may vary according to the school of family therapy followed. The prominent schools of family therapy and their utility in the treatment of emotional and behavioral disorders in children and adolescents are described in the following sections.

Format of Family Therapy

While conducting family therapy, therapists typically initiate with conjoint sessions and may decide to use either individual sessions with one family member or conjoint sessions where multiple family members are present, or a combination of both. The decision of the mode of therapy depends on various factors like therapeutic goals, family dynamics, specific issues being addressed, etc., as shown in **Table 2**.

TABLE 2: Schools of family therapy.[16]

School of family therapy	*Types of family therapy*	*Main areas of intervention*	*Indicated for*
System models	• Structural therapy • Strategic therapy • Bowenian therapy	• Hierarchy, boundaries and roles • Communication and cybernetics • Intergenerational patterns and differentiation of self	Internalizing and externalizing mental health conditions among adolescents including adolescent delinquency and substance use
Attachment perspective	• Attachment-based family therapy • Emotion-focused family therapy	• Emotional experiencing and expression • Intimacy • Trust	• Adolescent depression and self-harm • Eating disorders, anxiety, depression, and oppositional defiance problems among adolescents
Cognitive and behavioral models	• Cognitive behavioral therapy • Functional family therapy	• Beliefs • Sequence of actions • Interactional changes • Skills of communication, problem solving	Adolescent delinquency and substance use

Conjoint sessions are used for:

- *Improving communication:* The goal is to improve communication and interaction patterns among family members
- *Family dynamics:* Addressing issues that are rooted in family dynamics, such as conflict, roles, and boundaries
- *Shared goals:* Working on shared goals and improving the overall functioning of the family system
- *Conflict resolution:* Facilitating discussions to resolve conflicts or misunderstandings between family members
- *Behavioral changes:* Encouraging and reinforcing positive behavioral changes in the presence of the whole family.

Individual sessions are typically used for:

- *Confidentiality and safety:* A family member needs a safe space to discuss sensitive issues that they might not feel comfortable sharing in the presence of other family members.
- *Individual assessment:* The therapist needs to understand each family member's perspective, feelings, and behaviors independently.
- *Personal issues:* Addressing personal issues such as individual mental health concerns (e.g., depression, anxiety) that impact family dynamics.
- *Preparation:* Preparing a family member to handle or discuss difficult topics in conjoint sessions.
- *Skill development:* Helping an individual develop coping skills or strategies that they can later bring into family interactions.

Often, a combination of both individual and conjoint sessions is used. This approach allows the therapist to:

- *Gather comprehensive information:* Obtain a full picture of the family dynamics and individual issues.
- *Tailor interventions:* Tailor interventions to address both personal and relational aspects of the family's concerns.
- *Monitor progress:* Monitor individual and family progress over time, adjusting the therapeutic approach as needed.

SYSTEMIC SCHOOL OF FAMILY THERAPY

The systemic schools of family therapy developed as a result of a paradigm shift in the understanding of mental health issues. This approach is the cornerstone of family therapy and views individuals not in isolation but as part of interconnected systems within society, such as families, communities, and social networks. The school emphasizes the interdependence and impact of larger social systems on individual and family function and well-being.

Structural family therapy, strategic family therapy, and Bowen's intergenerational model fall under the systemic school of thought. Minuchin viewed families as systems operating through transactional patterns. A well-functioning family is "an open system in transformation, maintaining link with extrafamilial, possessing a capacity for development, and having an organizational structure composed of subsystems".[17]

Fundamental Concepts in Systemic Paradigm

A system: A system is a set of units, organized and interdependent, standing in interactional relation to each other. It is a set of interrelated subunits with capacity to adapt to the surrounding environment. These subunits work dynamically to ensure the survival of the total system.

A boundary: Rules that define "who participates and how much," and these can be physical as well as psychological.[16]

Circularity: Cause and effect are viewed as circular not as linear.

Neutrality: The therapist's ability to not align with or against any person.[18]

Feedback and homeostasis: Feedback loops are communicational pathways that circle across unit boundaries time and time again, signaling their level of stability or differences to the overall functioning of the unit. This stability is called homeostasis or system equilibrium which indicates the level of consistency with which the system functions.

STRUCTURAL FAMILY THERAPY

Introduction

A family is a system that operates through transactional patterns. Repeated transactions establish patterns of how, when, and with whom to relate, and these patterns underpin the system.

Minuchin[17] explains that an effective functioning family "is an open system in transformation, maintaining link with extrafamilial, possessing a capacity for development, and having an organizational structure composed of subsystems."

Goals of Structural Family Therapy

The overall goal of structural family therapy is reorganizing the family structure to promote effective interactions and adaptive family functioning. These are achieved by:

- Establishing clear and healthy boundaries
- Restoring healthy hierarchy
- Modifying maladaptive communication patterns.

Conceptualization of Pathology

Family is subjected to stress due to changes within its own members/outer pressure coming from the environment or both, which provides an opportunity to transform and maintain continuity.[17]

Failure in addressing stressors such as increased rigidity of their interaction cycle and boundaries within and outside the family system leads to dysfunctional behaviors.

Dysfunctional Boundaries (Figs. 1A and B)

- *Enmeshed:* Extreme sensitivity of the individual members in the system toward each other and to their primary subsystem. It is described as little interpersonal distance and blurring of subsystem boundaries. The behavior of an individual strongly affects others in the system and other subsystems as well and shows that the reverberating potential is high.
- *Disengaged:* Interpersonal distance is too great; the boundaries are too rigid in the system and reverberating potential is low.

Coalitions and Triangles (Figs. 2 to 6)

- *Conflict detouring or scapegoating:* Parents who express a total absence of conflict between themselves but are solidly united against an individual child or subunit of children. It reduces the stress on the spousal subsystem and shifts it on the children.

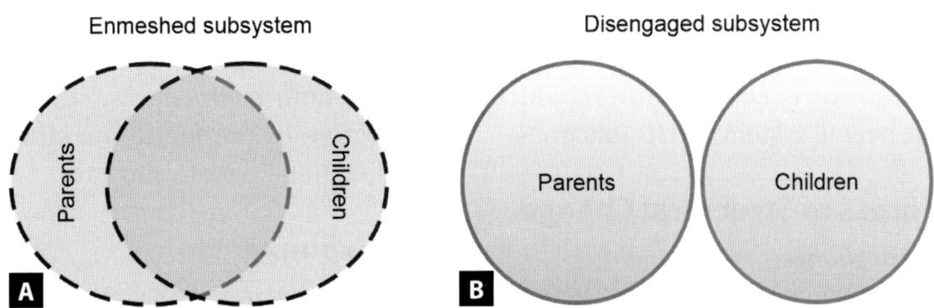

Figs. 1A and B: Dysfunctional boundaries.[19]

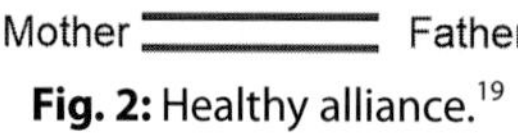

Fig. 2: Healthy alliance.[19]

Father Daughter

Fig. 3: Enmeshed or over involved affiliation.[19]

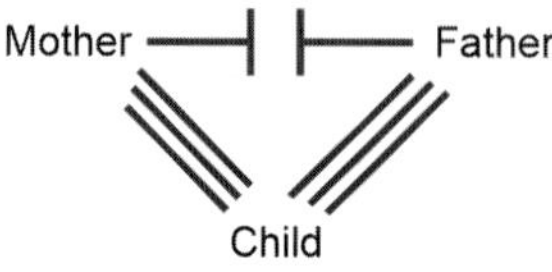

Fig. 4: Triangulation.[19]

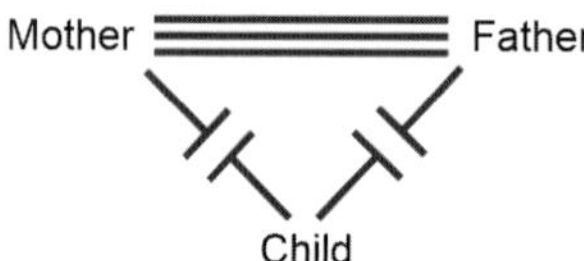

Fig. 5: Detouring—attacking.[19]

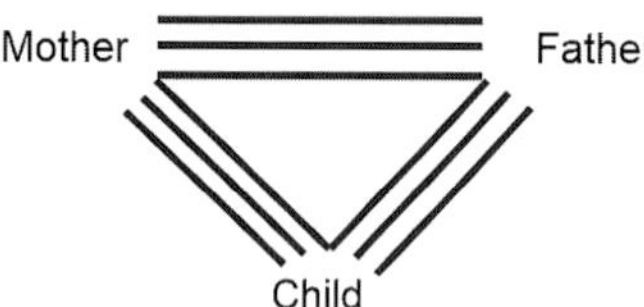

Fig. 6: Detouring—supportive.[19]

- *Inappropriate cross-generational coalitions:* When one parent and a child form a coalition against another parent

Hierarchies

Alterations in power hierarchies, such as a child becoming a part of the parental subsystem and assuming more executive power which imbalances the overall system and its functions.

Therapy Process of Structural Change

Steps of structural change:

1. Therapist intervenes with the existing homeostasis and creates a state of flux.
2. State of flux requires individuals in the system to behave in new ways to adapt.
3. New behavior allows members within the system to have new perspectives about each other.
4. These changes make it easy for emergence of new transactional sequences among family members.
5. Repetition of the new transactional sequences leads to a new set of structure and equilibrium.

Techniques

Enactment: Reconstruction of dysfunctional interpersonal transactions among family members where the therapist observes and intervenes to make modifications, initiating alternative transactions.

Joining: The therapist joins the system in different positions. Close position where the therapist affiliates with a family member. In median position, the therapist plays the role to help all the family members to tell their story. Disengaged position is where the therapist takes a position of an expert and directs the family members to engage with each other.

Boundary making: By changing the level of proximity and regulating the membership of the subsystem (making boundaries or diffusing boundaries).

Unbalancing: The therapist uses one's self to disequilibrate the family organization. This is done to disrupt an entrenched family hierarchical organization and introduce change.

Working with complementarity: Changing the perspective of the family members about the causality from linear to circular.

Case Example

Mr and Mrs Patel reported that their 15-year-old son Rohan has become increasingly defiant, skipping school and staying out late without informing them. These behaviors have led to frequent arguments and conflicts and an overall tense environment at home due to the lack of communication between family members. Rohan feels misunderstood and controlled by his parents, particularly his father. Rohan's younger sister, Anya, appears to be overlooked during these conflicts. The family was referred for family therapy.

Family assessment and conceptualization: During the initial sessions, the therapist observes the family dynamics and conducts individual interviews with each family member to gain a comprehensive understanding of the issues. The therapist notes that Mr Patel is authoritarian and often dominates family discussions, while Mrs Patel tends to remain passive and avoids confrontation. Rohan appears disengaged and resistant, frequently expressing anger and frustration toward his parents. Anya is quiet and tends to stay in the background, often ignored during family interactions.

Rohan is diagnosed with oppositional defiant disorder (ODD) based on symptoms including persistent defiance, argumentative behavior, and hostility toward authority figures. He exhibits a pattern of refusing to comply with rules, deliberately annoying others, and blaming others for his mistakes. Additionally, there are signs of underlying anxiety and depression, possibly exacerbated by family factors.

Therapeutic goals:

1. Reorganize family structure to establish clearer boundaries and improve communication.
2. Empower Mrs Patel to take a more active role in family decisions.
3. Help Mr Patel adopt a more collaborative and supportive approach.
4. Address Rohan's behavioral issues by improving family cohesion and support.
5. Ensure that Anya feels included and supported within the family.

Intervention:

Joining and accommodating: The therapist built a rapport with each family member, empathetically validating their perspectives, and worked toward reducing resistance and creating a safe space for open communication.

Mapping the family structure: The therapist created a visual representation of the family structure, highlighting subsystems (e.g., parental, sibling) and identifying dysfunctional hierarchies and boundaries. This mapping revealed that the parental subsystem is misaligned, with Mr Patel overly dominant and Mrs Patel overly passive, leading to enmeshed boundaries between Mr Patel and Rohan.

Reframing and enactment: The therapist reframed Rohan's defiance as a response to feeling controlled and misunderstood rather than just a behavioral problem. Through enactment, the therapist guided the family to role-play a recent conflict, allowing them to observe their interaction patterns and communication breakdowns.

Realigning subsystems and boundaries: The therapist worked with Mr and Mrs Patel to develop a more balanced co-parenting approach. Mr Patel was encouraged to share decision-making with Mrs Patel and to approach Rohan with empathy rather than authority. Mrs Patel was supported in asserting her views and actively participating in parenting decisions.

Improving communication: The therapist introduced communication skills training, teaching family members active listening, assertiveness, and conflict-resolution techniques. Family members practiced these skills during sessions to enhance their interactions.

Strengthening the sibling subsystem: The therapist ensured that Anya's needs are addressed by involving her in family activities and discussions. This helped in creating a more inclusive family environment and reducing her feelings of neglect.

Outcome: Over the sessions, Mr Patel learned to interact with Rohan with a more understanding and collaborative attitude, reducing conflicts and fostering mutual respect. Mrs Patel became more assertive, contributing to a balanced parental dynamic. Rohan started to feel heard and supported, leading to a decrease in his defiant behaviors and improved school attendance. Anya also became more engaged in family activities, strengthening her relationship with her parents and brother. The family's overall cohesion improved as they developed healthier boundaries and more effective communication patterns.

ATTACHMENT PERSPECTIVE

Fundamental Concepts in Attachment Perspective

Attachment theory: Children who experience their caregivers as sensitive, responsive, and available develop confident expectations of relational security. Attachment security which develops as a result of responsive parenting leads to learning of emotion regulation and self-reflection skills. When children do not have secure attachment with their parents, they develop defensive strategies that protect them from being hurt or disappointed.[20]

Emotional processing:[21,22] Activating a maladaptive emotional response to a meaningful event and accessing the avoided vulnerable emotions. Effective emotional processing is achieved when an individual is involved in accessing, expressing adaptive and often vulnerable emotions.

ATTACHMENT-BASED FAMILY THERAPY

Attachment-based family therapy (ABFT) treats adolescent depression, suicidality, and trauma with an attachment, trauma-informed approach. The framework ABFT provides by structuring sessions with the family as a whole and particular subsystem is one of its obvious strengths. By reducing the inherent complexity of family treatments, working with subsystems improves transparency and increases the likelihood of effective therapy.

Conceptualization

Attachment-based family therapy focuses on attachment ruptures, which are at the heart of family conflict. Discover the incidents (such as abuse) and interpersonal dynamics (such as excessive conflict and low warmth) that caused the attachment rupture and inhibited them from approaching their parents for assistance.

Goal of Therapy

The restoration of healthy caregiver–child relationships is accomplished via the "corrective attachment experience" and subsequent autonomy building conversations.

Process of Therapy

The process of therapy is breaking down into multiple phases, and each task has its unique goals and process through which it achieves the goals.

Task I: Engaging in therapy

This task focused on building relationships. To achieve this, the therapist focuses on caregivers who want to provide love and security to their child and on an adolescent's desire for support and protection from caregivers.

Task II: Individual sessions with adolescents

This task focused on assisting the adolescent's identity and articulating the felt injustices which they have experienced based on perceived caregivers' attachment failures.

Task III: Individual sessions with the caregivers

This task addressed the intergenerational attachment patterns of caregivers and how it affects their capacity to connect with their child. Building insight helps caregivers to understand and develop empathy for oneself and see its impact on the children as well. Developing empathy is crucial as it helps the caregiver to be more motivated to learn new parenting skills which develop more open, supportive, emotionally tuned relationships with their children.

Task IV: Bringing adolescent and caregiver together

Tsvieli et al.[23] describes a task that focuses on bringing the caregiver and the adolescent together and discusses how trust in their relationship is damaged due to relational failures. The adolescent's expressions of vulnerability motivate the caregivers to make amends.[24] The step to change happens when the caregivers acknowledge adolescents' experiences, which in turn helps the adolescent to be more open for discussion and emotionally regulated. Once mutual respect is recognized by both the caregivers and the adolescent, it leads to a "corrective attachment experience". With this new space, the therapist focuses on helping adolescents and caregivers to communicate adaptive and vulnerable emotions associated with unmet needs in the relationship. They helps the adolescents to identify, articulate, and regulate primary feelings and use family conversation as a learning opportunity.

The therapist helps the caregivers to respond to their children's concerns and experiences in an empathic and validating manner. These positive interactions serve as a foundation to develop a sense of security and trust in the relationship.[25]

Task V: Using a caregiver to build competency

These corrective attachment experiences and positive interaction cycles help adolescents build trust and are willing to seek comfort, advice, and support from their caregivers. This secure attachment with the caregiver becomes a resource and it assists the adolescents to explore and develop autonomy.

Case Example

The Singh family consists of parents Raj and Meera, their 17-year-old daughter, Anika, and their 14-year-old son, Arjun. The family sought therapy due to Anika's increasing withdrawal, low mood, and recent self-harming behavior. She was diagnosed with major depressive disorder due to persistent sadness, loss of interest in activities, and self-harm. The parents are concerned about her mental health but struggle to connect with her emotionally. Anika feels isolated and misunderstood by her parents. Arjun also shows signs of distress and feels neglected due to the attention given to Anika's issues.

Assessment: During the initial sessions, the therapist conducted individual interviews with the adolescents and their parents. Raj and Meera often focused on Anika's behavior rather than her emotional needs and appeared anxious and overprotective. Anika was emotionally withdrawn in sessions. She expressed her lack of trust in her parents. Arjun is quiet and seems to feel overlooked in the family dynamics. The therapist identified attachment issues within the family, noting that Anika's symptoms are partly a response to feeling emotionally disconnected from her parents.

Therapeutic goals:

- Rebuild and strengthen the emotional bonds between Anika and her parents.
- Help Raj and Meera understand and respond to Anika's emotional needs.
- Improve family communication to create a more supportive and empathetic environment.
- Address underlying attachment issues contributing to Anika's depressive symptoms.
- Ensure that Arjun feels included and supported within the family.

Intervention:

Creating a secure base: The therapist validated Anika's feelings and created a secure therapeutic environment where she feels safe to express her emotional needs and experiences to her parents.

Parental insight and empathy: The therapist helped Raj and Meera understand the impact of their behaviors and attitudes on their bond with Anika. Through guided discussions and reflective exercises, they learnt to empathize with her experiences and effectively respond to her needs.

Rebuilding the parent–child relationship: The therapist used emotion-focused interventions to help Anika and her parents identify and express their underlying emotions and communicate with each other. In role-playing activities, Anika was encouraged to express her feelings and needs, and her parents practiced responding with empathy and support.

Reframing and restructuring interactions: The therapist helped the family reframe their interactions, shifting from a focus on Anika's behavior to understanding and addressing her emotional needs. Restructuring family dynamics this way helped create more nurturing and supportive interactions.

Strengthening family bonds: Through attachment-based exercises, the therapist facilitates activities that promote emotional closeness and bonding. These included activities like shared storytelling, joint problem-solving tasks, and family rituals that fostered a sense of connection and security.

Inclusion of sibling: The therapist ensured that Arjun is included in the therapeutic process, addressing his feelings of neglect and promoting his role in the family.

Outcome: In the course of therapy, Raj and Meera became more attuned to Anika's emotional needs and learnt to respond with empathy and support. Anika started to feel more understood and connected to her parents, leading to a decrease in her depressive symptoms and self-harming behavior. The family developed healthier communication patterns, increased emotional openness, and mutual support. Arjun also felt more included and supported, improving his relationship with his parents and sister. The family was slowly able to function as a cohesive and supportive unit and provide a stable foundation for continued growth and well-being.

COGNITIVE BEHAVIORAL FAMILY THERAPY

The cognitive behavioral school of thought proposes that cognitive factors like beliefs, attitudes, expectations, thoughts, etc., influence individual behavior. Cognitive behavioral therapists believe that a person's experiences lead to the development of schemas or beliefs about the self. These schemas influence how the individual reacts to their environment. Experiences in the environment lead to negative automatic thoughts about the situation, which then leads to maladaptive assumptions and cognitive distortions that are in line with the person's underlying schema about themselves. In the process of therapy, the therapist helps the client modify these thoughts, eliminate cognitive distortions, and see the world more objectively. This process is called cognitive restructuring.

In cognitive behavioral family therapy (CBFT), the therapist engages in problem analysis to pinpoint the specific dysfunctions within the family and works toward resolving them and increasing positive interactions between the members.

Key Concepts

Information processing: It refers to the personal constructs through which individuals make sense of the world and categorize experiences as "good" or "bad". These constructs develop through children's early interactions with the world.

Schemas: These are irrational beliefs that people have about themselves. These beliefs are held onto and usually cause people to behave in a particular way.

Social learning theory: This theory explains how individuals incorporate responses they have observed in others into their schema of responses.

Individuals often model their family members' behaviors and patterns of interactions through social learning.

Conceptualization of Family Pathology

Cognitive behavioral family therapy focuses on the cognitive influences of family relationships, emotions, and behaviors. Because family members and their cognitions, emotions, and behaviors are interdependent, one family member's behavior triggers cognitions, emotions, and behaviors in other members, eliciting reactions in the first member.

Dattilio and Epstein[26] discussed how individuals have a set of schemas related to families in general and another set of schemas specific to their family of origin. When a family holds a dysfunctional set of schemas, it can lead to impaired functioning and unsatisfying relationships, contributing to the development of symptoms and mental health disorders in its members.

CBFT therapists conduct family assessments to:

- Identify strengths, vulnerabilities, and problem behaviors of the individual, family, and environment
- Understand these problems within the developmental context of the family and individual
- Identify the family interactions, cognitions, emotions, and behaviors that need to be targeted in therapy.[26]

Goals of Therapy

A CBFT therapist helps family members identify dysfunctional schemas and cognitive distortions and challenges them to help the family members improve the quality of their relationships. CBFT proposes that challenging faulty thought processes can help improve mood and promote behavior change. These changes affect the outcomes of family interactions and lead to new thought and behavior patterns.

Therapeutic Techniques

Cognitive behavioral family therapy therapists use different techniques to shift the focus from the child or adolescent with symptoms to the family system. This helps the family share responsibility and engage in therapy. Apart from cognitive restructuring, some such techniques include the following:

Modeling: The therapist engages the family in role-playing exercises to learn new responses to situations.

Guided discovery: The therapist guides the family through a scenario to help them understand any cognitive distortions that may affect their responses.

Cognitive rehearsal: The family recalls a problem situation that occurred in the past, and the therapist works with them to develop strategies to solve it if the situation occurs again in the future.

Validity testing: Family schemas and dysfunctional assessments are tested for their validity. The therapist discusses them with the family and if they cannot defend their schema, then they are considered invalid.

Contingency contract: A contract is drawn up with the family which details what each family member is to do in specific circumstances.

Systematic positive reinforcement: Family members are provided rewards or reinforcement for engaging in a desirable behavior.

Therapy Process

Phase 1: Joining and building rapport

The therapist conveys empathy, genuineness, and actively listens to and validates all family members and prepares them for assessment.

Phase 2: Understanding the present issue

The presenting issues are identified and understood in detail. The cognitions, emotions, and behaviors of all members are focused on and the problem is placed in the developmental and social context of the family.

Phase 3: Assessment of family dynamics

The therapist engages in functional analysis or behavior analysis to identify family schemas through identifying the automatic thoughts and assumptions.

Phase 4: Goals

In CBFT, the family decides on the therapeutic goals. The therapist helps them change their maladaptive thinking patterns to promote emotion and behavior change.

Phase 5: Amplifying change

The therapist continually evaluates the family's progress and amplifies change using therapeutic techniques and homework. Changes in each family member's emotion and behaviors are noted and inquiries about their thoughts and beliefs are made.

Phase 6: Termination

When the therapeutic goals are achieved, the therapist terminates therapy. Most therapists schedule regular follow-up sessions to help maintain progress.

Case Example

Rohit and Anjali sought therapy with their 15-year-old daughter, Neha. Neha has been experiencing increasing anxiety, frequent panic attacks, and academic decline. She has been diagnosed with generalized anxiety disorder (GAD). She feels overwhelmed by academic pressures and perceives her parents as overly critical. Rohit and Anjali are concerned about Neha's mental health and academic performance but feel frustrated by her lack of communication and avoidance behavior. During the initial sessions, the therapist notes that Rohit and Anjali have high expectations for Neha, which creates a pressure-filled environment. Neha appeared anxious and overwhelmed and reported negative thoughts about her self-worth and abilities.

Therapeutic goals:

- Reduce Neha's anxiety and improve her coping skills.
- Modify the critical and high-pressure environment created by Rohit and Anjali.
- Improve family communication and support.
- Address cognitive distortions and dysfunctional beliefs within the family.
- Change unhelpful family schemas that perpetuate stress and anxiety.

Intervention:

Rapport building and psychoeducation: The therapist empathetically listened to the various issues in the family and provided them with information about anxiety and its impact on Neha's functioning. The therapist also discussed the role of family factors in the occurrence and maintenance of anxiety symptoms.

Identifying and restructuring family schemas: The therapist helped the family identify and modify unhelpful family schemas that contribute to Neha's anxiety. The family held a schema that equates academic success with personal worth, leading to excessive pressure on Neha. By challenging and restructuring these schemas, the family could learn to adopt more supportive and flexible beliefs.

Family communication training: The therapist introduced communication skills training for the entire family, focusing on active listening, assertiveness, and expressing emotions constructively. This helps reduce misunderstandings and fosters a more supportive environment.

Modifying parental expectations: Rohit and Anjali were guided to recognize the impact of their high expectations and critical attitudes on

Neha's anxiety. The therapist works with them to set more realistic and supportive expectations, encouraging positive reinforcement and constructive feedback.

Outcome: Through family therapy, Rohit and Anjali became more aware of their impact on Neha and started to adopt a more supportive and encouraging approach. Family communication improved, with members expressing themselves more openly and constructively. The family's overall cohesion improved as supportive interactions increased, resulting in a more harmonious and balanced home environment.

SUMMARY AND CONCLUSION

To summarize, family members play a crucial role in the development of children and adolescents. Identifying various family factors which can predispose, precipitate, and perpetuate psychological and emotional disorders in children/adolescents and their family is crucial. By addressing vulnerability factors and protective factors, family therapy focuses on reducing distress and promoting well-being. Family therapy can be utilized in situations where family or relational factors play a role in the current symptomatology of the children or adolescent. Family therapy can be delivered through various modes such as individual session, conjoint, or both based on the nature of the present situation and overall goal of the therapy. Systemic perspective uses concepts such as hierarchy, boundaries and roles communication, and cybernetics to conceptualize and address the symptoms. Attachment perspectives utilize attachment and emotional processing theories to develop a secure attachment base between parents and offspring. Cognitive behavioral perspective addresses the maladaptive beliefs/schemas and communication patterns and brings changes by restructuring family beliefs, reinforcement strategies, and communication skills training.

In conclusion, one of the crucial factors affecting the mental health of children and adolescents is family, as they provide the environment and form the primary support systems for their growth and well-being. Family therapy is one of the empirically proven interventions to address emotional and behavioral issues of children and adolescents which incorporates the family members and working with them to reduce the symptoms and improve the children and adolescents' overall well-being. Building insight into how symptoms develop in a circular nature is paramount in all schools of family therapy. The modality of family therapy can be delivered through individual sessions, conjoint sessions, or both, depending on the family dynamics and goals of the stage of therapy. The principles of systemic perspective conceptualize the family as a system and the symptoms or changes as disequilibrium in the system. Restoring the equilibrium in the system is considered as the primary goal from a systemic perspective. The attachment perspective focused on interpersonal conflicts leading to attachment ruptures as the core reason for family conflicts and symptom development. Therapy focuses on providing corrective attachment experiences by rebuilding parent-child relationships, strengthening family bonds, and improving family functioning. Cognitive approaches focus on identifying dysfunctional schemas and cognitive errors among family members and utilize various techniques to challenge them to bring change and improve the quality of relationships.

REFERENCES

1. VanBergen AM, Love HA. Family-of-origin rejection on suicidal ideation among a sexual minority sample. J Marital Fam Ther. 2022;48(2):560-75.
2. Bagner DM, Rodríguez GM, Blake CA, Linares D, Carter AS. Assessment of behavioral and emotional problems in infancy: a systematic review. Clin Child Fam Psychol Rev. 2012;15(2):113-28.

3. Plant DT, Barker ED, Waters CS, Pawlby S, Pariante CM. Intergenerational transmission of maltreatment and psychopathology: the role of antenatal depression. Psychol Med. 2013; 43(3):519-28.
4. Brody GH, Murry VM, Kim S, Brown AC. Longitudinal pathways to competence and psychological adjustment among African American children living in rural single-parent households. Child Dev. 2002;73(5):1505-16.
5. Webster-Stratton C, Reid MJ, Hammond M. Treating children with early-onset conduct problems: intervention outcomes for parent, child, and teacher training. J Clin Child Adolesc Psychol. 2004;33(1):105-24.
6. Smeekens S, Riksen-Walraven JM, van Bakel HJ. Multiple determinants of externalizing behavior in 5-year-olds: a longitudinal model. J Abnorm Child Psychol. 2007;35(3):347-61.
7. Brendel KE, Maynard BR. Child–parent interventions for childhood anxiety disorders. Research on Social Work Practice. 2013;24(3): 287-95.
8. World Health Organization. (2021). Mental health of adolescents. [online] Available from https://www.who.int/news-room/fact-sheets/detail/adolescent-mental-health [Last accessed 20 November, 2025].
9. Seidel DH, Markes M, Grouven U, Messow CM, Sieben W, Knelangen M, et al. Systemic therapy in children and adolescents with mental disorders: a systematic review and meta-analysis. BMC Psychiatry. 2024;24:125.
10. Pine AE, Baumann MG, Modugno G, Compas BE. Parental involvement in adolescent psychological interventions: A meta-analysis. Clin Child Fam Psychol Rev. 2024;27(3):1-20.
11. Carr A. Family therapy and systemic interventions for child-focused problems: the current evidence base. J Family Ther. 2018;41(2):153-213.
12. Cottrell D, Boston P. Practitioner review: The effectiveness of systemic family therapy for children and adolescents. J Child Psychol Psychiatry. 2002;43(5):573-86.
13. Walrond-Skinner S. Indications and contra-indications for the use of family therapy. J Child Psychol Psychiatry. 1978;19(1):57-62.
14. Walrond-Skinner S. Family therapy: The treatment of family systems. London: Routledge & Kegan Paul; 1976.
15. Griffith JL, Slovik L. In: Tasman A, Kay J, Lieberman J (Eds). Psychiatry, 3rd edition. Hoboken, NJ: Wiley; 2008.
16. Satyanarayana VA, Das A, Shah A. Psychotherapy for Families with Adolescent Children: Clinical Practice Guidelines. J Indian Assoc Child Adolesc Ment Health. 2024;20(2):127-35.
17. Minuchin S. Families and Family Therapy. Cambridge, MA: Harvard University Press; 1974.
18. Selvini MP, Boscolo L, Cecchin G, Prata G. Hypothesizing—circularity—neutrality: three guidelines for the conductor of the session. Fam Process. 1980;19(1):3-12.
19. Minuchin S, Rosman BL, Baker L. Psychosomatic Families: Anorexia Nervosa in Context. Cambridge: Harvard University Press; 1978.
20. Bowlby J. Attachment and Loss: Attachment (vol. 1). New York: Basic Books; 1969.
21. Greenberg LS. Emotions, the great captains of our lives: their role in the process of change in psychotherapy. Am Psychol. 2012;67(8):697-707.
22. Pascual-Leone A, Greenberg LS. Emotional processing in experiential therapy: why "the only way out is through". J Consult Clin Psychol. 2007;75(6):875-87.
23. Tsvieli N, Lifshitz C, Diamond GM. Corrective attachment episodes in attachment-based family therapy: the power of enactment. Psychother Res. 2022;32(2):209-22.
24. Diamond G, Siqueland L, Diamond GM. Attachment-based family therapy for depressed adolescents: programmatic treatment development. Clin Child Fam Psychol Rev. 2003;6(2): 107-27.
25. Kobak R, Bosmans G. Attachment and psychopathology: a dynamic model of the insecure cycle. Curr Opin Psychol. 2019;25:76-80.
26. Dattilio FM, Epstein NB. Cognitive-behavioral couple and family therapy. In: Sexton TL, Lebow J (Eds). Handbook of Family Therapy. London: Routledge/Taylor & Francis; 2016. pp. 89-119.

Psychological Therapies for Neurodevelopmental Disorders (Speech-Language, Occupational, Sensory Integration, Special Education, and Related Therapies)

Vijaya Raman, Meghana Vijayanand

INTRODUCTION

Neurodevelopmental disorders (NDDs) are developmental variations that alter the trajectory of the child's social, cognitive, adaptive, and academic functioning. Owing to the fact that they are developmental in their etiologies and present with unique challenges all through their lifespan, the primary treatment would be consistent and systematic therapeutic intervention.[1,2] Most NDDs have various therapeutic techniques that are recommended based on the presentation of the child's strengths and deficits. These interventions serve as a means to foster their skills and improve their quality of life.

The common NDDs that require intervention are autism spectrum disorder (ASD), attention-deficit/hyperactivity disorder (ADHD), intellectual developmental disorder (IDD), specific learning disabilities (SLDs), communication disorders, motor disorders, and other disorders that cause developmental delays.[3] These disorders can present significant challenges in communication, behavior, social interaction, and learning. In the absence of appropriate support and training, these challenges can cause functional impairments that impact a child's quality of life and their ability to reach their full potential.[4]

Therapeutic interventions offer a range of strategies and techniques designed to address specific needs.[5] By providing targeted support, these interventions can help children to develop essential skills, improve their overall well-being, and enhance their ability to participate fully in society.[6]

Intervention is usually targeted for specific symptom deficits. These deficits are not circumscribed to particular disorders, like speech difficulties are present in autism and communication disorders, while motor challenges can be present in ASD, motor difficulties, cerebral palsy, with nuanced difficulties in those with dysgraphia or ADHD. This heterogeneity in presentation indicates that the challenges experienced by children with NDDs are myriad, while co-occurring or comorbid diagnoses is the norm rather than an exception.[7] Hence, targeting these difficulties symptomatically is clinically prudent, and also beneficial for the child.

This chapter will explore the various therapeutic interventions available for children with NDDs. We will discuss the rationale for these interventions, the common issues they address, and the evidence supporting their effectiveness. By understanding the benefits and applications of therapeutic interventions, parents, educators, and healthcare professionals can work together to develop personalized treatment plans that meet the unique needs of each child. The common intervention techniques are discussed below based on the symptomatic difficulties the child experiences.

COMMUNICATION DIFFICULTIES

Communication difficulties are more often the primary concern the parents present with for a child with autism. Depending on the age and severity of the difficulty, the child's speech can vary from having an absence of nonverbal/gestural communication or absence of using words, selective or limited usage of words, or inability to narrate or have a to-and-fro communication. The disorders enlisted in the communication disorders section of the Diagnostic and Statistical Manual (DSM) also require speech-language therapy as its primary treatment modality. The primary intervention strategy for these various presentations is speech-language therapy.

Speech-language Therapy

Speech-language therapy helps people with difficulties in communication and language skills–both verbal and nonverbal. Speech-language pathologists (SLPs) work with people across age ranges beginning from infancy. Their primary areas of focus are with improving articulation (making clear and understandable sounds), fluency (speaking smoothly without stuttering), language (using vocabulary, grammar, and syntax, and comprehending it), and voice (quality, pitch, and loudness of a voice).

Children with NDDs often have significant challenges with communication. It is usually the foremost presenting complaint of parents when they seek help for their children, especially for those children who do not have a global developmental delay (GDD). Communication difficulties have far-reaching consequences as they impede socialization, learning, and participation in daily activities. Without adequate communication skills, it is difficult for the child to learn and understand what is being taught, and form and maintain social relationships.

The indications for speech therapy are diverse and encompass a wide range of communication difficulties. The common reasons why speech therapy is recommended for the child are delayed acquisition of language milestones, language disorders like expressive language disorders or aphasia, mispronunciation or misarticulation, difficulties with fluency, and social-communication or pragmatic language disorders.

It is common for children with communication disorders and GDD to avail of speech therapy, but those with other NDDs also benefit from it. Children with ASD often have difficulties and differences in language acquisition, social communication, and pragmatic language skills. Speech therapy helps them to develop these essential skills, enabling them to express their thoughts and feelings more effectively. Adequate communication is essential for the child's cognitive, social, and emotional development.

Speech therapy additionally helps children with NDDs by improving articulation and teaching them to produce sounds accurately. It addresses language delays by working on their lexical vocabulary and improving syntax and grammar. They work on social communication skills by teaching them to initiate conversations, maintain eye contact, and use body language appropriately. Speech therapy addresses challenges by improving listening skills, reducing impulsivity, and enhancing language organizational skills.[8]

Techniques used in therapy for children with NDDs vary depending on the specific needs and the goals set. Some of the common strategies include *speech sound therapy*, which works on the production of sounds of individual syllables. They target specific sounds like /r/, /l/ and so on to help with the correct articulation. *Language therapy* enhances comprehension and expression through exercises that expand vocabulary, improve sentence structure, and develop narrative skills. *Social communication skills* improve social understanding, interaction, and overall pragmatic skills. They also focus on initiating conversations, maintaining eye contact, and understanding social cues. Speech therapists may also use *augmentative and alternative communication (AAC)* methods for children with limited verbal skills. These can include picture boards [picture exchange communication system (PECS)], communication devices (AWAZ), or sign language, that provide alternative means of communication.

Speech and language therapy is one of the core intervention methods for children with NDDs. Targeted speech-language interventions can significantly improve communication skills, decrease behavioral issues, enhance academic performance, have better social relationships, and have a better overall quality of life for individuals with NDDs.

Key Points

- Speech-language therapy is a core intervention method for children with NDDs.
- It is the most studied and recommended technique for speech delay and communication difficulties.
- Speech-language therapy can help children with speech delay learn to verbalize beginning from syllables to naming and communication in phrases/sentences.
- For children with fluency and pragmatic difficulties, higher-order techniques are used.
- In the case of minimally verbal or nonverbal children, augmented techniques are used.

DIFFICULTIES WITH REGULATING MOVEMENT AND ACTIVITY LEVELS

Motor disorders, such as developmental coordination disorder, stereotypic movement disorder, and tic disorder, in addition to children with ASD and ADHD, have difficulties regulating their body movements. They either have an increased physical activation or decreased physical ability. For both scenarios, occupational therapy (OT)-based therapies can be used to increase or regulate gross motor and fine motor skills. Several sensory systems also are related to how the body interprets stimuli from the outside world or from within one's body. Helping children regulate their sensory systems is also part of OT-based therapies.

Occupational Therapy

Occupational therapy, commonly known as OT, plays a crucial role in assisting individuals of all ages to gain independence and engage fully in daily activities that matter to them by addressing physical limitations as well, as cognitive and emotional challenges they may face.

Adequate daily living skills are often a deficit in children with NDDs and other developmental delays. It impacts their self-care skills that require independent toileting, bathing, dressing, and eating. Fine motor skill deficits can impact writing, using educational aids, and classroom independence. Motor skill deficits can impact the child's ability to complete household chores and daily routines and participate in age-appropriate play/leisure activities with peers. As a specialized form of therapy focused on improving daily living skills, OT plays a vital role in supporting children with NDDs, including those with ASD, ADHD, dysgraphia, and IDD. They address sensory processing, fine motor skills, and adaptive functioning to facilitate children participating more fully in life's activities and achieve greater independence.[9]

Occupational therapy intervention is often necessitated for a myriad set of symptoms or skill deficits the child presents with. Some of the common indications for OT include motor difficulties—both fine motor and gross motor, difficulties with processing sensory information, difficulties making sense of visual-spatial inputs, and those requiring to better their adaptive living skills.

Techniques used in OT for children with NDDs vary depending on the specific needs and the goals set. Some of the common strategies include *gross motor therapy* which works on the child's balance, running, jumping, and climbing skills while *fine motor skills therapy* develops the small muscles in the hands and fingers, that are essential for coloring, writing, buttoning, and using cutlery or tools. *Sensory integration therapy* (SIT) addresses sensory processing difficulties. It involves controlling sensory input to help children learn to regulate their responses to the environment. Common activities include swinging, rocking, or engaging in tactile activities to improve sensory awareness and integration.

Occupational therapy is another core intervention strategy for children with NDDs. By addressing functional challenges using targeted strategies, OT can significantly improve motor skills and daily living skills and thus enhance independence for children with ASD, ADHD, IDD, and others with motor difficulties.

Physical Therapy

Physical therapy (PT) helps people to recover their movement and function of physical skills. Traditionally, physical therapists work with people of all ages who have physical impairments or disabilities. They use various techniques to restore function and improve mobility and strength after injuries or illnesses. They work to prevent disability by maintaining or improving physical health and function. In children with NDDs, especially motor disorders, GDD/IDD and some children with ASD, PT addresses physical limitations and improves motor skills.

Children with NDDs often experience physical challenges that can impact their development and daily activities. PT helps children to improve motor skills by developing or enhancing gross motor skills (walking, running, and jumping) and fine motor skills (using cutlery and other household objects, cutting, pasting, and writing). It helps to increase strength and endurance by building muscle strength and improving stamina. They work on improving balance and coordination by enhancing core strength to prevent falls and injuries. They also manage pain associated with physical conditions, such as joint stiffness or muscle tightness.

Indications for initiating PT include muscle weakness, low muscle tone, spasticity, postural difficulties, and physical pain. These physical difficulties need to be dealt with before more functional aspects are targeted with OT. Methods to deal with these symptoms vary based on the deficit and motor profile of the child. Some of the common strategies are *balance and coordination therapy* which involves activities to improve balance, coordination, and spatial awareness, using exercises on balance beams, stability balls, or other equipment. *Therapeutic exercises* help using targeted exercises to improve strength, flexibility, balance, and coordination while *manual therapy* uses hands-on techniques, such as massage and mobilization, to improve joint mobility and reduce pain. Other techniques involve using heat and cold to augment exercises or recovery.

It is important to note that PT is an intervention that is usually used in combination with OT or is incorporated within OT.

Sensory Integration Therapy

Sensory processing is the ability to interpret and respond to sensory information from the environment. SIT is a specialized form of OT that focuses on improving sensory processing. This therapeutic approach helps children to improve their ability to process sensory information, such as touch, sight, sound, smell, and movement. It is based on the theory that the brain needs to organize and integrate sensory input in order to function effectively.[9]

Children with NDDs often have difficulties processing sensory information (touch, sounds, sights, smells, or movements). This is one of the core symptoms of ASD, which comes under the restrictive repetitive behaviors (RRBs) section. It can lead to a range of challenges, which present as *sensory hypersensitivity* where they are overly sensitive to sensory input, which can lead to anxiety, avoidance, or meltdowns, *sensory hyposensitivity* where they are under-sensitive to sensory input, which can lead to seeking out excessive sensory stimulation. They have *sensory seeking* where they have a strong desire for sensory input, which can result in behaviors such as fidgeting, chewing, or rocking. *Visual-spatial challenges* where they have difficulties with understanding spatial relationships and navigating the environment, and *auditory processing difficulties* where they have challenges with processing auditory information, such as understanding speech or following directions are also part of the sensory processing deficits. Indications for SIT can be any feature mentioned above or any combination thereof.

Sensory integration therapy helps children with NDDs by improving sensory processing by enhancing the brain's ability to organize and integrate sensory information. It helps to develop motor skills by improving coordination, balance, and fine motor skills. This, in turn, enhances social and emotional skills by fostering better social interactions, emotional regulation, and self-esteem. It also decreases behavioral issues by decreasing meltdowns due to sensory overload, and ultimately, increasing independence and full participation in everyday activities.[10]

Methods used in SIT vary depending on the child's specific needs and therapy goals. However, several core strategies are commonly employed. *Sensory input activities* are used to provide controlled sensory stimulation. This teaches the child to process and integrate sensory information better. It involves activities such as swinging, rocking, or engaging in tactile activities. A *sensory diet* is a personalized plan of sensory activities and experiences that help children to regulate their sensory input throughout the day. It includes activities that are calming or improve alertness, depending on the child's needs. *Environmental modifications* are used to create a sensory-friendly environment if the child has several sensory sensitivities or if they cause severe overwhelm. It may involve adjusting lighting, sound levels, or temperature to reduce sensory overload.

Sensory integration therapy typically involves a variety of activities that provide sensory input, such as swinging, rocking, bouncing, playing in a sensory room, and engaging in sensory-based crafts. The therapist works with the child to gradually introduce new sensory experiences and help them to develop the skills they need to process and integrate sensory information effectively.

Key Points

- OT-based therapies can be used to increase or regulate gross motor and fine motor skills.
- Hyper- or hyposensitivity to various sensory modalities is moderated by SIT.
- Gross motor and fine motor deficits are worked with in OT.
- PT entails more strength work and handling pain

ACADEMIC DIFFICULTIES

Children with SLDs have significant challenges in learning grade-appropriate academics. They can have difficulties with learning languages (dyslexia), learning mathematical concepts (dyscalculia), difficulties with writing and fine motor tasks (dysgraphia), or learning through listening (auditory processing disorder). Specialized techniques to teach children with each of these symptom profiles are what special education techniques are made of. Children with autism and ADHD additionally require special education sessions to help them to cope with grade-expected academics (if their cognitive capacity permits them to acquire it). Special education is also provided in many schools as part of the inclusive education program.

Special Education

Special education is a specialized form of education designed to meet the unique needs of students with disabilities. It provides individualized support, accommodations, and modifications to help students with academic difficulties, access education.[11]

Children with NDDs face several challenges in learning or keeping up with academic expectations. Common symptoms that necessitate special education inputs are difficulties with core academic tasks such as reading and writing and particular challenges with math and spelling. Other difficulties, such as issues with attention, impulsivity, emotional regulation, instruction-following, sensory processing, and poor receptive language skills, can also impact learning and classroom behavior.

Children with SLD require regular and consistent special education sessions to help them with their academic difficulties. Children with ASD have difficulties in communication, social interaction, and behavior, requiring specialized instruction to foster progress. Students with ADHD struggle with attention, impulsivity, and hyperactivity, all of which impact academic performance. Special education provides these children with the necessary accommodations and support to help them succeed. Children with NDDs often require *specialized support* to meet their educational needs in the form of *individualized instruction,* that uses tailored teaching methods and materials to address specific learning styles and challenges, *accommodations* that provide modifications to the learning environment or curriculum to help students succeed, *support services* providing additional assistance, such as speech therapy or OT, to address other symptomatic needs, and ultimately providing *inclusive education,* where the opportunities to learn alongside their peers in a general education setting is a legal right.[12]

Indications for special education vary depending on the nature and severity of a student's disability. The specific services provided will depend on the student's individual needs. Common techniques used in special education[11] for children with SLD, ASD, IDD, and ADHD vary depending on their specific needs and goals. However, several core strategies are frequently employed. Every child who avails of special education sessions is provided with an *individualized education programs (IEPs).* These are developed for each student with a disability, outlining their unique needs and goals. IEPs are created in collaboration with parents, teachers, and other professionals involved in the student's education. *Specialized instruction* is provided to address the specific challenges faced by students with ASD and ADHD. This may involve using specialized teaching techniques that are adapted to the student's learning style and pace, adapted materials, or assistive technology including tools and devices that help students to access education and communicate. *Small group instruction* and using *visual schedules* can also be beneficial for students who require more individualized attention. *Behavior management techniques* address challenging behaviors and promote more positive behavior. *Accommodations* are provided to help them to access education and participate fully in classroom activities. These accommodations may include extended time for assignments, preferential seating, or the use of assistive technology. *Modifications* may also be made to the curriculum to make it more accessible to students with disabilities and ensure *inclusive settings* that provide opportunities to learn alongside peers in general education classrooms, with appropriate supports in place, and other related support services, such as speech therapy or OT, that address related needs. The key to a robust plan is *collaboration* between parents, teachers, and other professionals which is essential in providing effective special education services.

Key Points

- Special education is a choice of therapy modality when the child has difficulty in academics.
- Special education focuses on preacademic skills and prerequisite skills for younger children. For older children, special education services help more with IEPs, accommodations, and assistance.
- It usually entails a highly IEP, with extra support with resource room settings and trained special educators in schools.

MULTIMODAL THERAPIES

Multimodal refers to the combined use of other disparate intervention techniques to create a new comprehensive framework. Some therapy techniques are a combination of the above-discussed techniques.

Early Intervention

Early intervention (EI) is a comprehensive combination of services designed to help very young children with developmental delays by playing a vital role in supporting their growth and development.[13] There are several models of early intervention like the Com Deall model (founded by Dr Prathibha Karanth, in Bangalore),[14] other internationally formulated models of early intervention include the Early Start Denver model,[15] TEACCH,[16] and early intensive behavioral intervention (EIBI).[17]

Early intervention programs typically involve a multidisciplinary team of professionals including special education teachers, speech-language therapists, occupational therapists, physical therapists, and developmental psychologists. Early intervention is ideally provided from birth to age 3 and is designed to address developmental needs in areas such as:

- *Cognitive development:* Thinking, learning, and problem-solving skills.
- *Physical development:* Gross motor skills (like walking and running) and fine motor skills (like using utensils and writing).
- *Communication and language development:* Speech, language, and social skills.
- *Adaptive development:* Self-help skills, such as dressing and eating.

Early intervention is crucial for children with NDDs because it provides the support and resources they need to develop essential skills at an early age. Early intervention aims to decrease the adverse effects on cognition, motor, language, and emotional delays in young children.[18] Thus, improving developmental outcomes and preventing secondary disabilities by addressing the delays and preventing them from becoming more severe. It also supports families by providing them with the information and resources they need to help their children thrive. Indications for early intervention usually encompass a wide range of developmental challenges. One of the indications for early intervention is when very young children (around a year) are diagnosed with a delay, and present with a combination of deficits—delayed communication, socialization, and/or cognition.

Early intervention is a team-based approach that involves collaboration between families, educators, therapists, and healthcare providers. The goal is to provide a comprehensive and coordinated approach to support the child's development.

Group Therapy

Group therapy is a form of psychotherapy that involves a group of individuals meeting together under the guidance of a therapist, for a particular goal. It provides a supportive environment where participants can share their experiences, learn from each other, and develop coping strategies. Group therapy is used as a therapy modality for children to practice their communication and social skills in a supportive and collaborative environment.

Group therapy is particularly beneficial for children with NDDs to improve social skills, where children can learn and practice social skills in a safe and supportive environment. They learn from peer support, where children benefit from the support and understanding of peers who share similar experiences. Role modeling helps them through which children can observe and learn from the positive behaviors of their peers. Group settings help to generalize the skills learned in other therapies and strategies from group therapy can be applied to other settings, such as school or home. This improves the child's learning as they learn to apply the skills learned.

Common methods used in group therapy for children with ASD and ADHD vary depending on the specific needs and goals of the group. They *practice* the skills learned in other forms of therapy like speech-language therapy and OT. *Social skills training* is another important component of group therapy for children with ASD and ADHD. This involves teaching children how to initiate conversations, maintain eye contact, and understand social cues. By interacting with their peers in a group setting, children can practice these skills and receive feedback from others. *Play therapy* is a valuable technique for younger children, as it allows them to express their emotions and experiences through play. In a group setting, children can learn to share, cooperate, and resolve conflicts. Group therapy for older children also provides a sense of belonging and support for children who may feel isolated or misunderstood. By connecting with others who share similar experiences, children can develop a sense of community and reduce feelings of loneliness. Additionally, group therapy can help children develop empathy and understanding for others, fostering positive relationships and social skills.

It is important to note that group therapy may not be suitable for all children, and individual factors should be considered when determining if group therapy is the right approach. However, for many children with ASD and ADHD, group therapy can offer a valuable and effective form of support.

BEHAVIORAL CHALLENGES

Children with NDDs have several behavioral challenges that are part of their symptomatology. These behavioral issues interfere in their learning process and most often are the reason schools refer children for assessments. More severe behavioral challenges include self-injurious behaviors (SIBs), severe disruptive behaviors, and aggression.[19] It is important to understand the reason or the etiology of challenging behaviors, as they always serve a purpose—either to communicate distress, dissent, as a response to sensory overwhelm, or as a stubborn habit. It is important to understand why a behavior occurs before setting out to intervene. Behavioral issues can be dealt with using the following methods.

Behavior Therapy

Originally, behavior therapy (BT) was a type of psychotherapy that focused on changing unwanted behaviors through learning new skills and developing healthy coping mechanisms. It is based on the principle that behaviors are learned and can be unlearned (classical conditioning and operant conditioning principles). BT is often used to treat a variety of mental health conditions including anxiety, depression, and substance abuse. The basic premise of BT is that behaviors have a cause, have patterns, and can be modified or altered.

With challenging behaviors being one of the primary concerns of parents and teachers of children with NDDs, BT becomes a crucial therapy method. Almost all the NDDs—ASD, ADHD, IDD, and GDD, have children who display some behavioral challenges or the other. They often exhibit challenging behaviors that impact their home, school, and social functioning. By identifying and addressing unwanted behaviors while reinforcing desired ones, BT makes it easier to manage and teach children with NDDs.

Behavior therapy is a very valuable tool to reduce challenging behaviors and teach new skills. New coping mechanisms will replace unwanted behaviors which can have far-reaching impacts including improving social skills, enhancing communication, cooperation, and empathy; improving academic performance; increasing independence and developing self-care and daily living skills, and enhance overall well-being by improving emotional regulation and reducing stress.[20]

Common issues addressed in BT for children with IDD, ADHD, and ASD include aggression (physical or verbal aggression toward others or objects), self-injury (hurting oneself, such as biting, scratching, or head-banging), property destruction (damaging objects or property), tantrums (intense emotional outbursts), meltdowns (intense reactions to intolerance of sensory overload), defiance and stubbornness (refusing to follow rules or cooperate), stereotyped behaviors (repetitive or ritualistic behaviors), social withdrawal (avoiding social interactions or activities), and anxiety (excessive fear or worry).

Techniques for BT vary depending on the child's specific needs and the type of NDD. However, several core methods are frequently employed. *Applied behavior analysis (ABA)* is a method based on BT principles. It is widely used for children with ASD. ABA involves breaking down complex behaviors into smaller, more manageable steps and providing positive reinforcement for desired behaviors.[21] This can help to teach new skills, reduce problem behaviors, and improve communication. However, it is also important to note that there have been some controversies with regard to the use of ABA for NDD children in recent times.[22,23]

There are some key concepts from BT that are used to formulate and explain a child's behavior. They include *positive reinforcement*, which is rewarding desired behaviors to increase their frequency. Positive reinforcers can be tangible reward, such as praise, stickers, or preferred activities. *Extinction* is used to reduce problem behaviors. It involves withholding reinforcement for a previously reinforced behavior, which can lead to a decrease in the behavior over time. *Token economies* are often used to motivate desired behaviors. In a token economy, children earn tokens for positive behaviors, which can later be exchanged for reward. *Shaping* is used to gradually teach new behaviors. It involves reinforcing successive approximations of the desired behavior, leading to the development of the target behavior over time.

Behavior therapy is a valuable therapy technique for children with NDDs to reduce challenging behaviors, improve social skills, and enhance overall functioning.

Cognitive Behavior Therapy

Cognitive behavior therapy (CBT) is a type of psychotherapy that focuses on changing negative thought patterns and problem behaviors to improve emotional and psychological well-being. It is based on the premise that our thoughts, feelings, and behaviors are interconnected, and by modifying our thoughts, we can change our feelings and behaviors. While CBT is very commonly used with adolescents and adults, it can also be adapted for children, providing them with valuable tools to navigate the challenges they may face.

Children with NDDs often experience difficulties with social interactions, emotional regulation, and problem-solving. CBT can help children with these difficulties by improving social skills and developing strategies for initiating and maintaining social interactions. It helps them to manage emotions by learning to identify and regulate emotions effectively. It enhances problem-solving skills by developing strategies to navigate challenging situations. For older and more aware children with NDDs, it reduces anxiety and depression by addressing negative thought patterns and developing coping mechanisms. By teaching children to identify and challenge negative thought patterns, CBT helps them to develop healthier coping mechanisms.

Methods used in CBT for children involve a variety of techniques aimed at helping them understand and modify their thoughts, feelings, and behaviors. One key technique is *cognitive restructuring*, which involves identifying and challenging negative thoughts, and replacing the negative thoughts with more positive and realistic alternatives. While this works on the cognitions, the other important aspect of CBT is *behavioral techniques*. These techniques focus on changing behaviors through positive reinforcement and exposure therapy. Positive reinforcement involves rewarding desired behaviors, while exposure therapy involves gradually exposing children to feared situations or stimuli in a safe and controlled environment. This can help them overcome anxiety and develop more adaptive coping mechanisms. CBT also emphasizes the importance of *emotion regulation*, where children are taught to identify and manage their emotions effectively. This may involve mindfulness techniques, relaxation exercises, or problem-solving strategies.

Cognitive behavior therapy for children combines individual therapy sessions and parent training, using techniques such as cognitive restructuring, exposure therapy, relaxation techniques, problem-solving skills training, and social skills training. These techniques help the child identify and challenge negative thought patterns, manage stress and anxiety through gradual and systematic exposure and relaxation exercises, develop problem-solving strategies, and initiate/maintain social interactions. The goal is to help the child overcome anxiety and improve their overall well-being.

Parent Management Training

Parent management training (PMT) is a form of therapy that focuses on equipping parents with effective strategies to manage their child's behavior.[24] It is often used in conjunction with other interventions, such as BT, to address behavioral challenges in children. PMT helps parents to understand the underlying causes of their child's behavior, develop positive parenting techniques, and create a supportive home environment.[25]

With children, especially those with NDDs, it is important for the parents to be involved in therapy. Since several skills are being taught in sessions, it is important for the parents to know how to continue to foster development in home settings. Oftentimes, parents are involved as *cotherapists* to help to enforce therapy principles outside therapy sessions. In some cases, parents are given strategies to help them work with a child with behavioral challenges, to make them more amenable to work in therapy.

The challenging behaviors of children with NDDs can strain family relationships and make it difficult for parents to manage their child's behavior effectively. PMT provides parents with the tools and support they need to improve parent-child relationships. They focus on reducing challenging behaviors through implementing effective strategies to manage problem behaviors by establishing consistent rules, expectations, and consequences. This helps to regulate emotions and develop positive interactions and strengthen bonds that create a positive home environment.

Parents of children with ASD and IDD may face difficulties managing aggression, tantrums, or self-injury. Similarly, parents of children with ADHD may struggle with their child's impulsivity, hyperactivity, or inattention. PMT can help parents to develop effective strategies to manage these symptoms and create a more structured and supportive home environment.[26] For children with ADHD, PMT is known to be a more efficacious adjunct to pharmacological methods than the latter in isolation.[27]

Common methods used in PMT involve teaching parents a variety of behavioral management techniques. One of the core principles of PMT is *positive reinforcement*. Parents learn to identify and praise positive behaviors while minimizing attention to negative behaviors. Another important technique is *consequence management*, which involves implementing consistent predecided consequences for undesirable behaviors. This can include natural consequences, time-outs, or loss of privileges. PMT also emphasizes the importance of *clear communication* and *consistent expectations*. Parents learn to set clear expectations for their child's behavior and to communicate them. Additionally, parents develop *effective problem-solving skills* to address challenging situations. By teaching parents how to identify the underlying causes of behavioral problems and develop strategies to address them, PMT equips parents to be ready to handle challenges.

Parent management training typically involves several sessions with a trained therapist who provides parents with information, guidance on strategies, and support. Common components of PMT include, teaching parents about the principles of behavior modification, such as positive reinforcement and extinction, fostering better problem-solving skills, where parents are helped to identify and address specific behavioral challenges, teaching parents how to communicate effectively with their child and setting clear expectations, introduce conflict resolution skills by helping parents manage disagreements and resolve conflicts peacefully, and have better stress management techniques by providing parents with strategies to cope with stress and maintain their own well-being.

Parent management training is a collaborative process that involves ongoing communication and support between parents and the therapist. By providing parents with the tools and techniques they need to manage their child's behavior effectively, PMT can empower parents and create a more positive and supportive home environment for both the child and the family.

Behavioral interventions have been established to improve cognition, language skills, and behavior.[28] Most of the features and symptoms that indicate the use of BT or CBT with the child are similar to the need for PMT. The difference between PMT and BT/CBT has to do with the ability of the child. PMT is indicated when the child is younger, has lower cognitive skills, or has significant delays in language or adaptive functioning. Whereas CBT and BT are more successful with children who are amenable to psychotherapy, and who are older and with adequate cognitive skills. PMT principles are also used for older children/adolescents in addition to individual therapy.

SKILL-BASED DIFFICULTIES

Children with ASD, ADHD, and IDD have difficulties in learning skills in keeping with the trajectory of typical peers.[29] These skills will need to be broken down into smaller steps (with a task analysis) and be taught repeatedly. Two intervention methods that can be employed.

Adaptive and Self-help Skill Training

Adaptive and self-help skills training focuses on developing essential life skills in children by teaching them how to perform everyday tasks independently. This helps them to achieve independent living skills which is usually a worry for parents as children with NDDs grow older. Some of these skills can include:

- *Personal self-care:* Dressing, grooming, and bathing.
- *Household chores:* Cleaning, cooking, and laundry.
- *Community living:* Skills needed to navigate the community, such as using public transportation, shopping, and managing money.
- *Vocational skills:* Skills needed for employment, such as job search, interviewing, and workplace communication.

Adaptive skills training is crucial for children with NDDs for several reasons such as developing *independence* as adaptive skills help children become more independent and reduce their reliance on others, *quality of life* where improved adaptive skills can enhance a child's overall quality of life and well-being, *social inclusion* as mastery of adaptive skills can facilitate social interactions and integration into the community, and *future success* as developing adaptive skills can prepare children for future education, employment, and independent living.

Common methods used in adaptive and self-help skills training for children with NDDs vary based on cognitive ability and symptom profile. Children with IDD and/or ASD will require adaptive skill training from basic self-care, while a child with ADHD or SLD will require adaptive skill training specific to their difficulty or deficit.

Many of the techniques used in BT and PMT are utilized here. Some specific several core approaches are frequently employed. *Task analysis* is a common technique that involves breaking down complex tasks into smaller and more manageable steps. This helps children learn and practice each step individually before combining them to complete the entire task. *Visual supports* are often used to assist children with ASD in understanding and completing tasks. These supports may include visual schedules, picture prompts, or social stories. *Social skills training* is another important component of adaptive and self-help skills training, particularly for children with ASD. This therapy involves teaching children how to interact with others, understand social cues, and express their emotions appropriately.

Adaptive and self-help skills training is conducted in various settings including schools, homes, therapy centers, and community centers. It often involves a multidisciplinary approach, with input from therapists, educators, and family members. The therapy is often individualized to meet the unique needs of each child. By providing targeted interventions and support, adaptive and self-help skills training can significantly improve independence, self-esteem, and overall quality of life for individuals with NDDs.

Social Skills Training

Social skills training is a therapeutic approach formulated to help children and adolescents to develop and improve their social communication skills. It involves teaching them how to interact effectively with others, express themselves clearly, and understand social cues.[30] It empowers them to connect with others more effectively and build meaningful relationships.

Children with NDDs tend to face challenges in social interactions. These challenges can impact their ability to connect with peers and build meaningful relationships. They have difficulty in expressing their thoughts and feelings clearly along with understanding and interpreting nonverbal communication and social situations. They struggle to participate and engage in age-appropriate social activities and events. This causes them difficulty in coping and managing social anxiety and discomfort in navigating difficult social situations.

Indications for social skills training include a wide range of social and communication difficulties like difficulty initiating and maintaining conversations, struggling to start conversations, problems understanding social cues and interpreting nonverbal communication, difficulty expressing emotions and needs, difficulty in sharing and taking turns and challenges with group dynamics, and difficulties participating in group activities and following rules.

Social skills training can help children with NDDs by focusing on goals like *improving social communication* by teaching them how to initiate conversations, maintain eye contact, and use appropriate body language, *developing empathy* by helping them understand and respond to the emotions of others, *enhancing social problem-solving skills* by teaching them how to navigate social situations, resolve conflicts, and make appropriate decisions, *reducing social anxiety* by helping them to overcome their fear of social interactions and build confidence, *promoting social inclusion* by encouraging them to participate in social activities and form friendships.

Common methods used in social skills training for children with ASD and ADHD vary depending on the specific needs and goals. However, several core approaches are frequently employed like *modeling* that involves demonstrating appropriate social behaviors for children to observe and imitate. *Role-playing* is a popular technique that involves practicing social situations in a safe and supportive environment. This allows children to experiment with different responses and receive feedback from the therapist. *Social stories* are another effective tool for teaching social skills. These stories provide visual and textual information about social situations, helping children understand expectations and appropriate behaviors. *Group therapy* sessions can be used to have the child practice their skills within a safe environment.

Social skills training typically involves a combination of individual therapy sessions, group therapy, and role-playing exercises. It is a process that requires ongoing practice and reinforcement. It is important for parents and caregivers to support their child's social skills development at home and in the community. The ultimate aim of social skills training is the ability of the child or adolescent to generalize the skills learnt to lead a functional life.

SUMMARY AND CONCLUSION

To summarize: Effective interventions often involve a multidisciplinary approach consisting of a team of professionals including therapists, educators, and healthcare providers. Individualized treatment plans are vital as each child with a NDD has unique needs, requiring tailored treatment plans. Early intervention is crucial as early diagnosis and intervention can significantly improve outcomes for children with NDDs. Speech therapy and OT (including SIT) are vital therapy techniques that are highly recommended. Behavioral therapy is indicated for children with highly challenging behaviors, aggression, or self-harm tendencies. It is also indicated for children who have difficulty with attention and executive functioning.

Special education is intended for children who have difficulties with academics, where they require to learn the foundational skills, or they have particular difficulties with reading, writing, spelling, or math. Older children can present with difficulties in comprehension rather than reading. Common techniques for teaching children with NDDs across therapy techniques include breaking complex tasks into smaller, more manageable steps, using visual aids, such as pictures or checklists, to help children understand and remember tasks, positive reinforcement, modeling desired behavior, and practice and repetition. Various therapeutic techniques are recommended based on the presentation of the child's strengths and deficits.

Periodic assessments are necessary to understand the child's difficulties and challenges to provide adequate intervention at the appropriate time.

In conclusion, therapeutic intervention plays a vital role in supporting children with NDDs, enhancing their quality of life, and fostering their development. By addressing specific challenges and providing tailored support, these interventions empower children to reach their full potential to lead functional lives.

The effectiveness of therapeutic intervention lies in its ability to address the unique needs of each child. From behavioral therapies that target specific behaviors to educational interventions that support academic growth, these therapies offer a comprehensive approach to addressing the multifaceted challenges faced by children with NDDs.

Furthermore, therapeutic interventions often involve a collaborative effort between families, therapists, educators, and healthcare providers. This collaborative approach ensures that children receive the necessary support and resources to thrive. By working together, these professionals can create personalized treatment plans that address the child's individual needs and goals.

It is also important to note that periodic re-evaluation is required as therapy can train the child and facilitate the learning of specific skills. As the child grows, the demands on the child increase. Continued revision of therapy goals is necessary to keep up with the increasing demands of a growing child and their transitional ages.

In summary, therapeutic intervention are necessary and indispensable methods of improving the functional outcomes for children with NDDs.

REFERENCES

1. Myers SM, Johnson CP; American Academy of Pediatrics Council on Children With Disabilities. Management of children with autism spectrum disorders. Pediatrics. 2007;120(5):1162-82.
2. Kodak T, Carroll RA. Substantiated and unsubstantiated interventions for individuals with ASD. In: Matson JL (Ed). Handbook of Treatments for Autism Spectrum Disorder. Berlin: Springer International Publishing; 2017. pp. 17-40.
3. American Psychiatric Association. Diagnostic and Statistical Manual of Mental Disorders, 5th edition. Washington DC; 2013.
4. Bitta M, Kariuki SM, Abubakar A, Newton CRJC. Burden of neurodevelopmental disorders in low and middle-income countries: A systematic review and meta-analysis. Wellcome Open Res. 2017;2:121.
5. Boivin MJ, Kakooza AM, Warf BC, Davidson LL, Grigorenko EL. Reducing neurodevelopmental disorders and disability through research and interventions. Nature. 2015.527(7578): S155-S160.
6. Accardo J, Shapiro BK. Neurodevelopmental Disabilities: Beyond the Diagnosis. Semin Pediatr Neurol. 2005;12(4):242-9.
7. Thapar A, Cooper M, Rutter M. Neuro-developmental disorders. Lancet Psychiatry. 2017;4(4):339-46.
8. Lord C, Risi S, Pickles A. Trajectory of language development in autistic spectrum disorders. In: Rice ML, Warren SF (Eds). Developmental Language Disorders. New York: Psychology Press; 2004. pp. 18-41.

9. Schaaf RC, Miller LJ. Occupational therapy using a sensory integrative approach for children with developmental disabilities. Ment Retard Dev Disabil Res Rev. 2005;11(2):143-8.
10. Baranek GT. Efficacy of Sensory and Motor Interventions for Children with Autism. J Autism Dev Disord. 2002;32(5):397-422.
11. Hornby G. Inclusive Special Education. New York: Springer; 2014.
12. Murphy K. Psychosocial treatments for ADHD in teens and adults: A practice-friendly review. J Clin Psychol. 2005;61(5):607-19.
13. Cioni G, Inguaggiato E, Sgandurra G. Early intervention in neurodevelopmental disorders: underlying neural mechanisms. Dev Med Child Neurol. 2016;58(S4):61-6.
14. Karanth P. Shaista S. Srikanth N. Efficacy of Communication DEALL—An indigenous early intervention program for children with autism spectrum disorders. Indian J Pediatr. 2010;77:957-62.
15. Fuller EA, Oliver K, Vejnoska SF, Rogers SJ. The Effects of the Early Start Denver Model for Children with Autism Spectrum Disorder: A Meta-Analysis. Brain Sci. 2020;10(6):368.
16. Mesibov GB, Shea V. The TEACCH program in the era of evidence-based practice. J Autism Dev Disord. 2010;40(5):570-9.
17. Reichow B, Barton EE, Boyd BA, Hume K. Early intensive behavioral intervention (EIBI) for young children with autism spectrum disorders (ASD): A systematic review. Campbell Syst Rev. 2014;10(1):1-116.
18. Guralnick MJ. Why Early Intervention Works: A Systems Perspective. Infants Young Child. 2011;24(1):6-28.
19. Guinchat V, Cravero C, Lefèvre-Utile J, Cohen D. Multidisciplinary treatment plan for challenging behaviors in neurodevelopmental disorders. Handb Clin Neurol. 2020;174:301-21.
20. Horner RH, Carr EG, Strain PS, Todd AW, Reed HK. Problem behavior interventions for young children with autism: a research synthesis. J Autism Dev Disord. 2002;32(5):423-46.
21. Bregman JD, Zager D, Gerdtz J. Behavioral interventions. In: Volkmar FR, Rogers SJ, Paul R, Pelphrey KA (Eds). Handbook of Autism and Pervasive Developmental Disorders, Assessment, Interventions, and Policy. Hoboken, NJ: John Wiley & Sons; 2014.
22. Wilkenfeld DA, McCarthy AM. Ethical Concerns with Applied Behavior Analysis for Autism Spectrum "Disorder." Kennedy Inst Ethics J. 2020;30(1):31-69.
23. Leaf JB, Cihon JH, Leaf R, McEachin J, Liu N, Russell N, et al. Concerns About ABA-Based Intervention: An Evaluation and Recommendations. J Autism Dev Disord. 2022;52(6):2838-2853. Erratum in: J Autism Dev Disord. 2022;52(6):2854.
24. Leaf JB, Cihon JH, Weinkauf SM, Oppenheim-Leaf ML, Taubman M, Leaf R. Parent training for parents of individuals diagnosed with autism spectrum disorder. In: Matson JL (Ed). Handbook of Treatments for Autism Spectrum Disorder. Berlin: Springer International Publishing; 2017. pp. 109-25.
25. Cullenward J, Curtin M, Santos VD. Characteristics of effective parent-mediated interventions for parents of children with neurodevelopmental disorders in rural areas: a systematic review protocol. BMJ Open. 2024;14(8):e083464.
26. Ge D, Wei H, Wang Y, Li Y, Luo J, Liu X, et al. Effectiveness of caregiver-mediated intervention: a pilot study for children with neurodevelopmental disorders. Prim Health Care Res Dev. 2022;23:e63.
27. Daly BP, Creed T, Xanthopoulos M, Brown RT. Psychosocial Treatments for Children with Attention Deficit/Hyperactivity Disorder. Neuropsychol Rev. 2007;17(1):73-89.
28. Dawson G, Burner K. Behavioral interventions in children and adolescents with autism spectrum disorder: a review of recent findings. Curr Opin Pediatr. 2011;23(6):616-20.
29. Weiss MJ, Harris SL. Teaching social skills to people with autism. Behav Modif. 2001;25(5):785-802.
30. Reichow B, Steiner AM, Volkmar F. Social skills groups for people aged 6 to 21 with autism spectrum disorders (ASD). Campbell Syst Rev. 2012;8(1):1-76.

CHAPTER 27

Psychopharmacology in Children and Adolescents-I: General Principles

Harshini Manohar, Dhamodhara Pandian

INTRODUCTION

Psychopharmacology is an essential part of the multimodal intervention approach to treating children and adolescents* with mental health and neurodevelopmental conditions.[1] There are significant gaps between research and clinical practice in pediatric psychopharmacology, despite evident advancements. For instance, methylphenidate has been shown to be effective in treating attention-deficit/hyperactivity disorder (ADHD) in >100 placebo-controlled trials; however, the long-term effects of this medication have only been assessed in a small number of methodologically rigorous studies.[2] Selective serotonin reuptake inhibitors (SSRIs) have been shown to be safe and effective in treating obsessive-compulsive disorder (OCD) in children; however, existing research does not inform the required duration of long-term prophylaxis and its effectiveness in this age group.[3] Over the past 20 years, there has been a significant increase in the prescription of psychotropic drugs to pediatric population, despite the fact that empirical basis for pediatric psychopharmacology is still developing.[4] However, in the last 10 years, a number of controlled clinical trials have been undertaken for various prevalent psychiatric disorders in children, forming the groundwork for development of evidence-based treatment guidelines, thereby impacting the rate of advancement in this field.[5]

*Here on referred to as children (<18 years of age).

WHAT DOES THIS CHAPTER OFFER?

This chapter aims to provide an overview of clinical psychopharmacology's broad concepts for pediatric population. This chapter examines and evaluates the psychotropic drugs currently used to treat children based on their pharmacology, side effects, therapeutic uses, empirical support that is available, and their clinical applications. Pharmacokinetic principles such as medication interactions, mechanisms of action, and pharmacodynamic concerns are briefly discussed. Pharmacotherapeutic management of specific disorders is beyond the scope of this chapter. The readers may refer to the specific chapters and clinical practice guidelines for the same.

INTERPLAY OF DEVELOPMENT, NEUROBIOLOGY, AND TREATMENT

Child development is profoundly influenced by the quality of caregiver-child relationships, as well as familial, child care, community, and cultural contexts, all of which can impact the clinical presentation, case formulation, and treatment plan.[6] Regardless of the setting, developing a rational treatment plan requires thorough history-taking and mental status examination to establish a *comprehensive biopsychosocial formulation* that will inform an individualized treatment plan. Pharmacotherapy is one of the aspects of the multimodal approach that can assist in addressing the critical biopsychosocial factors, informed by biological underpinnings of mental health conditions and target symptom dimensions.

Key elements of practicing pediatric psychopharmacology include understanding the impact on the developing brain, neurobiology of mental health conditions, differential mechanisms on brain function in children, and the target symptom dimensions (goals of intervention). The interaction among these factors determines the potential benefits and risks of treatment. Ethical and regulatory considerations are particularly important when treating young patients, in both clinical care and research. Extrapolating findings from studies involving adult population is not sufficient for guiding pediatric pharmacotherapy. It is crucial to understand the differences in how drugs are processed in a developing body (pharmacokinetics), how the developing brain responds to them (pharmacodynamics), and how mental health conditions present during specific developmental stages all impact the safety, tolerability, and effectiveness of treatment, both in the short and the long-term. Beyond research studies on stimulants for ADHD, SSRIs for OCD, major depression, and childhood anxiety disorders, risperidone for behavioral disturbances in children with autism, much of clinical practice is supported by limited controlled studies and relies heavily on findings from adult literature, case reports, and clinical experience. Additionally, there is a lack of literature examining medication therapies for comorbid conditions, and the justification for research-supported co-pharmacy[#] is essentially nonexistent.[7]

SECULAR TRENDS IN PRESCRIPTION PRACTICES

A new era has begun in child psychiatry sparked by an increased demand for comprehensive and credible evidence supporting the use of medications in youth.[8] In the last decade, dramatic increases in psychotropic prescriptions to children and adolescents have expanded ongoing concerns about safety and efficacy to include criticisms of evidence supporting their use.[9]

Pharmacoepidemiology studies assessing disorder-specific prescription patterns have provided critical insights. A study assessing prescription patterns over a 12 year period (1999–2010) in the US, reported the prevalence of any-class and multiclass psychotropic polypharmacy grew steadily from 21.2% and 18.8% in 1999–2000 to 27.3% and 24.4% in 2009–2010, respectively, with higher estimates for older adolescents.[10] A Canadian study assessing prescription patterns from 2012 to 2016 reported prescriptions for antipsychotics decreased by 10% from 2010 to 2016, in contrast to a 114% increase observed between 2005 and 2009. Prescriptions for psychostimulants and antidepressants rose by 35% and 27%, respectively, prescriptions for antipsychotics for autism increased by 34% over the study period.[11] A meta-analysis of 59 studies across 23 countries reported a pooled prevalence of 15.3% for ADHD medications, 6.4% antidepressants, and 5.5% for antipsychotics. Large increases were found in the prevalence of ADHD medications in most countries, a U-shaped trend for antidepressants with the lowest prevalence in 2007–2009 and rise more recently, and increases in the prevalence of antipsychotics until 2011, with declining trends found recently.[12] Prescription patterns for ADHD and pediatric bipolar disorders were the subject of intense debate.

Prescription patterns are practice and experience-informed and are related to effects and side effects, availability of new agents, and

[#]Co-pharmacy is different from polypharmacy. Co-pharmacy is essential in cases where there is high severity or high comorbidity. Polypharmacy (use of multiple medications to manage the same problem) must be avoided.

acceptability among the families. These contextual factors are crucial in addition to treatment guidelines and practice parameters. There is paucity of data in the Indian context regarding prescription patterns and experiences of (child and adolescent) psychiatrists.

GENERAL PRINCIPLES IN PEDIATRIC PSYCHOPHARMACOLOGY

- Pharmacotherapy is rarely a standalone treatment. Pharmacotherapy is effective for indicated conditions, alongside psychological, psychosocial and developmental interventions, focusing on the child and the family. Combination treatment is "gold standard" in child psychiatric disorders, and practice guidelines such as National Institute for Health and Care Excellence (NICE), American Academy of Child and Adolescent Psychiatry (AACAP) strongly recommend the same.
- Target symptom-focused, dimensional approach may be helpful. While having a working diagnosis can aid in setting expectations and communicating with patients and parents, it is important to recognize that the mental health conditions in children may evolve over time. Comorbidities present additional challenges in diagnostic ascertainment.
- Regarding prescribing medications to children, it is essential for healthcare providers to ensure that sufficient evidence supports the safety, efficacy, and intended use of the drug, even if it involves off-label use.
- Considering developmental aspects is crucial, starting with lower doses (lower than minimal effective doses for adults) and gradually increasing while closely monitoring for both effectiveness and adverse reactions, which are more common in young people, compared to adults. Additional caution should be considered in children and youth atypical neurodevelopment (intellectual disability, autism, and neurological disorders).
- Assess for comorbid conditions, and the influence of comorbid conditions on the illness course and response to medications. Preference for a particular drug is to be considered keeping in mind the comorbidity, e.g., a child with ADHD and comorbid mood disorder may be started on methylphenidate after substantive management of mood disorder (sequential management).
- Though monotherapy is preferred, in cases of resistant or refractory illness, a combination of medications may be necessary, and has to be planned with due consideration. Management of comorbidities or multiple symptom dimensions with different medication classes may be required, and is referred to as co-pharmacy. Co-pharmacy is essential in cases where there is high severity or high comorbidity. Polypharmacy (use of multiple medications to manage the same problem) must be avoided.
- Adequate trial at an optimal dose is required, before considering nonresponse. Standard guidelines recommend 8 weeks for depression and schizophrenia, 12 weeks for OCD.
- Combining psychological and psychosocial interventions with medication is essential at all stages.
- Patience is key, as children may require longer treatment periods before responding, and changes to medication should be made one at a time whenever possible. Combination of higher doses of medications should be avoided.
- It is important to monitor treatment outcomes across different settings, as symptoms may vary. Providing education to patients and families about their medications, potential side effects, adherence, and open communication regarding treatment adjustments is crucial,

especially considering that some patients may require long-term medication management.[13]

- Informed consent from parents and assent from children should be taken. Actively involving children in the decision-making process regarding pharmacotherapy is crucial.
- Consider the child's developmental activities such as school timings, while planning the medication regimen, e.g., medications with sedating effects can be avoided during school hours or during therapy sessions.

Pharmacokinetics

It is important to understand the pharmacokinetic and pharmacodynamic principles that are operating in the given developmental stage. As children develop, the processes of drug absorption, distribution, metabolism, and excretion undergo significant changes. This means that simply extrapolating medication doses and administration frequencies from adult data can result in inappropriate treatment for children. Despite children having smaller bodies overall, their liver and kidney tissue, relative to body weight, is proportionally greater than that of adults.[14] Children also exhibit relatively higher proportions of body water, lower levels of fat, and reduced plasma albumin, which serves as a binding site for drugs. Consequently, the volume of distribution of medications typically tends to be larger in children compared to adults. Due to these variances, children experience greater drug extraction during the initial passage through the liver, leading to lower bioavailability, and undergo faster metabolism and elimination processes. Therefore, merely reducing adult doses based on a child's weight may lead to inadequate treatment.

During adolescence, alongside significant increases in body size, there are notable shifts in the distribution of body compartments. In males, the proportion of total body water increases while body fat decreases, whereas the reverse happens in females. This leads to various pharmacokinetic differences between children and adults (**Table 1**).

TABLE 1: Pharmacokinetic characteristics in children relative to adults.

Liver and kidney mass adjusted for body weight	Greater	Higher doses recommended
Metabolism and elimination	Faster	Frequent doses recommended
Dosing	Higher and more frequent	–
Elimination half-life	Shorter	Frequent doses recommended
Plasma steady-state	Achieved sooner	–
Withdrawal symptoms	More likely	Frequent doses recommended

Following absorption, most drugs undergo biotransformation, or metabolism, which converts the parent compound into more polar metabolites that are easier to eliminate. Phase I oxidative processes are facilitated by cytochrome P450 (CYP450) microsomal enzymes, primarily located in the liver. At birth, the CYP450 system is underdeveloped, but it matures rapidly, reaching about 20% of its adult capacity by one month of age and achieving full maturity by 3 years. Children, having proportionally more liver tissue than adults, possess a higher weight-adjusted metabolic capacity, and hence higher rates of metabolism.

In pediatric psychopharmacology, the most crucial CYP450 enzymes are CYP3A4 and CYP2D6, responsible for metabolizing many psychotropic drugs, along with CYP2C9 and CYP2C19. Certain psychotropic medications can also function as inhibitors of these enzymes, leading to reduced metabolism and higher drug concentrations in the body when administered concurrently with other drugs that are substrates for the enzyme. For instance, fluoxetine or fluvoxamine can inhibit CYP3A4 enzymes.

Concurrent use of fluvoxamine (a 3A4 inhibitor) with quetiapine or aripiprazole (metabolized by 3A4) may result in elevated levels of quetiapine or aripiprazole, potentially prolonging the QTc interval. Furthermore, some medications such as carbamazepine and phenobarbital can induce CYP3A4 activity, thereby enhancing its metabolic capacity. When administered together with a medication metabolized by CYP3A4, such as various anticonvulsants, antipsychotics, tricyclic antidepressants (TCAs), clonazepam, and oral contraceptives, carbamazepine can lead to lower blood levels of these drugs.

The primary method of drug elimination is through the kidneys. While absolute clearance tends to be lower in children compared to adults, when adjusted for weight, clearance is typically greater in children. Due to faster elimination rates, the drug plasma half-life in children can be shorter than that in adults.[15] A shorter elimination half-life indicates that plasma steady-state is achieved more rapidly with repeated drug administration and increases the likelihood of withdrawal symptoms upon discontinuation. To prevent such symptoms between doses, more frequent administration may be necessary to maintain consistent therapeutic levels. Additionally, for certain medications, both the dose and duration of treatment can impact pharmacokinetics. For example, in adolescents, the mean half-life of sertraline is approximately 27 hours after a single 50 mg dose, but with repeated administration, it decreases to around 15 hours.[16] Furthermore, when administering lower doses (50 mg/day) of sertraline, it is advisable to give them twice a day to maintain consistent treatment and minimize withdrawal symptoms. In contrast, higher doses (100–150 mg) can be administered once daily. Research on the pharmacokinetics of many psychotropic medications, including escitalopram, aripiprazole, quetiapine, risperidone, and lithium, has shown similar profiles in children and adolescents compared to adults.[17]

Nevertheless, significant intersubject variability has been noted, leading to major individual differences in the pharmacological effects over time in clinical settings. Methylphenidate and amphetamines, with their short half-lives necessitating multiple daily administrations, have prompted the development of various extended-release formulations. Practitioners must remain updated to effectively manage the diverse needs of patients.

Pharmacodynamics

Majority of psychotropic medications exert their effects by targeting neurotransmitters such as dopamine, serotonin, glutamate, gamma-aminobutyric acid (GABA), and norepinephrine, whose receptors undergo significant alterations throughout development. Receptor density typically peaks during the preschool years and gradually decreases toward adult levels by late adolescence.[18]

The effects of developmental changes on drug activity, efficacy, and safety remain incompletely understood **(Table 2)**. However, disparities observed between children and adults in terms of efficacy and safety indicate that development can substantially impact the effects of psychotropic medications. For instance, while TCAs have been established as effective in treating adult depression, they do not demonstrate antidepressant effects in children.[19] Amphetamine-based stimulants are more prone to inducing euphoria in adults than in children. Antipsychotic medications exert stronger metabolic effects in youth compared to adults;[20] serotonergic antidepressants elevate the risk of suicidal ideation in children, adolescents, and young adults, but not in middle-aged or elderly individuals.[21]

The response to various psychotropic medications is influenced by the developmental stage. For instance, methylphenidate's tolerability and efficacy in children with ADHD between 3 and

TABLE 2: *Psychotropic drug groups:* Pharmacodynamic differences between children and adults.

Drug group	*Children*	*Adults*
Serotonergic antidepressants	Increase the risk of suicidal Ideation (black box warning)	Do not increase the risk after age 25
Antipsychotics	Relatively greater metabolic side effects	Relatively lower metabolic side effects
Amphetamine-based stimulants	Less likely to induce euphoria	More likely to induce euphoria
Methylphenidate	Lower tolerability and efficacy in children with ADHD aged 3–5 years	Higher tolerability and efficacy in adults and children with ADHD above the age of 5 years
Lithium	Comparatively lesser efficacy in pediatric BPAD	Better efficacy in adult onset BPAD
Tricyclic antidepressants	Not effective for pediatric depression	Effective for adult depression

(ADHD: attention-deficit/hyperactivity disorder; BPAD: bipolar affective disorder)

5 years old are lower compared to older children.[2,22,23] Evidence regarding the effectiveness of SSRIs for treating compulsive and repetitive behaviors in children with autism is mixed. However, there is some support for using SSRIs to address repetitive behaviors in adults with autism spectrum disorder (ASD) based on a small number of studies.[24] This highlights the necessity for research tailored to specific patient population.

Pharmacogenomics

Genetic polymorphisms have been identified for CYP450 enzymes, with about 7–10% of Caucasians, 1–8% of Africans, and 1–3% of East Asians being poor CYP2D6 metabolizers of specific medications. Poor metabolizers tend to have higher drug concentrations in plasma and other body tissues. For example, the elimination half-life of atomoxetine is around 5 hours in fast metabolizers but can extend to 22 hours in poor metabolizers, whether children or adults.[25] While genetic testing for polymorphism is not typically standard in current child psychiatry practice, it could be considered for specific patients who fail to respond to appropriate medication doses or exhibit unusual reactions to drugs metabolized by enzymes with genetic variability, such as 2D6 and 2C19. An Indian study on pharmacogenetics of lithium response among individuals with early-onset bipolar disorder reported preliminary findings of association with specific single nucleotide polymorphisms, however, requires replication in larger samples.[26]

GOOD PRACTICE PARAMETERS IN PEDIATRIC PSYCHOPHARMACOLOGY

This section describes the guiding principles in choosing a particular molecule for a condition/indication, factors, and processes that require due consideration.

Choosing a Molecule

Disorder-specific versus Target Symptom-Specific Approach

For disorders such as the early-onset bipolar disorder, schizophrenia, and OCD, the phenomenology and the clinical diagnosis inform treatment approach and an algorithm for pharmacotherapy that is evidence based.[27] In some cases, clinicians may feel pressured by parental or societal expectations to pursue nonevidence-based interventions or treatments in a desperate attempt to alter the course of a neurodevelopmental or psychiatric condition.

In disorders such as ASD, the core features such as sociocommunication cannot be addressed by pharmacotherapeutic interventions, however, symptoms dimensions such as hyperactivity, irritability, stereotypies, aggression, self-injurious behavior, and comorbid disorders such as depression and obsessive-compulsive behaviors respond to effective and judicious use of pharmacotherapy.[28] Stimulants have been employed to address attentional difficulties, while SSRIs are used for obsessional thoughts and repetitive behaviors. Additionally, atypical antipsychotics, anticonvulsants, and mood stabilizers, have been utilized to manage aggression observed in ASD, though supported by limited evidence.[4,28]

The following situations support the adoption of a target-symptom focused approach—(1) when the presentation exhibits multiple phenotypes, and/or when its underlying cause is poorly understood, target-symptom approaches become advantageous. For instance, mood dysregulation, a transdiagnostic phenomenon, characterized by symptoms like irritability, can serve as a target for pharmacological treatment, irrespective of the diagnostic categories.[4,29] (2) When the mechanism of action of a psychopharmacologic medication in a particular disorder is poorly understood and does not directly align with the underlying disorder, employing a target-symptom approach becomes more beneficial.[4,30] Clinical trials evaluating risperidone and aripiprazole for irritability associated with neurodevelopmental disorders like autism have led to the acceptance of target-symptom focused approach.[30]

Evidence-based Practice in Children

- *Stimulants:* The efficacy of stimulants for short-term treatment of ADHD is extensively documented and represents the most substantial body of evidence in pediatric psychopharmacology.[2] Research consistently demonstrates positive responses in core ADHD symptoms, with some studies also reporting improvement in comorbid externalizing disorders and reduction in aggression. Controlled studies also provide evidence supporting the efficacy of mixed amphetamine salts, however, amphetamines are not available in India.[31-33] Methylphenidate is FDA approved for use in individuals aged 6 years and older, safety and efficacy supported by the Preschool ADHD Treatment Study (PATS).[23] Dextroamphetamine is approved for use in those aged 3 years and older.
- *Alternative to stimulant medications:* Atomoxetine, a noradrenergic reuptake inhibitor, has demonstrated efficacy in treating ADHD in both pediatric and adult populations.[34] Noteworthy benefits of atomoxetine include its ability to provide round-the-clock coverage with once-daily dosing and its nonabuse potential. Additionally, it holds FDA approval for the treatment of ADHD in children aged 6 years and older, and contraindicated in children <6 years in view of potential hepatotoxicity. Clonidine and guanfacine are approved for ADHD in children.[35]
- Antidepressants
- *SSRIs:* The strongest evidence indicates that SSRIs and clomipramine are the most effective treatments for OCD. Fluvoxamine and sertraline obtained FDA approval for pediatric OCD treatment in 1997, with indications extending to children as young as 8 and 6 years of age, respectively. Additionally, there is research supporting the efficacy of SSRIs in treating various depression and other anxiety disorders.[36]
- *Heterocyclic antidepressants:* Although bupropion and TCAs have not demonstrated efficacy in treating anxiety or mood disorders

aside from OCD, they have been found effective for ADHD. Concerns about TCAs, particularly their side effect profile, especially regarding cardiotoxicity, is not commonly considered in children. Additionally, controlled studies indicate the efficacy of TCAs for enuresis,[37] although their effect is solely symptomatic and not curative.

- *Antipsychotics:* There is a scarcity of studies investigating the efficacy of antipsychotics in early-onset psychotic disorders. Atypical antipsychotics are reported to be effective in pediatric bipolar disorders.[38] A multicenter study coordinated through the Research Units on Pediatric Psychopharmacology (RUPP) network found risperidone beneficial in managing aggression and self-injurious behaviors in children with ASD.[30] Similar positive responses have been observed in children with intellectual disabilities and externalizing behaviours.[39] Historically, antipsychotic agents were frequently overprescribed in individuals with intellectual disabilities and developmental disorders. Low-dose regimens, over a shorter time-duration (6–12 weeks), with careful monitoring of side effects, are recommended over higher doses.[39]
- *Mood stabilizers:* Despite the absence of controlled trials, there has been a significant rise in the use of mood stabilizers in youth within clinical settings,[40] partly attributed to the growing number of youths diagnosed with bipolar disorder, a subject of considerable controversy. Currently, only a limited number of studies have investigated the efficacy of lithium in youths with mania.[41] Valproate, as a second line, often recommended as monotherapy or with an atypical antipsychotic, demonstrate effectiveness, but it poses risks such as weight gain, polycystic ovarian disease, impaired male fertility, and teratogenic risk through paternal exposure to valproate.[42] Despite its potential to reduce aggression, especially in young individuals with bipolar disorder, cautious deliberation is necessary regarding its utilization due to possible adverse outcomes.[42,43] Presently, there is insufficient high-quality data concerning the efficacy and acceptability of oxcarbazepine in treating acute bipolar disorder.[43] Lamotrigine (LAM) is safe and efficacious for treating mood disorders in children, however, there is a dearth of data concerning the ideal therapeutic dosage range for LAM in this demographic.[44]
- *α-adrenergic agonists:* Although α-adrenergic agonists are commonly prescribed for ADHD and behavioral issues, there are only a limited number of small controlled studies supporting the effectiveness of clonidine for ADHD. An Indian study reported, clonidine as the primary choice for 84% of children due to factors such as affordability and comorbid conditions where methylphenidate is contraindicated.[45] Sedation although reported as the most common adverse effect, it was well tolerated in preschool children. One multicentered controlled trial discovered that clonidine, both alone and in combination with methylphenidate, improved both tics and ADHD symptoms, with combined therapy showing the best outcomes for ADHD symptoms.[46]
- *Long-acting injectables in the Indian context:* Limited research indicates promising effectiveness and acceptable safety and tolerability of long-acting injectable antipsychotics in adolescents with severe mental illness (SMI). However, there is a notable absence of research investigating their usage in children under the age of 12.[47] A 10-year review of first-generation depot antipsychotic utilization in youth at a tertiary care center in India demonstrated positive treatment response, although nearly half of the subjects (47.4%) encountered at least one

acute adverse event such as tremors, rigidity, excessive salivation, and bradykinesia. Indications for the use of LAIA were failure or partial response to multiple oral medication trials (65.8%), severe, current aggression, resistant to oral or short-acting antipsychotics (34.2%), and noncompliance with oral medication (31.6%).[48]

Use of FDA Approved/Guideline Recommended Drugs versus Off-label Use

The majority of medications are approved for marketing based on favorable benefit-to-risk assessments from clinical trial data in adults. Pediatric medical practice has largely relied on off-label use, meaning that the drug was not specifically indicated for this age group or condition in the FDA-approved product label. Off-label use of drugs is widespread, accounting for approximately 50–75% of pediatric medication use.[49] Off-label use does not mean use despite contraindications, but use of a drug for indications apart from approved ones, based on the clinician's judgment of its appropriateness.

Being off-label does not prohibit the use of the molecule in children, allowing practitioners to prescribe the drug as they see fit. Nonetheless, clinicians should be aware that despite their widespread use, such off-label treatments may be perceived as standard treatments, potentially leading individuals who are wary of experimental treatments in clinical trials to prefer these inadequately evaluated but commonly used treatments **(Table 3)**.[50]

Pre-treatment Assessments and Discussions

Informed consent and assent: In pediatric psychopharmacology, the prescription of psychotropic medication is a contentious issue due to legal and ethical differences in consent between children and adults. Children cannot legally consent to treatment, leaving the decision-making responsibility to their parents, which can present challenges for psychiatrists. Children should be educated about their condition and potential treatments according to their cognitive and emotional capabilities, and actively involved in the decision making. Psychiatrists often face pressure from various parties, including parents and community members, who may have differing opinions on medication use, and therapeutic misconception is an important phenomenon.[52] Despite the myriad challenges, psychiatrists are tasked with integrating information from various sources to formulate appropriate treatment plans and often serve as "advocates" for the child. Stigma associated with psychiatric treatment, particularly medication, is a concern for patients and families. Educating children and parents about the diagnosis, target symptoms for suggested medication, is beneficial, but if resistance to medication arises and the issues are not acute, allowing families to pursue treatment methods they are comfortable with, may be advisable. It is the prescribing clinician's duty to inform the child and the parents about the anticipated benefits and risks associated with medication, and aid in informed decision making. Additionally, parents play a crucial role in facilitating pharmacotherapy by ensuring the proper administration of prescribed medication and promptly reporting any treatment-related adverse effects.

Discussions related to initiating and continuing pharmacotherapy should be considered as a "process" that needs to be revisited, especially in the context of long-term prophylaxis or maintenance treatment. The informed parental consent and child's assent should be documented in the case notes. Similarly, in case of dissent, the psychiatrist should document the reasons, and the plan to revisit the discussion with the child and the family if deemed necessary.[53]

Operationalizing outcomes: Before initiating psychotropic medications, it is essential to conduct a comprehensive assessment of the individual's

TABLE 3: Psychotropic drug use by their FDA approved and off-label status.[51]

Class/subclass	*Drug*	*Age (in years)*	*Indication*	*Off-label use in pediatric population*
Stimulants	Amphetamines*	3+	ADHD; narcolepsy	Treatment-resistant depression in adults
	Methylphenidate	6+	ADHD	
	Modafinil	16+	Narcolepsy, OSA	ADHD
	Atomoxetine	6+	ADHD	Treatment-resistant depression
Antipsychotics: Typical	Chlorpromazine		Severe behavior problems*, hyperactivity*, aggression, intractable hiccups	Psychosis, agitation, delirium
	Haloperidol		Tourette syndrome, severe behavior problems,* hyperactivity*	
	Pimozide	8+	Tourette syndrome	
	• Trifluoperazine • Fluphenazine	–	–	Psychotic disorders, aggression
Antipsychotics: Atypical	Aripiprazole	13+	Schizophrenia	• Other psychotic disorders, behavioral dysregulation in children, disorders associated with impulse control, aggression • Depression/OCD—adjunct • Maintenance in schizophrenia and BPAD • Quetiapine and olanzapine—maintenance for bipolar depression
		10+	Acute and mixed mania (BPAD I)	
		6+	Irritability in autism, Tourette syndrome	
	Risperidone	13+	Schizophrenia	
		10+	Acute and mixed mania	
		5+	Irritability in autism	
	Olanzapine	13+	BPAD type 1, Schizophrenia	
		10+	Bipolar depression (in combination with fluoxetine)	
	Quetiapine	13+	Schizophrenia	
		10+	Acute and mixed mania (BPAD I)	
	Asenapine	10+	Acute and mixed mania (BPAD I)	
	Paliperidone	12+	Schizophrenia	
	Clozapine			Treatment-resistant schizophrenia, reduction of suicidal risk in schizophrenia, treatment resistant BPAD, aggression

Contd...

Contd...

Class/subclass	*Drug*	*Age (in years)*	*Indication*	*Off-label use in pediatric population*
	Lurasidone	13+ 10+	• Schizophrenia • Bipolar depression	Bipolar disorder
Antidepressants: SSRIs and SNRIs	Fluoxetine	8+	Depression	Treatment-resistant depression, bulimia nervosa, anxiety disorders
		7+	OCD	
		10+	Bipolar depression (in combination with olanzapine)	
	Fluvoxamine	8+	OCD	Depression, anxiety disorders
	Sertraline	6+		
	Escitalopram	12+	Depression	OCD, anxiety disorders
	• Citalopram • Duloxetine • Paroxetine			Depression, dysthymia, anxiety disorders
	Bupropion	-	-	Depression, anxiety, ADHD
	Venlafaxine			Depression, OCD, ADHD
	Mirtazapine			Depression, sleep
Antidepressants: TCA	Clomipramine	10+	OCD	
	Imipramine	6+	Enuresis	
		12+	Depression	
	Lithium			Acute mania (BPAD), maintenance treatment for BPAD
Mood stabilizers	Divalproex, carbamazepine, oxcarbazepine.	–	–	Bipolar disorder; aggression
	Lamotrigine			
Alpha-2 agonist	Clonidine, guanfacine	6+	ADHD	Sleep, aggression in ODD and CD, Tourette's syndrome, substance withdrawal, anxiety, PTSD

Note: *Second line

(ADHD: attention-deficit/hyperactivity disorder; BPAD: bipolar affective disorder; CD: conduct disorder; ODD: oppositional defiant disorder; OSA: obstructive sleep apnea; PTSD: post-traumatic stress disorder; SNRIs: serotonin and norepinephrine reuptake inhibitors; SSRIs: selective serotonin reuptake inhibitors; TCA: tricyclic antidepressant)

health status, including symptom severity and impairment ratings. "Operationalizing outcomes" is an essential aspect of treatment planning as symptoms are contributed and maintained by various environmental factors and comorbidities as well, e.g., (1) in a child with bipolar affective disorder (BPAD) and comorbid ADHD, treatment of mood disorder with antipsychotic should be followed by targeted treatment for ADHD symptoms based on severity and functional impairment. (2) In a child with ID and comorbid OCD, SSRIs may help reduce the severity of OCD alone and not result in overall reduction in functional impairment that is attributed to intellectual abilities.

Baseline and follow-up assessments of symptom severity and outcome measures will aid in making decisions related to pharmacotherapy.

Periodic monitoring of treatment-emergent side effects: Following the initiation of drug therapy, regular safety and tolerability assessments are important to monitor the continued effects of medication use **(Table 4)**. Adjustments to dosage and changes in concurrent drug therapy may prompt biological status checks, including laboratory assessments and vital sign

TABLE 4: Recommended pretreatment evaluation and periodic monitoring.

Drug class	*Drug*	*Adverse events*	*Specific comments on pretreatment evaluation and periodic monitoring*
Alpha-agonists	Clonidine Guanfacine	Bradycardia; hypo-tension; and heart block	Rule out congenital heart disease; ECG, blood pressure and heart rate at baseline and follow-up
Stimulants	Amphetamines, methylphenidate	Serious cardiovascular risk[54]	Blood pressure and heart rate; ECG where there is a question of congenital heart disease
Anticonvulsant-mood stabilizer	Divalproex; valproic acid	Polycystic ovaries in girls; malformation rate of 11.1% compared with 3.1% in nondrug exposed fetuses; hepatotoxicity; pancreatitis[42,55,56]	Discuss risks and provide written information before initiating therapy; close laboratory monitoring of liver enzymes and coagulation tests in the first 6 months; clinical monitoring for vomiting and apathy; blood levels.[42] Should be avoided in women of child bearing age; should be counseled regarding birth control if valproate is considered
	Lamotrigine	Rash requiring hospitalization, possible Stevens–Johnson syndrome or hypersensitivity syndrome; serum concentrations doubled when divalproex was added in adjunctive treatment of epilepsy or as a mood stabilizer	Indication in those younger than 16 is restricted to Lennox–Gastaut syndrome. Black box warning for potentially life-threatening rashes. Careful dose titration as per prescribed guidelines and monitoring for rashes (benign rash and SJS)
Antidepressants	SSRIs	Activation syndrome, suicidality[57]	A written diary by the parent of target symptoms and selected adverse events is useful. Regular contact to review information when drug or dose is initiated or changed. Monitor side effects and response regularly
	TCAs	Dose-dependent cardiac conduction delays; asystole	Baseline and follow-up ECG at therapeutic dose, blood levels
	Bupropion	Dose-dependent risk of seizure	Consider alternatives in youth with a history of seizure disorders or bulimia

Contd...

Contd...

Drug class	*Drug*	*Adverse events*	*Specific comments on pretreatment evaluation and periodic monitoring*
Atypical antipsychotics	Olanzapine, risperidone, quetiapine, ziprasidone	Relatively greater weight gain in youth than in adults, extrapyramidal side effects (EPS), hyperprolactinemia, thyroid dysfunction (quetiapine)	Baseline and repeat weight, height and waist circumference, serum fasting lipid and hepatic enzyme levels, and thyroid panel (for quetiapine). Fasting glucose level monitoring for the risk of diabetes; diet and exercise management. Monitor quarterly or as indicated for movement disorders with the Abnormal Involuntary Movement Scale (AIMS). Prolactin blood level monitoring in the presence of amenorrhea, galactorrhea, headache, visual disturbances, etc.
	Clozapine	Relatively greater risk tachycardia, orthostatic shifts and QTc interval prolongation was noted in some patients necessitating cautious titration. Although risk of neutropenia is found to be higher that adults incidence of agranulocytosis remained low	Before starting clozapine treatment, conduct liver function tests, an electrocardiogram, and a general physical exam, including a baseline cardiac assessment. Maintain ANC levels above 1,500/mm^3. Monitor for myocarditis, especially during the first 6 weeks, with baseline and weekly troponin and CRP measurements. Discontinue clozapine if troponin levels exceed twice the upper limit of normal or if CRP levels exceed 100 mg/L. Consider annual echocardiograms to monitor for cardiomyopathy. Conduct metabolic tests before initiation, with closer monitoring in children and adolescents. Monitor weight gain against expected growth using pediatric height/weight charts. After initiation, perform monthly BMI measurements for 3 months, then quarterly. Monitor fasting triglycerides monthly for several months to detect metabolic changes early
Lithium	Lithium	Thyroid abnormalities; nephrotoxicity; renal concentration diminution; lithium toxicity	Lithium levels, baseline thyroid panel, serum creatinine, and urinalysis. Repeat periodically, and when dose or regimen changes or symptoms suggest toxicity

(ANC: absolute neutrophil count; BMI: body mass index; CRP: C-reactive protein; ECG: electrocardiography; SSRI: selective serotonin reuptake inhibitor; TCA: tricyclic antidepressant)

measurements, in addition to evaluating drug-specific adverse events.

Assessing school performance and social development provides insight into the effectiveness of treatment on overall functioning, with the child's and parent's report of adherence being crucial for evaluation and reflecting changes in outcome measures. When cognitive or emotional symptoms do not improve or worsen, examining the temporal pattern of drug usage, dosage adjustments, and potential drug interactions can help determine if iatrogenic psychiatric symptoms, is a probable cause, e.g., (1) paradoxical worsening of irritability and hyperactivity after initiation of methylphenidate, clonidine, and atomoxetine and (2) activation with SSRIs are common treatment-emergent adverse events. In such cases, discontinuation of the psychotropic medication responsible for adverse behavioral events may be necessary.

Response—adequate trial, adequate duration: In child psychiatry, it is crucial to ensure that patients receive an adequate trial of treatment and that the duration of treatment is sufficient. This means allowing enough time for the treatment to take effect and for any potential benefits to become apparent. Rushing to conclusions or prematurely discontinuing treatment may result in missed opportunities for improvement or effective intervention. Therefore, clinicians must carefully monitor progress and make adjustments as necessary to optimize outcomes for their young patients. Guidelines such as NICE and AACAP recommend 6–8 weeks trial for depression and psychosis and 12 weeks for OCD.

Addressing nonadherence: Multiple meta-analyses indicate that nonadherence to psychotropic medication among youth with SMI is prevalent, and certain variables related to patient adherence can be identified.[58] These variables include comorbid conditions, interpersonal care processes, illness severity, and adherence to psychotherapy, although some heterogeneity remains. Patient demographics and the class of prescribed medication have less predictive value for adherence. In research studies, the primary diagnosis and methodological factors moderate predictors of adherence.[58] Some variables that influence adherence include other improvement in symptoms, school performance and family relationships, and reduced level of parenting stress while variables such as adverse side effects, social stigma, lack of response, fears of addiction, and changing the child's personality reduce adherence.[59]

Tapering medications: The plan for tapering medications or trial discontinuation depends on multiple factors. Stable dose of medications is continued based on response in target symptoms. To determine the need for ongoing treatment in a child receiving long-term pharmacotherapy, the following factors need to be considered:

- Severity of illness, e.g., BPAD—duration of the illness, severity of the current episode, time taken to achieve remission, etc.
- Presence of comorbidities that could impact the course of illness or developmental engagement, e.g., ADHD in a child with ASD, whose engagement in therapy had improved with addressing ADHD.
- Anticipated stressful events, e.g., exams, which can precipitate an episode.
- If there is no objective improvement in symptoms, despite appropriate dosage adjustments over an 8 week period, treatment should be discontinued, and alternate treatments/augmentation may be tried.
- Developmental phase, e.g., trial discontinuation of stimulant medications for ADHD during late adolescence

Trials off treatment should be scheduled at times least disruptive to the child's academic and social functioning, such as during periods without major commitments like exams. Warning signs of relapse of symptoms and dysfunction have to be discussed with the parent and the child. The child's mental state should be assessed and documented before and during the trial off treatment. Regular monitoring every 3 months for 1 year is beneficial. Treatment should be reinitiated at the previously effective dose, if there is a significant reemergence of symptoms, or if symptom reemergence is observed during follow-up visits.

Role of interdisciplinary professionals: It is important for the child psychiatrist to have a network with a team of professionals, pediatrician, endocrinologists, cardiologists, neurologists, etc., for systemic evaluation and to take expert opinions in case of comorbid disorders, relative contraindications to certain medications where expert evaluation and clearance may be required. Written referral with specifications will be helpful. Discussing with families before initiating referrals and maintaining appropriate documentation is important.

Networking and having an open dialogue with psychotherapists and interventionists who are assisting the child are equally important. Discussions regarding how pharmacotherapy is helping bring down specific symptom dimensions, challenges in participating in therapy sessions owing to medications, etc. will help the psychiatrist plan a child-centric approach to pharmacotherapy.

FUTURE DIRECTIONS

To date, the majority of randomized trials in pediatric psychopharmacology, including comparative effectiveness studies, have been conducted within research settings, and have critical limitations such as small sample sizes, restrictive diagnostic criteria, and short treatment durations, not accounting for comorbidities,[7] thereby limiting the generalizability of their findings. Given the significant burden of mental illness in childhood, high prevalence of comorbidities, and the growing use of psychotropic medications, there is a notable absence of practical trials in pediatric psychopharmacology.[60] Practical trials are essential for evaluating the comparative effectiveness of pharmacological treatments under real-world practice conditions. These trials should incorporate measures beyond symptom scores, including developmentally appropriate assessments of functioning and objective outcomes such as school attendance, academic performance, suicide attempts, emergency room visits, hospitalizations, and healthcare costs. Future research should focus on studying transdiagnostic phenotypes instead of disorder-specific response and outcomes in the context of pharmacotherapy.

SUMMARY AND CONCLUSION

Pharmacotherapy is an essential part of the multimodal intervention approach to treating children and adolescents with mental health and neurodevelopmental conditions. Using a multimodal approach, integrating pharmacotherapy with psychological, psychosocial, and developmental interventions tailored to the child and family, is emphasized. Challenges such as variability in drug response, comorbidities, and developmental considerations underscore the need for evidence-based guidelines to guide clinical decision-making, along with close monitoring and need of personalized treatment plans tailored to each child's unique characteristics and needs. Additionally, comorbid conditions can complicate treatment strategies, requiring careful assessment and consideration of potential interactions between medications.

Understanding pharmacokinetic and pharmacodynamic principles in children is paramount for safe and effective medication management. Children exhibit distinct physiological differences, such as changes in drug absorption, distribution, metabolism, and excretion, compared to adults. Additionally, developmental stages influence drug response, with factors such as liver and kidney function, body composition, and receptor density impacting pharmacological effects. Individual variations in drug metabolism and response necessitate close monitoring of treatment outcomes and regular adjustments to medication regimens in order to optimize therapeutic efficacy and minimize adverse effects. Informed consent and assent, with active involvement of the child in the decision-making process is crucial.

Moving forward, further research is imperative to address existing gaps and develop evidence-based guidelines. Collaboration between researchers, clinicians, and regulatory bodies is essential to enhance integration of research-informed practice and practice-informed research toward providing targeted and comprehensive care to pediatric patients.

REFERENCES

1. Cortese S, Purper-Ouakil D, Apter A, Arango C, Baeza I, Banaschewski T, et al. Psychopharmacology in children and adolescents: unmet needs and opportunities. Lancet Psychiatry. 2024;11(2):143-54.
2. A 14-Month Randomized Clinical Trial of Treatment Strategies for Attention-Deficit/Hyperactivity Disorder. Arch Gen Psychiatry. 1999;56(12):1073.
3. MTA Cooperative Group. National Institute of Mental Health Multimodal Treatment Study of ADHD Follow-up: Changes in Effectiveness and Growth After the End of Treatment. Pediatrics. 2004;113(4):762-9.
4. Vitiello B, Davico C. Twenty years of progress in paediatric psychopharmacology: accomplishments and unmet needs. Evid Based Ment Health. 2018;21(4):e10.
5. Vitiello B. Research in child and adolescent psychopharmacology: recent accomplishments and new challenges. Psychopharmacology (Berl). 2007;191(1):5-13.
6. Seifer R, Dickstein S, Sameroff AJ, Magee KD, Hayden LC. Infant Mental Health and Variability of Parental Depression Symptoms. J Am Acad Child Adolesc Psychiatry. 2001;40(12):1375-82.
7. McCellan JM, Werry JS. Evidence-Based Treatments in Child and Adolescent Psychiatry: An Inventory. J Am Acad Child Adolesc Psychiatry. 2003;42(12):1388-400.
8. Pappadopulos EA, Tate Guelzow B, Wong C, Ortega M, Jensen PS. A review of the growing evidence base for pediatric psychopharmacology. Child Adolesc Psychiatr Clin N Am. 2004;13(4):817-55.
9. Zito JM, Safer DJ, dosReis S, Gardner JF, Magder L, Soeken K, et al. Psychotropic Practice Patterns for Youth: A 10-Year Perspective. Arch Pediatr Adolesc Med. 2003;157(1):17.
10. Soria Saucedo R, Liu X, Hincapie-Castillo JM, Zambrano D, Bussing R, Winterstein AG. Prevalence, Time Trends, and Utilization Patterns of Psychotropic Polypharmacy Among Pediatric Medicaid Beneficiaries, 1999–2010. Psychiatr Serv. 2018;69(8):919-26.
11. Pringsheim T, Stewart DG, Chan P, Tehrani A, Patten SB. The Pharmacoepidemiology of Psychotropic Medication Use in Canadian Children from 2012 to 2016. J Child Adolesc Psychopharmacol. 2019;29(10):740-5.
12. Piovani D, Clavenna A, Bonati M. Prescription prevalence of psychotropic drugs in children and adolescents: an analysis of international data. Eur J Clin Pharmacol. 2019;75(10):1333-46.
13. Gorman DA. Pediatric Psychopharmacology: Principles and Practice, Second Edition. J Can Acad Child Adolesc Psychiatry. 2011;20(4):325.
14. Milsap RL, Jusko WJ. Pharmacokinetics in the infant. Environ Health Perspect. 1994;102(suppl 11):107-10.
15. Daviss WB, Perel JM, Rudolph GR, Axelson DA, Gilchrist R, Nuss S, et al. Steady-State Pharmacokinetics of Bupropion SR in Juvenile Patients. J Am Acad Child Adolesc Psychiatry. 2005;44(4):349-57.
16. Axelson DA, Perel JM, Birmaher B, Rudolph GR, Nuss S, Bridge J, et al. Sertraline Pharmacokinetics and Dynamics in Adolescents. J Am Acad Child Adolesc Psychiatry. 2002;41(9):1037-44.
17. Findling RL, Landersdorfer CB, Kafantaris V, Pavuluri M, McNamara NK, McClellan J, et al. First-Dose Pharmacokinetics of Lithium Carbonate in Children and Adolescents. J Clin Psychopharmacol. 2010;30(4):404-10.
18. Chugani DC, Muzik O, Juhász C, Janisse JJ, Ager J, Chugani HT. Postnatal maturation of human GABA A receptors measured with positron emission tomography. Ann Neurol. 2001;49(5):618-26.
19. Hazell P, O'Connell D, Heathcote D, Robertson J, Henry D. Efficacy of tricyclic drugs in treating

child and adolescent depression: a meta-analysis. BMJ. 1995;310(6984):897-901.
20. Correll CU. Cardiometabolic Risk of Second-Generation Antipsychotic Medications During First-Time Use in Children and Adolescents. JAMA. 2009;302(16):1765.
21. Hammad TA, Laughren T, Racoosin J. Suicidality in Pediatric Patients Treated With Antidepressant Drugs. Arch Gen Psychiatry. 2006;63(3):332.
22. Greenhill L, Kollins S, Abikoff H, Mccracken J, Riddle M, Swanson J, et al. Efficacy and Safety of Immediate-Release Methylphenidate Treatment for Preschoolers With ADHD. J Am Acad Child Adolesc Psychiatry. 2006;45(11):1284-93.
23. Vitiello B, Lazzaretto D, Yershova K, Abikoff H, Paykina N, McCracken JT, et al. Pharmacotherapy of the Preschool ADHD Treatment Study (PATS) Children Growing Up. J Am Acad Child Adolesc Psychiatry. 2015;54(7):550-6.
24. Williams K, Brignell A, Randall M, Silove N, Hazell P. Selective serotonin reuptake inhibitors (SSRIs) for autism spectrum disorders (ASD). Cochrane Database Syst Rev. 2013;2013(8):CD004677.
25. Sauer JM, Ring BJ, Witcher JW. Clinical Pharmacokinetics of Atomoxetine: Clin Pharmacokinet. 2005;44(6):571-90.
26. Selvarajan S, Srinivasan A, Sakkarabani P, Verma A, Rajendran P, Kandasamy P. Genetic polymorphisms influencing response to lithium in early-onset Bipolar disorder from south India. Asian J Psychiatr. 2022;70:103018.
27. Vitiello B. (2012). Principles in using psychotropic medication in children and adolescents. [online] Available from https://www.semanticscholar.org/paper/Principles-in-using-psychotropic-medications-in-and-Vitiello/1c48c6565b00b11c61977bc75703424c5a0bb694 [Last accessed November, 2025].
28. Carrasco M, Volkmar FR, Bloch MH. Pharmacologic Treatment of Repetitive Behaviors in Autism Spectrum Disorders: Evidence of Publication Bias. Pediatrics. 2012;129(5):e1301-10.
29. Brotman MA, Kircanski K, Stringaris A, Pine DS, Leibenluft E. Irritability in Youths: A Translational Model. Am J Psychiatry. 2017;174(6):520-32.
30. Howes OD, Rogdaki M, Findon JL, Wichers RH, Charman T, King BH, et al. Autism spectrum disorder: Consensus guidelines on assessment, treatment and research from the British Association for Psychopharmacology. J Psychopharmacol Oxf Engl. 2018;32(1):3-29.
31. McCracken JT, Biederman J, Greenhill LL, Swanson JM, McGough JJ, Spencer TJ, et al. Analog classroom assessment of a once-daily mixed amphetamine formulation, SLI381 (Adderall XR), in children with ADHD. J Am Acad Child Adolesc Psychiatry. 2003;42(6):673-83.
32. Pelham WE, Aronoff HR, Midlam JK, Shapiro CJ, Gnagy EM, Chronis AM, et al. A comparison of ritalin and adderall: efficacy and time-course in children with attention-deficit/hyperactivity disorder. Pediatrics. 1999;103(4):e43.
33. Pliszka SR, Browne RG, Olvera RL, Wynne SK. A double-blind, placebo-controlled study of Adderall and methylphenidate in the treatment of attention-deficit/hyperactivity disorder. J Am Acad Child Adolesc Psychiatry. 2000;39(5):619-26.
34. Kratochvil CJ, Heiligenstein JH, Dittmann R, Spencer TJ, Biederman J, Wernicke J, et al. Atomoxetine and methylphenidate treatment in children with ADHD: a prospective, randomized, open-label trial. J Am Acad Child Adolesc Psychiatry. 2002;41(7):776-84.
35. Mechler K, Banaschewski T, Hohmann S, Häge A. Evidence-based pharmacological treatment options for ADHD in children and adolescents. Pharmacol Ther. 2022;230:107940.
36. Birmaher B, Axelson DA, Monk K, Kalas C, Clark DB, Ehmann M, et al. Fluoxetine for the treatment of childhood anxiety disorders. J Am Acad Child Adolesc Psychiatry. 2003;42(4):415-23.
37. Geller B, Reising D, Leonard HL, Riddle MA, Walsh BT. Critical Review of Tricyclic Antidepressant Use in Children and Adolescents. J Am Acad Child Adolesc Psychiatry. 1999;38(5):513-6.
38. Singh MK, Ketter TA, Chang KD. Atypical Antipsychotics for Acute Manic and Mixed Episodes in Children and Adolescents with Bipolar Disorder. Drugs. 2010;70(4):433-42.
39. de Kuijper GM, Lenderink AW. Antipsychotic Drug Prescription and Behavioral Problems in Individuals with Intellectual Disability. In: Riederer P, Laux G, Nagatsu T, Le W, Riederer C (Eds). NeuroPsychopharmacotherapy. Philadelphia: Springer International Publishing; 2020. pp. 1-21.

40. Ryan ND, Bhatara VS, Perel JM. Mood Stabilizers in Children and Adolescents. J Am Acad Child Adolesc Psychiatry. 1999;38(5):529-36.
41. Findling RL, Robb A, McNamara NK, Pavuluri MN, Kafantaris V, Scheffer R, et al. Lithium in the acute treatment of bipolar I disorder: a double-blind, placebo-controlled study. Pediatrics. 2015;136(5):885-94.
42. Medicines and Healthcare products Regulatory Agency. (2023). Valproate: review of safety data and expert advice on management of risks. GOV. UK. [online] Available from https://www.gov.uk/government/publications/valproate-review-of-safety-data-and-expert-advice-on-management-of-risks [Last accessed November, 2025].
43. Vasudev A, Macritchie K, Vasudev K, Watson S, Geddes J, Young AH. Oxcarbazepine for acute affective episodes in bipolar disorder. Cochrane Database Syst Rev. 2011;(12):CD004857.
44. Kumar R, Garzon J, Yuruk D, Hassett LC, Saliba M, Ozger C, et al. Efficacy and safety of lamotrigine in pediatric mood disorders: A systematic review. Acta Psychiatr Scand. 2023;147(3):248-56.
45. Vaidyanathan S, Rajan TM, Chandrasekaran V, Kandasamy P. Pre-school attention deficit hyperactivity disorder: 12 weeks prospective study. Asian J Psychiatry. 2020;48:101903.
46. Tourette's Syndrome Study Group. Treatment of ADHD in children with tics: a randomized controlled trial. Neurology. 2002;58(4):527-36.
47. Baeza I, Fortea A, Ilzarbe D, Sugranyes G. What Role for Long-Acting Injectable Antipsychotics in Managing Schizophrenia Spectrum Disorders in Children and Adolescents? A Systematic Review. Pediatr Drugs. 2023;25(2):135-49.
48. Jacob P, Shere S, Kommu JVS. The use of first-generation long-acting injectable antipsychotics in children and adolescents—A retrospective audit from India. Asian J Psychiatry. 2021;61:102663.
49. Roberts R, Rodriguez W, Murphy D, Crescenzi T. Pediatric Drug Labeling: Improving the Safety and Efficacy of Pediatric Therapies. JAMA. 2003;290(7):905.
50. Fost N. Ethical issues in research and innovative therapy in children with mood disorders. Biol Psychiatry. 2001;49(12);1015-22.
51. Stahl SM. Prescriber's Guide-Children and Adolescents: Stahl's Essential Psychopharmacology. Cambridge: Cambridge University Press; 2021.
52. Pruett KD, Joshi SV, Martin AN. Thinking about prescribing: the psychology of psychopharmacology. Pediatric psychopharmacology: Principles and practice. New York: Oxford University Press; 2010. pp. 422-33.
53. Tosyali MC, Greenhill LL. Child and Adolescent Psychopharmacology: Important Developmental Issues. Pediatr Clin North Am. 1998;45(5):1021-35.
54. Nissen SE. ADHD Drugs and Cardiovascular Risk. N Engl J Med. 2006;354(14):1445-48.
55. Swann AC. Major system toxicities and side effects of anticonvulsants. J Clin Psychiatry. 2001;62 Suppl 14:16-21.
56. Grauso-Eby NL, Goldfarb O, Feldman-Winter LB, McAbee GN. Acute pancreatitis in children from Valproic acid: case series and review. Pediatr Neurol. 2003;28(2):145-8.
57. Brown R, James A. Practical pharmacotherapy in child psychiatry: an update. BJPsych Adv. 2015;21(6):387-95.
58. Edgcomb JB, Zima B. Medication Adherence Among Children and Adolescents with Severe Mental Illness: A Systematic Review and Meta-Analysis. J Child Adolesc Psychopharmacol. 2018;28(8):508-20.
59. Hamrin V, McCarthy EM, Tyson V. Pediatric psychotropic medication initiation and adherence: a literature review based on social exchange theory. J Child Adolesc Psychiatr Nurs. 2010;23(3):151-72.
60. Vitiello B. Practical Clinical Trials in Psychopharmacology: a Systematic Review. J Clin Psychopharmacol. 2015;35(2):178-83.

Psychopharmacology in Children and Adolescents-II: Evidence-based Use of Psychotropics

Akhilesh Sharma, Mirza Sarwar Baig, Pranshu Sharma

INTRODUCTION

Pediatric psychopharmacology lies at the intersection of child psychiatry, neurology, pediatrics, and pharmacology. As children are in constant developmental flux, the drug metabolism is more dynamic. Prescribing psychotropic medications in youth is akin to aiming at a constantly moving target. Children metabolize drugs differently than adults, often more efficiently, despite their smaller size. Clinicians must rely on external observations, as younger children are unable to precisely describe their symptoms.

Selecting a pharmacotherapeutic agent depends on the robustness of evidence supporting its efficacy and safety for the specific illness or condition, as well as the child's age. The highest standard of evidence is derived from having at least one systematic review encompassing multiple well-designed randomized controlled trials (RCTs) (Type I). A step below this is evidence drawn from at least one RCT (Type II). Then comes evidence drawn from rigorously conducted studies lacking randomization, such as single-group, pre-post designs, cohort or time-series analyses, or matched case-control studies (Type III). A level below that are findings from well-executed nonexperimental investigations conducted across multiple centers or research teams (Type IV). The lowest level of evidence is expert consensus or authoritative opinion grounded in clinical experience, descriptive research, or reports from expert panels (Type V).[1]

The general principles of psychopharmacology in children and adolescents and the off-label use of psychotropic medications in children and adolescents are dealt with in separate chapters in this book. This chapter starts with a nonexhaustive list of Food and Drug Administration (FDA)-approved psychotropics for various child and adolescent psychiatric conditions along with the level of evidence for each drug **(Table 1)**. This will be followed by a disorder-wise description of the existing evidence base and the prescribing strategies for the psychotropics used for that particular disorder.

EVIDENCE-BASED PSYCHOPHARMACOLOGY FOR VARIOUS CHILD AND ADOLESCENT PSYCHIATRIC DISORDERS

Autism Spectrum Disorder

Pharmacotherapy in autism is used to target a specific symptom or for treating a comorbidity. Comorbidities such as anxiety and depression, and other symptoms such as irritability, self-injurious behavior, and hyperactivity are the targets of pharmacotherapy. Risperidone and aripiprazole are approved by the FDA for managing irritability in children and adolescents with autism spectrum disorder (ASD).[2] Depression is common in higher-functioning children and adolescents with ASD.[3]

TABLE 1: Nonexhaustive list of psychotropic medications and level of evidence for efficacy in children and adolescents younger than 18 years.[1]

Medication	*Indications*	*Evidence level*	*FDA-approved pediatric indications (with age in years)*
Methylphenidate/ dexmethylphenidate	ADHD	I	ADHD (6+)
Amphetamines	ADHD	I	ADHD (3+)
Atomoxetine	ADHD	I	ADHD (6+)
Clonidine	ADHD; Tourette's disorder	I	ADHD (6+); Tourette's
Guanfacine	ADHD	I	ADHD (6+)
Fluoxetine	Major depression; OCD; GAD/SP	I (MDD); II (OCD); II (GAD/SP)	MDD (8+); OCD (7+)
Sertraline	OCD; MDD; GAD/SP	I (OCD, GAD/SP); II (MDD)	OCD (6+)
Escitalopram	MDD	I	MDD (12+)
Fluvoxamine	OCD; GAD/SP	II (OCD); I (GAD/SP)	OCD (7+)
Bupropion	ADHD; MDD	II (ADHD); V (MDD)	–
Clomipramine	OCD	II	OCD (10+)
Haloperidol	Tourette's; psychosis; severe behavioral issues	I (Tourette's); II (others)	3+ for all listed
Pimozide	Tourette's	I	12+
Risperidone	Schizophrenia; bipolar; aggression in autism; Tourette's	I (aggression, Tourette's, bipolar); II (schizophrenia)	Schizophrenia (13+); bipolar (10+); autism irritability (5–16)
Quetiapine	Schizophrenia; bipolar	II	Schizophrenia (13+); bipolar (10+)
Aripiprazole	Schizophrenia; bipolar; aggression in autism	I (aggression); II (others)	Schizophrenia (13+); bipolar (10+); autism irritability (6+)
Olanzapine	Schizophrenia; bipolar	II	Schizophrenia (13+); bipolar (10+)
Lithium	Bipolar; aggression	III (bipolar); II (aggression)	Bipolar (7+)
Valproate	Bipolar; aggression	II	(Epilepsy approval from infancy)

(ADHD: attention-deficit/hyperactivity disorder; FDA: Food and Drug Administration; GAD: generalized anxiety disorder; MDD: major depressive disorder; OCD: obsessive-compulsive disorder; SP: social phobia)

Risperidone is approved for children and adolescents from the age of 5–16 years with autism. Aripiprazole is approved for children and adolescents with autism from 6 to 17 years of age. While no medications are currently approved for treating the core symptoms of ASD, medications such as memantine and oxytocin are being investigated for this purpose. Pharmacotherapy in

TABLE 2: FDA-approved psychotropic medications in children and adolescents with autism spectrum disorder.[2,3]

Drug	*Approved age range*	*Typical dosage*	*Common side effects*
Risperidone	5–16 years	0.25–3 mg/day	Weight gain, sedation, drowsiness
Aripiprazole	6–17 years	2–15 mg/day	Sedation, weight gain, irritability

ASD is intended to improve how the child engages with the nonpharmacological intervention.[1,4] Psychopharmacology in ASD is geared toward addressing symptom clusters, such as irritability, stereotypy, and hyperactivity **(Table 2)**.

Families of children with ASD often also resort to complementary and alternative medicine, such as supplements and chelating agents, and it is important to enquire about this as these may interact with the prescribed medications.[3] Carnosine supplementation in mice has been shown to normalize autistic-like behavioral deficits in animal studies. However, a systematic review and meta-analysis from 2021 looked at the effect of L-Carnosine in children with ASD and concluded that the current evidence does not support using L-Carnosine in the management of children with ASD.[5] Inappropriate sexual behaviors are common in children and adolescents with ASD, and there are a few case reports about the off-label use of mirtazapine in such patients.[6] Sulforaphane, a broccoli-derived antioxidant, has also been studied for use in ASD and is already being marketed in India, as a 30 mg capsule formulation.[3]

Attention-deficit/Hyperactivity Disorder

Landmark trials such as the Multimodal Treatment Study of Children with ADHD (MTA) and the Preschool ADHD Treatment Study (PATS) helped generate evidence for the psychopharmacological treatment of attention-deficit/hyperactivity disorder (ADHD).

The most effective options for managing the core symptoms of ADHD are methylphenidate and amphetamines, with 65–75% of patients responding positively to psychostimulants, whereas only 4–30% show improvement with a placebo.[4,7]

Methylphenidate and amphetamines are the preferred first-line treatments for managing ADHD in school-aged children. Immediate-release methylphenidate is typically prescribed at a daily dose ranging from 0.3 to 1 mg/kg of body weight, divided into one to three doses—two-thirds in the morning and one-third at midday. Treatment typically starts with a 5 mg dose in the morning, with an optional additional 5 mg at midday if needed. The daily dose may be increased by 5–10 mg after 1 week. In the MTA study, an average daily dose of 32 mg (ranging from 15 to 50 mg) of immediate-release methylphenidate, administered in three divided doses, was found to be effective in reducing ADHD symptoms. The maximum permissible daily dose of methylphenidate is 60 mg. The final dose of the day is recommended no later than 4 PM to prevent prolonged sleep latency.[4]

As per the AACAP guidelines, psychostimulants are the first-line treatment for managing ADHD. Immediate-release formulations of methylphenidate and amphetamine take effect quickly; however, due to their short duration of action, optimal symptom control often requires administering two to three doses per day.[4] Various long-acting preparations of methylphenidate and amphetamine were designed to enable once-daily dosing through diverse mechanisms that prolong their effects. These options include a transdermal patch and an oral system utilizing osmotic-release technology.[4]

Lisdexamfetamine (Vyvanse) is a prodrug of dextroamphetamine that is approved by the FDA for children 6 years and older with ADHD. As a long-acting stimulant, it provides symptom control for up to 10–12 hours and is administered once daily. Because it requires enzymatic conversion in the blood to become active, it has a lower potential for misuse or diversion compared with immediate-release stimulants. Its efficacy and side-effect profile are similar to other stimulant medications, with common adverse effects including appetite loss, insomnia, and irritability.[7]

The most commonly reported short-term adverse effects of psychostimulants are decreased appetite, headaches, and disturbances in sleep. Additionally, the MTA study found that stimulants slowed growth velocity over time. The diminished growth in height was in the range of 1–2 cm.[7]

Atomoxetine may be used when there is a risk of drug abuse or diversion by the patient.[7,8] It is also preferred for patients with co-occurring anxiety or tic disorders. It is also preferred if psychostimulants produce severe side effects in a patient.[4] Atomoxetine is initially prescribed twice daily during the first week to minimize side effects such as nausea and sedation. Starting from the second week, a single dose of the medication is given in the morning. The recommended dosage begins at 0.5 mg/kg of body weight per day during the first week and is increased to 1.2 mg/kg/day thereafter.[4]

Extended-release forms of the α2-adrenoceptor agonists, clonidine and guanfacine, have received FDA approval for the treatment of ADHD in children and adolescents between the ages of 6 and 17 years, as monotherapy or as adjunctive to other treatments.[4,7]

Prior to starting pharmacological therapy, baseline assessments of height, weight, heart rate, and blood pressure should be recorded. In cases with a family history of sudden cardiac death or a personal history of structural heart abnormalities, a cardiac evaluation—including ECG and echocardiography—is recommended.[4,7]

The American Academy of Pediatrics (AAP) clinical practice guidelines advocate for parent training in behavior management and classroom-based behavioral strategies as the first-line approach for preschool-aged children, with methylphenidate recommended as a second-line option.[7] Psychostimulants should be considered for preschool children only when symptoms are significantly impairing and behavioral interventions have proven ineffective. In this age group, methylphenidate dosage should be titrated with particular caution. A recommended approach is to begin with 2.5 mg of an immediate-release formulation and then increase to 5 mg daily for 8 days, administered with breakfast. Subsequent dose adjustments should be individualized, titrating in 2.5 mg increments—the equivalent of a quarter of a 10 mg tablet or half of a 5 mg tablet.[4] See **Table 3** for FDA-approved psychotropics for ADHD.

Anxiety Disorders and Phobias

The landmark Child/Adolescent Anxiety Multimodal Study (CAMS) provided robust evidence for combining cognitive behavioral therapy (CBT) and a selective serotonin reuptake inhibitor (SSRI) in treating pediatric anxiety disorders.

The use of psychopharmacological agents for anxiety disorders in children and adolescents should be carefully considered and time-bound. The dosage should be slowly titrated. See **Table 4** for a list of psychotropics used in children and adolescents for anxiety disorders.

If there is no benefit at all after 8 weeks of an SSRI, a different SSRI should be started. After 4–6 months of monitoring the symptoms under treatment, the dosage should be gradually reduced, and an effort may be made to withdraw the SSRI.[4]

TABLE 3: FDA-approved psychotropic medications in children and adolescents with ADHD.[4,7]

Drug	Approved age range	Typical dosage	Common side effects
Methylphenidate	≥6 years	0.3–1 mg/kg/day (up to 60 mg/day)	Appetite loss, insomnia, abdominal pain
Amphetamine salts	≥6 years	5–40 mg/day	Headache, insomnia, decreased appetite
Lisdexamfetamine	≥6 years	30–70 mg/day	Appetite loss, insomnia, irritability, abdominal pain
Atomoxetine	≥6 years	0.5–1.2 mg/kg/day	Nausea, fatigue, mood swings
Guanfacine XR	6–17 years	1–7 mg/day	Fatigue, dizziness, dry mouth
Clonidine XR	6–17 years	0.1–0.4 mg/day	Sedation, constipation, hypotension

(ADHD: attention-deficit/hyperactivity disorder; FDA: Food and Drug Administration)

TABLE 4: FDA-approved psychotropic medications in children and adolescents with anxiety disorders.[10]

Drug	Approved age range	Typical dosage	Common side effects	Black box warning
Sertraline	≥6 years (OCD)	25–200 mg/day	Nausea, insomnia, tremor	Suicidality in youth
Fluvoxamine	≥8 years (OCD)	25–300 mg/day	Sedation, GI distress, agitation	Same as above
Fluoxetine	≥8 years	10–60 mg/day	Headache, restlessness, insomnia	Same as above
Escitalopram	≥12 years	10–20 mg/day	Nausea, drowsiness, sweating	Same as above

(GI: gastrointestinal)

Discontinuation of benzodiazepines should start within 4–6 weeks because of the risk of dependence. Weekly reduction of 25% of the dosage at the start of withdrawal should be done.[4]

Panic disorder, separation anxiety disorder: Among psychotropics, SSRIs are the first choice for these disorders.[4,9]

Social phobia: SSRIs, such as paroxetine, sertraline, escitalopram, and fluoxetine, are the medications of first choice in social phobia.[4,9]

When symptoms such as nervousness, shaking, muscular tension, sweating, and palpitations accompany social phobia, or in the case of "stage fright," β-blockers, such as propranolol, are prescribed. In anxiety-provoking social situations, benzodiazepines such as clonazepam or alprazolam can be helpful on a short-term basis.[4]

Generalized anxiety disorder (GAD): In several RCTs, SSRIs have been found to be superior to placebo and hence are medications of first choice in the treatment of GAD.[4,9]

In case of acute anxiety, benzodiazepines such as diazepam, alprazolam, and clonazepam can be considered in the short term. When benzodiazepines are contraindicated—for example, due to the risk of respiratory depression—buspirone, which is a less sedative pharmacological alternative, may be considered for the treatment of GAD.[4]

Post-traumatic stress disorder (PTSD): Various SSRIs, including sertraline (which is FDA-approved for PTSD in adults), are used for treating children and adolescents with PTSD, although none of the pharmacological agents are FDA-approved for treating PTSD in children and adolescents.[4] Excessive agitation may be treated with clonidine and propranolol, especially in cases with tachycardia and intrusion symptoms, where they are used for about 7 days and then slowly stopped.[4] Anxiolytics are used in the treatment of chronic PTSD for up to 12–24 months.[4]

DEPRESSION

Two important studies—TADS (Treatments for Adolescents with Depression Study) and TORDIA (Treatment of SSRI-Resistant Depression in Adolescents Study)—were done in children and adolescents with depression. TADS provided evidence supporting the use of antidepressants for childhood depression. In this study, the drug treatments were significantly more effective than placebo or psychotherapy alone. This emphasized the benefits of combining medication treatment with psychotherapy.[11,12] TORDIA is the only RCT of youth with treatment-refractory depression. In this, combination of CBT and antidepressant was found to be more efficacious than the antidepressant alone (54.8% vs. 40.5%). There was no major difference between the antidepressants used (fluoxetine, citalopram, venlafaxine).[13] The AACAP (American Academy of Child and Adolescent Psychiatry) recommends using SSRIs for moderate-to-severe cases of major depressive disorder (MDD) in children and adolescents, especially fluoxetine (but not paroxetine).[14] Fluoxetine (approved for ages 8 years and older) and escitalopram (approved for ages 12 years and older) are the only antidepressants with FDA approval for treating depression in youth. However, all antidepressants prescribed to children and adolescents—including SSRIs, serotonin-norepinephrine reuptake inhibitors (SNRIs), and clomipramine—carry an FDA black box warning regarding the potential risk of suicidal thoughts. A meta-analysis, including both published and unpublished trials (13 MDD, 6 OCD, 6 anxiety), found that the antidepressant benefits outweigh risks. The benefit-risk ratio was better for SSRIs than for non-SSRIs.[10,12] After successful acute treatment, treatment with the same dosage of antidepressants and psychotherapy (e.g., CBT) should continue for 6–12 months to prevent relapses. The maintenance treatment with antidepressants and/or psychotherapy for 1 year or longer should be reserved for the youth with severe depression or frequent recurrence. For some, treatment may go on for several years. In these cases, medications should be stopped for a short while to observe whether the patient needs further treatment.[12,13] **Table 5** lists FDA-approved psychotropics for depression in children and adolescents.

Obsessive-compulsive Disorder

The Pediatric OCD Treatment Study (POTS) was conducted in 2004 across multiple centers which

TABLE 5: FDA-approved psychotropic medications in children and adolescents with depression.[10,14]

Drug	*Approved age range*	*Typical dosage*	*Common side effects*	*Black box warning*
Fluoxetine	≥8 years	10–60 mg/day	Nausea, insomnia, headache	Suicidality in youth
Escitalopram	≥12 years	10–20 mg/day	Nausea, drowsiness, sweating	Same as above

(FDA: Food and Drug Administration)

TABLE 6: FDA-approved psychotropic medications in children and adolescents with OCD.[10,16]

Drug	*Approved age range*	*Typical dosage*	*Common side effects*	*Black box warning*
Sertraline	≥6 years	50–200 mg/day	Diarrhea, insomnia, fatigue	Suicidality in youth
Fluvoxamine	≥8 years	50–300 mg/day	Drowsiness, nausea, insomnia	Same as above
Clomipramine	≥10 years	50–200 mg/day	Sedation, dry mouth, weight gain	Same as above

(FDA: Food and Drug Administration; OCD: obsessive-compulsive disorder)

found that the best way to treat OCD in children is to start with CBT alone or CBT combined with an SSRI.[10,15,16] The AACAP recommends starting with CBT for children with mild-to-moderate OCD. For moderate-to-severe cases, medications should be added along with CBT. SSRIs are the first-line medications.[16] Sertraline and fluvoxamine are the only FDA-approved SSRIs for the treatment of OCD from age 6 and 8 years. respectively **(Table 6)**. Clomipramine, a tricyclic antidepressant with potent serotonergic effect, has also got FDA approval for use in children and adolescents from the age of 10 years. In treatment-resistant cases, medication augmentation strategies are utilized. Adding clomipramine to an SSRI has been found to be helpful. In cases of treatment-resistant OCD, some children may benefit from cautious augmentation with neuroleptic agents—particularly those with comorbid tic disorders, poor insight, mood instability, or pervasive developmental disorder symptoms. Studies in adults have demonstrated that augmentation with risperidone or haloperidol provides a significant advantage over placebo, with especially favorable outcomes observed in individuals with co-occurring tic disorders.[16-18] Emerging augmentation strategies have also been explored using agents such as stimulants, gabapentin, pindolol, inositol, N-acetylcysteine, St. John's wort, and glutamate modulators like memantine. However, current evidence for these interventions remains insufficient to support their routine clinical use.[16]

Schizophrenia

Antipsychotic medications form the cornerstone of treatment for schizophrenia spectrum disorders in children and adolescents, with second-generation antipsychotics (SGAs) generally being the treatment of first choice. These medications should ideally be used along with psychotherapy and other supportive interventions.[19,20] The TEOSS (Treatment of Early-Onset Schizophrenia Spectrum Disorders Study) utilized a randomized, double-blind methodology to evaluate and compare the effectiveness of olanzapine, risperidone, and molindone in treating children and adolescents diagnosed with schizophrenia. The three treatment groups showed comparable response rates and symptom reduction. However, olanzapine was associated with significantly greater weight gain. There were no meaningful differences in extrapyramidal symptoms across treatment groups; however, all individuals receiving molindone were prophylactically given benztropine.[10,20,21] The FDA has approved aripiprazole, risperidone, olanzapine, quetiapine, and lurasidone for ages 13–17 years and paliperidone for ages 12–17 years **(Table 7)**. For youth with treatment-resistant schizophrenia spectrum disorders, a trial of clozapine is an option.[10,19,20,22] Studies show that these SGAs often cause significant weight gain in youth, increasing the risk for heart disease and metabolic problems later on. Therefore, regular monitoring of metabolic health is essential and

TABLE 7: FDA-approved psychotropic medications in children and adolescents with schizophrenia.[4,10]

Drug	*Approved age range*	*Typical dosage*	*Common side effects*
Aripiprazole	13–17 years	10–30 mg/day	Sedation, weight gain, dizziness
Risperidone	13–17 years	2–6 mg/day	Weight gain, increased appetite, drowsiness
Olanzapine	13–17 years	5–20 mg/day	Significant weight gain, sedation
Quetiapine	13–17 years	400–600 mg/day	Sedation, dry mouth, dizziness
Paliperidone	12–17 years	3–12 mg/day	Weight gain, prolactin elevation, tremor
Lurasidone	13–17 years	40–80 mg/day	Nausea, somnolence, restlessness

TABLE 8: FDA-approved psychotropic medications in children and adolescents with pediatric bipolar disorder.[4,10]

Drug	*Approved age range*	*Typical dosage*	*Common side effects*
Lithium	≥7 years	600–1,800 mg/day	Tremor, hypothyroidism, polyuria
Risperidone	10–17 years	0.5–6 mg/day	Weight gain, sedation, metabolic changes
Aripiprazole	10–17 years	2–30 mg/day	Sedation, akathisia, restlessness
Olanzapine	13–17 years	5–20 mg/day	Weight gain, increased appetite, sedation
Quetiapine	10–17 years	400–600 mg/day	Drowsiness, orthostatic hypotension
Lurasidone	10–17 years	20–80 mg/day	Nausea, fatigue, agitation

should include assessments of body mass index, fasting glucose, triglycerides, cholesterol levels, waist circumference, high-density lipoprotein/low-density lipoprotein (HDL/LDL) ratios, blood pressure, and signs or symptoms indicative of diabetes.[10,20,23,24]

Pediatric Bipolar Disorder

In children, the diagnosis of bipolar disorder is often delayed, which can lead to poor outcomes. Its recognition remains a topic of ongoing debate, as the presentation in pediatric cases is frequently complex, with rapid-cycling patterns and mixed affective states. Irritability is a hallmark symptom in both depressive and manic episodes, further complicating the diagnostic process. Additionally, significant symptomatic overlap between mania and ADHD poses challenges in distinguishing the two conditions. Features such as excessive energy, distractibility, and overtalkativeness are common to both disorders. However, key differentiating signs of bipolar disorder include euphoria, a decreased need for sleep, and hypersexuality, which should be carefully assessed to ensure an accurate diagnosis.[25] Several FDA-approved treatments are available for bipolar disorder in youth, starting from the age of 13 years in most cases and, in some instances, from the age of 10 years **(Table 8)**. The majority of these treatments are SGAs, which, while serving as the first-line therapy for childhood-onset bipolar disorder, are associated with significant metabolic side effects. Lithium is approved by the FDA for pediatric bipolar disorder from the age of 7 years, and evidence from research indicates that both lithium and lamotrigine are effective in managing bipolar depression in adolescents. Additionally, pediatric bipolar disorder is often accompanied by comorbid conditions such as ADHD, anxiety disorders, ASD, oppositional defiant disorder (ODD), and conduct disorder (CD).

Once mood symptoms—mania and depression—are effectively stabilized, it becomes crucial to address these co-occurring conditions.[6,26]

The TEAM (Treatment of Early Age Mania) study, conducted by Geller et al., looked at the comparative efficacy of risperidone, valproic acid, and lithium in an 8-week RCT involving pediatric patients experiencing manic or mixed episodes of bipolar disorder. The findings revealed that risperidone was more effective than both valproic acid and lithium for the initial management of mania, though it was associated with significant metabolic side effects.[27]

CASE VIGNETTES AND CLINICAL APPLICATIONS

CASE VIGNETTE 1

A 9-year-old girl, living with her paternal aunt, presented with persistent sadness, irritability, restlessness, and dissociative episodes. Her history revealed maternal abandonment, father's cannabis use, and ongoing family discord. Management included escitalopram (2.5–7.5 mg/day), and clonazepam (0.25 mg TDS). SSRIs were chosen for their proven efficacy in pediatric depression and anxiety, while clonazepam was used short-term for its anxiolytic effect, with psychoeducation aimed at reducing reinforcement of dissociation.

CASE VIGNETTE 2

A 14-year-old boy presented with intrusive fears of contamination and repetitive handwashing rituals that occupied several hours each day. These symptoms led to distress, school absenteeism, and family conflict. He was started on CBT with exposure and response prevention, which produced only partial improvement. Fluoxetine (20–40 mg/day) was then added and gradually titrated, resulting in further reduction of obsessions and compulsions. As significant symptoms persisted, low-dose risperidone (0.5–1 mg/day) was introduced as augmentation. Over the next 2 months, he showed marked functional improvement, with reduced ritualistic behavior and regular school attendance.

This case highlights the stepwise management of pediatric OCD—beginning with CBT, using SSRIs when symptoms remain impairing, and adding risperidone augmentation in partial responders. The approach reflects evidence from the Pediatric OCD Treatment Study (POTS).

CASE VIGNETTE 3

A 16-year-old girl with moderate-to-severe MDD was treated with fluoxetine (20–40 mg/day) for 10 weeks with only partial improvement. Her depressive symptoms persisted with low energy, anhedonia, and school refusal. Based on TORDIA trial evidence, she was switched to escitalopram (10–20 mg/day) and simultaneously started on CBT sessions. Over 12 weeks, she showed significant improvement.

This case illustrates evidence-based management of SSRI-resistant depression in adolescents and highlights the superiority of combined pharmacotherapy and psychotherapy.

CASE VIGNETTE 4

A 10-year-old boy presented with inattention, hyperactivity, and academic underperformance. After baseline cardiovascular assessment, he was started on methylphenidate immediate release (5 mg twice daily), gradually titrated to 20 mg/day. Appetite suppression and mild insomnia were noted, so it was switched to a long-acting methylphenidate preparation [osmotic-release oral system (OROS)]. The new regimen provided sustained symptom control throughout the school day with fewer side effects and improved adherence.

This case emphasizes the evidence for stimulant use in ADHD and the rationale for choosing long-acting formulations when once-daily dosing and smoother pharmacokinetics are desired.

CASE VIGNETTE 5

A 12-year-old girl presented with a 6-month history of social withdrawal, decline in academic performance, and suspiciousness toward peers. Over the past 2 months, she developed auditory hallucinations in the form of voices commenting on her actions, along with disorganized speech and poor self-care. Following baseline medical and metabolic workup, she was started on aripiprazole at 5 mg/day and gradually titrated to 15 mg/day. Over 8 weeks, there was a significant reduction in hallucinations and improvement in social interaction. Psychoeducation and family interventions were provided alongside medication.

This case highlights the evidence-based role of SGAs, such as aripiprazole, as first-line treatment for early-onset schizophrenia with combined psychosocial interventions to support recovery.

SUMMARY AND CONCLUSION

To summarize, evidence-based psychopharmacology in children and adolescents aims to use medications that are supported by robust clinical data, guideline-based recommendations, and careful monitoring for efficacy and safety. Stimulants such as methylphenidate and amphetamine remain first line, supported by large trials showing improvement in attention and impulsivity. All prescriptions must consider developmental stage, comorbidities, psychosocial context, and the increased susceptibility to adverse effects.

In conclusion, psychopharmacologic treatment in children and adolescents significantly improves functioning when guided by evidence, safe prescribing principles, and ongoing monitoring. Clinicians must remain vigilant about side-effect profiles, informed consent, and the need for regular review as the child develops.

REFERENCES

1. Lorberg B, Davico C, Martsenkovskyi D, Vitiello B. Principles in using psychotropic medication in children and adolescents. In: Rey JM (Ed). IACAPAP e-Textbook of Child and Adolescent Mental Health. Geneva: International Association for Child and Adolescent Psychiatry and Allied Professions; 2019.
2. Volkmar F, Siegel M, Woodbury-Smith M, King B, McCracken J, State M. Practice parameter for the assessment and treatment of children and adolescents with autism spectrum disorder. J Am Acad Child Adolesc Psychiatry. 2014;53(2):237-57.
3. Accordino RE, Kidd C, Politte LC, Henry CA, McDougle CJ. Psychopharmacological

interventions in autism spectrum disorder. Expert Opin Pharmacother. 2016;17(7):937-52.

4. Gerlach M, Warnke A, Greenhill L (Eds). Psychiatric Drugs in Children and Adolescents: Basic Pharmacology and Practical Applications. Vienna: Springer; 2014.
5. Abraham DA, Undela K, Narasimhan U, Rajanandh MG. Effect of L-carnosine in children with autism spectrum disorders: a systematic review and meta-analysis of randomized controlled trials. Amino Acids. 2021;53(4):575-85.
6. Chen F, Grandjean C, Richard S. Pharmacological management of inappropriate sexual behaviors in youth with autism spectrum disorder: a case study and review of the literature. Neuropsychiatr Enfance Adolesc. 2016;64(3):163-7.
7. Wolraich ML, Hagan JF, Allan C, Chan E, Davison D, Earls M, et al. Clinical practice guideline for the diagnosis, evaluation, and treatment of attention-deficit/hyperactivity disorder in children and adolescents. Pediatrics. 2019;144(4):e20192528.
8. Bolea-Alamañac B, Nutt DJ, Adamou M, Asherson P, Bazire S, Coghill D, et al. Evidence-based guidelines for the pharmacological management of attention deficit hyperactivity disorder: update on recommendations from the British Association for Psychopharmacology. J Psychopharmacol. 2014;28(3):179-203.
9. Walter HJ, Bukstein OG, Abright AR, Keable H, Ramtekkar U, Ripperger-Suhler J, et al. Clinical practice guideline for the assessment and treatment of children and adolescents with anxiety disorders. J Am Acad Child Adolesc Psychiatry. 2020;59(10):1107-24.
10. March JS, Silva S, Petrycki S, Curry J, Wells K, Fairbank J, et al. The Treatment for Adolescents With Depression Study (TADS): long-term effectiveness and safety outcomes. Arch Gen Psychiatry. 2007;64(10):1132-43.
11. Bridge JA, Iyengar S, Salary CB, Barbe RP, Birmaher B, Pincus HA, et al. Clinical response and risk for reported suicidal ideation and suicide attempts in pediatric antidepressant treatment: a meta-analysis of randomized controlled trials. JAMA. 2007;297(15):1683-96.
12. Brent D, Emslie G, Clarke G, Wagner KD, Asarnow JR, Keller M, et al. Switching to another SSRI or to venlafaxine with or without cognitive behavioral therapy for adolescents with SSRI-resistant depression: the TORDIA randomized controlled trial. JAMA. 2008;299(8):901-13.
13. Walter HJ, Abright AR, Bukstein OG, Diamond J, Keable H, Ripperger-Suhler J, et al. Clinical practice guideline for the assessment and treatment of children and adolescents with major and persistent depressive disorders. J Am Acad Child Adolesc Psychiatry. 2023;62(5):479-502.
14. McVoy M, Stepanova E, Findling RL (Eds). Clinical Manual of Child and Adolescent Psychopharmacology, 4th edition. Washington, DC: American Psychiatric Association Publishing; 2024.
15. Pediatric OCD Treatment Study (POTS) Team. Cognitive-behavior therapy, sertraline, and their combination for children and adolescents with obsessive-compulsive disorder: the Pediatric OCD Treatment Study (POTS) randomized controlled trial. JAMA. 2004;292(16):1969-76.
16. Geller DA, March J. Practice parameter for the assessment and treatment of children and adolescents with obsessive-compulsive disorder. J Am Acad Child Adolesc Psychiatry. 2012;51(1):98-113.
17. McDougle CJ, Epperson CN, Pelton GH, Wasylink S, Price LH. A double-blind, placebo-controlled study of risperidone addition in serotonin reuptake inhibitor–refractory obsessive-compulsive disorder. Arch Gen Psychiatry. 2000;57(8):794-801.
18. Dold M, Aigner M, Lanzenberger R, Kasper S. Antipsychotic augmentation of serotonin reuptake inhibitors in treatment-resistant obsessive-compulsive disorder: a meta-analysis of double-blind, randomized, placebo-controlled trials. Mol Psychiatry. 2013;18(2):159-74. doi:10.1038/mp.2011.183
19. Kumra S, Oberstar JV, Sikich L, Findling RL, McClellan JM, Vinogradov S, et al. Efficacy and tolerability of second-generation antipsychotics in children and adolescents with schizophrenia. Schizophr Bull. 2008;34(1):60-71.
20. McClellan J, Stock S. Practice parameter for the assessment and treatment of children and adolescents with schizophrenia. J Am Acad Child Adolesc Psychiatry. 2013;52(9):976-90.

21. Sikich L, Frazier JA, McClellan J, Findling RL, Vitiello B, Ritz L, et al. Double-blind comparison of first- and second-generation antipsychotics in early-onset schizophrenia and schizoaffective disorder: findings from the Treatment of Early-Onset Schizophrenia Spectrum Disorders (TEOSS) study. Am J Psychiatry. 2008;165(11):1420-31.
22. Shaw P, Sporn A, Gogtay N, Overman GP, Greenstein D, Gochman P, et al. Childhood-onset schizophrenia: a double-blind, randomized clozapine-olanzapine comparison. Arch Gen Psychiatry. 2006;63(7):721-30.
23. De Hert M, Vancampfort D, Correll CU, Mercken V, Peuskens J, Sweers K, et al. Guidelines for screening and monitoring of cardiometabolic risk in schizophrenia: systematic evaluation. Br J Psychiatry. 2011;199(2):99-105.
24. Mitchell AJ, Delaffon V, Vancampfort D, Correll CU, De Hert M. Guideline-concordant monitoring of metabolic risk in people treated with antipsychotic medication: systematic review and meta-analysis of screening practices. Psychol Med. 2012;42(1):125-47.
25. Wozniak J, O'Connor H, Iorini M, Ambrose AJH. Pediatric bipolar disorder: challenges in diagnosis and treatment. Pediatr Drugs. 2025;27(2):125-42.
26. Gautam S, Jain A, Gautam M, Gautam A, Jagawat T. Clinical practice guidelines for bipolar affective disorder in children and adolescents. Indian J Psychiatry. 2019;61(8):294-305.
27. Geller B. A randomized controlled trial of risperidone, lithium, or divalproex sodium for initial treatment of bipolar I disorder, manic or mixed phase, in children and adolescents. Arch Gen Psychiatry. 2012;69(5):515-28.

CHAPTER 29

Psychopharmacology in Children and Adolescents-III: Off-label Use

Nidhi Chauhan, Himani Adarsh

INTRODUCTION

The term "off-label drug use" describes medications that do not comply with the product license terms regarding dose, patient age, administration route, indications, and contraindications.[1] Drugs are given marketing permission based on their effectiveness and safety for specific usages, as evidenced by positive benefit–risk ratios in clinical studies. It is almost impossible to determine all the potential uses for a drug during the approval process, making it difficult to approve the drug for all indications, in all dosage forms, routes of administration, and age groups, especially for children. Drugs may be used either unlicensed, i.e., used in the age group in which it is not approved, or off-label i.e., outside the terms of the product license or marketing authorizations. Drug preparations that are not approved for use in children usually carry statements on the product label regarding inadequate data/warnings about potential dangers if used in this population. However, being an off-label drug is not an absolute contraindication per se for use in children, and thus, practitioners prescribe off-label drugs to children. However, the danger of using frequent off-label drugs in children comes from the fact that over time, these are assumed to be "standard treatments", leading to a preferential use of these inadequately evaluated but commonly used drugs.

Besides the level of evidence for medications, as clinicians, we should understand the process and the regulatory body that approves a drug for commercial usage. Some organized regulatory bodies, such as the Food and Drug Administration (FDA) and the European Medicines Agency (EMA), exist in high-income countries like the United States and Europe. The FDA has approved some essential psychotropic medications that can be used in children, like methylphenidate for attention-deficit/hyperactivity disorder (ADHD), 6 years or above. The rest of the psychotropics, which are not approved for specific indications, are used as "off-label." If we look at the controlled clinical trials of methylphenidate use in ADHD for preschoolers (3–6 years of age), research has demonstrated efficacy in this population; however, methylphenidate is still not approved for ADHD under 6 years of age.[2] Some older psychotropics, like haloperidol, have evidence-based approval processes but have shown less efficacy. Some medications, like sertraline, were already made generic in the United States before it was studied in children with generalized anxiety disorder. After a medication is labeled as generic, there is no point in the pharmaceutical companies going through the costly and cumbersome process of approval from the FDA for a particular indication. Due to all these factors, different medications, both in general medicine and in psychiatry, are used off-label in essentially all age groups. While FDA approval provides a drug safety and efficacy standard, off-label prescribing often relies on emerging research, case studies, and clinical experience.

Even though it is often insufficiently supported by solid scientific data, off-label drug use is rather prevalent in psychiatric practice. The testing and assessment required before a medication is approved for marketing have yet to be applied to off-label applications. Along with physicians and pharmaceutical companies, patients and regulatory agencies also take part in off-label medicine usage. It is necessary to note that the phrase "off-label" does not signify an inappropriate, unlawful, contraindicated, or investigational use. Sometimes, it is impossible to avoid using prescription pharmaceuticals off-label, as a lot of marketed drugs do not have child-specific labeling indications. At times, off-label usage can offer patients the best available intervention and standard of care for a specific health issue for which there is no relief from the conventional medications that are principally prescribed for managing it.

EMERGENCE FOR THE NEED OF OFF-LABEL MEDICATIONS IN CHILD PSYCHIATRY

The role of pharmacology in the pediatric population has always been a topic of debate and controversy. When we try to understand the historical underpinnings of how psychotropic usage started in children, it is found that most psychotropics were first developed and researched in the adult population. After the clinical trials demonstrated safety and efficacy in adults with various psychiatric disorders, the use of these agents gradually shifted toward the adolescent population. Later, it was extended to children. However, one important thing to note here is that the scenario is slightly different in the case of medications for ADHD. The drug benzedrine was first used in 1937 by Charles Bradley, a psychiatrist in the United States, in "problem" children to alleviate headaches. During follow-ups, it was noticed that these children started to perform better in school and social domains, and there was an improvement in their emotional issues. This was an important landmark and contributed to future research in ADHD medication development.[2]

However, for the rest of the psychotropics used in different disorders, the evidence-based treatment guidelines were first approved in the adult population. The efficacy, dosing, administration, and side-effect profiles from adult studies have been used to understand off-label pediatric drug use. When we talk about the pediatric population, many ethical, practical, and clinical issues need to be considered before planning for any pharmacologically based intervention or clinical trial. The lack of clinical trials and, thus, evidence base leads to dilemmas in decision-making and uncertainties while initiating pharmacotherapy in children. Also, it is now clear that children are more vulnerable to the side effects of medications and respond differently compared to adults. Due to a variety of factors, including barriers to pharmaceutical therapies and the lack of evidence-based treatment alternatives for children, psychotropic medication usage is frequently not explored in younger patients. This has led to very few options when it comes to the treatment of childhood psychiatric disorders using pharmacotherapy. Sometimes, the term "therapeutic orphan" is used in infants and children where research on safety and efficacy is lacking.[3]

In clinical trials, including those of the pediatric population, the sample sizes are generally small, limiting the generalizability of results. Also, issues related to taking assent/consent, ensuring that parents are willing to continue with the trials, safety concerns, and the need for age-appropriate formulations are to be considered. In the realm of psychopharmacology, off-label use is widespread due to limited research on the use of medications in pediatric populations. In child and adolescent psychiatry, off-label prescriptions are widespread, approximately 50% for antidepressants (ADs) and up to 95% for antipsychotics, as reported in European studies.[4] A few Indian-based studies showed that up to 42% of prescriptions included off-label psychotropic usage.[5]

CONCERNS REGARDING OFF-LABEL PSYCHOTROPIC USE IN CHILDREN AND ADOLESCENTS

Despite being legal and frequently used in medical practice, off-label prescription raises important safety, effectiveness, and ethical concerns—particularly concerning vulnerable groups such as children and adolescents. There are almost no prospective drug safety studies in child and adolescent psychiatry, and the risks of side effects, especially with prescribing off-label psychotropic drugs to minors, are unclear.[6]

A historical example is the use of pemoline in the treatment of ADHD. In adults, it was known that pemoline can be hepatotoxic. Due to its minimal use in children, its safety profile was not studied. However, as the off-label use of pemoline in children with ADHD continued for decades, cases of hepatotoxicity and even fatalities were reported. Finally, in 1996, a black box warning was given, and over the years, the drug was voluntarily withdrawn from the US market.[7]

The decision to use specific medications can be complex and sometimes controversial for families, patients, and psychiatrists, as practice guidelines may only consider some of the details needed to make a clinical decision. Some important points are to be considered before initiating pharmacotherapy in children and adolescents, which are as follows:

- The quality of the research literature involves methodological rigor, sampling considerations (such as diversity in samples), and comprehension of long-term results.
- The extent to which psychotropic medication prescription in community settings aligns with the standard of psychotropic medication prescription in the randomized controlled trials (RCTs)/trials where it was researched.
- The psychiatric as well as medical comorbidities of the index patient can alter the drug pharmacokinetics.
- The extent to which treatment decision-making can be aided by various modes, like involving a multidisciplinary team
- Exploring the attitudes, acceptability, and satisfaction of patients and their families toward medications, which could impact adherence and ongoing help-seeking
- Trying to establish an equilibrium between the advantages and side effects in the context of the "First, Do No Harm" principle in medical ethics
- The availability and easy access to medications and professional healthcare in case of any adverse drug reactions.

One of the primary concerns with off-label psychotropic use in children and adolescents is the lack of comprehensive research and clinical trials supporting its safety and efficacy in this population.

Another concern is the potential for adverse effects and long-term consequences associated with off-label psychotropic use. Side effects like weight gain, metabolic changes, hormonal imbalances, and a higher risk of suicidal thoughts may be more common in children and adolescents. Furthermore, the effect of psychotropic drugs on cognitive growth, school achievement, and social skills is still a significant issue, given their importance in the overall health of young people.

Ethical concerns are also a factor to be considered while prescribing psychotropic drugs off-label to children and adolescents. In this group, informed consent is more complicated because they might not grasp the possible consequences and dangers of taking medication. Furthermore, there is a possibility of excessive medication or incorrect prescribing methods, as medical professionals might resort to using medications off-label because of restricted treatment choices or demands from parents and caregivers for immediate answers to behavioral or emotional issues.

Additionally, the impact of pharmaceutical marketing and relationships with the industry on prescription practices must be considered. There have been cases where psychotropic medications for pediatric use have been promoted off-label despite limited evidence of safety and effectiveness in children. This raises worries about potential conflicts of interest, the transparency of research, and the importance of impartial information to help with clinical decision-making.

Addressing the Concerns

To deal with the issues related to the off-label use of psychotropic drugs in young people, a comprehensive approach is required. Above all, it is crucial to conduct further thorough research and clinical trials that specifically examine the safety and effectiveness of psychotropic medications in children. Long-term studies are vital for evaluating the effects of these medications on neurodevelopment, mental health outcomes, and overall well-being.

Furthermore, healthcare professionals need to prioritize evidence-based practices and follow set guidelines when contemplating the use of psychotropic medications in young patients. This involves a comprehensive evaluation and diagnosis, exploration of nondrug treatments, and careful observation of medication outcomes and adverse reactions. Healthcare professionals, parents, educators, and mental health advocates must work together to provide comprehensive and patient-focused care for young people.

Education and awareness campaigns are essential for empowering parents, caregivers, and adolescents to make informed choices regarding mental health treatments. Offering resources, assistance, and psychoeducational information can ease worries and promote open dialogue among individuals involved in caring for children and teenagers with mental health requirements.

FACTORS TO CONSIDER WHEN IT COMES TO PRESCRIBING OFF-LABEL PSYCHOTROPICS

While prescribing psychotropic medications, psychiatrists must take into account the unique patient characteristics, therapeutic objectives, and potential dangers, in addition to the helpful insights provided by evidence-based reviews for the use of psychotropic drugs in children and adolescents. Off-label prescribing requires careful consideration of the following:

- *Risk–benefit analysis:* Professionals need to weigh the possible advantages of medication against the risks involved, considering variables like the severity of mental illness, how it affects functioning, and any potential side effects. Relying on good-quality scientific evidence rather than label indications can help decision-making.
- *Developmental considerations:* Children and adolescents may react to psychotropic drugs differently than adults due to developmental aspects like metabolism and neurobiology. Individual factors such as age, comorbidities, genetic predispositions, and medication history must be meticulously assessed.
- *Psychiatric diagnoses and symptomatology* also shape off-label prescribing choices. Clinicians must consider the severity and nature of the patient's symptoms, responsiveness to previous treatments, and the potential for drug interactions. Tailoring treatment to address specific symptoms while minimizing adverse effects is essential for optimizing patient outcomes.
- *Monitoring and follow-up:* When prescribing psychiatric drugs off-label, it is critical to do routine monitoring, which includes

evaluations of symptom response, adverse effects, and treatment compliance.

- *Legal and ethical ramifications* underscore off-label prescribing practices. Clinicians must adhere to regulatory frameworks, balancing patient needs with legal obligations and professional standards of care. Diligent rationale documentation, informed consent discussions, and ongoing monitoring are imperative to mitigate legal risks and uphold ethical principles.
- *Informed consent:* Professionals must participate in collaborative decision-making with patients and their families, including unambiguous and thorough details regarding the justification for off-label prescriptions, possible hazards, and substitute therapeutic alternatives.

In conclusion, prescribing off-label psychotropics necessitates a multifaceted approach that considers evidence-based practice, patient characteristics, informed consent, legal and ethical considerations, and ongoing monitoring. By carefully balancing these factors, clinicians can optimize treatment outcomes while prioritizing patient safety and well-being.

VARIOUS PSYCHOTROPICS USED OFF-LABEL IN CHILD PSYCHIATRY

Antidepressants

Antidepressants have been used for neurotic disorders for decades. Concerns from regulatory authorities about a possible link between AD use and suicidal behavior in minors caused a reduction in its use. Nonetheless, this decrease was only momentary, and research conducted in various nations noticed a rise in use among children and adolescents with time. Some ADs are approved by the Food and Drug Administration, like fluoxetine for major depressive disorder. Other types of ADs, such as serotonin–norepinephrine reuptake inhibitors (SNRIs), norepinephrine dopamine reuptake inhibitors (NDRIs), and tetracyclic antidepressants (TCAs), are being used off-label to treat depression and anxiety in children and adolescents as shown in **Box 1 and Table 1**.

Antipsychotics

In children, antipsychotic medications have been approved for mental health conditions such as schizophrenia, bipolar disorder, Tourette syndrome, and autism spectrum disorder. Nevertheless, in clinical practice, antipsychotics are often given to this group for various mental health disorders lacking US FDA approval. The rise in off-label antipsychotic use during the late 1990s and early 2000s was the main reason for the increase in antipsychotic usage. Multiple recommendations have been issued since 2011 regarding the common off-label utilization of antipsychotic medications.

The American Academy of Child and Adolescent Psychiatry (AACAP) practice parameter on the use of atypical antipsychotic medications in children and adolescents recommends that second-generation antipsychotics (SGAs) be considered the initial treatment option for FDA-approved conditions in children

BOX 1: Disorders in which antidepressants are used off-label in children and adolescents.

- Depression
- Anxiety disorders
- Obsessive-compulsive disorder (OCD)
- Dysthymia
- Bipolar disorder
- Mixed anxiety and depressive disorder
- Posttraumatic stress disorder (PTSD)
- Attention-deficit/hyperactivity disorder (ADHD)
- Tic disorder
- Autism spectrum disorders (ASDs)
- Somatoform disorders
- Sleep disorders
- Eating disorders
- Personality disorders
- Dissociative disorder
- Elimination disorders

TABLE 1: List of some commonly used antidepressants in child psychiatric clinical practice, along with potential side effects.

ADs	*Off-label use in*	*Side effects*[8]	*Dose range*
Escitalopram	• SAD[8] • Specific phobia • Panic disorder[8] • Separation anxiety disorder • Bipolar depression • PMDD[8] • PTSD[8]	• Gastrointestinal (decreased appetite, nausea, diarrhea, constipation, dry mouth) • Central nervous system (insomnia but also sedation, agitation, tremors, headache, dizziness) • Behavioral activation (rarely)	2.5–20 mg
Fluoxetine	• GAD[8] • SAD • Panic disorder • PTSD[8]	• Gastrointestinal (decreased appetite, nausea, diarrhea, constipation, dry mouth) • Central nervous system (insomnia but also sedation, agitation, tremors, headache, dizziness) • Behavioral activation	5–40 mg
Sertraline	• Depressive disorders • Bipolar depression • GAD[8] • SAD • PMDD • PTSD • Borderline personality disorder	• Decreased appetite, nausea, diarrhea, constipation, dry mouth • Insomnia but also sedation, agitation, tremors, headache, dizziness • Autonomic (sweating) • Bruising and rare bleeding • Behavioral activation	25–150 mg
Paroxetine	• GAD • SAD • Panic disorder • PTSD	• Decreased appetite, nausea, diarrhea, constipation, dry mouth • Insomnia but also sedation, agitation, dose-dependent tremors, headache, dizziness	12.5–37.5 mg
Duloxetine	• Somatoform disorders • Chronic pain[8]	• Nausea, diarrhea, decreased appetite, dry mouth, constipation • Insomnia, sedation, dizziness	10–40 mg
Venlafaxine	• Depressive disorders • SAD • PTSD[8] • PMDD[8]	• Headache, nervousness, insomnia, sedation • Nausea, diarrhea, decreased appetite • Asthenia, sweating • SIADH (syndrome of inappropriate antidiuretic hormone secretion) • Hyponatremia • Dose-dependent increase in blood pressure	37.5–200 mg
Bupropion	• ADHD[8] • Depressive disorders • Bipolar disorder[8] • Anxiety disorders	• Dry mouth, constipation, nausea, weight loss, anorexia, myalgia • Insomnia, dizziness, headache, agitation, anxiety, tremor, abdominal pain, tinnitus • Sweating, rash • Hypertension	50–200 mg

Contd...

Contd...

ADs	Off-label use in	Side effects[8]	Dose range
Mirtazapine	• Depressive disorders • Panic disorder[8] • GAD[8] • PTSD[8] • Insomnia • Anorexia nervosa • ADHD	• Dry mouth, constipation, increased appetite, weight gain • Sedation, dizziness, abnormal dreams, confusion • Flu-like symptoms (may indicate low white blood cell or granulocyte count) • Hypotension	6.25–30 mg
Amitriptyline	• Headache[8] • Somatoform disorders[8] • Enuresis • Depression • Anxiety disorders[8] • Insomnia[8]	• Sedative effects, dry mouth, constipation, and blurred vision • Weight gain • Dizziness, sedation, and hypotension • Cardiac arrhythmias and seizures	5–20 mg
Clomipramine	• OCD • Anxiety disorders[8] • Depressive disorders[8]	• Blurred vision, constipation, urinary retention, increased appetite, dry mouth, nausea, diarrhea, heartburn, unusual taste in the mouth, weight gain • Fatigue, weakness, dizziness, sedation, headache, anxiety, nervousness, restlessness	10–150 mg

(ADs: antidepressants; ADHD: attention-deficit/hyperactivity disorder; GAD: generalized anxiety disorder; OCD: obsessive-compulsive disorder; PMDD: premenstrual dysphoric disorder; PTSD: post-traumatic stress disorder; SAD: social anxiety disorder)

and adolescents aged 5–18 years.[9] **Box 2** gives a list of disorders in which antipsychotics are used off-label in children and adolescents. **Table 2** gives the uses and side effects of antipsychotics used in this population.

BOX 2: Disorders in which antipsychotics are used off-label in children and adolescents.

- Attention-deficit/hyperactivity disorder (ADHD)
- Disruptive behavior disorders (DBDs)
- Unspecified mood disorder
- Depression
- Bipolar disorder
- Anxiety
- Psychotic disorders
- Schizophrenia
- Tourette's syndrome
- Autism spectrum disorders

Antiepileptics

The use of anticonvulsants for psychiatric disorders in children and adolescents has significantly increased all over the world. **Box 3** gives a list of disorders in which anti-epileptic drugs (AEDs) are used off-label and **Table 3** gives the usual dose range and side effects of various AEDs.

Hypnotics and Sedatives

Sleep disturbances are commonly reported in children and adolescents, either primary sleep disorders or secondarily due to other disorders. In children with NDDs such as ADHD and ASD, parents are generally worried about the poor quality of their sleep. Neurotypical children also suffer from various sleep-related issues, impairing their quality of life. The use of hypnotics in children has always been a topic of controversy. Still, these are widely used in various childhood psychiatric as well as medical illnesses **(Table 4)**. Melatonin is considered a safe choice, and it is the only medicine approved in individuals aged 2–18 years with autism spectrum disorder and Smith–Magenis syndrome.[10]

TABLE 2: List of some commonly used antipsychotics in child psychiatric clinical practice, along with potential side effects.

Antipsychotic	*Off-label use in*	*Side effects*[8]	*Dose range*
Aripiprazole	• Depression (adjunct) • Acute agitation associated with schizophrenia or bipolar disorder [intramuscular (IM)] • Bipolar depression[8] • Behavioral disturbances in children and adolescents[8] • Disorders associated with problems with impulse control[8] • PTSD • Obsessive-compulsive disorder (adjunct to SSRIs)	• Extrapyramidal side effects (EPS, also called drug-induced parkinsonism), akathisia, sedation, tremor, headache, dizziness, insomnia • Nausea, vomiting • Salivary hypersecretion • Increased appetite, weight gain • Orthostatic hypotension, occasionally during initial dosing	1.25–20 mg
Clozapine	• Treatment-resistant COS • Reduction in the risk of recurrent suicidal behavior in patients with schizophrenia or schizoaffective disorder • Other psychotic disorders • Treatment-resistant bipolar disorder[8] • Violent, aggressive patients with psychosis and other brain disorders not responsive to other treatments[8] • Pervasive developmental disorders	*Limited data on children:* • Tachycardia • Increased appetite • Abnormal movements and EPS • Hypertension • Sedation/fatigue • *Hematological side effects:* Reduction in absolute WBC counts or ANC • Dizziness and hypotension • Sialorrhea • Enuresis • Constipation • QTc prolongation • Headache • Eosinophilia • Abnormal metabolic parameters—fever	50–300 mg
Haloperidol	• Bipolar disorder[8] • Delirium[8] • Violent, aggressive patients with psychosis	• EPS • NMS • Galactorrhea, amenorrhea (girls) • Gynecomastia (boys) • Sedation • Dizziness • Dry mouth, constipation, blurred vision, urinary retention • Decreased sweating • Hypotension, hypertension • Tardive dyskinesia, tardive dystonia (risk is higher in children than in adults) • Rare tachycardia	*Oral:* Initial 0.5 mg/day; target dose 0.05–0.15 mg/kg/day for psychotic disorders; 0.05–0.075 mg/kg/day for nonpsychotic disorders[8]

Contd...

Contd...

Antipsychotic	*Off-label use in*	*Side effects*[8]	*Dose range*
Olanzapine	• Treatment-resistant depression (in combination with fluoxetine) • Other psychotic disorders[8] • Behavioral disturbances in children and adolescents[8] • Disorders associated with problems with impulse control[8] • Anorexia nervosa • Borderline personality disorder[8] • Pervasive developmental disorders • Trichotillomania	• Increased appetite • Abnormal movements and EPS • Hypertension • Sedation/fatigue • Dizziness and hypotension • Headaches • Dyslipidemia and hyperglycemia • Deranged LFTs	2.5–20 mg
Quetiapine	• Bipolar depression • Childhood depression • Other psychotic disorders[8] • Mixed mania[8] • Behavioral disturbances in children and adolescents[8] • Disorders associated with problems with impulse control • Severe treatment-resistant anxiety[8]	• Weight gain, increased appetite • Dizziness, sedation, fatigue • Nausea, vomiting • Dry mouth • Dyslipidemia • Tachycardia • Orthostatic hypotension, usually during initial dose titration • The risk of tardive dyskinesia may be higher in children than it is in adults	12.5–400 mg
Risperidone	• Bipolar maintenance (monotherapy) • Bipolar depression[8] • Other psychotic disorders • Behavioral disturbances in children and adolescents[8] (except autism) • Pediatric delirium • Disorders associated with problems with impulse control[8] • Borderline personality disorder • Complex PTSD • Obsessive-compulsive disorder (adjunct to SSRIs) • Trichotillomania	• Dose-dependent extrapyramidal symptoms • Dose-dependent hyperprolactinemia • Dose-dependent dizziness, anxiety, sedation, tremor, akathisia • Nausea, vomiting, constipation, • Abdominal pain • Weight gain, increased appetite • The risk of tardive dyskinesia may be higher in children than it is in adults • Galactorrhea/amenorrhea (girls) • Gynecomastia (boys) • Dyslipidemia	0.25–6 mg

(ANC: absolute neutrophil count; COS: childhood-onset schizophrenia; EPS: extrapyramidal symptoms; LFTs: liver function tests; NMS: neuroleptic malignant syndrome; PTSD: post-traumatic stress disorder; SSRIs: selective serotonin reuptake inhibitors; WBC: white blood cell)

Psychostimulants

Psychostimulant medications, such as methylphenidate and amphetamine derivates, have long been a cornerstone in the treatment of children and adolescents with ADHD. Numerous studies have highlighted their effectiveness in enhancing attention span, impulse control, and overall behavioral regulation, facilitating better classroom performance and interpersonal relationships. **Table 5** provides a list of psychostimulants used in children and adolescents.

Drugs-addictive Disorder

Apart from buprenorphine, which is approved for opioid-use disorder from 16 years of age, there are currently no FDA-approved drugs for substance-use disorder in adolescents.[11]

Studies have shown preliminary evidence for the use of disulfiram and acamprosate for the treatment of adolescents with alcohol dependence. Also, naltrexone has been shown to reduce cravings in this population.

BOX 3: Disorders in which antiepileptics are used off-label in children and adolescents.

- Autism spectrum disorders (ASDs)
- Disruptive behavior disorders (DBDs)
- Aggression, agitation in neurodevelopmental disorders (NDDs)
- Intermittent explosive disorder
- Bipolar disorder
- Depression
- Anxiety disorders
- Gaming disorder

N-acetylcysteine (NAC) is used off-label for cannabis dependence syndrome in adolescents.

For the treatment of methamphetamine dependence, bupropion has been tried in adolescents.[12]

Miscellaneous

Apart for the drugs mentioned above, there are other drugs used off-label in this population **(Table 6)**.

SUMMARY AND CONCLUSION

To summarize, the significance of recognizing and managing mental health disorders in children and adolescents has gained more attention in recent years. The treatment of a variety of mental illnesses in this population depends extensively on psychopharmacology, the study of how medications affect mood, behavior, and cognition. Nonetheless, some difficulties and factors need to be considered when using psychotropic drugs in children and adolescents, especially when doing so off-label as in such circumstances adequate research and review process have not happened for approval.

TABLE 3: List of some commonly used antiepileptics in child psychiatric clinical practice, along with potential side effects.

Antiepileptics	*Off-label use*	*Side effects*[8]	*Dose range*
Valproate	• Acute mania • Maintenance treatment of bipolar disorder[8] • Bipolar depression[8] • Schizophrenia (adjunctive)[8] • Aggression/agitation in neurodevelopmental disorders • Treatment-resistant depression • Borderline personality disorder	• Sedation, dose-dependent tremor, dizziness, ataxia, asthenia, headache • Abdominal pain, nausea, vomiting, diarrhea, reduced appetite, constipation, dyspepsia, weight gain • Alopecia • Hyperandrogenism, hyperinsulinemia, lipid dysregulation	150–800 mg
Lamotrigine	• Bipolar depression[8] • Major depressive disorder (adjunctive)[8] • Schizophrenia (adjunctive)[8]	• Benign rash • Blurred or double vision, dizziness, ataxia • Sedation, headache, tremor, insomnia, poor coordination, fatigue • Nausea, vomiting, dyspepsia, rhinitis • Pharyngitis, asthenia	25–200 mg

TABLE 4: List of some commonly used hypnotics in child psychiatric clinical practice, along with potential side effects.

Medication	*Off-label use in*	*Side effects*[8]	*Dose range*
Melatonin	• Sleep disturbances in ADHD • Primary insomnia • Secondary insomnia • Pediatric delirium	• Headaches • Increased bedwetting • Dizziness • Morning grogginess	1.5–6 mg
Clonazepam	• Acute mania (adjunctive)[8] • Acute psychosis (adjunctive)[8] • Primary insomnia[8] • Catatonia[8] • Panic disorder[8] • Other anxiety disorders • Aggression/agitation in children with NDDs	• Sedation, fatigue • Dizziness, ataxia, slurred speech, weakness • Forgetfulness, confusion • Hyperexcitability, nervousness • Hypersalivation, dry mouth • Long-term effects of clonazepam in children/adolescents are unknown • For anxiety, children and adolescents should generally receive lower doses and be more closely monitored	0.25–2 mg
Lorazepam	• Catatonia[8] • Acute mania (adjunctive)[8] • Acute psychosis (adjunctive)[8] • Primary insomnia[8] • Panic disorder • Other anxiety disorders • Rapid tranquilization of the agitated patient • Aggression/agitation in children with NDDs • Delirium[8]	• Sedation, fatigue, depression • Dizziness, ataxia, slurred speech, weakness • Forgetfulness, confusion • Hyperexcitability, nervousness • Pain at the injection site	0.5–8 mg

(ADHD: attention-deficit/hyperactivity disorder; NDDs: neurodevelopmental disorders)

TABLE 5: Psychostimulants used in children and adolescents.

Medication	*Off-label use in*	*Side effects*[8]	*Dose range*
Methylphenidate	• Treatment-resistant depression[8] • Hyperactivity/inattention in ASD • Hyperactivity in intellectual disability	• Insomnia, headache, exacerbation of tics, nervousness, irritability, overstimulation, tremor, dizziness • Anorexia, nausea, abdominal pain, weight loss • Can temporarily slow average growth in children • Blurred vision	5–30 mg
Modafinil	• ADHD[8] • Major depressive disorder (adjunctive)[8] • Bipolar depression[8]	• Headache (dose-dependent) • Anxiety, nervousness, insomnia • Dry mouth, diarrhea, nausea, anorexia • Pharyngitis, rhinitis, infection • Hypertension • Palpitations	100–200 mg

(ADHD: attention-deficit/hyperactivity disorder; ASD: autism spectrum disorder)

TABLE 6: Other drugs used off-label.

Medication	*Off-label use*	*Side effects*[8]	*Dose range*
Lithium	• Major depressive disorder (adjunctive)[8] • Bipolar depression[8] • Neutropenia[8] • Aggression/agitation in neurodevelopmental disorders	• Ataxia, dysarthria, delirium, tremor, memory problems • Polyuria, polydipsia (nephrogenic diabetes insipidus) • Diarrhea, nausea • Weight gain • Euthyroid goiter or hypothyroid goiter • Acne, rash, alopecia	150–600 mg

Overall in the field of child and adolescent psychiatry, off-label prescriptions are widespread. However, there is not enough evidence to support the off-label use of medications in this population. Treatment during a stage of life when the patient experiences significant changes in neurobiology, hormones, and development frequently necessitates dosage schedules that differ from those of adults and can cause substantial and potentially severe adverse drug reactions. Therapeutic options may be limited in pediatric populations without the off-label prescription. This presents challenges and opportunities for psychiatrists as we must navigate between available evidence, clinical guidelines, and individual patient needs.

REFERENCES

1. Choonara I, Conroy S. Unlicensed and off-label drug use in children: implications for safety. Drug Saf. 2002;25(1):1-5.
2. Lorberg B, Davico C, Martsenkovskyi D, Vitiello B. Principles in using psychotropic medication in children and adolescents. In Rey JM, Martin A (Eds), IACAPAP e-Textbook of Child and Adolescent Mental Health. Geneva: International Association for Child and Adolescent Psychiatry and Allied Professions; 2019.
3. Bell JS, Richards GC. Off-label medicine use: Ethics, practice, and future directions. Aust J Gen Pract. 2021;50(5):329-31.
4. Dörks M, Langner I, Dittmann U, Timmer A, Garbe E. Antidepressant drug use and off-label prescribing in children and adolescents in Germany: results from a large population-based cohort study. Eur Child Adolesc Psychiatry. 2013;22(8):511-8.
5. Sridharan K, Arora K, Chaudhary S. Off-label drug use in psychiatry: A retrospective audit in a tertiary care hospital. Asian J Psychiatr. 2016;24:124.
6. Egberts KM, Gerlach M, Correll CU, Plener PL, Malzahn U, Heuschmann P, et al. Serious Adverse Drug Reactions in Children and Adolescents Treated On- and Off-Label with Antidepressants and Antipsychotics in Clinical Practice. Pharmacopsychiatry. 2022;55(5):255-65.
7. Zito JM, Derivan AT, Kratochvil CJ, Safer DJ, Fegert JM, Greenhill LL. Off-label psychopharmacologic prescribing for children: History supports close clinical monitoring. Child Adolesc Psychiatry Ment Health. 2008;2:24.
8. Stahl SM. Stahl's Essential Psychopharmacology, Prescriber's Guide, Antipsychotics, 6th edition. Cambridge University Press; 2018.
9. Findling R, Drury S, Jensen P, Rapoport J. (2011). Practice parameter for using atypical antipsychotic medications in children and adolescents. AACAP. [online] Available from https://www.aacap.org/ App_Themes/AACAP/docs/practice_parameters/Atypical_antipsychotic_Medications_Web.pdf [Last accessed 20 November, 2025].
10. European Medicines Agency. [online] Available from https://www.ema.europa.eu/en/medicines/human/EPAR/slenyto. [Last accessed November, 2025].
11. Squeglia LM, Fadus MC, McClure EA, Tomko RL, Gray KM. Pharmacological Treatment of Youth Substance Use Disorders. J Child Adolesc Psychopharmacol. 2019;29(7):559-72.
12. Courtney DB, Milin R. Pharmacotherapy for Adolescents with Substance Use Disorders. Curr Treat Options Psych. 2015;2(3):312-25.

CHAPTER 30

Somatic Therapies

Shivani Gusain, Shrinidhi Pratinidhi, Nishant Goyal

INTRODUCTION

The mainstays of treatment for psychiatric diseases continue to be medications and psychotherapies. Even with advances in basic neurosciences, 20–60% of these patients still do not respond well to these kinds of therapy. Additionally, a lack of adherence to the prescribed treatment methods adds to the expense of healthcare. Thus, the need for developing novel ways of treatment has emerged.

Prior to the development of pharmacology, new somatic treatments for psychiatric diseases were subject of intense interest in the 1930s and 1940s.[1] Insulin coma and malarial fever therapy, e.g., were intensely studied and clinically used. Convulsive therapies (chemical and electrical) also initially appeared in that era. After the advent of antidepressant medications and other pharmacologic treatments, only electroconvulsive therapy (ECT) remained the earliest and one of the most effective treatment modalities to treat altered brain activity through electrical activity modification. Since its origin, ECT, the "gold standard" intervention, has withstood the test of time and is still regarded as one of the most effective "interventions", being used in both the West and India. Utilizing the "Ediswan system", created by Wilcox and Friedman, it was first employed in India in 1953 at the Central Institute of Psychiatry (CIP). Today, nonpharmacological somatic treatments are making a comeback. This may be due to the fact that many patients cannot benefit from pharmacotherapy and psychotherapy, as well as the fact that advancements in engineering have made it possible to use previously unheard-of noninvasive neuromodulation techniques.[2] There is currently an explosion of knowledge about brain functioning and neurocircuitry thanks to the US Government's Brain Research Through Advancing Innovative Neurotechnologies (BRAIN) initiative and the Defense Advanced Research Projects Agency's $70 million project called Systems-Based Neurotechnology and Understanding for the Treatment of Neuropsychological Illnesses (SUBNETS). The goal of SUBNETS is to create closed-loop, intelligent neuromodulation technologies that can be used to alter malfunctioning circuits in neuropsychiatric illnesses.[3] Our understanding of the brain has changed as a result of these research initiatives, and many newer modalities are being employed to modulate neuronal functioning, including noninvasive brain stimulation (NIBS) methods such as repetitive transcranial magnetic stimulation (rTMS), transcranial direct current stimulation (tDCS), and invasive ones such as vagus nerve stimulation (VNS), epidural cortical stimulation, and deep brain stimulation (DBS) **(Flowcharts 1 and 2)**. The basic differences are further briefed in **Table 1**.

Flowchart 1: Methods of noninvasive brain stimulation.

- **Brain stimulation** → Noninvasive
  - Transcranial electric stimulation
    - Electroconvulsive therapy (ECT)
    - Low-intensity transcranial electrical stimulation
      - Transcranial direct current stimulation (tDCS)
      - Transcranial alternate current stimulation (tACS)
      - Transcranial random noise stimulation (tRNS)
  - Transcranial magnetic stimulation
    - Deep transcranial magnetic stimulation (dTMS)
    - Magnetic seizure therapy
    - Repetitive transcranial magnetic stimulation (rTMS)
      - *Standard protocols:* High and low frequency rTMS
      - *Theta burst protocol:* Intermittent TBS (iTBS) and continuous TBS (cTBS)

Flowchart 2: Methods of invasive brain stimulation.

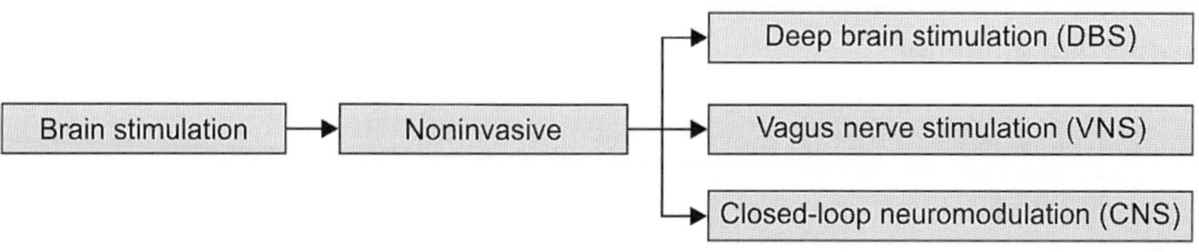

TABLE 1: Brain stimulation methods—human interventions.

Intervention	*Convulsive*	*Implanted*	*Magnetic*
Transcranial magnetic stimulation (TMS)	–	–	Yes
Transcranial electrical stimulation (tDCS, tACS, and tRNS)	–	–	–
Transcranial pulsed ultrasound stimulation (tPUS)	–	–	–
Vagus nerve stimulation (VNS)	–	Yes	–
Deep brain stimulation (DBS)	–	Yes	–
Closed-loop or responsive DBS	–	Yes	–
Electroconvulsive therapy (ECT)	Yes	–	–
Magnetic seizure therapy (MST)	Yes	–	Yes
Focal electrically applied seizure therapy (FEAST)	Yes	–	–

(tACS: transcranial alternating current stimulation; tDCS: transcranial direct current stimulation; tRNS: transcranial random noise stimulation)

ELECTROCONVULSIVE THERAPY

Electroconvulsive therapy is somatic treatment that is based on conducting an electrical current through the brain to stimulate it and trigger generalized convulsive activity with therapeutic outcomes. It is highly proven modality for various psychiatric disorders. Ladislas J Meduna suggested that seizures could be used to treat mental illness in 1934. Ugo Cerletti and Lucio Bini developed a faster, less adverse seizure induction method using dogs. With advancements in their techniques, the first human study was conducted in 1938 on a 39-year-old man with schizophrenia and disorganization. Holmberg and Thesleff introduced "modified" (anesthetized) ECT in 1952, which significantly improved patient comfort and tolerance.[4]

Indications

In **Table 2**, there is a list of conditions where ECT is recommended in children and adolescents according to different guidelines.

Procedure

Electrode Placement (Fig. 1)

- *Bilateral:* Bitemporal and bifrontal
- *Unilateral*
  - *Right unilateral:* This is shown to have lesser cognitive adversities.
  - *Left unilateral:* This placement can be chosen when sparing nonverbal and visual memory is needed more than sparing verbal memory. It is also considered in those having the right dominant brain function.[6]

The pediatric psychiatrist may choose a right unilateral or bifrontal position over the classic bitemporal position to reduce post-ECT language, cognitive, or retrograde amnestic complications in some children. ECT is generally administered twice or thrice a week.[7] If there is a total clinical improvement or remission, ECT can be stopped at any moment. Before considering the lack of response to ECT, at least 8–12 ECT sessions should be given in acute courses if adequate clinical

TABLE 2: Common indications for use of ECT in children and adolescents population.[5]

	NIH/NICE	*AACAP*	*APA*
General indications	Severe symptoms after an adequate trial of other treatment options have been ineffective and/or considered to be potentially life-threatening	Failure to respond to at least 2 adequate trials of appropriate psychopharmacological agents accompanied by other appropriate treatment modalities	Other viable treatments have been ineffective or if other treatments cannot be administered safely
Mood disorders	Yes, for major depression or prolonged and/or severe manic episode	Yes, severe persistent major depression or mania with/ without psychotic features	Yes, major depressive disorder or mania
Schizophrenia	Not recommended	Yes, schizoaffective disorder, or, less often, schizophrenia	Yes
Catatonia	Yes	Yes	Yes
ID	Not recommended	Not recommended	Not recommended
SIB and aggression	Not recommended	Not recommended	Not recommended
Others		NMS	NMS

(AACAP: American Academy of Child and Adolescent Psychiatry; APA: American Psychological Association; ID: intellectual disabilities; NIH: National Institute of Health; NICE: National Institute for Health and Care Excellence; SIB: self-injurious behavior)

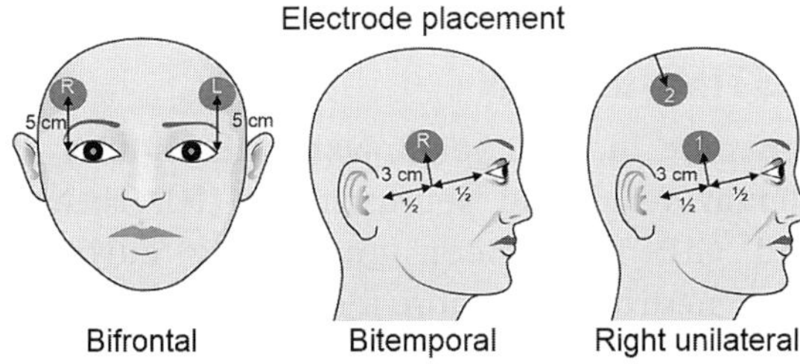

Fig. 1: Various electrode placements for ECT.
Source: Adapted from Tirthalli et al. (2023).

improvement is not seen.[6] Children with severe neuropsychiatric disorders characterized by extreme self-injury and aggression may require 12 or more treatments. Modified ECT is given under general anesthesia.

Mechanism of Action of Electroconvulsive Therapy

Electroconvulsive therapy possesses several key therapeutic actions, having antimanic, antidepressants, and antipsychotic effects by modulating various neuronal functions as well as neuroplasticity. The exact mechanism **(Table 3)** by which ECT produces favorable outcomes in certain pediatric psychiatric diseases is unknown, but most theories suggest that major neurotransmitter, neuroendocrine, and neurotrophic changes occur within the central nervous system after a series of treatments. **Table 3** shows some proposed neuronal changes leading to therapeutic effects of ECT.

TABLE 3: Various proposed mechanisms of ECT.[8]

Neurotransmitter	*Neuroendocrine*	*Neurotropic*
Increased serotonin	Increased ACTH	Neurogenesis (Hippocampus, prefrontal cortex, and limbic structures)
Increased dopamine	Increased cortisol	Gliogenesis
Increased norepinephrine	Increased prolactin	Alteration of dendritic/axonal arborization
Increased GABA	Increased arginine/vasopressin	
Increased glutamate		
Decreased glutamate/GABA ratio		

Regulatory Issues and Ethics

Mental Healthcare Act (MHCA) 2017 prohibits unmodified ECT in Section 95(1) for mental illness patients without muscle relaxants and anesthesia, and for minors. However, it allows for ECT for minors with informed consent and prior Board permission, as per WHO recommendations. This exception allows for ECT for minors. Section 94 of the MHCA 2017 allows emergency treatment for persons with mental illness (PMI) for 72 hours or until assessed at a mental health establishment. Treatment is only given to prevent death, irreversible harm, serious harm, or property damage.[9]

Safety

Electroconvulsive therapy is infrequently used in adolescents and children due to concerns about adverse effects on maturing nervous systems; however, in clinical conditions that are life-threatening such as psychotic depression and catatonic states, ECT is considered beneficial and safe.[10]

Attitude (and Stigma) Toward Electroconvulsive Therapy

Despite its importance in treating life-threatening mental illnesses, ECT is often misunderstood and feared due to its negative portrayal in films and television shows where it is often administered without consent, under duress, or without anesthesia. Despite recent improvements in media portrayal of people with mental illnesses, realistic depictions of ECT remain difficult to find. Differences in perceptions between patients and clinicians regarding the benefits and drawbacks of ECT remain a concern in contemporary psychiatry.[11]

Adverse Effects

- General adverse effects include headache, nausea, and generalized myalgia. These adverse effects generally resolve by themselves.
- *Cognitive impairment:* This includes small deficits in processing speed, spatial problem-solving, global cognition, episodic memory, and medium-to-large short-term (up to 3 days post-ECT) deficits in executive functioning and episodic memory. All deficits start to improve within 15 days of completion of ECT and intellectual ability deficiency is not reported.
- *Anterograde and retrograde amnesia:* Anterograde and retrograde amnesia cumulate across the ECT course; that is, it increases with the number of ECTs administered. Anterograde amnesia attenuates days to weeks after ECT, and return of learning abilities to the pre-ECT baseline (or better, especially, if the illness has remitted) is substantially complete within a month. Retrograde amnesia slowly attenuates weeks to months after ECT. However, many patients experience long-lasting, patchy memory deficits, particularly for events during and around the ECT course. Some patients may have difficulty in recalling events that occurred years before the treatment.[10]

TRANSCRANIAL MAGNETIC STIMULATION

For more than 15 years, National Institute of Mental Health and Neurosciences (NIMHANS) and CIP have been employing cutting-edge neuromodulation techniques, such as transcranial magnetic stimulation (TMS), for a range of diagnostic and therapeutic applications. They have lately included more modern brain stimulation techniques, including hybrid and direct current stimulation. These neuromodulations and neuroinvestigative research are conducted at the CIP and NIMHANS-run Translational Psychiatry Laboratory and the Center for Cognitive Neurosciences, respectively. These facilities use techniques such as functional magnetic resonance imaging (MRI), volumetric MRI, diffusion tensor imaging, high-resolution EEG, and infrared spectroscopy, which continuously provide translational inputs for further delineating the brain's physiology derangement. A Centre for Advanced Research and Excellence in Neuromodulation (CARE) grant has been given to AIIMS, New Delhi, by the ICMR to strengthen the work.[12]

The number of rTMS studies, including clinical trials, has increased significantly over the past ten years and has been found to be a promising noninvasive treatment for a variety of neuropsychiatric conditions.[13-17] TMS is safe if appropriate guidelines and precautions are followed.[18] TMS can be used to explore brain-behavior relations, map sensory, motor, and higher-order cognitive functions[19] and examine the excitability, connectivity, and plasticity of different cortical regions from newborns to the elderly.[20] Depending on the stimulation parameters, particularly frequency and pattern of stimulation, cortical reactivity is potentiated or depressed.

Repetitive Transcranial Magnetic Stimulation

Basic Principle of Transcranial Magnetic Stimulation

Transcranial magnetic stimulation works on the principle of electromagnetic induction **(Fig. 2)**, which was first discovered by Michael Faraday in 1831. A wire on the scalp generates a magnetic field that penetrates the cranium, causing an eddy current in the brain. This current then penetrates neuron membranes, triggering an action potential or excitatory/inhibitory postsynaptic potential **(Fig. 3)**.

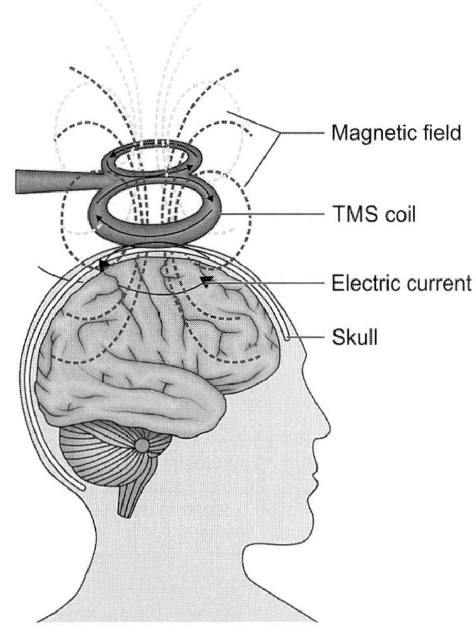

Fig. 2: Basic principle of transcranial magnetic stimulation (TMS).

Mechanism of Action

The differences between ECT and TMS are listed in **Table 4**.

Types of Repetitive Transcranial Magnetic Stimulation

Types of rTMS are as follows:

- *Low frequency:* ≤1 Hz—decreases cortical excitability
- *High frequency:* ≥5 Hz—increases cortical excitability
- *Patterned rTMS:* Theta burst stimulation (TBS)—continuous, intermittent and intermediate
- *Quadripulse stimulation (QPS)*

This variability is based on intensity and duration of stimulation and baseline excitability. **Figure 4** illustrates the various types of rTMS.

Types of Coil

The simplest TMS coil type, circular or round, produces an annulus-shaped E-field pattern. Figure-8 coils produce a more focused pattern, with significant cortex stimulation. There is a trade-off between stimulation focality and depth, with larger coils having a deeper but less focal E-field.[21-23]

Double-cone coils are larger versions of figure-8 coils, angled toward the subject's head to increase magnetic field strength and electrical efficiency, resulting in a deeper E-field and less focality.[24] They have been utilized to target brain regions [such as the leg motor area, medial prefrontal cortex (PFC), insula, and cerebellum] difficult to reach with standard coil.[25-27] Similarly, H-coils also designed to penetrate deeper in the brain than typical figure-8 coils at the expense of reduced focality.[28-31]

Investigations are being conducted into a number of protocols, including once daily, twice or more daily (sometimes known as intense or accelerated protocols),[32] 3–5/week, once weekly, fortnightly, or even once a month maintenance program. Researchers are exploring the effects of rTMS on psychiatric disorders using new brain regions, such as supplementary motor area, cerebellum, and orbitofrontal cortex in addition to traditional target sites such as temporoparietal cortex (TPC), and the dorsolateral prefrontal cortex (DLPFC).[33]

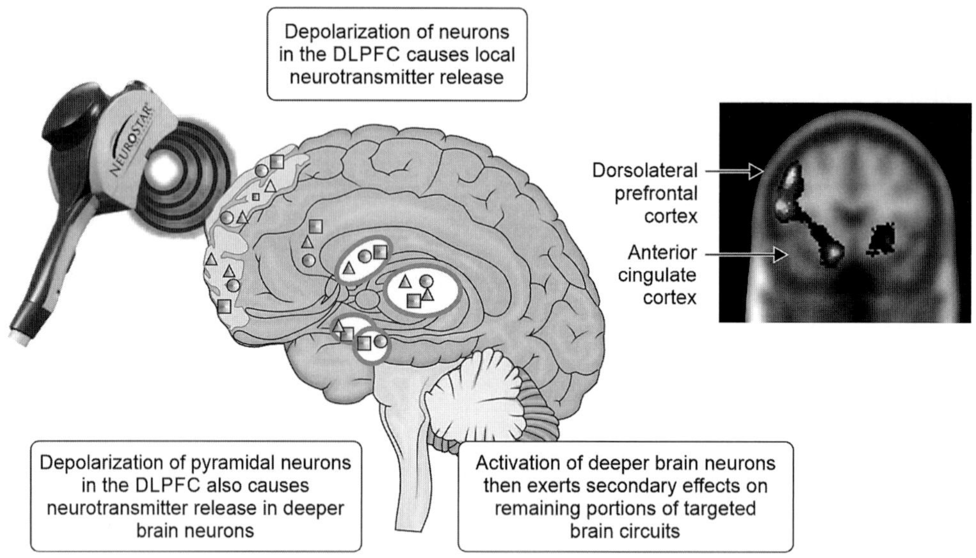

Fig. 3: Mechanism of action of transcranial magnetic stimulation (TMS). (DLPFC: dorsolateral prefrontal cortex)

TABLE 4: Differences between ECT and TMS.

	ECT	*TMS*
Direction of induced current	Radial	Tangential
Current reaches deep structures	Yes	No
Anesthesia required	Yes	No
Seizure induced	Yes	No

(ECT: electroconvulsive therapy; TMS: transcranial magnetic stimulation)

It has been suggested that using image-guided navigation without or with a robot to hold the coil will increase the reproducibility and dependability of TMS coil positioning.[34-36]

TMS has been used more frequently in children and adolescents throughout the past 10 years, particularly in the last 2 years, which calls for special consideration of how they are used in developing brains. During development, the brain undergoes extensive neuronal changes, making it more susceptible to neuroplastic changes, potentially beneficial in pediatric populations, but raising safety and ethical concerns about stimulation parameters.[37]

Clinical Application of Repetitive Transcranial Magnetic Stimulation

Clinical applications of rTMS include the following:

- *Major depressive disorder:*
    - Donaldson et al.[38] suggested that TMS may be an effective and well-tolerated treatment for treatment-resistant depression in adolescents.[28]
    - Sun et al.[39] have also suggested the efficacy, tolerability, and safety of rTMS as an adjunct treatment for adolescents (12–18 years) with first episode of major depressive disorder and also found it to be effective not only in improving depressive symptoms but also neurocognitive functioning in the patients. High-frequency TMS (10 Hz) over the left DLPFC is the most commonly used protocol in such studies.

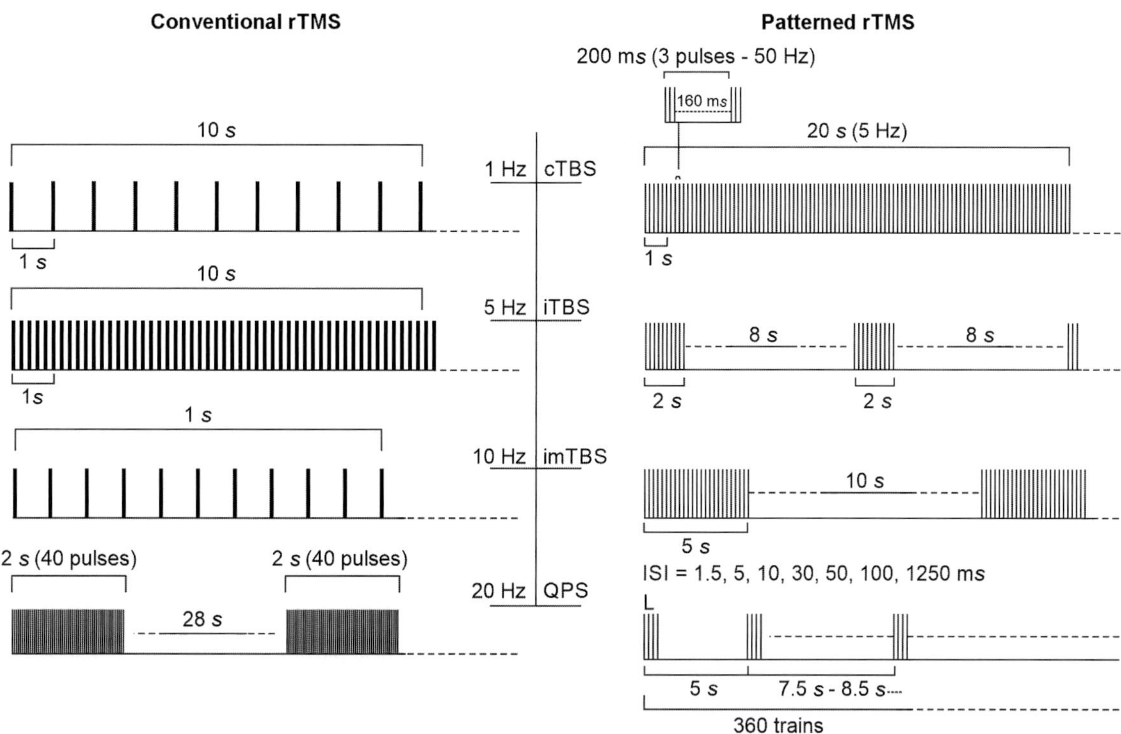

Fig. 4: Various types of rTMS used for therapeutic purposes.[18] (cTBS: continuous theta burst stimulation, iTBS: intermittent TBS, imTBS: intermediate TBS, QPS: quadripulse stimulation; rTMS: repetitive transcranial magnetic stimulation)

- *Autism spectrum disorder (ASD):* Smith et al.[40] have suggested the role of low frequency (1 Hz) rTMS over DLPFC in the treatment of restricted and repetitive behaviors and improving deficits in executive functioning in patients of ASD. One study by Ni et al.[41] has shown promise for improvement in social symptoms by targeting to the posterior superior temporal sulcus (pSTS) via TBS. High-frequency TBS protocols have been applied to the motor cortex in high functioning autism for the same.[42]
- *Tourette disorder:* Low-frequency TMS (at 1 Hz, 110% MT, 10–20 sessions) applied over bilateral supplementary motor area has been shown to improve symptoms for up to 6 months but more controlled research is required in these group of patients.[43]
- *Attention-deficit/hyperactivity disorder (ADHD):* In a study of 9 subjects (age 15–20 years), high-frequency TMS applied to the right PFC (100% MT, 10 sessions) showed no difference between active and sham groups. Adults with ADHD have benefited most from TMS use, which has been shown to improve hyperactivity but not attention.[44]
- *Schizophrenia:* Numerous research studies have demonstrated the efficacy of low-frequency rTMS (LF-rTMS), which targets the left temporoparietal cortex (LTPC), in reducing auditory hallucinations in individuals with schizophrenia in adults. However, the results have been less clear when it comes to other psychotic and negative symptoms or cognitive function. The high-frequency rTMS (HF-rTMS) localized at the

L-DLPFC has been utilized in several research to relieve unpleasant symptoms.[45]

- *Cerebral palsy:* The most current review study examined the safety of noninvasive brain stimulation (rTMS and tDCS) for children with cerebral palsy's upper extremities and concluded that both methods were reasonably certain to be safe and practicable.[46]

Deep Transcranial Magnetic Stimulation

Studies have been done to modulate orbitofrontal cortex with the use of deep TMS (dTMS) in improvement of obsessive–compulsive disorder (OCD) symptomatology.[47] In another study, dTMS was applied for 15 sessions over 3 weeks to the right PFC in adults with ADHD, which showed improvement in inattention/memory symptom severity.[44] Another study by Garg et al., showed that high-frequency dTMS over cerebellar vermis can be used as an effective adjunct to treat negative and affective symptoms of schizophrenia.[48]

Quadripulse stimulation: The QPS was invented to induce robust long-term potentiation (LTP) or long-term depression (LTD) effects in human brain using monophasic magnetic/electric pulses.[49-51]

Side Effects

The most frequent side effects are mild and include headaches, tingling, warmth, twitching of the face muscles, and lightheadedness, which resolve soon after stimulation. Studies using paired and single pulse TMSs demonstrate minimal harm to children. The most serious risk of rTMS, particularly with HF-rTMS, is theoretically the induction of seizures, but this is rare. It is highly recommended to use child-sized well-fitting earplugs during TMS application (especially, HF-rTMS) as loud clicking noises (up to 120 dB) can also induce hearing deficiencies.[37]

Safety and Tolerability

Many systematic reviews have confirmed that rTMS poses little risk to children and adolescents, especially, when the specific safety guidelines for the application of rTMS are followed.[37,52]

TRANSCRANIAL ELECTRICAL STIMULATION

Unlike TMS, in which electrical current is induced via electromagnetic induction, in transcranial electrical stimulation (TES), electrical current transfers directly through electrodes. Here, a weak electrical current is applied to the scalp, typically via two (or more) electrodes in different modalities, impacting neuroplasticity and other neuronal functions. If the electrical current is applied directly between electrodes mounted on the head, it is called tDCS, which is the most popular variant of TES.[53] It can depolarize or hyperpolarize resting membrane potential, with anodal polarity having excitatory effects and cathodal polarity having inhibitory effects. Transcranial alternating current stimulation (tACS) is another modality that uses oscillatory electrical current to facilitate neuronal activity in specific frequency bands.[54] Transcranial random noise stimulation (tRNS) is a mix of frequencies of alternating electrical current, which can be delivered at low (between 0.1 and 100 Hz) or high (between 101 and 640 Hz) frequencies.[55] tDCS is a more portable, economical, and tolerable NIBS technique as compared to TMS, offering a safer profile and potential to reach a broader population[56] **(Figs. 5A to D)**.

Transcranial direct current stimulation has been increasingly researched for potential in treating severe psychiatric disorders in childhood and adolescence and can be combined with other therapeutic tools such as psychotherapy, physical therapy, cognitive rehabilitation, and pharmacotherapy to enhance clinical effects.[56,57]

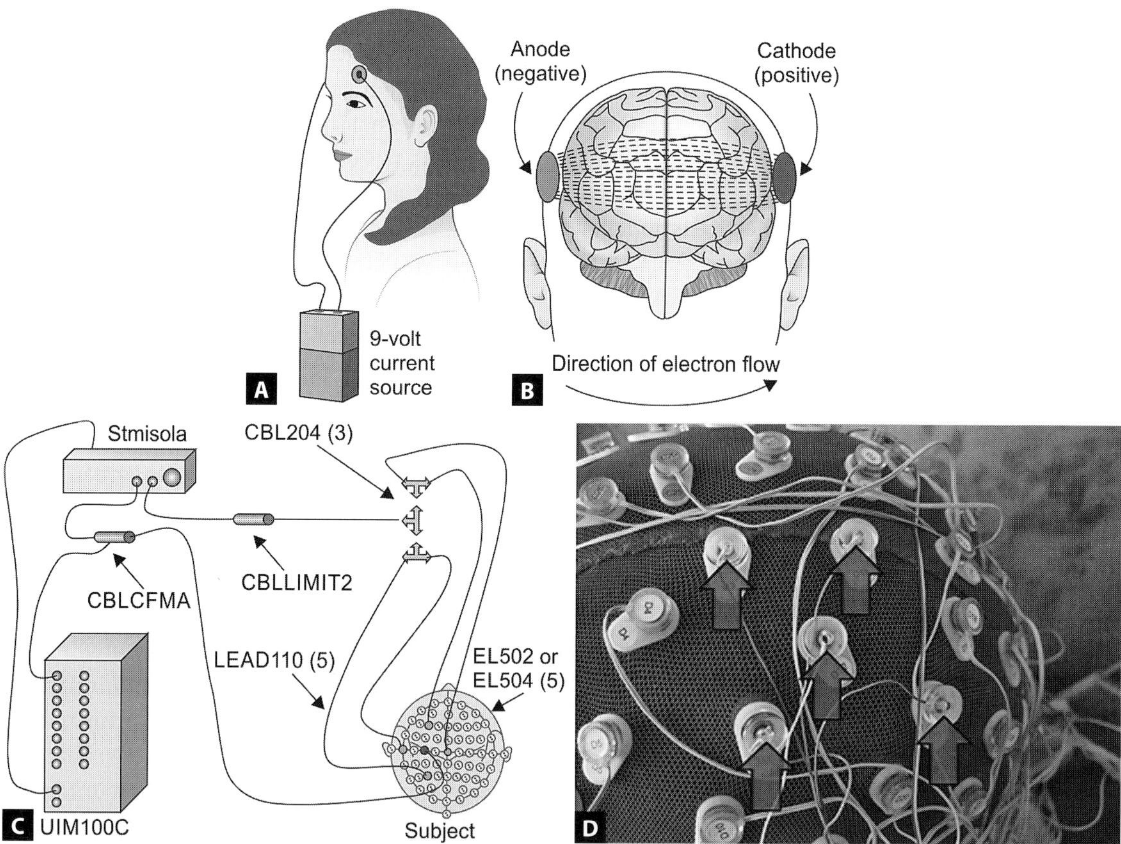

Figs. 5A to D: Transcranial direct current stimulation (tDCS) setup.

Clinical Applications of Transcranial Electrical Stimulation

- *Autism spectrum disorder:*
    - Anodal tDCS over the left DLPFC[58-60] was the most often applied protocol in ASD, for improvement in behavioral and social functioning in such patients. Other recent studies also have reported improving effects of frontocerebellar tDCS on behavioral symptoms,[61] and anodal stimulation over the primary motor cortex showing improvement in motor skills in children with ASD.[62]
    - These studies raise the possibility of the use of tDCS as a therapeutic tool for core autistic symptoms.
- *Attention-deficit/hyperactivity disorder:* 10 studies have shown partial improvement in cognitive deficits (response inhibition, working memory, attention, and cognitive flexibility) or clinical symptoms (e.g., impulsivity and inattention) with good tolerability of tDCS, targeting the left and right DLPFC. Anodal tDCS is most commonly applied, with a smaller intensity of 1 mA in children and adolescents.[63,64] Additional cortical regions such as the medial PFC, right inferior frontal gyrus, and right DLPFC are also being investigated.
- *Dyslexia:* Reading performance and abilities were primary outcome measures in 5 of 7 tDCS randomized controlled trials (RCTs) in

developmental dyslexia[65-67] and in all of them, a significant improvement was observed in reading components (e.g., reading accuracy, word frequency, reading speed, and reading fluency).

- *Emotional regulation in adolescents:* Abend et al.[68] have suggested that subjective emotional experiences may be modulated by tDCS, this effect has been found to be linked with mPFC and limbic activation.
- *Addictive behaviors:* tDCS have been found to modulate craving, impulsivity, and executive functions, improving inhibitory control over addiction-related distractors and influencing control and reward systems[69,70] in internet gaming disorders and food addiction.

Side Effects

The most common adverse effects of TES include mild tingling, fatigue, itching, headache, nausea, and insomnia, similar in children. These mild effects disappear soon after stimulation, indicating good tolerability in existing study samples.[37] There were no serious side effects or adverse events. A previous study[52] also reported great tolerability of NIBS (tDCS and TMS) in children and adolescents with neurological and psychiatric conditions. **Figure 6** illustrates the safety considerations in children and adolescents.

Regulatory Issues and Ethics

It is crucial to take into account the possible effects of the neurological or psychiatric condition being treated, the effects of concurrent medications, and the chronicity of exposure in order to comprehend the unique safety and ethical challenges raised by therapeutic uses of TMS. Utilizing TMS in patient populations is different from using it in basic neuroscience because the individual getting TMS has a neurological or psychiatric condition already, and they are probably on a variety of concurrent treatments that involve CNS acting medications (e.g., antidepressants, antipsychotics, anxiolytics, analgesics, and anticonvulsants), which may impact the effectiveness of TMS and alter seizure risk. The increasing use of NIBS in pediatric populations necessitates careful consideration and ethical and safe implementation of these methods. Pediatric TMS safety may be influenced by some physical developmental processes, such as (a) cortical excitability maturation, (b) fontanelle closure, and (c) external auditory canal expansion.

Three fundamental ethical and regulatory considerations that apply to all studies involving human participants have been fully agreed upon and should guide research and therapeutic uses of TMS:

1. *Informed consent:* The choice to participate by the subject (or legal representation in the event of a minor or mentally challenged person) must be voluntary and founded on the disclosure of all pertinent information and potential hazards. The methods, hazards, and discomforts of the research must be explained to volunteers in a way that they can comprehend in order for their permission to be considered validly informed. The creation of standard consent language that outlines the risks associated with various types or uses of TMS and provides a lay description of common procedures can help investigators and reassure members of local ethics committees or the Institutional Review Board (IRB) that TMS is properly disclosed and discussed.
2. *Risk benefit ratio:* An impartial evaluation must determine that the research's possible benefits exceed the risks. Merely having the subject agree to take on the risk is insufficient, and there needs to be no way to get the needed data without putting the subjects in danger. The possibility of a therapeutic benefit must likewise exceed the possible dangers in the event of a clinical application.

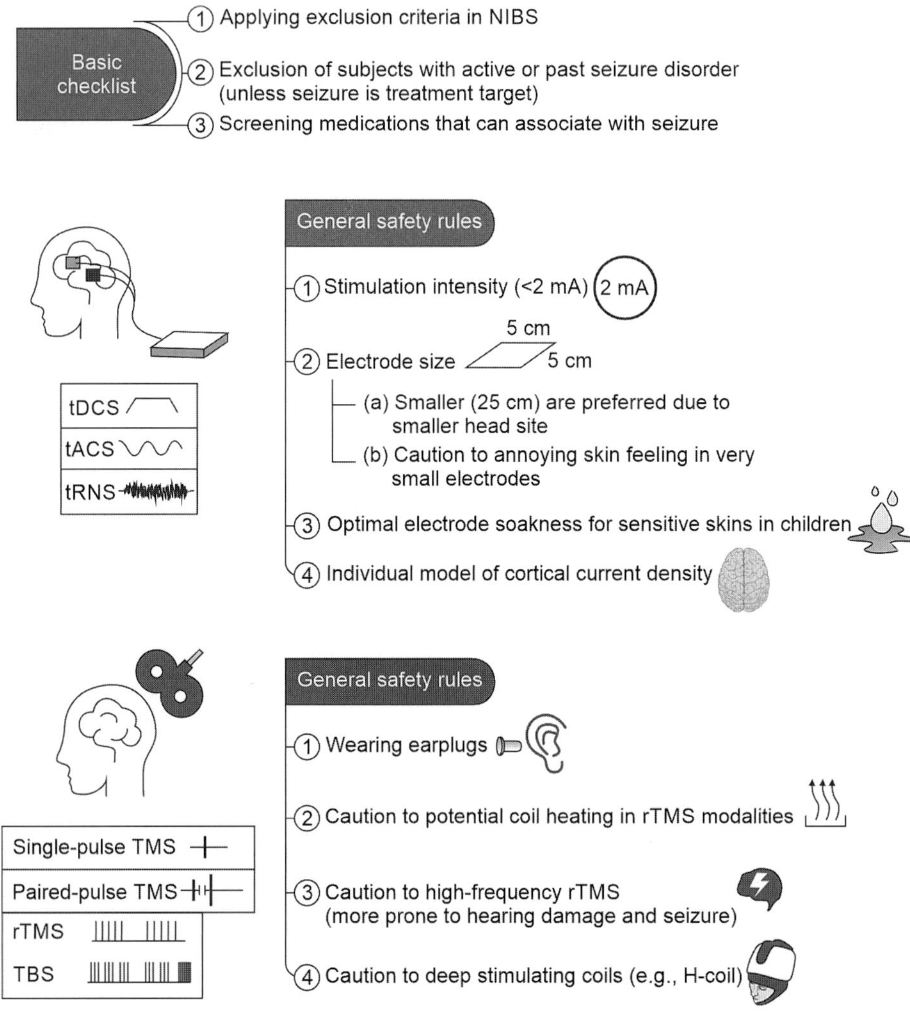

Fig. 6: Safety considerations for TMS/tDCS studies in children and adolescents. (NIBS: noninvasive brain stimulation; rTMS: repetitive transcranial magnetic stimulation; TBS: theta burst stimulation; tACS, transcranial alternating current stimulation; tDCS, transcranial direct current stimulation; TMS, transcranial magnetic stimulation; tRNS, transcranial random noise stimulation)
Source: Adapted from Salehinejad et al. (2024).

3. *Equal distribution of the burdens and benefits of research:* When studies are done on patient groups that are susceptible due to social, medical, or economic circumstances and who are most likely to experience solely the negative effects of the illness, this requirement is violated.[18]

Our knowledge of brain circuitry will surely grow quickly over the next 20 years, and it will be critical that the ethical concerns raised by these developments be addressed concurrently with the creation of well planned, hypothesis-driven clinical trials.

MAGNETIC SEIZURE THERAPY

Magnetic seizure therapy is the deliberate use of TMS to induce seizures, under general anesthesia, for treating depression or other serious neuropsychiatric conditions, allowing for increased control over stimulation site and sparing brain regions related to ECT-induced adverse events, thereby resulting in a safer way of administering seizure therapy.[71,72] It is usually given at 100% of maximal stimulator output, at a frequency of 25–100 Hz, in a single train lasting up to 10 seconds. To date, MST has been studied in patients with clinical conditions requiring ECT, mainly major depressive disorder,[73-75] bipolar disorder,[76,77] and to a lesser extent, schizophrenia.[78] Cognitive side effects were evaluated using a neurocognitive test battery, showing no significant change.[79]

DEEP BRAIN STIMULATION

In DBS, an invasive procedure of brain stimulation, electrodes are surgically inserted into particular brain locations to administer continuous or intermittent electrical stimulation via an implanted battery source. DBS has revolutionized the understanding and treatment of brain illnesses by directly interfering with abnormal neural networks. When used as a surgical instrument, DBS can precisely quantify abnormal brain activity and provide therapeutically tunable stimulation for neurological and psychiatric conditions associated with malfunctioning circuitry.[80]

Mechanism of Action

The proposed mechanisms are: Direct excitation or inhibition of neural activity and synaptic filtering **(Fig. 7)**. Improvements in symptoms are produced by the stimulating effects that cause this disruption at the cellular, network, ionic, and protein levels.[80] The effects of DBS are often delayed and progressive and sometimes take months to achieve maximal benefit in a variety of disorders, including dystonia, depression and epilepsy.

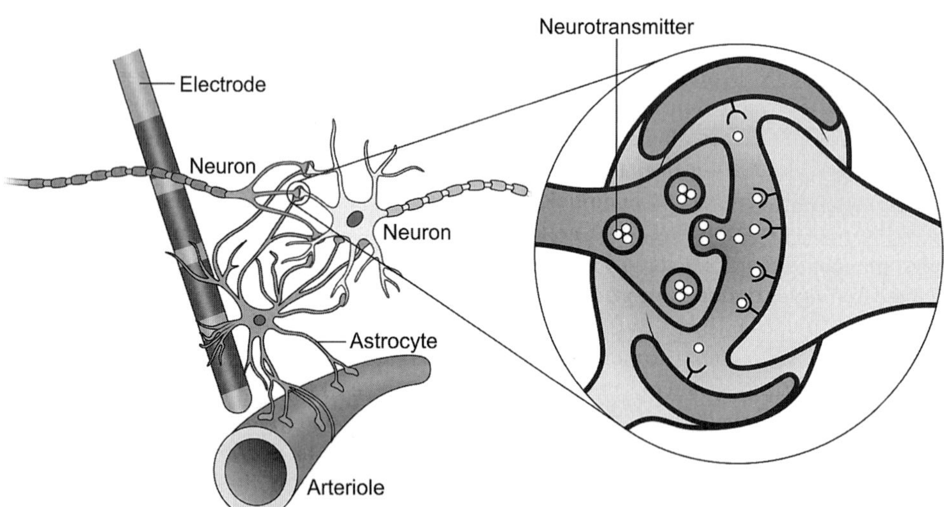

Fig. 7: Mechanism of action of deep brain stimulation (DBS).
Source: Adapted from Lozano et al. (2019).

TABLE 5: The common indications and their corresponding target sites.[81]

Condition	*Target sites*
Gilles de la Tourette syndrome	Globus pallidus internal, thalamus, internal capsule, and nucleus accumbens
Obsessive–compulsive disorder	Ventral anterior limb of internal capsule, anteromedial subthalamic nucleus, nucleus accumbens, and ventral striatum
Treatment-resistant depression	Ventral striatum and superolateral medial forebrain bundle
Anorexia nervosa	Nucleus accumbens and subcingulate gyrus
Aggressive and self-harm behaviors	Posterior hypothalamus
Resistant epilepsy	Posterior hypothalamus
Dystonia	Globus pallidum, subthalamic nucleus, and thalamus

Clinical Applications of Deep Brain Stimulation

Table 5 provides a list of disorders where DBS is beneficial.

Advances in Deep Brain Stimulation

Advances in DBS include:

- *Closed loop DBS:* Stimulation can be on demand, e.g., triggering of thalamic DBS by arm movement in essential tremors or during seizure activity in epilepsy.
- *Phase-controlled DBS:* Stimulation will be delivered at specific phases/timings that either alter or decrease oscillations, e.g., in tremors.
- *Model-based control:* DBS parameters are customized according to model of the underlying neurocircuitry.
- *High resolution electrodes:* Multicontact electrodes to provide better control of the stimulation field and high-resolution readouts of neural circuit dysfunction
- *Efficient rechargeable batteries:* To increase battery life and reduce the risks associated with surgical battery changes
- *Miniaturized implanted pulse generators:* Small enough to be embedded in the skull[80]

Ethical Considerations

The ethical implications of implanting electrodes into deep brain structures, particularly in new indications for DBS, are significant because although minimally invasive, it is a neurosurgical procedure that is associated with serious surgical risk, high capital costs, and the need for a multidisciplinary team to provide patient programs and troubleshoot issues.[80]

VAGAL NERVE STIMULATION

Vagal nerve stimulation is an invasive neuromodulatory procedure in which an electrical stimulator implanted in the body stimulates the vagus nerve, the cranial nerve's tenth nerve.[82]

Mechanism of Action

The precise processes that underlie VNS's therapeutic benefits are yet unknown. In summary, the vagus nerve transmits data from many organ systems in the human body to the brainstem's nucleus tractus solitarii (NTS), from where it is transmitted both directly and indirectly to various brain regions. Key regions involved in affect/emotion control, pain modulation, or memory and attention functions have their neuronal activity variably modulated by synaptic projections from the NTS[83] **(Figs. 8A and B)**.

Types

Vagal nerve stimulation is of two types: Invasive and noninvasive [transcutaneous VNS (tVNS)].

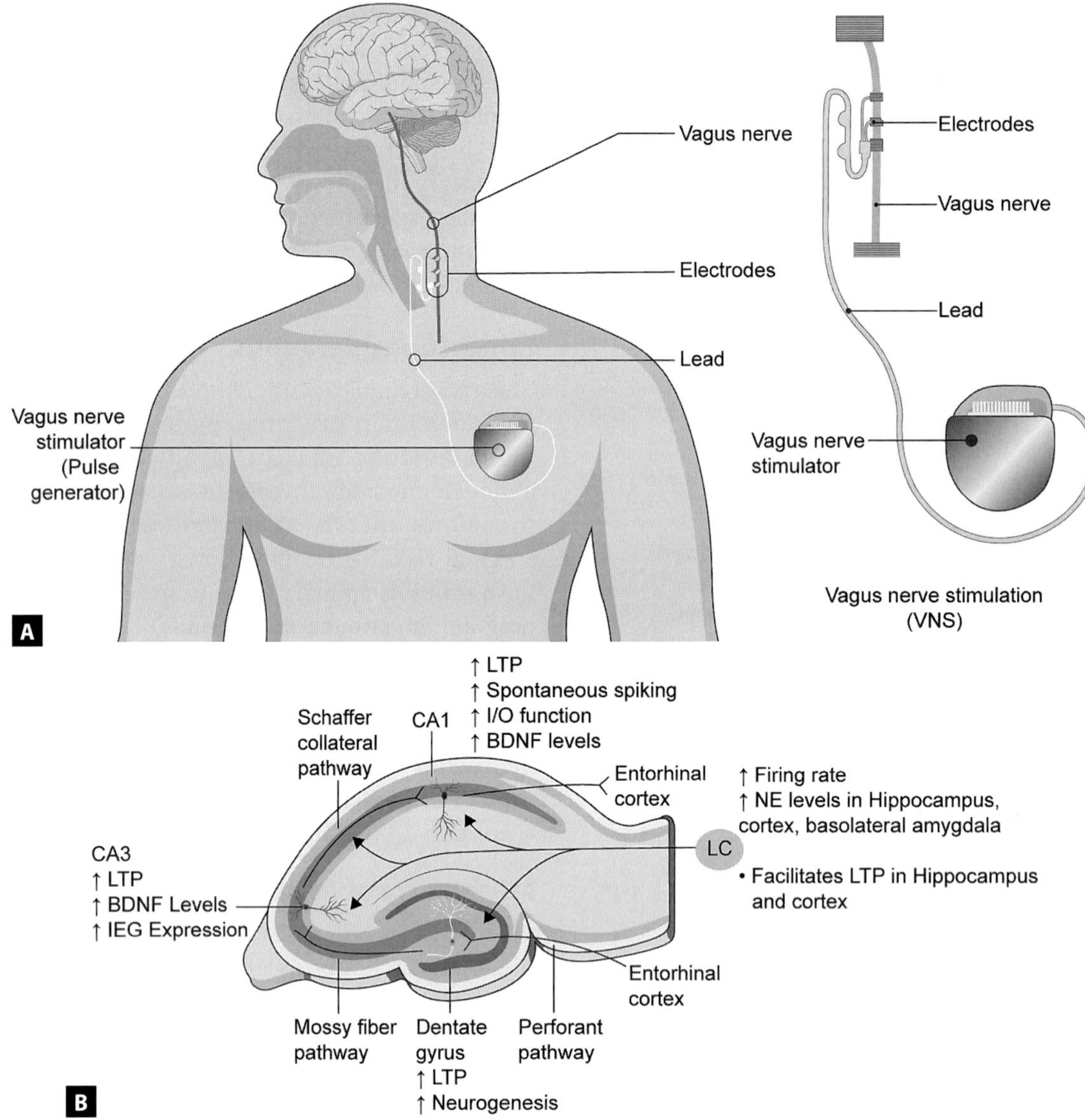

Figs. 8A and B: (A) Placement of VNS apparatus and (B) Proposed mechanisms of actions.[84] (BDNF: brain-derived neurotrophic factor; I/O: input/output; IEG: immediate early gene; LC: locus coeruleus; LTP: long-term potentiation; NE: norepinephrine; VNS: vagal nerve stimulation)

Current forms of tVNS can include both transcutaneous auricular VNS (applied to the external surface of the ear, in the areas innervated by the auricular branch of the vagus) and transcutaneous cervical VNS (applied to the surface of the neck over the cervical vagus nerve).[85]

Clinical Applications

- Vagal nerve stimulation is most commonly used in treatment of intractable epilepsy and treatment-resistant depression, where it is Food and Drug Administration (FDA) approved in adolescents over 12 years of age.[86]

- *Transcutaneous VNS:* Pediatric patients with a variety of clinical problems, primarily epilepsy, depression, and tinnitus, have been treated using tVNS. The usage of tVNS in children and adolescents with various ailments including Prader–Willi syndrome, eating issues, or opioid withdrawal syndrome is being studied in registered and ongoing trials.[85]

Side Effects

Side effects are frequent but often bearable. Procedure-related problems, such as infection, fluid accumulation around the stimulator, dyspnea, and hoarseness, were frequent adverse effects. Additional adverse effects included hardware malfunctions connected to the device and aspiration caused by malfunctioning vocal cords during the stimulation period, which were related to the stimuli. Delayed consequences were identified as arrhythmias.[82]

TRIGEMINAL NERVE STIMULATION

In trigeminal nerve stimulation (TNS), mild electrical signals stimulate branches of the trigeminal nerve (the largest cranial nerve) in order to modulate the activity of targeted brain regions.

Mechanism of Action

Trigeminal nerve stimulation has therapeutic potential due to its unique connections to key brain regions such as the cerebrovasculature, limbic system, entorhinal cortex, trigeminal mesencephalic nucleus, and medullary dorsal horn. TNS has been observed to induce cerebral vasodilation, regulate metabolism and neurotransmission, reduce neuroinflammation, and indirectly influence the autonomic nervous system, peripheral vasoconstriction, and cardiac performance.[86-88]

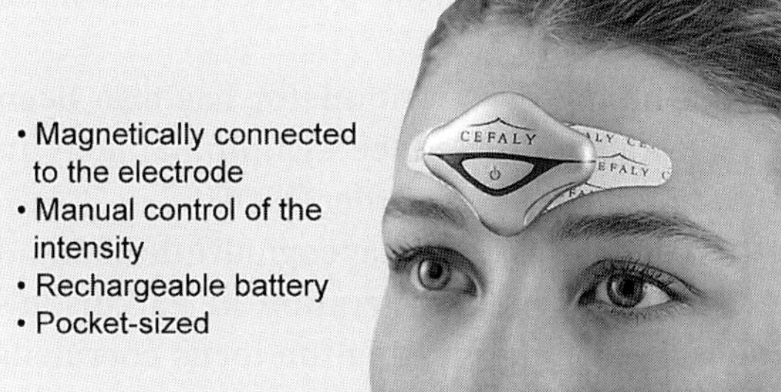

Fig. 9: Self-adhesive external trigeminal nerve stimulator (e-TENS) device.

External Trigeminal Nerve Stimulator

External trigeminal nerve stimulator (e-TNS) is an intervention that stimulates the supraorbital branch of the trigeminal nerve with the aim of reducing the frequency and length of migraine attacks. The self-adhesive e-TNS electrode, placed on the forehead, targets the supraorbital nerve. A battery-operated electrical pulse generator connects to the electrode, conducting micropulses **(Fig. 9)**.

Indications

- The US FDA issued its first approval of a nonpharmacological, device-based treatment for ADHD among children ages 8–12 years in April 2019. TNS stimulates the V1 branch of the trigeminal nerve and activates the anterior cingulate cortex, inferior and middle frontal gyri, and other brain areas implicated in executive function and ADHD.[89]
- External trigeminal nerve stimulator has been shown to reduce seizure frequency, symptoms of depression, and quality of life, in people with epilepsy.[90,91]
- The e-TNS can be used for migraine prevention through daily sessions or for acute treatment as a 60 or 120-minute intervention. The pulse width and intensity remain the same, but the preventive mode has a pulse frequency of

60 Hz, while the acute treatment mode has a frequency of 100 Hz.[92,93]

- Trigeminal nerve stimulator has also been investigated to reduce symptomatology in major depressive disorder (MDD).[94]
- It has been found to delay cognitive decline and dopaminergic degeneration in Parkinson's disease via modulating the locus coeruleus (LC)-noradrenergic system.[95]
- In trigeminal neuralgia, studies have been conducted but clinical relevance is found to be limited.

Side Effects

The most common side effects reported were anxiety, headache, and skin irritation. No serious side effects were reported.

SUMMARY AND CONCLUSION

Repetitive transcranial magnetic stimulation and tDCS have shown potential in treating various psychiatric and neurological disorders in children, such as major depressive disorder, autism spectrum disorder, and ADHD. rTMS and tDCS have been found to be safe and effective for children and adolescents when safety guidelines are strictly followed. Common side effects of tDCS and rTMS in children include mild tingling, headache, and fatigue, which are generally well-tolerated and temporary.

In conclusion, neuromodulation techniques (rtMS and tDCS) are newer therapeutic strategies for management of various psychiatric and neurological disorders in children and adolescents. These are found to be safe and effective with minor adverse effects. However, while employing such treatment modalities, it is important to adhere to ethical considerations, including informed consent and risk–benefit ratio. Also, equitable distribution of research burdens and benefits is crucial for the safe and ethical use of these technologies in pediatric populations. New protocols and brain regions are being explored for neuromodulation, potentially expanding their applicability and improving outcomes for various disorders.

REFERENCES

1. Shorter E, Healy D. Shock therapy: A history of electroconvulsive treatment in mental illness. New Brunswick, NJ: Rutgers University Press; 2007.
2. Wassermann EM, Zimmermann T. Transcranial magnetic brain stimulation: Therapeutic promises and scientific gaps. Pharmacol Ther. 2012;133(1):98-107.
3. Williams NR, Taylor JJ, Kerns S, Short EB, Kantor EM, George MS. Interventional psychiatry: Why now? J Clin Psychiatry. 2014;75(8):895-7.
4. Suleman R. A brief history of electroconvulsive therapy. Am J Psychiatry. 2020;16(1):6.
5. Døssing E, Pagsberg AK. Electroconvulsive therapy in children and adolescents: A systematic review of current literature and guidelines. J ECT. 2021;37(3):158-70.
6. Thirthalli J, Sinha P, Sreeraj VS. Clinical practice guidelines for the use of electroconvulsive therapy. Indian J Psychiatry. 2023;65(2):258-69.
7. Charlson F, Siskind D, Doi SA, McCallum E, Broome A, Lie DC. ECT efficacy and treatment course: A systematic review and meta-analysis of twice vs thrice weekly schedules. J Affect Disord. 2012;138(1-2):1-8.
8. Franklin AD, Sobey JH, Stickles ET. Anesthetic considerations for pediatric electroconvulsive therapy. Paediatr Anaesth. 2017;27(5):471-9.
9. Narayan CL, Deepanshu M. Electroconvulsive therapy: A Closer look into legal provisions in the MHCA, 2017. Indian J Psychol Med. 2022;44(3):293-6.
10. Andrade C, Arumugham SS, Thirthalli J. Adverse effects of electroconvulsive therapy. Psychiatr Clin North Am. 2016;39(3):513-30.
11. Sienaert P. Based on a True Story? The portrayal of ECT in International Movies and television programs. Brain Stimul. 2016;9(6):882-91.
12. Singh OP. Need to develop "Interventional Psychiatry" as a subspecialty in India. Indian J Psychiatry. 2020;62(1):1-2.

13. Wassermann EM, Lisanby SH. Therapeutic application of repetitive transcranial magnetic stimulation: A review. Clinical Neurophysiol. 2001;112(8):1367-77.
14. Rossi S, Rossini PM. TMS in cognitive plasticity and the potential for rehabilitation. Trends Cogn Sci. 2004;8(6):273-9.
15. George MS, Nahas Z, Borckardt JJ, Anderson B, Foust MJ, Burns C, et al. Brain stimulation for the treatment of psychiatric disorders. Current Opin Psychiatry. 2007;20(3):250-4.
16. Devlin JT, Watkins KE. Stimulating language: Insights from TMS. Brain. 2007;130(3):610-22.
17. Ridding MC, Rothwell JC. Is there a future for therapeutic use of transcranial magnetic stimulation?. Nat Rev Neurosci. 2007;8(7):559-67.
18. Rossi S, Hallett M, Rossini PM, Pascual-Leone A; Safety of TMS Consensus Group. Safety, ethical considerations, and application guidelines for the use of transcranial magnetic stimulation in clinical practice and research. Clin Neurophysiol. 2009;120(12):2008-39.
19. Hallett M, Di Iorio R, Rossini PM, Park JE, Chen R, Celnik P, et al. Contribution of transcranial magnetic stimulation to assessment of brain connectivity and networks. Clin Neurophysiol. 2017;128(11):2125-39.
20. Pascual-Leone A, Freitas C, Oberman L, Horvath JC, Halko M, Eldaief M, et al. Characterizing brain cortical plasticity and network dynamics across the age-span in health and disease with TMS-EEG and TMS-fMRI. Brain Topogr. 2011;24(3-4):302-15.
21. Deng ZD, Lisanby SH, Peterchev AV. Electric field depth-focality tradeoff in transcranial magnetic stimulation: Simulation comparison of 50 coil designs. Brain Stimul. 2013;6(1):1-3.
22. Peterchev AV, Deng ZD, Goetz SM. Advances in transcranial magnetic stimulation technology. In: Reti IM (Ed). Brain stimulation: Methodologies and interventions. New Jersey, US: John Wiley & Sons; 2015. pp. 165-89.
23. Gomez LJ, Goetz SM, Peterchev AV. Design of transcranial magnetic stimulation coils with optimal trade-off between depth, focality, and energy. J Neural Eng. 2018;15(4):046033.
24. Deng ZD, Lisanby SH, Peterchev AV. Coil design considerations for deep transcranial magnetic stimulation. Clin Neurophysiol. 2014;125(6):1202-12.
25. de Andrade DC, Galhardoni R, Pinto LF, Lancelotti R, Rosi Jr J, Marcolin MA, et al. Into the island: A new technique of non-invasive cortical stimulation of the insula. Neurophysiol Clin. 2012;42(6):363-8.
26. Kreuzer PM, Schecklmann M, Lehner A, Wetter TC, Poeppl TB, Rupprecht R, et al. The ACDC pilot trial: Targeting the anterior cingulate by double cone coil rTMS for the treatment of depression. Brain Stimul. 2015;8(2):240-6.
27. Fernandez L, Major BP, Teo WP, Byrne LK, Enticott PG. Assessing cerebellar brain inhibition (CBI) via transcranial magnetic stimulation (TMS): A systematic review. Neurosci Biobehav Rev. 2018;86:176-206.
28. Huang YZ, Chen RS, Fong PY, Rothwell JC, Chuang WL, Weng YH, et al. Inter-cortical modulation from premotor to motor plasticity. J Physiol. 2018;596(17):4207-17.
29. Guadagnin V, Parazzini M, Fiocchi S, Liorni I, Ravazzani P. Deep transcranial magnetic stimulation: Modeling of different coil configurations. IEEE Trans Biomed Eng. 2015;63(7):1543-50.
30. Tendler A, Barnea Ygael N, Roth Y, Zangen A. Deep transcranial magnetic stimulation (dTMS)–beyond depression. Expert Rev Med Devices. 2016;13(10):987-1000.
31. Parazzini M, Fiocchi S, Chiaramello E, Roth Y, Zangen A, Ravazzani P. Electric field estimation of deep transcranial magnetic stimulation clinically used for the treatment of neuropsychiatric disorders in anatomical head models. Med Eng Phys. 2017;43:30-8.
32. Thomson AC, Sack AT. How to design optimal accelerated rTMS protocols capable of promoting therapeutically beneficial metaplasticity. Front Neurol. 2020;11:599918.
33. Ferrarelli F, Phillips ML. Examining and modulating neural circuits in psychiatric disorders with transcranial magnetic stimulation and electroencephalography: Present practices and future developments. Am J Psychiatry. 2021;178(5):400-13.
34. Lancaster JL, Narayana S, Wenzel D, Luckemeyer J, Roby J, Fox P. Evaluation of an image-guided,

robotically positioned transcranial magnetic stimulation system. Hum Brain Mapp. 2004;22(4):329-40.
35. Ginhoux R, Renaud P, Zorn L, Goffin L, Bayle B, Foucher J, et al. A custom robot for transcranial magnetic stimulation: first assessment on healthy subjects. Annu Int Conf IEEE Eng Med Biol Soc. 2013;2013:5352-5.
36. Richter L, Trillenberg P, Schweikard A, Schlaefer A. Stimulus intensity for hand held and robotic transcranial magnetic stimulation. Brain Stimul. 2013;6(3):315-21.
37. Salehinejad MA, Siniatchkin M. Safety of noninvasive brain stimulation in children. Curr Opin Psychiatry. 2024;37(2):78-86.
38. Donaldson AE, Gordon MS, Melvin GA, Barton DA, Fitzgerald PB. Addressing the needs of adolescents with treatment resistant depressive disorders: a systematic review of rTMS. Brain Stimulation. 2014;7(1):7-12.
39. Sun CH, Mai JX, Shi ZM, Zheng W, Jiang WL, Li ZZ, et al. Adjunctive repetitive transcranial magnetic stimulation for adolescents with first-episode major depressive disorder: A meta-analysis. Front Psychiatry. 2023;14:1200738.
40. Smith JR, DiSalvo M, Green A, Ceranoglu TA, Anteraper SA, Croarkin P, et al. Treatment response of transcranial magnetic stimulation in intellectually capable youth and young adults with autism spectrum disorder: A systematic review and meta-analysis. Neuropsychol Rev. 2023;33(4):834-55.
41. Ni HC, Chen YL, Chao YP, Wu CT, Wu YY, Liang SH, et al. Intermittent theta burst stimulation over the posterior superior temporal sulcus for children with autism spectrum disorder: A 4-week randomized blinded controlled trial followed by another 4-week open-label intervention. Autism. 2021;25(5):1279-94.
42. Jannati A, Block G, Ryan MA, Kaye HL, Kayarian FB, Bashir S, et al. Continuous theta-burst stimulation in children with high-functioning autism spectrum disorder and typically developing children. Front Integr Neurosci. 2020;14:13.
43. Grados M, Huselid R, Duque-Serrano L. Transcranial magnetic stimulation in Tourette syndrome: A historical perspective, its current use and the influence of comorbidities in treatment response. Brain Sci. 2018;8(7):129.
44. Bleich-Cohen M, Gurevitch G, Carmi N, Medvedovsky M, Bregman N, Nevler N, et al. A functional magnetic resonance imaging investigation of prefrontal cortex deep transcranial magnetic stimulation efficacy in adults with attention deficit/hyperactive disorder: A double blind, randomized clinical trial. Neuroimage Clin. 2021;30:102670.
45. Bejenaru AM, Malhi NK. Use of repetitive transcranial magnetic stimulation in child psychiatry. Innov Clin Neurosci. 2022;19(4-6): 11-22.
46. Metelski N, Gu Y, Quinn L, Friel KM, Gordon AM. Safety and efficacy of non-invasive brain stimulation for the upper extremities in children with cerebral palsy: A systematic review. Dev Med Child Neurol. 2024;66(5):573-97.
47. Nauczyciel C, Le Jeune F, Naudet F, Douabin S, Esquevin A, Vérin M, et al. Repetitive transcranial magnetic stimulation over the orbitofrontal cortex for obsessive-compulsive disorder: A double-blind, crossover study. Transl Psychiatry. 2014;4(9):e436.
48. Garg S, Sinha VK, Tikka SK, Mishra P, Goyal N. The efficacy of cerebellar vermal deep high frequency (theta range) repetitive transcranial magnetic stimulation (rTMS) in schizophrenia: a randomized rater blind-sham controlled study. Psychiatry Res. 2016;243:413-20.
49. Hamada M, Hanajima R, Terao Y, Okabe S, Nakatani-Enomoto S, Furubayashi T, et al. Primary motor cortical metaplasticity induced by priming over the supplementary motor area. J Physiol. 2009;587(20):4845-62.
50. Hamada M, Terao Y, Hanajima R, Shirota Y, Nakatani-Enomoto S, Furubayashi T, et al. Bidirectional long-term motor cortical plasticity and metaplasticity induced by quadripulse transcranial magnetic stimulation. J Physiol. 2008;586(16):3927-47.
51. Hamada M, Ugawa Y. Quadripulse stimulation–a new patterned rTMS. Restor Neurol Neurosci. 2010;28(4):419-24.
52. Krishnan C, Santos L, Peterson MD, Ehinger M. Safety of noninvasive brain stimulation in children and adolescents. Brain Stimul. 2015;8(1):76-87.

53. Nitsche MA, Paulus W. Excitability changes induced in the human motor cortex by weak transcranial direct current stimulation. Journal Physiol. 2000;527(Pt 3):633.
54. Wischnewski M, Alekseichuk I, Opitz A. Neurocognitive, physiological, and biophysical effects of transcranial alternating current stimulation. Trends Cogn Sci. 2023;27(2):189-205.
55. Van der Groen O, Potok W, Wenderoth N, Edwards G, Mattingley JB, Edwards D. Using noise for the better: The effects of transcranial random noise stimulation on the brain and behavior. Neurosci Biobehav Rev. 2022;138:104702.
56. Fregni F, Nitsche MA, Loo CK, Brunoni AR, Marangolo P, Leite J, et al. Regulatory considerations for the clinical and research use of transcranial direct current stimulation (tDCS): review and recommendations from an expert panel. Clin Res Regul Aff. 2015;32(1):22-35.
57. Lefaucheur JP, Antal A, Ayache SS, Benninger DH, Brunelin J, Cogiamanian F, et al. Evidence-based guidelines on the therapeutic use of transcranial direct current stimulation (tDCS). Clin Neurophysiol. 2017;128(1):56-92.
58. Amatachaya A, Jensen MP, Patjanasoontorn N, Uvichayapat N, Suphakunpinyo C, Janjarasjitt S, et al. The short-term effects of transcranial direct current stimulation on electroencephalography in children with autism: A randomized crossover controlled trial. Behav Neurol. 2015;2015:928631.
59. Qiu J, Kong X, Li J, Yang J, Huang Y, Huang M, et al. Transcranial direct current stimulation (tDCS) over the left dorsal lateral prefrontal cortex in children with autism spectrum disorder (ASD). Neural Plast. 2021;2021:6627507.
60. Sun C, Zhao Z, Cheng L, Tian R, Zhao W, Du J, et al. Effect of transcranial direct current stimulation on the mismatch negativity features of deviated stimuli in children with autism spectrum disorder. Front Neurosci. 2022;16:721987.
61. Toscano E, Sanges V, Riccio MP, Bravaccio C, de Bartolomeis A, D'Urso G. Fronto-cerebellar tDCS in children with autism spectrum disorder. L'Encéphale. 2019;45:S79-80.
62. Mahmoodifar E, Sotoodeh MS. Combined transcranial direct current stimulation and selective motor training enhances balance in children with autism spectrum disorder. Percept Mot Skills. 2020;127(1):113-25.
63. Salehinejad MA, Wischnewski M, Nejati V, Vicario CM, Nitsche MA. Transcranial direct current stimulation in attention-deficit hyperactivity disorder: A meta-analysis of neuropsychological deficits. PloS one. 2019;14(4):e0215095.
64. Salehinejad MA, Ghayerin E, Nejati V, Yavari F, Nitsche MA. Domain-specific involvement of the right posterior parietal cortex in attention network and attentional control of ADHD: A randomized, cross-over, sham-controlled tDCS study. Neuroscience. 2020;444:149-59.
65. Costanzo F, Rossi S, Varuzza C, Varvara P, Vicari S, Menghini D. Long-lasting improvement following tDCS treatment combined with a training for reading in children and adolescents with dyslexia. Neuropsychologia. 2019;130:38-43.
66. Rahimi M, Heidari A, Naderi F, Makvandi B, Bakhtiyarpour S. Comparison of cognitive training method and transcranial direct current stimulation (tDCS) on the visual attention processes in the students with special learning disorders. Int J Behav Sci. 2019;12(4):162-8.
67. Lazzaro G, Costanzo F, Varuzza C, Rossi S, De Matteis ME, Vicari S, et al. Individual differences modulate the effects of tDCS on reading in children and adolescents with dyslexia. Sci Stud Read. 2021;25(6):470-85.
68. Abend R, Sar-El R, Gonen T, Jalon I, Vaisvaser S, Bar-Haim Y, et al. Modulating emotional experience using electrical stimulation of the medial-prefrontal cortex: A preliminary tDCS-fMRI study. Neuromodulation. 2019;22(8):884-93.
69. Wu LL, Potenza MN, Zhou N, Kober H, Shi XH, Yip SW, et al. Efficacy of single-session transcranial direct current stimulation on addiction-related inhibitory control and craving: a randomized trial in males with Internet gaming disorder. J Psychiatry Neuroscience. 2021;46(1):E111-8.
70. Sauvaget A, Trojak B, Bulteau S, Jiménez-Murcia S, Fernández-Aranda F, et al. Transcranial direct current stimulation (tDCS) in behavioral and food addiction: A systematic review of efficacy, technical, and methodological issues. Front Neurosci. 2015;9:349.

71. Lisanby SH. Update on magnetic seizure therapy: A novel form of convulsive therapy. J ECT. 2002;18(4):182-8.
72. Lisanby SH, Luber B, Schlaepfer TE, Sackeim HA. Safety and feasibility of magnetic seizure therapy (MST) in major depression: Randomized within-subject comparison with electroconvulsive therapy. Neuropsychopharmacology. 2003;28(10): 1852-65.
73. Fitzgerald PB, Hoy KE, Herring SE, Clinton AM, Downey G, Daskalakis ZJ. Pilot study of the clinical and cognitive effects of high-frequency magnetic seizure therapy in major depressive disorder. Depress Anxiety. 2013;30(2):129-36.
74. Sun Y, Farzan F, Mulsant BH, Rajji TK, Fitzgerald PB, Barr MS, et al. Indicators for remission of suicidal ideation following magnetic seizure therapy in patients with treatment-resistant depression. JAMA psychiatry. 2016;73(4):337-45.
75. Daskalakis ZJ, Dimitrova J, McClintock SM, Sun Y, Voineskos D, Rajji TK, et al. Magnetic seizure therapy (MST) for major depressive disorder. Neuropsychopharmacology. 2020;45(2):276-82.
76. Cretaz E, Brunoni AR, Lafer B. Magnetic seizure therapy for unipolar and bipolar depression: A systematic review. Neural Plast. 2015;2015: 521398.
77. Kayser S, Bewernick B, Axmacher N, Schlaepfer TE. Magnetic seizure therapy of treatment-resistant depression in a patient with bipolar disorder. J ECT. 2009;25(2):137-40.
78. Tang AD, Bennett W, Hadrill C, Collins J, Fulopova B, Wills K, et al. Low intensity repetitive transcranial magnetic stimulation modulates skilled motor learning in adult mice. Scientific reports. 2018;8(1):4016.
79. Polster JD, Kayser S, Bewernick BH, Hurlemann R, Schlaepfer TE. Effects of electroconvulsive therapy and magnetic seizure therapy on acute memory retrieval. J ECT. 2015;31(1):13-9.
80. Lozano AM, Lipsman N, Bergman H, Brown P, Chabardes S, Chang JW, et al. Deep brain stimulation: Current challenges and future directions. Nat Rev Neurol. 2019;15(3):148-60.
81. Ashkan K, Mirza AB, Tambirajoo K, Furlanetti L. Deep brain stimulation in the management of paediatric neuropsychiatric conditions: Current evidence and future directions. Eur J Paediatr Neurol. 2021;33:146-58.
82. Doruk Camsari D, Kirkovski M, Croarkin PE. Therapeutic applications of invasive neuromodulation in children and adolescents. Psychiatr Clin North Am. 2018;41(3):479-83.
83. Sigrist C, Torki B, Bolz LO, Jeglorz T, Bolz A, Koenig J. Transcutaneous auricular vagus nerve stimulation in pediatric patients: A systematic review of clinical treatment protocols and stimulation parameters. Neuromodulation. 2023;26(3):507-17.
84. Olsen LK, Solis E Jr, McIntire LK, Hatcher-Solis CN. Vagus nerve stimulation: Mechanisms and factors involved in memory enhancement. Front Hum Neurosci. 2023;17:1152064.
85. Edwards CA, Kouzani A, Lee KH, Ross EK. Neurostimulation devices for the treatment of neurologic disorders. Mayo Clin Proc. 2017;92(9):1427-44.
86. Shah KA, White TG, Powell K, Woo HH, Narayan RK, Li C. Trigeminal nerve stimulation improves cerebral macrocirculation and microcirculation after subarachnoid hemorrhage: An exploratory study. Neurosurgery. 2022;90(4):485-94.
87. Nash C, Powell K, Lynch DG, Hartings JA, Li C. Nonpharmacological modulation of cortical spreading depolarization. Life Sci. 2023;327:121833.
88. Xu J, Wu S, Huo L, Zhang Q, Liu L, Ye Z, et al. Trigeminal nerve stimulation restores hippocampal dopamine deficiency to promote cognitive recovery in traumatic brain injury. Prog Neurobiol. 2023;227:102477.
89. Loo SK, Salgari GC, Ellis A, Cowen J, Dillon A, McGough JJ. Trigeminal nerve stimulation for attention-deficit/hyperactivity disorder: Cognitive and electroencephalographic predictors of treatment response. J Am Acad Child Adolesc Psychiatry. 2021;60(7):856-64.e1.
90. DeGiorgio CM, Shewmon A, Murray D, Whitehurst T. Pilot study of trigeminal nerve stimulation (TNS) for epilepsy: A proof-of-concept trial. Epilepsia. 2006;47(7):1213-5.
91. Ginatempo F, Fois C, De Carli F, Todesco S, Mercante B, Sechi G, et al. Effect of short-term transcutaneous trigeminal nerve stimulation on

EEG activity in drug-resistant epilepsy. J Neurol Sci. 2019;400:90-6.

92. Stanak M, Wolf S, Jagoš H, Zebenholzer K. The impact of external trigeminal nerve stimulator (e-TNS) on prevention and acute treatment of episodic and chronic migraine: A systematic review. J Neurol Sci. 2020;412:116725.
93. Westwood SJ, Conti AA, Tang W, Xue S, Cortese S, Rubia K. Clinical and cognitive effects of external trigeminal nerve stimulation (eTNS) in neurological and psychiatric disorders: A systematic review and meta-analysis. Mol Psychiatry. 2023;28(10):4025-43.
94. Shiozawa P, Duailibi MS, da Silva ME, Cordeiro Q. Trigeminal nerve stimulation (TNS) protocol for treating major depression: An open-label proof-of-concept trial. Epilepsy Behav. 2014;39:6-9.
95. Ozdemir K. Next-generation cranial nerve stimulation and neuromodulation techniques: Potential and clinical applications in Parkinson's disease treatment. Authorea Preprints. 2023.

SECTION 5

Special Circumstances

CHAPTER 31

Disability Certification and Related Acts in India

Smita Neelkanth Deshpande, Ram Pratap Beniwal

INTRODUCTION

Society, it is hoped, has moved ahead of the old beliefs due to which the disabled were stigmatized and discriminated against. Worse still, disability was considered a curse or punishment. This led to people with disabilities (PWD) being banished into distant, closed institutions, leading to deprivation of their human rights and denial of their novel ways of perceiving. Humanity is indebted to several unique disabled individuals who stood up and resisted this discrimination.

HISTORY OF DISABILITY ADVOCACY IN INDIA AND INDIAN LEGISLATIONS

Disabled individuals joined hands with various movements for civil and human rights in the early 20th century. All groups including those of the minority, women, disabled, or disadvantaged demanded equal treatment, equal access, and equal opportunity to societal resources. Parents and caregivers of disabled children became their advocates, demanding educational, occupational, and social opportunities for their children. During World War II, Hitler had tried to decimate the population of German disabled persons, along with Jews and gypsies. But after the war, disabled soldiers returning home demanded social recognition of their conditions.

In India, lobbying, petitions, and protests for disabled rights—led mainly by parents, caregivers, and nongovernmental organization (NGOs) in the 1980s—finally resulted in the enactment of the Persons with Disabilities (Equal Opportunities, Protection of Rights and Full Participation) Act, 1995 (or PWD Act).[1] When India ratified the United Nations Convention on the Rights of Persons with Disability (UNCRPD), in 2007, it became legally bound to implement its provisions.[2] The two subsequent legislations—the Rights of Persons with Disability Act (RPWD) 2016 and the Mental Health Care (MHC) Act 2017—naturally followed.[3,4] **Table 1** provides a list of Indian Acts concerning disability in force in 2024.

Questions about the number of citizens with disability began to be included in the Indian national census from 2001 onward. In 2011 (when the last nationwide census was conducted), the population of India was about 121 crore (12,00,00,000) out of which 2.21% (2.68 crore) were disabled. There was no separate data concerning mental or neurodevelopmental disabilities, but 20% suffered with motor disabilities, 19% visual disability, 19% hearing disability, and 8% had multiple disabilities. Almost one-fourth (23%) of young children (0–6 years of age) had a hearing disability, 30% visual disability, and 7% multiple disabilities.[9] Again, neurodevelopmental or mental disabilities are not mentioned separately. **Box 1** shows the objectives of the National Trust Board.

GLOBAL SITUATION AND UNITED NATIONS RESOLUTIONS

The United Nations Sustainable Development Goal 3 (SDG 3) aims to "Ensure healthy lives and

TABLE 1: Indian Acts concerning disability in force in 2024.

Year	*Name*	*Purpose*
1992	Rehabilitation Council of India Act[5]	To regulate special education, training, and certification of rehabilitation professionals, encourage education and research in rehabilitation, and maintain a Central Rehabilitation Register
1999	National Trust for the Welfare of Persons with Autism, Cerebral Palsy, Mental Retardation and Multiple Disabilities Act[6]	To establish the National Trust a statutory body to create and provide for capacity development of persons with autism, mental retardation, cerebral palsy and multiple disabilities and their families, realization of their rights, facilitating and promoting the creation of an enabling environment and an inclusive society, establishing Guardianship rules, etc.
2016	Rights of Persons with Disabilities Act[7]	An Act to give effect to the United Nations Convention on the Rights of Persons with Disabilities and connected issues
2017	Mental Health Care Act[8]	Provide healthcare and protect rights of persons with mental illness (PWMI), aligned to United Nations Convention on the Rights of Persons with Disability (UNCRPD)

BOX 1: Objectives of National Trust Board.

- To enable and empower PWD to live as independently and as fully as possible within and as close to the community to which they belong
- To strengthen facilities to provide support to PWD to live within their own families
- To extend support to registered organizations to provide need-based services
- To deal with problems of PWD who do not have family support
- To promote measures for the care and protection of PWD in the event of death of their parents or guardians
- To evolve the procedure for the appointment of guardians and trustees
- To facilitate the realization of equal opportunities, protection of rights, and full participation of PWD
- To do any other act which is incidental to the aforesaid objects

The National Trust supports programs which promote independent community living by:

- Supporting daycare centers for those with ID, autism spectrum disorders, or cerebral palsy through its Samarth and Vikas schemes
- Setting up adult training units
- Setting up individual and group homes

It preferably funds:

- Women with disability or
- Persons with severe disability and
- Senior citizens with disability

(ID: intellectual disability; PWD: people with disabilities)

promote well-being for all at all ages".[10] Its Target 3.8 aims to "Achieve universal health coverage, including financial risk protection, access to quality essential healthcare services and access to safe, effective, quality and affordable essential medicines and vaccines for all." Nations must ensure the inclusion of PWD into all spheres of public life.

Worldwide, the inclusion of children with disabilities (CWD) is hampered by a lack of data. The UNICEF undertook this task using existing data.[11] Over the world, nearly 240 million (24 crore) children are estimated to be disabled. This estimate includes children who lack psychosocial well-being as well. Such disabilities include sensory disabilities, intellectual disability (ID), epilepsy, cerebral palsy, autism spectrum disorder (ASD), or attention-deficit/hyperactivity disorder. While most children are disabled in only one functional domain, psychosocial difficulties are faced by almost all such children. Along with their disability, such children face malnutrition, infections, lack of schooling, and discrimination with little hope of better conditions. This UNICEF report states that in South Asia as a whole, 4% of children aged 0–4 years, 13% aged 5–17 years, and a total of 11% of children and adolescents from 0 to 17 years (64.4 million) are affected by disabilities. **Table 2** highlights the United Nations and its agencies' resolution for CWD.

Similarly, the World Health Organization (WHO) published a Call for Action for Rehabilitation 2030 in 2017.[12,13] Based on the SDG described in the preceding text, the WHO aims to include rehabilitation as an integral part of healthcare services similar to prevention, promotion, treatment, and palliation. It described 10 areas for action. These areas include, among others, developing a strong multidisciplinary rehabilitation workforce, collecting data, and encouraging research.

The SDGs were adopted by the UN General Assembly on September 25, 2015.[15] They envisaged well-being and an optimal developmental trajectory, inclusive quality education and healthcare for all children, especially marginalized and disabled. They will be difficult to achieve unless governments pitch in with adequate funding and capacity building for healthcare and rehabilitative services for CWD. **Box 2** shows the general principles of the UNCRPD, 2007.

TABLE 2: United Nations and its agencies' resolutions for children with disabilities.

Year	*Resolution*	*Description*
1946	UNICEF Mission Statement	Most disadvantaged children to be prioritized
1990	UN Convention on the Rights of the Child (UNCRPD) Article 23[2]	Access to education, training, healthcare services, rehabilitation services, preparation for employment and recreation opportunities in a manner conducive to the child's achieving the fullest possible social integration and individual development, including his or her cultural and spiritual development
2002	Special UN Resolution on A World Fit for Children: Plan of Action, A:21	Full and equal enjoyment of all human rights and fundamental freedoms
2006	UN Convention on the Rights of Persons with Disabilities, Article 25	Early identification and intervention as appropriate, and services designed to minimize and prevent further disabilities, including among children and older persons
2011	WHO World Report on Disability (service delivery)	Early identification and intervention through community-based workers, strengthening community-based rehabilitation services within the existing health infrastructure
2013	Resolution of the World Health Assembly on Disability [WHA66.9 Disability, Resolution 2(6)]	WHO to provide required technical assistance
2013	UNICEF State of the World's Children	Immediate implementation of disability inclusiveness measures rather than waiting for comprehensive data
2015	United Nations Sustainable Development Goal 3	"Ensure healthy lives and promote well-being for all at all ages."
2015	UN Sustainable Development Goals no. 4	Ensure inclusive and equitable quality education and promote lifelong learning opportunities for all
2017	World Health Organization Rehabilitation 2030: Call for Action	Statistics on children with disabilities, work toward strengthening services and the scope, availability and accessibility of rehabilitation

Source: Adapted from Olusanya et al.[14]

BOX 2: General principles of UNCRPD, 2007.

- Enjoyment of Rights on equal terms as others
- Respect for inherent dignity, individual autonomy, freedom to make own choices
- Nondiscrimination
- Full and effective participation and inclusion in society
- Respect for difference and acceptance of persons with disabilities as part of human diversity and humanity
- Equality of opportunity
- Accessibility to facilities and services which are open or provided to the public
- Equality between men and women
- Respect for evolving capacities of CWDs and their right to preserve their identities

Note: India signed in October 2007, and Indian disability legislation follows the principles of the UNCRPD (CWDs: children with disabilities; UNCRPD: United Nations Convention on the Rights of Persons with Disability)

ABLEISM AND THE ROLE OF HEALTHCARE WORKERS

Ableism is a system of discrimination and social prejudice against people with physical or mental disabilities. Almost since civilization began to be recorded, able-bodied individuals were considered the "norm". Able-bodied individuals were viewed as superior to the disabled, with an expectation that disabled individuals would strive toward "normalcy". Rather than societal empathy, disabled individuals were stigmatized and discriminated against. Unfortunately, this prejudice extends to doctors and other healthcare occupations in today's times as well. Beliefs and norms and even social-political-physical environments are shaped by these ableist attitudes. Stereotyping of disabilities (e.g., that all disabled people want to be "normal") is a result of such attitudes. **Box 3** depicts the models of disability.

As disabled activism grew, beginning in the West and spreading globally, it became increasingly evident that the experiences of disabled individuals were unique and could lend value to societal growth. Thus, while the growing discipline of disability studies focused on the social aspects of disability, the consequent impairment was a medical field. Increasingly, the line between the two has been becoming blurred. The International Classification of Functioning, Disability and Health (ICF)[16] attempts to consider all the major models of disability and includes environmental factors, associated health conditions, and their effects. Recognized by the United Nations as a social classification, it can be used to measure the human rights of disabled people, for formulating national legislation and policy, and as a universal language by all healthcare workers for health-related states in disability. However, in India, at least for mental and behavioral as well as neurodevelopmental disorders, the ICF is still a work in progress. Instruments used for disability evaluation, diagnosis, etc., are often copyrighted and need to be purchased. This is not possible for an entire country like India. Hence, we have adopted a different set of measures for disability evaluation.

BOX 3: Models for disability.

- *Medical model of disability:*
  - People are disabled by their impairments or differences
  - Looks at what is "wrong" with the person, not what the person needs
- *Social model of disability:*
  - People are disabled by barriers in society, such as buildings not having a ramp or accessible toilets
  - People's attitudes are responsible, like assuming people with disability cannot do certain things
- *Disability is:*
  - Injustice, not tragedy
  - Unequal treatment not inherent inequality

WHY CERTIFY CHILDREN WITH DISABILITIES: THE DUTY OF MEDICAL PROFESSIONALS

Among PWD, CWD are even more vulnerable to abuse of their rights. They are more at risk of health and social neglect. By recognizing their disabled status, we can identify their needs, provide them opportunities for self-realization, and improve their life.

Children with neurodevelopmental disabilities frequently suffer from multiple disabilities. By identifying their needs separately for each disability and avoiding "diagnostic overshadowing" (all symptoms being attributed to impairment alone without considering other causes), denying required care can be avoided.[17] Identifying their disability enables more accurate diagnosis of other ailments that such children may suffer along with better satisfaction, and better health outcomes.

Healthcare providers must work toward removing barriers that prevent disabled children from realizing their potential.[17] Hidden disabilities (primarily developmental) are significant barriers to inclusive care in healthcare institutions, as are ableist attitudes of healthcare personnel themselves.[18] Adequate research must be undertaken wherein disabled children are not specifically excluded.

As healthcare professionals, we must prevent the abuse of disabled children and enable their inclusion into society. The United Nations Convention on the Rights of the Child (UNCRC), 1989 detailed several Rights of Children. Pertinent to disabled children, these include the right of the child to health and education and a full and decent life and access to special care as required for their disability, preferably free of cost.[19] Most importantly, the best interests of the child must always be considered primary. We must recognize that disability is not a "problem" for the individual; rather, it is a societal responsibility.[20]

In our vast country, the simplest method to identify children with special needs/disability is certification. As healthcare professionals, we must protect the dignity and improve the quality of life of our vulnerable children—those with disabilities. As you will see below, there are several specific and tangible advantages of obtaining a certificate of disability for the PWD/CWD. Central and state governments provide educational, occupational, and other benefits for PWD/CWD.

There are intangible benefits for the PWD as well. They no longer have to hide their specific requirements. Rather, they can demand as citizens that society provide them inclusivity and empower them to develop equitably. The government can evaluate the extent of demand and the prevalence of disability by the number of certificates issued. As their number increases, PWD will feel the power of togetherness and this reduces stigma. By encouraging PWD and CWD to apply and help them to obtain Disability Certificates, we ourselves become advocates of disabled people.

INDIAN RULES FOR DISABILITY CERTIFICATION

In this chapter, as mental health professionals, we will focus on four groups of disabilities and describe their certification procedures briefly.

In India, Acts are implemented through their Rules which lay out specific ways and means for implementing a law. After the RPWD Act was passed in 2016, various committees were notified. They formulated Rules which were then discussed and evaluated by various organs of the Government. These Rules were notified on January 4, 2018. The first author (SND) Chaired the Committees which determined the Rules for Mental and Neurological Disabilities and the Committee for Multiple Disabilities. The Rules were revised and notified on March 12, 2024.[21] The notification describes each certification including the instruments to be used and how to calculate disability in detail. **Table 3** shows the list of disabilities in RPWD, 2024.

PROCEDURES OF CERTIFICATION

The Disability Certificate is a legal document with implications for education, employment,

TABLE 3: List of disabilities.

Ministry of Social Justice and Empowerment [Department of Empowerment of Persons with Disabilities (Divyangjan)]: Notification, New Delhi, 12th March, 2024, SO 1338(E)[@21] List of disabilities	
• Locomotor disability • Visual impairment • Hearing impairment and speech and language disability • Blood disorder (s)	• Intellectual disability, specific learning disability and autism spectrum disorder • Mental illness • Multiple disorder (s) • Chronic neurological disorder[#]

[@]This document provides all details about disability certification, including transcripts of some of the tests to be used.
[#]These Rules were not separated from mental illness in the Rules notified in 2018, now they have a separate Certification Committee.

social benefits, and several other benefits. Hence, a detailed procedure must be followed to obtain such a certificate. That said, the applicant and their family should not be unduly harassed. The Department of Empowerment aims to make certification available at every district hospital.

We present below a brief run-through of disabilities a mental health professional comes across and the procedure for assessment and certification.

Unique Disability ID (UDID) and disability assessment and certification (the Swavlamban card): PWD need a one-click appliance to make the process of applying for a disability card.[22] The UDID website not only eases the process of applying for a Unique Disability Identity Card to every Indian PWD but also aims to develop a National Database for PWDs. Presently, seven disabilities are included in this portal but will increase over time.

The UDID portal facilitates online application and filing for a disability certificate. PWD can also update their own information on this portal. Healthcare workers can calculate the percentage of disability as well. If disability conditions are not fulfilled, a nondisability certificate should be provided to the applicant.

Steps for applying for a disability certificate:

1. *Log into the UDID portal and register*. Once registered, they can apply for a disability certificate and UDID card, track their application once registered at the eligible place for certification, and renew/apply for a duplicate card (if their certificate/card is lost). The concerned government officers are the CMO Office/Medical Authority for the assessment of disability and the District Welfare Officer for other assistance and PWD schemes.
2. *Attend the medical institution for assessment procedures*. Once registration/application is complete, the CMO/Medical Authority assigns the applicant to the concerned Medical Board. Due assessment is completed and Disability Certificate/UDID card is issued electronically. The documents can be downloaded and printed from the same portal.
3. This portal can also be used during camps for disability certification.

The dedicated portal has facilitated and shortened the process of application. However, receiving the certificate may still take considerable time, because the certificates are issued only at empaneled medical facilities, many of which do not have the personnel, the tests, or the certification facilities required by the Rules.

BENEFITS OF THE UDID CARD

The possessor of a UDID card can avail all benefits that PWD are entitled to as shown in **Box 4**. These change from time to time, with more and more facilities becoming available as advocacy grows (see below; also see Philip et al.[23]).

One UDID card replaces the multiple certificates, papers, etc., that PWD have to carry. It acts as a document for identification as well as verification of the PWD concerned. For the government administration, benefits such as financial grants provided to the PWD can be reliably tracked and verified.

BOX 4: Benefits after disability certification.

Entitlements after disability certification:
- Income tax deduction under Section 80U
- Disability pension for BPL PWD
- Train travel concession for PWD and accompanying caregiver for up to 75%
- 4% quota in government jobs; employee cannot be dismissed based on their disability
- Right to inclusive education
- Various concessions by education boards
- Punishment for discrimination against disabled
- In government housing schemes, the disabled have a special quota

Educational concessions:[24]
- Some concessions may differ among various state and central boards of education
- The National Institute of Open Schooling offers concessions described below, as well as vocational training courses
- Special scholarships for PWD
- Inclusive education with mainstreaming
- Students with "benchmark" (i.e., 40% or higher) disability with certificates issued by recognized entities and recommended by the head of the educational institution are entitled to:
  - Facilities of a scribe/reader and compensatory time
  - Specific schools as examination centers with trained teachers as invigilators
  - Answer sheets to mention disability
  - Use of aids such as calculators
  - Relaxation in attendance at school in specified cases up to 50%
  - Exemption from third language
  - Flexibility in choice of subjects
  - Alternate/separate question papers in specified cases

Principles of inclusive education (as per the CBSE circular above):
- Ensure that no child with special needs is denied admission to mainstream education
- Monitor enrolment of disabled children in schools
- Schools to provide support through assistive devices and the availability of trained teachers
- Modify the existing physical infrastructure and teaching methodologies to meet the needs of all children including children with special needs
- Ensure that the school premises are made disabled-friendly by 2020 and all educational institutions including hostels, libraries, laboratories, and buildings have barrier-free access for the disabled
- Ensure availability of study material for the disabled and talking textbooks, reading machines, and computers with speech software
- Ensure an adequate number of sign language interpreters, transcription services, and a loop induction system for students with speech language disability
- Revisit classroom organization required for the education of children with special needs
- Ensure regular in-service training of teachers in inclusive education at the elementary and secondary levels

Contd...

Contd...

Employment:
Every appropriate government shall appoint in every government establishment, not less than 4% of the total number of vacancies in the cadre strength in each group of posts meant to be filled with persons with benchmark disabilities of which 1% each shall be reserved for persons with benchmark disabilities under clauses (*a*), (*b*), and (*c*) and *1% for persons with benchmark disabilities under clauses (d) and (e)*, namely:
- (*a*) Blindness and low vision; (*b*) deaf and hard of hearing
- (*c*) Locomotor disability including cerebral palsy, leprosy cured, dwarfism, acid attack victims, and muscular dystrophy
- (*d*) Autism, intellectual disability, specific learning disability, and mental illness
- (*e*) Multiple disabilities from amongst persons under clauses (*a*) to (*e*)

For applying a government job in the disability quota, all 21 disabilities need certification for benchmark disability (≥40%)
- Fewer disabilities are included for reservation in government jobs, depending on the special requirements of the job
- The format of the certificate may need to be modified to incorporate two disability scores, one for all multiple disabilities and another for multiple disabilities for job applications if needed.

CERTIFICATION FOR "NEURODEVELOPMENTAL DISORDERS"

The law recognizes these as a diverse group of chronic, lifelong disorders, beginning at any time during the development process (even prenatally) up to 22 years of age. PWD affected with these disorders can have difficulty with memory and learning, behavior, speech and language, and motor skills. The law includes ID, specific learning disorder (SLD), and ASD in these disorders for certification. Other mental disorders specific to development are NOT included.

Intellectual disability (above 5 years)/global developmental delay (GDD) (below 5 years of age): For assessing GDD, the Vineland Social Maturity Scale (VSMS) needs to be used while for assessing ID, several different scales can be used **(Box 5)**.

BOX 5: Tests recommended for assessment of intellectual disability.

- *Tests for global developmental delay (<5 years):* Vineland Social Maturity Scale
- *Tests for intellectual disability (>5 years):* VSMS/Binet-Kamat Test (BKT)/Wechsler Intelligence Scale for Children (WISC)- IV/Malin's Intelligence Scale for Indian Children (MISIC)/WISC/NIEPID Indian Test of Intelligence

A certificate can be applied for, only after the child attains 1 year of age. For all children, preliminary screening for hearing, vision, locomotor impairments, epilepsy, or any other associated comorbidity should be conducted.

Children below 5 years receive a temporary certificate for "Global Developmental Delay", valid till the child attains 5 years of age or for 3 years, whichever is earlier.[25] Certificates will need to be renewed at 10 and 18 years for children above 5 years of age with less than 80% disability. For children above 5 years with more than 80% disability, the certificate will be renewed at 18 years of age. Once renewed at 18 years, for both groups, the certificate will be valid lifelong.

Disability scores are to be calculated on the basis of VSMS score alone. A chart with VSMS scores and degree of disability, as well as constituents of the Medical Board for certification, is provided. Some scales, made by government institutions for use regarding disability certification, are produced as such in these Rules for ease of administration.

Specific learning disability (SLD): This is defined as a mixed group affected by deficits in processing language, spoken or written, which are observable as difficulty in understanding, speaking, reading, writing, spelling, and/or mathematics. Medically, these conditions manifest as perceptual disabilities, dyslexia, dysgraphia, dyscalculia, dyspraxia, and developmental aphasia.

Certification can be done only at 8 years of age, with repeat assessments during the academic years of classes X and XII if required. The certificate issued at 18 years old will be permanent.

Every school needs to organize a screening committee with the teacher/s and the principal. Teachers are tasked with screening the children, talking to parents to ascertain their willingness for referral, and discussing anomalies with the screening committee. A footnote mentions that the member of this board can also be a private practitioner. The principal, along with the screening committee endorsement, needs to refer the child to a pediatrician if the parents are willing and motivated.

The pediatrician who receives the referred child needs to check for visual or hearing abnormalities or other associated comorbidities. Then the child or clinical psychologist needs to conduct IQ assessment using the same IQ tests as for ID. SLD assessment is carried out only if IQ is >85. The NIMHANS (National Institute for Mental Health and Neurosciences) battery or the Grade Level Assessment Device (GLAD) can be used (provided in the notification). These tools will be used across all ages till such time until new scales are developed and validated for older children and adults. The criteria for certification are given in **Box 6**.

BOX 6: SLD certification criteria.

All need to be fulfilled:
- IQ ≥ 85
- No vision and/or hearing impairment which is likely to affect learning
- No emotional and behavioral disorders mimicking SLD
- Presence of adequate opportunity for learning with proper motivation
- The child is functioning at 3 standard deviations below the current class on NIMHANS battery or his/her GLAD score is below 40%, for the child's current class level

(SLD: specific learning disorder)

Autism spectrum disorder: This lifelong condition may be noticed in the first 3 years of life. There are impairments in social skills and communication, which may be accompanied by hyper or hyporeactivity to sensory input, unusual interests, and repetitive, stereotypical rituals or behaviors. It may occur along with intellectual impairment.

For the diagnosis of ASD, the DSM-5-based AIIMS-modified INCLEN diagnostic tool for ASD needs to be used.[26] The Indian Scale of Assessment of Autism (ISAA) will be utilized for calculating disability among children ≥ 6 years.[27] A short 10-item binary short form of ISAA has been tested and can be utilized for community-based screening for ASD [Indian Autism Screening Questionnaire (IASQ)] as shown in **Figure 1**.[28-30]

All children with an ASD in the age group below 6 years will be assessed and given a disability of 60–79% (moderate autism). They will be re-assessed at the age of ≥6 years for severity-based disability calculation as per the Indian Scale of Assessment of Autism. A table for ascribing disability levels is also provided.

Mental illness: The RPWD Act defines mental illness as "a substantial disorder of thinking, mood, perception, orientation, or memory that grossly impairs judgment, behaviour, capacity to recognise reality or ability to meet the ordinary demands of life but does not include mental retardation which is a condition of arrested or incomplete development of mind of a person, specially characterised by sub-normality of intelligence".

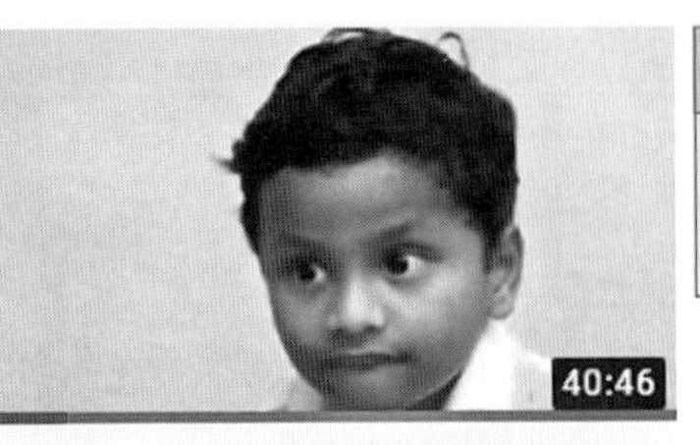

YouTube guide to IASQ and ISAA Administration

✓ ISAA : https://www.youtube.com/watch?v=kz-rddmCEQQ&t=25s
✓ IASQ : https://www.youtube.com/watch?v=Wrooa5lDcso
Search on YouTube – ISAA OR Smita Deshpande

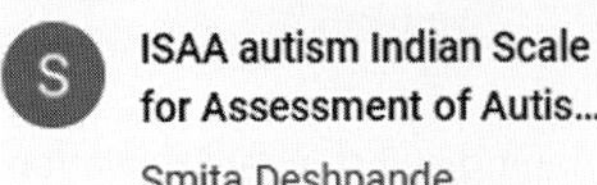

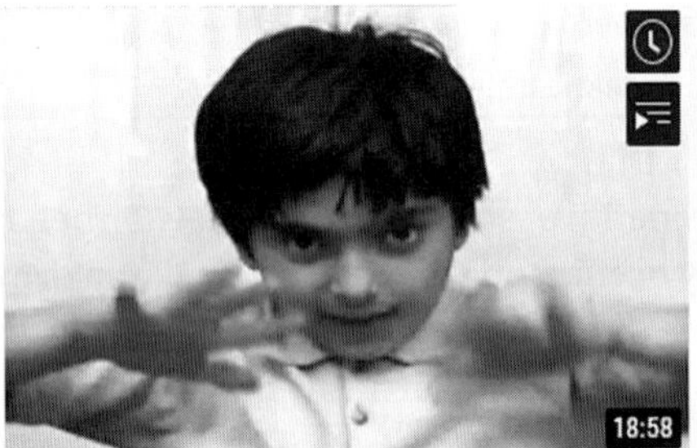

Indian autism screening questionnaire (IASQ) 2021
135 views • 2 months ago
S Smita Deshpande
Indian community screening tool for **autism** tested in persons from 3-18 years of age. Ten items, ten minutes to administer.

Fig. 1: Tests used for disability assessment in autism spectrum disorder (ASD).

A certificate for mental illness will need clinical assessment, applying the Indian Disability Evaluation and Assessment Scale (IDEAS) instrument and/or IQ assessment. Where applicants are suspected to have ID or additional intellectual evaluation is required for any reason, the IQ tests mentioned in the ID guidelines may be used. Where only IDEAS is required with no suspicion of intellectual deficits, then only IDEAS may be applied and disability scored as per these guidelines.

Persons who have both benchmark ID and mental illness disability are to be issued a certificate for multiple disabilities.

From the onset of the mental illness as related by the person/caregivers, if the duration is over 2 years then a permanent disability can be certified. If the duration is less than 2 years, a certificate with time validity may be allowed, the degree depending on the extent of disability. If the disability is severe or profound, the medical board may consider permanent certification.

For persons with mental illness (PWMI), who have not received standard-of-care treatment, a disability certificate with a time validity of up to 2 years may be issued by the board.

The disability board can recommend treatment for an adequate duration from a recognized mental health institution. Subsequently, it may issue a permanent disability certificate.

Thus, this board assesses the person on residual disability after adequate "evidence-based treatment" as documented on medical records. Treatment naïve disabled or their caregivers must be advised to seek appropriate treatment and advised to seek certification of disability only after or despite adequate treatment. For PWMI who have obtained psychiatric treatment but do not have any treatment records, a disability certificate with time validity may be issued with advice to seek appropriate psychiatric treatment, preserve medical records, and repeat disability certification after 2 years.

Chronic neurological disability: The impairment due to neurological conditions should last for at least 3 months. The effect of the neurological condition on general functional capacity rather than on occupation, trade, or work and employment should be assessed.

The effects on activities such as locomotion, vision, or hearing due to neurological conditions are evaluated and certified by experts in the respective specialties. If IQ assessment is required, the person is evaluated based on ID disability evaluation, using the same tests. Disability due to dementia is to be assessed on the IDEAS scale.[31]

A temporary certificate is for 2 years only. Neurologically disabled children are to be provided temporary certificates and re-assessed every 3–5 years. A permanent certificate can be provided for genetic conditions which are not expected to improve and which may even deteriorate. A psychiatrist and trained psychologist are included in the Neurology Assessment Board. A duly qualified expert from the private sector may be included if a government member is not available.

Multiple disabilities: Combination of two or more disabilities: For people with multiple disabilities, each disability has to be evaluated as per Rules, 2024 (each condition should cause at least 25% disability). Thereafter, all disabilities are classified from least to greatest based on their disability scores. If in scoring disabilities, a range is provided (as with IDEAS), then the mid-point of that range is considered. The formula is given in **Box 7**.

BOX 7: Formula for calculating disability score for multiple disability.

a—disability #1
b—disability #2
c—disability #3

$$\frac{a + b\,(100 - a)}{100} = x$$

This (*x*) becomes (*a*) for calculating disability 3 (c)

$$\frac{x + c\,(90 - x)}{90} = y$$

Maximum: Not more than 100%

UNMET NEEDS AND FUTURE REQUIREMENTS

Since 2002 when the IDEAS scale was accepted by the government for certification of mental illness to the 2024 Rules, we have come a long way. Yet lacunae remain for the assessment and certification of neurodevelopmental and mental disabilities in children and adults.[32]

While we do have Indian scales or adaptations of scales for assessing ID and ASDs, the same is not true for SLD.[33] There is a multiplicity of education boards, curricula, and languages in which the child needs to be assessed. Far greater research needs to be conducted all over the country to develop a test for SLDs which can be uniformly applied to every Indian child.

The IDEAS was developed only for four major disorders (schizophrenia, bipolar affective disorders, obsessive-compulsive disorders, and dementia), which were chronic and had caused significant disability over 2 years. With the expansion of the definition of mental illnesses in the Rules, we need a much bigger canvas of evaluation. Another significance with IDEAS is that it provides a range of scores, while the UDID portal and Courts under Motor Accidents Claim Tribunal accept only an exact number.

In short, we need nationally acceptable instrument/s that are available in several large Indian languages, valid and reliable, easy, brief, and free for use. Medical specialists even at the district level should be able to apply the instrument after limited training. They should be tested in varied parts of India for their science through collaborative work all over the country.

Most importantly, just as Rules 2024 for neurological disabilities state, we should be able to look beyond the diagnosis to the dysfunction leading to a specified amount of disability. Due to finite resources, a "cutoff point" for "legal disability" will probably always be necessary. Hence, we will need instruments which measure disability, not diagnosis, accurately providing a number and not a range. To achieve this goal, a lot more work needs to be undertaken on the ground.

SUMMARY AND CONCLUSION

To summarize, disability is not a tragedy, curse, or stigma. It is due to injustice and unequal treatment, not inherent inequality. India has four major legislations to empower and include Persons with Disability into mainstream society, based on the UNCRPD, which India signed in October, 2007. While the Rehabilitation Council of India regulates special education, training, and certification of rehabilitation professionals, the National Trust focuses on specified disabilities to aid, mainstream, and provide guardianship. For availing of disability benefits, a disability certificate is essential. Certificate issuance is regulated by the RPWD Act 2016 and subsequent Rules. Rules for issuing Disability Certificates for benchmark disabilities (≥40%) are available at the website of the UDID: https://www.swavlambancard.gov.in/. Certificates can be permanent (for disabilities from which recovery is not possible) or temporary (for developmental disabilities which may change over time). Children should be evaluated for disability early on to enable inclusive education, to make available all possible assistive technologies, and special assistance if required. Permanent certificates are generally made available only at 18 years of age for childhood neurodevelopmental disabilities. Disability certificate is a right, not a favor and every healthcare professional must work to integrating and mainstreaming CWD.

One can conclude that all human beings are equal and have equal rights to lead a fulfilling life. Among humans, children have a greater right to assistance and care. CWD need greater protection and help from society, their families, and healthcare professionals. As children are more prone to being misunderstood and disregarded in their preferences, this may result in discrimination and inadequate, sparse care facilities. Although Indian laws follow the UNCRPD, lack of resources and ignorance hamper the development of facilities for children with neurodevelopmental disabilities and mental illnesses.

A legal method of recognizing their existence and need for special care is by certifying them for their disability. All healthcare workers need to learn the enabling laws for disability and benefits that disability certification ensures. We should inform families and caregivers at every encounter. If such certification facilities are not available within easy access, we must advocate for them to be set up. As mental healthcare personnel, we must ensure that CWD with neurodevelopmental and mental disabilities receive due benefits and rehabilitation facilities.

ACKNOWLEDGMENTS

We acknowledge the efforts of Professor Pankaj Verma, Head, Department of Psychiatry, VMMC and Safdarjung Hospital, New Delhi, for his support. We thank Dr Triptish Bhatia for her help with referencing.

We acknowledge the bravery and dedication of persons with disability and their caregivers and advocates. This chapter is dedicated to them.

REFERENCES

1. Math SB, Gowda GS, Basavaraju V, Manjunatha N, Kumar CN, Philip S, et al. The Rights of Persons with Disability Act, 2016: Challenges and opportunities. Indian J Psychiatry. 2019;61:S809-15.

2. United Nations. Convention on the rights of persons with disabilities. New York: United Nations, 2006.
3. Ministry of Social Justice and Empowerment. Rights of Persons with Disability Act; Act No. 49 of 2016. In: Ministry of Social Justice and Empowerment and India Go. New Delhi: Government of India; 2016.
4. Ministry of Health and Family Welfare. The Mental Health Care Act No. 10 of 2017. In: India Go. New Delhi: Government of India; 2017.
5. Department of Empowerment of Persons with Disabilities (Divyangjan). Rehabilitation Council of India (a statutory body of Ministry of Social Justice and Empowerment). [online] Available from rehabcouncil.nic.in. [Last accessed 22 November, 2025].
6. India Go. The National Trust Act 1999. New Delhi: Government of India; 1999.
7. Thomas Kishore M, Maru R, Seshadri SP, Kumar D, Vijay Sagar JK, Jacob P, et al. Specific learning disability in the context of current diagnostic systems and policies in India: Implications for assessment and certification. Asian J Psychiatr. 2021;55:102506.
8. Ministry of Law and Justice. New Delhi: Government of India; 2017.
9. Department of Empowerment of Persons with Disabilities (Divyangjan). Office of Chief Commissioner for Persons with Disabilities https://share.google/ew9Piyas8us7mqzFm. [Last accessed 22 November, 2025].
10. United Nations. Department of Economic and Social Affairs, Sustainable Development. [online] Available from https://sdgs.un.org/goals/goal9 [Last accessed 22 November, 2025].
11. UNICEF for Every Child. Division of Data Analytics Planning and Monitoring Annual Report.
12. World Health Organization. (2017). Rehabilitation 2030: A call for action. [online] Available from https://www.who.int/publications/m/item/rehabilitation-2030-a-call-for-action [Last accessed 22 November, 2025].
13. World Health Organization. (1976). World Health Organisation: International Classification of Diseases (ICD) https://share.google/l6DWu3Kb0fmHrjPXO [Last accessed 22 November, 2025].
14. Olusanya BO, Cheung VG, Hadders-Algra M, Breinbauer C, Smythe T, Moreno-Angarita M, et al. Sustainable Development Goals summit 2023 and the global pledge on disability-focused early childhood development. Lancet Glob Health 2023;11:e823-5.
15. United Nations Department of Economic and Social Affairs. (2015). Transforming our world: the 2030 Agenda for sustainable development. [online] Available from https://sdgs.un.org/2030agenda [Last accessed 22 November, 2025].
16. World Health Organization. (2001). International classification of functioning, disability and health (ICF) https://share.google/2cusKA7Wk8tLs0RWr [Last accessed 22 November, 2025].
17. Picton-Howell Z. The human rights of children with disabilities: How can medical professionals better fulfil rather than breach them? Dev Med Child Neurol. 2023;65:1429-35.
18. Ayoub MC, Rava J, Lewis Hunter A, Kuo AA. Facilitators and Barriers to Care for Patients with Disabilities in Primary Pediatrics. Pediatr Ann. 2022;51:e243-53.
19. United Nations Human Rights. (1989). Convention on the rights of the child. [online] Available from https://www.ohchr.org/en/instruments-mechanisms/instruments/convention-rights-child [Last accessed 22 November, 2025].
20. Ladds E, Darbyshire JL, Bakerly ND, Falope Z, Tucker-Bell I. Cognitive dysfunction after covid-19. BMJ. 2024;384:e075387.
21. Gazette of India E. Gazette of India. Latest Notified Guidelines for assessing the extent of specified disabilities dated 14.03.2024|Department of Empowerment of Persons with Disabilities (DEPwD)|Home| India https://share.google/u0d27vctK0GTUWLVd [Last accessed 22 November, 2025].
22. Ministry of Social Justice and Empowerment. UDID https://share.google/c3Fuw7whn8pjvlMvU [Last accessed 22 November, 2025].
23. Philip SJP, Sharda A, Allam A, Singh A, Seralathan M. Psychiatric rehabilitation in routine Indian mental health practice: A review of social protections for persons with mental health conditions. Indian J Psychiatry. 2024;66:235-46.
24. Bhardwaj S. (2018). Exemptions/concessions extended to Persons with Benchmark Disabilities

for Class X & XII Examinations conducted by the CBSE and Standard Operating Procedure. CBSE/COORD/112233/2018. [online] Available from https://www.cbse.gov.in/cbsenew/Examination_Circular/2018/3_CIRCULAR.pdf [Last accessed 22 November, 2025].

25. Juneja M, Gupta A, Sairam S, Jain R, Sharma M, Thadani, et al. Diagnosis and Management of Global Development Delay: Consensus Guidelines of Growth, Development and Behavioral Pediatrics Chapter, Neurology Chapter and Neurodevelopment Pediatrics Chapter of the Indian Academy of Pediatrics. Indian Pediatr. 2022;59:401-15.
26. Gulati S, Kaushik JS, Saini L, Sondhi V, Madaan P, Arora NK, et al. Development and validation of DSM-5 based diagnostic tool for children with Autism Spectrum Disorder. PLoS One. 2019;14:e0213242.
27. Indian Scale for Assessment of Autism. Report on assessment tool for autism. Ministry of Social Justice & Empowerment, Government of India, New Delhi.
28. Chakraborty S, Bhatia T, Sharma V, Antony N, Das D, Sahu S, et al. Psychometric properties of a screening tool for autism in the community-The Indian Autism Screening Questionnaire (IASQ). PLoS One. 2021;16:e0249970.
29. Chakraborty S, Bhatia T, Sharma V, Antony N, Das D, Sahu S, et al. Protocol for Development of the Indian Autism Screening Questionnaire: The Screening Version of the Indian Scale for Assessment of Autism. Indian J Psychol Med. 2020;42:S63-7.
30. Chakraborty S, Bhatia T, Antony N, Roy A, Shriharsh V, Sahay A, et al. Comparing the Indian Autism Screening Questionnaire (IASQ) and the Indian Scale for Assessment of Autism (ISAA) with the Childhood Autism Rating Scale-Second Edition (CARS2) in Indian settings. PLoS One. 2022;17:e0273780.
31. IDEAS. (2002). Guidelines for evaluation and assessment of mental illness and procedure for certification.. [online] Available from https://punarbhava.in/images/images1/RCI_programme/publications/eval_ment.pdf
32. Government of India. Guidelines for evaluation and assessment of mental illness and procedure for certification. In (Divyangjan) DoEoPwD (Eds). New Delhi: Government of India, February 27; 2002.
33. Sahu S, Shriharsh V, Bhatia T, Goel P. A Comparative Pilot Study of Curriculum-Based vs. Skill-Based Assessment for Dyslexia. Asia Pacific J Develop Differ. 2022;9. DOI:10.3850/S2345734122000113.

CHAPTER 32

Laws Related to Child Mental Healthcare

Shivender Singh, Lakshmi Sravanti, Rajendra KM, Suresh Bada Math

INTRODUCTION

India is home to one of the youngest populations in the world. Adequate physical and mental healthcare is crucial for children and adolescents' development and overall well-being. While providing mental healthcare, mental health professionals need to be familiar with the relevant legal aspects of this population. Some legal issues involving minors, such as custody disputes, do not have adult parallels. There are differences even when similar legal issues arise, such as the need to consider minors' developmental levels and hold them to a lesser degree of responsibility. The legal provisions for child mental healthcare in India encompass the protection, treatment, and rehabilitation of vulnerable children, as well as the evaluation and rehabilitation of young offenders. The Mental Health Care Act (MHCA), 2017,[1] which was passed on 7th April 2017, to provide mental healthcare and services for persons with mental illness, also includes specific provisions for minors. The Rights of Persons with Disabilities (RPwD) Act, 2016,[2] came into force on 19th April 2017 to ensure that all persons with disabilities can lead their lives with dignity, without discrimination, and enjoy their rights equally with others. The Protection of Children from Sexual Offences (POCSO) Act, 2012,[3] was passed to protect children from offenses of sexual assault, sexual harassment, and pornography and provide for the establishment of special courts with a child-friendly atmosphere for speedy trials of such offenses. The Juvenile Justice (Care and Protection of Children) Act, 2015, consists of the setting up of Juvenile Justice Boards (JJB), Child Welfare Committees (CWC), a description of procedures concerning children in need of care and protection, and children in conflict with the law. Finally, there are various religion-based child custody laws in India, relevant details of which, along with the approach to child custody evaluation, have been briefly discussed in the chapter. This chapter offers insights into these laws related to child mental healthcare and the approaches to assessment in various clinical situations relevant to these laws. We discuss the applied aspects of the Mental Healthcare Act, 2017; the Rights of Persons with Disabilities Act, 2016; the Protection of Children from Sexual Offences Act, 2012; the Juvenile Justice (Care and Protection of Children) Act, 2015; and the laws governing custody and guardianship in India under Child Custody Evaluations (CCE) in the context of child mental health.

MENTAL HEALTHCARE ACT, 2017[1]

The MHCA, 2017, was passed on 7th April 2017 to provide mental healthcare and services for persons with mental illness and to protect, promote, and fulfil the rights of such persons during the delivery of healthcare. The act includes specific provisions for minors concerning advanced directives, nominated representatives, admission, treatment, and discharge, which are detailed below.

Sections Relevant to Child Mental Healthcare

Definitions

Section 1(2)s: "Mental illness" means a substantial disorder of thinking, mood, perception, orientation, or memory that grossly impairs judgment, behavior, capacity to recognize reality, or ability to meet the ordinary demands of life, mental conditions associated with the abuse of alcohol and drugs, but does not include mental retardation which is a condition of arrested or incomplete development of mind of a person, mainly characterized by subnormality of intelligence.

Section 1(2)t: "minor" means a person who has not completed the age of 18 years.

Advance Directive

Section 11(4): The legal guardian shall have the right to make an advance directive in writing with respect to a minor.

Nominated Representative

Section 15: Nominated representative of a minor

- The legal guardian shall be the nominated representative.
- However, the concerned board may appoint any other nominated representative if it is of the opinion that the legal guardian is either not fit or is not acting in the minor's best interests.
- Suppose no individual is available for appointment as a nominated representative. In that case, the Board shall appoint the Director of the Department of Social Welfare of the State or his nominee as the nominated representative of the minor with mental illness.

Rights of Persons with Mental Illness

Section 21(2):

- A child <3 years of age shall not be separated from the mother who is receiving care, treatment, or rehabilitation at a mental health establishment.
- The child shall be temporarily separated from the mother if there is a risk of harm to the child; however, she shall continue to have access to the child under the supervision of the staff or family.

Section 21(3):

- The need to separate the child from the mother shall be reviewed every 15 days.
- The separation shall be terminated as soon as conditions that required the separation no longer exist.
- If separation exceeds 30 days at a stretch, it shall be required to be approved by the respective authority.

Admission, Treatment, and Discharge

Section 87: Admission of a minor

- The minor may be admitted to the mental health establishment if:
    - Two psychiatrists, or
    - One psychiatrist and one mental health professional, or
    - One psychiatrist and one medical practitioner have independently examined the minor on the day of admission or in the preceding 7 days, and both independently conclude that:
        - The mental illness is of a severity requiring admission.
        - The admission shall be in the best interests of the minor.
        - The mental healthcare needs of the minor cannot be fulfilled unless he is admitted.
        - All community-based alternatives have failed or are unsuitable.
- A minor shall be accommodated separately from adults in an environment considering his age and developmental needs.
- The nominated representative or an attendant appointed by the nominated representative

shall, under all circumstances, stay with the minor for the entire duration of the admission.

- A minor shall be given treatment with the informed consent of his nominated representative.
- If the nominated representative no longer supports the minor's admission or requests the minor's discharge, the minor shall be discharged.
- Admission of a minor shall be informed by the medical officer or mental health professional in charge of the mental health establishment to the concerned board within 72 hours.
- The concerned board can visit and interview the minor or review the medical records if needed.
- Any minor's admission that continues beyond 30 days shall be immediately informed to the concerned board.
- The concerned board shall carry out a mandatory review within 7 days of being informed of all admissions of minors continuing beyond 30 days and every 30 days after that.

Section 88: Discharge of independent patients
Where a minor admitted under section 87 attains the age of 18 years during his stay in the mental health establishment, he shall be classified as an independent patient under section 86 and all provisions of the Mental Healthcare Act, 2017, as applicable to an independent patient who is not a minor, shall apply to such person.

Section 95: Prohibited procedures
Electroconvulsive therapy for minors is a prohibited procedure. However, suppose the psychiatrist in charge of a minor's treatment is of the opinion that electroconvulsive therapy is required. In that case, such treatment can be done with the guardian's informed consent and prior permission of the concerned board.

RIGHTS OF PERSONS WITH DISABILITIES ACT, 2016[2]

Overview

The Rights of Persons with Disabilities (RPwD) Act, 2016, was enacted on 28th December 2016 and came into force on 19th April 2017. The act provides for effective measures to ensure that persons with disabilities enjoy their rights equally with others. It defines and covers 21 specified disabilities. The act also provides additional benefits for persons with benchmark disabilities and penalties for offenses committed against such persons.

Guidelines for the Purpose of Assessing the Extent of Specified Disability in a Person Included under the Rights of Persons with Disabilities Act, 2016

Intellectual Disability

Intellectual disability is defined as a condition characterized by significant limitations both in intellectual functioning (reasoning, learning, and problem-solving) and in adaptive behavior, with onset in the developmental period, and which covers a range of daily social skills and skills required for activities of daily living. This term is used for children with age 5 years and above (≥5 years). The term "Global Developmental Delay" is used for children aged <5 years with a similar disability. Disability assessment for GDD/IDD has been mentioned in **Flowchart 1**.

Specific Learning Disability

It refers to developmental learning disorders with deficit in processing spoken or written language resulting in difficulty in comprehension, reading, writing, spelling, or mathematical calculations. Disability assessment for "Specific Learning Disability" has been described in **Flowchart 2**.

Flowchart 1: Disability assessment for global developmental delay (GDD)/intellectual disability (IDD).

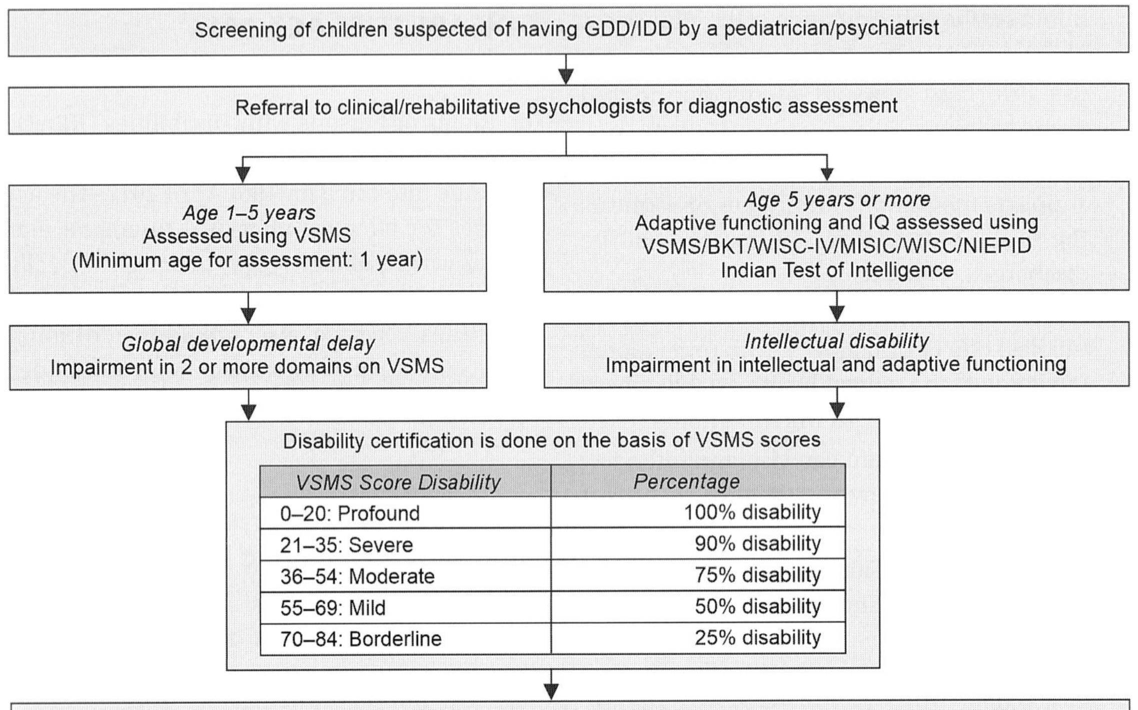

VSMS Score Disability	Percentage
0–20: Profound	100% disability
21–35: Severe	90% disability
36–54: Moderate	75% disability
55–69: Mild	50% disability
70–84: Borderline	25% disability

Medical authority
- Medical Superintendent or Chief Medical Officer or Civil Surgeon or any other equivalent authority as notified by the State Government (head of the Medical Board)
- Pediatrician or Pediatric Neurologist (where available) or Developmental Pediatrician (where available) or physician (if age >18 years)
- Psychiatrist or Child and Adolescent Psychiatrist (wherever available)
- Clinical or Rehabilitation Psychologist

The chairperson may, if required due to shortage of the specialist doctors, include private medical practitioner(s) (qualified in the respective medical domain) as a board member.

Validity of certificate

For children aged 1–5 years: Temporary certificate valid till age of 5 years

For children aged >5 years:
- *If disability is 80% or more:* Reassessment and recertification at 18 years of age
- *If disability is <80%:* Certificate will have to be renewed at 10 and 18 years of age

Certificate issued at age of 18 years or more will be valid lifelong

Autism Spectrum Disorder

Usually appears in the first 3 years of life, characterized by impairments in the social skills, communication, and restricted repetitive behaviors. Disability assessment for "Autism Spectrum Disorders" has been mentioned in **Flowchart 3**.

Mental Illness

Means a substantial disorder of thinking, mood, perception, orientation, or memory that

Flowchart 2: Disability assessment for "Specific Learning Disability".

Screening
- At eight years of age or in Class III, whichever is earlier
- Screening test (Form A) performed by teachers of the public and private schools if poor understanding or drop in academic performance is noted
- If an anomaly is detected, the teacher informs the principal and screening committee of the school
- Child is referred for specific learning disability assessment by the screening committee with a referral letter and teacher's screening report

↓

Clinical Assessment
Initial assessment by pediatrician (or pediatric Neurologist or developmental pediatrician, where available):
- Detailed clinical examination including neurological examination,
- Vision and hearing assessment

Assessment by psychiatrist to rule out associated comorbidities, emotional and behavioral disorders that may mimic "Specific Learning Disability (SLD)"

IQ Assessment
- Performed by child/ clinical psychologists using MISIC/ WISCIV/NIEPID Indian Test of Intelligence/BKT/VSMS
- If IQ>85, perform SLD assessment

↓

Specific learning disability assessment
Assessed using National Institute for Mental Health and Neurosciences (NIMHANS) battery or Grade Level Assessment Device (GLAD)

Diagnosed as SLD if all of the following criteria are fulfilled:
- IQ 85 or more
- No vision and /or hearing impairment which are likely to affect learning
- No emotional and behavioral disorders mimicking SLD
- Presence of adequate opportunity for learning with proper motivation
- The child is functioning at 3 standard deviations below the current class on NIMHANS battery or his/ her GLAD score is below 40%, for the child's current class level

Medical authority
- The Medical Superintendent or Chief Medical Officer or Civil Surgeon or any other equivalent authority as notified by the State Government (head of the Medical Board)
- Pediatrician or Pediatric Neurologist (where available) or Developmental Pediatrician (where available)
- Psychiatrist or Child and Adolescent Psychiatrist (wherever available)
- Clinical or Rehabilitation Psychologist (line)

The chairperson may, if required due to shortage of the specialist doctors, include private medical practitioner(s) (qualified in the respective medical domain) as a board member

Validity of certificate
- The certification is done for children aged eight years and above only
- Repeat certification during the academic year of Class X and academic year of Class XII, if required
- The certificate issued at 18 years or more is valid life-long

grossly impairs judgment, behavior, capacity to recognize reality or ability to meet the ordinary demands of life but does not include mental retardation which is a condition of arrested or incomplete development of mind of a person, specially characterized by subnormality of intelligence. Persons with schizophrenia, bipolar disorder, obsessive-compulsive disorder, and dementia with 2 years of illness can be assessed using the IDEAS scale. Disability assessment for mental illness has been mentioned in **Flowchart 4**.

Flowchart 3: Disability assessment for "Autism Spectrum Disorders".

Diagnosis
- Assessed by AIIMS-modified INCLEN diagnostic tool for ASD
- The Indian Scale of Assessment of Autism (ISAA) will be used for the calculation of disability among children ≥6 years

Disability calculation
Children <6 years with ASD:
- Disability of 60–79%(Moderate autism) is given to all
- Reassessed at the age of 6 years or more for severity-based disability calculation as per ISAA

Children aged 6 years or more with ASD:
- The severity-based disability calculation will be based on the ISAA
- Disability levels will be as shown below:

Indian Scale of Assessment of Autism Score	*Disability Percentage*
• Mild autism (ISAA score 70–106)	40–59%
• Moderate autism (ISAA score (107–153)	60–79%
• Severe autism (ISAA score >153)	≥80%

Medical authority
- The Medical Superintendent, Chief Medical Officer, Civil Surgeon, or any other equivalent authority, as notified by the State Government (Head of the Medical Board)
- Pediatrician or Pediatric Neurologist (where available) or Developmental Pediatrician (where available) or physician if aged >18 years (MD Internal Medicine or Family Medicine)
- Psychiatrist or Child and Adolescent Psychiatrist (where available)
- Psychologist (Clinical/rehabilitation)

The chairperson may, if required due to shortage of the specialist doctors, include private medical practitioner(s) (qualified in the respective medical domain) as a board member

Validity of certificate
Children <6 years:
- The certificate will be temporary.
- These children will need reassessment between the age of 6 and 7 years for recertification and calculation of disability

Children aged 6 years or more but <18 years:
Disability of > 40%: Reassessment and recertification will be done at the age of 18 years

Age ≥18 years:
Disability certificate issued after the age of 18 years will be permanent

THE PROTECTION OF CHILDREN FROM SEXUAL OFFENCES ACT, 2012[3]

Overview

The act came into force on 14th November 2012, intending to protect children from offenses of sexual assault, sexual harassment, and pornography and provide for the establishment of Special Courts with child-friendly atmosphere for speedy trial of such offenses. The act defines a child as any person below the age of 18 years. Furthermore, it describes various forms of sexual offenses against children, which include sexual harassment, sexual assault, penetrative sexual assault, and pornography. Sexual assault and penetrative sexual assault are defined as "aggravated"; for example, when the victim is below 12 years of age, the victim has a mental or physical disability, or when a person is in a position of trust or authority over a child, such as a parent, police, or hospital staff, commits the offense.

The POCSO Act was amended in 2019 to make it more effective in dealing with cases of child sexual abuse. The Amendment Act introduced

Flowchart 4: Disability assessment for mental illness.

Diagnosis
- The examination involves clinical assessment, IDEAS scale and/or IQ assessment
- Indian Disability Evaluation and Assessment Scale (IDEAS) administration is to be used for degree of disability certification in mental illness (If required)
- In cases, where there is suspicion of intellectual deficits Standardised IQ test may be carried out as per prescribed standards in Intellectual Disability Guidelines
- In cases wherein, there is both intellectual disability and mental illness disability, the person may be classified as having multiple disability and certificate issued accordingly
- The duration of the mental illness should be determined from the onset of the mental illness. For certifying permanent disability, a minimum duration of at least two years of mental illness is required

Validity of certificate
- For any mental illness with duration of less than two years, only certificate with time validity may be provided. In case of severe or profound disability, the medical board may consider permanent certification
- For persons with mental illness (PWMI), who have not received standard of care treatment only disability certificate with time validity up to two years may be issued by the board
- The disability board may recommend for treatment from any mental health establishment (MHE) and then may issue permanent disability certificate based on assessment of the residual disability only after the PWMI has received the treatment for adequate duration as determined by the Board
- Treatment naïve patients of Mental Illness/their caregivers must be advised to seek appropriate treatment to empower them and advised to seek disability certification of disability despite adequate treatment
- For persons with Mental Illness who have taken psychiatric treatment but do not have any treatment records, disability certificate with time validity may be issued with advice to seek appropriate psychiatric treatment, preserve medical records and repeat disability certification after 2 years

Medical authority
- Medical Superintendent, or Chief Medical Officer, or Civil Surgeon or any other equivalent authority as notified by the State Government (head of the Medical Board)
- Psychiatrist
- Psychiatrist/Physician or RCI registered Clinical Psychologist/Rehab Psychologist/Psychiatric social worker (wherever required Psychological Assessment report from RCI registered Psychologist obtained in last three months)

The chairperson may, if required due to shortage of the specialist doctors, include private medical practitioner(s) (qualified in the respective medical domain) as a board member

more stringent punishments, such as an increase in the imprisonment period, and included the death penalty in extreme cases of aggravated penetrative sexual assault. The procedure for reporting offenses under this act is described in Chapter V of the act. The health professionals need to be familiar with the procedure, as a victim child may be brought by parents or caregivers or referred by other agencies for management.

Chapter V: Procedure for Mandatory Reporting of Cases

19. Reporting of offenses:

- As per subsection (1), any person (including the child) who has apprehension that an offense under this act is likely to be committed or has knowledge that such an offense has been committed shall provide such information to (a) the Special Juvenile Police Unit or (b) the local police.
- As per subsection (6), the Special Juvenile Police Unit or local police shall report the matter to the CWC and the Special Court, or where no Special Court has been designated, to the Court of Session within a period of 24 hours.
- As per subsection (7), no person shall incur any civil or criminal liability for giving the information in good faith for the purpose of subsection (*l*).

21. Punishment for failure to report or record a case:

- As per subsection (1), any person who fails to report the commission of an offense under this act shall be punished with imprisonment for up to 6 months or with a fine or both.
- As per subsection (2), any person who is in charge of any company or an institution who fails to report the commission of an offense under this act, in respect of a subordinate under his control, shall be punished with imprisonment for up to 1 year and with fine.

The approach to assessment of a victim of child sexual abuse is outlined in **Table 1**.

Guidelines for Interviewing Children in Sensitive Situations[4]

Phase 1: Preparation and Establishing Rapport

- Approach with extreme sensitivity to the child's experience and its potential impact on their responses.
- Try to establish rapport and a neutral, nonjudgmental environment without distractions before beginning the interview.
- Clarify confidentiality limits and inform the child who will access their shared information.
- Provide interview instructions; if you do not understand, correct me.
- Event narration practice
- Gather information about the child's verbal skills and cognitive maturity.
- Assess the child's developmental level; young children may not fully understand the concept of time and numbers, and their vocabulary may be limited. If needed, consider doing a developmental or intelligence assessment.

Phase 2: Conducting the Interview

- If a support person is needed for the child, he should be seated out of the child's line of vision and instructed not to interrupt the child's account.
- Use drawings, toys, dolls, puppets, etc., carefully to assist young children in communication, as these items may sometimes distract the child.
- Provide breaks as needed during the interview.

Phase 3: Questioning Techniques

- Begin with broad and open-ended questions.
- Use prompts while repeating the relevant child's words to elicit details.
- Use direct questioning when the open-ended questioning has been exhausted.
- Avoid leading questions and complex questions.
- Maintain objectivity and refrain from suggesting answers.
- Avoid lengthy interviews.
- Avoid asking the child why they behaved in a certain way; they may have difficulty answering such questions.

Phase 4: Conclusion and Postinterview Support

- Before ending the interview, ensure the child understands that the interview is concluding soon and ask if there is anything else they would like to share or clarify.
- Provide closure by summarizing the interview process and offering feedback on the child's participation, acknowledging their courage and contribution.

Practical Tips to Psychiatrist for Doing Forensic Interview with Children

Forensic interview in children requires a structured, sensitive, and patient-centered approach. Children often disclose information gradually, in bits and pieces, and across multiple sessions, making it essential for the psychiatrist to allow time for a full understanding of events. Interviews should be conducted in a safe, private, and nonthreatening environment, ensuring the child feels secure.

TABLE 1: Psychosocial and mental health assessment for victims of child sexual abuse.

Background details	• Name, age, gender, and address • Date and time of assessment • Informants
Referral details	*Referral from CWC, other medical specialists* • Request a referral letter including: – The date and time – Circumstances of referral – Whether a case has been filed, if yes: - Status of the case - Copy of the first information report (FIR) *Self-referral by child's parents* • Note the presence of informants (parent or primary caregiver) • Contact details of the accompanying person • Whether a case has been filed, if yes: – Copy of the first information report (FIR)
Details of the incident	• What happened? • Who was the accused? • Which place of incident? • When was the first time it happened? • How many times has it happened? • What are circumstances of disclosure? • What happened after the disclosure? • Is the child safe currently? • Was any help sought previously, e.g., from the police, CWC, etc.? • What is collateral information from other sources
Assessment of psychiatric symptoms following the incident	• Irritability and aggression • Fearfulness, anxiety, depressive features, and self-harm • Clingy behavior and separation anxiety • Sleep disturbances, nightmares, flashbacks, and avoidance behavior • Bedwetting • School refusal and academic decline • Sexualized behavior • Substance use
Family history	Support and family reaction
Personal history	Strengths and academics
Physical examination	• In the presence of a parent or any other person in whom the child reposes trust or confidence or a woman nominated by the Head of the Medical Institution • Consent of child (12 years and above) and consent from parent • In case the victim is a girl child, the medical examination shall be conducted by a woman doctor
Medical evaluation and treatment	As per the state or central government guidelines

Inpatient care should be considered for comprehensive interview and 360° assessments, particularly if the child presents with significant trauma, emotional distress, or risk factors such as self-harm, aggression, or unsafe home environments. Admission also allows for detailed family and environmental evaluations, ensuring that external influences do not interfere with the child's ability to provide reliable information.

Rapport-building is crucial, beginning with neutral conversations before moving to sensitive topics. Open-ended and nonleading questions should be used to elicit responses, avoiding suggestions that may influence their statements. Since children's accounts may vary across sessions, validation through multiple sittings, serial assessments, collateral information, and consistency checks is necessary. A thorough forensic interview requires close observation of both verbal and nonverbal cues, such as inconsistencies, emotional distress, or avoidance behaviors. Given that traumatic experiences can impact recall, multiple sessions may be required to gather complete and coherent information. The assessment process should remain neutral and evidence-based, avoiding bias, assumptions, or speculation about guilt or victimhood.

What to Report?[5]

The report should describe in detail what happened to the child, the abuse details, and the involved parties. It should be specific, and unnecessary details must be avoided.

Drafting a child abuse report for forensic purposes invariably needs IP care for following reasons. First, children who have experienced abuse often disclose information gradually and in fragmented episodes due to trauma, fear, or confusion. Inpatient care provides a safe, structured, and supportive environment where trained professionals can build rapport and facilitate disclosure over time. Second, many children experience severe emotional distress, including anxiety, depression, dissociation, and post-traumatic stress symptoms, which require continuous monitoring and intensive psychological intervention. Third, if the abuse involved close family members, returning home may place the child at high risk of further harm, necessitating temporary separation from the perpetrator. Fourth, inpatient care allows for comprehensive forensic evaluation, including medical, psychological, and legal assessments, to document evidence systematically without external pressure or interference. Lastly, inpatient care supports family counseling and stabilization, ensuring that nonoffending caregivers are equipped to provide a safe and supportive environment postdischarge.

The report should begin with identifying information, including the child's name, parents' name, child's age, gender, hospital registration number, and the date of admission. Details about the parent or guardian, including their relationship with the child and their contact information, should also be recorded. The reason for assessment and accompanying letters from the authorities and requestion should be noted in the report. Providing a brief but precise statement about the circumstances leading to hospitalization ensures clarity in the report.

The history of abuse should be recorded based on the child's disclosure and collateral sources. The child's account must be documented as accurately as possible, preferably using their own words, while ensuring that leading questions are avoided. The report should detail the type of abuse (physical, sexual, emotional, or neglect), the frequency and timeline of incidents, and descriptions of specific abusive acts. Information about the perpetrator(s) and their relationship to the child, as well as the locations where the abuse occurred, should also be included. Collateral information from caregivers, teachers, or social workers can help to validate the child's disclosure and provide additional context. Structured forensic interviewing should be conducted in a child-friendly manner to ensure legally admissible documentation. If sexual abuse is suspected, a forensic medical examination should be performed promptly to preserve crucial evidence. The examination of child sexual abuse should be done by all registered medical practitioners and also, they should know how to collect evidence. Additionally, the report should document the mandatory reporting process, law enforcement, and relevant child protection agencies.

The clinical assessment should include a thorough physical examination to document injuries, scars, malnutrition, or signs of neglect. A Mental Status Examination (MSE) should assess the child's cognitive, emotional, and behavioral state. The assessments should focus on signs of trauma, such as flashbacks, nightmares, avoidance behaviors, and emotional withdrawal. Developmental assessments, including IQ evaluations, should be conducted only if there are suspected delays in cognitive or emotional development.

The treatment and intervention plan should address both medical and mental health needs. Medical management should focus on treating physical injuries, infections, or other health concerns. Psychological therapy should be trauma-focused, incorporating evidence-based interventions such as cognitive-behavioral therapy (CBT) to help the child process their experiences. Family counseling should also be included to educate caregivers on trauma-informed care and enhance protective factors. Furthermore, legal and social support must be coordinated with child protection agencies to ensure ongoing safety and justice for the child.

The report should conclude with a follow-up and discharge plan. Ongoing mental health support should be arranged postdischarge, ensuring continued therapy and monitoring of the child's well-being. A safety plan should be put in place to prevent re-exposure to the perpetrator, including legal safeguards where necessary. Efforts should also be made to support the child's educational and social reintegration, ensuring that their schooling and peer relationships are not disrupted.

In summary, the report should be fact-based, specific, and legally sound, avoiding unnecessary details that could dilute the core issues. Inpatient care is justified because it ensures a safe space for gradual disclosure, allows for intensive psychological support, prevents re-exposure to perpetrators, facilitates forensic assessment, and prepares the child for legal testimony. Lastly, the report should highlight the importance of legal coordination to ensure the child's safety, justice, and long-term recovery.

THE JUVENILE JUSTICE (CARE AND PROTECTION OF CHILDREN) ACT, 2015[6]

It is an act concerned with children alleged and children in need of care and protection and/or found to be in conflict with the law. It has provisions for care, protection, development, treatment, rehabilitation, and social reintegration, which can be achieved by adopting a child-friendly approach and acting in the children's best interest.

The act came into force on 15th January 2016 and repealed the Juvenile Justice (Care and Protection of Children) Act of 2000. The act includes setting up JJB, CWC, and a description of procedures concerning children in conflict with the law and children in need of care and protection. Furthermore, this act also has sections on rehabilitation and adoption.

As per the Juvenile Justice Act (JJA), 2015

- *Child* means a person below 18 years of age.
- *Child in conflict with the law* means a child who is alleged or found to have committed an

offense and has not completed 18 years of age on the commission of such offense.

- *Child in need of care and protection* means a child.
    - Who is found without any support, without any home, begging, living on the street, or working in contravention of labor laws.
    - Any child who resides with a person who has either threatened or injured, exploited, abused, or neglected the child.
    - Who is abandoned, surrendered, missing, or run away a child.
    - Who is at risk of harm such as by drug abuse, sexual abuse, or illegal acts.
- *Heinous offenses:* Offenses with a minimum punishment of imprisonment for 7 years or more under the Bharatiya Nyaya Sanhita (IPC) or any other law.
- *Petty offenses:* Offenses with a maximum punishment of imprisonment for up to 3 years.
- *Serious offenses:* Offenses for which the punishment is imprisonment between 3 and 7 years.

General Principles of Care and Protection of Children (as per JJA, 2015)

Some of the fundamental principles that guide the provisions of this act are listed below.

- *Principle of presumption of innocence:* Any child shall be presumed to be innocent of any criminal intent up to the age of 18 years.
- *Principle of participation:* The child shall have a right to participate in all processes and decisions affecting his interest under this act.
- *Principle of best interest:* All decisions regarding the child shall be taken in the child's best interest.
- *Principle of safety:* All measures shall be taken to ensure the child is safe from harm, abuse, or maltreatment.
- *Principle of nonwaiver of rights:* No waiver of the child's rights is permissible or valid.
- *Principle of right to privacy and confidentiality:* Privacy and confidentiality of every child shall be protected throughout the judicial process.
- *Principle of institutionalization as a measure of last resort:* A child shall be placed in institutional care as a last resort after making a reasonable inquiry.
- *Principle of fresh start:* Any child's past records under this act should be erased except in special circumstances.
- *Principle of diversion:* Measures for dealing with children in conflict with the law without resorting to judicial proceedings shall be promoted unless it is in the best interest of the child or the society.

Systems in Place for Children in Need of Care and Protection and Children in Conflict with Law are the Juvenile Justice Board (Box 1) and Child Welfare Committee (Box 2).

The CWC has the authority to dispose of cases related to the care, protection, treatment, development, and rehabilitation of children who need care and protection.

BOX 1: Juvenile Justice Board (JJB).

JUVENILE JUSTIC BOARD
(One or more for every district)

Members:

- *Metropolitan Magistrate/Judicial Magistrate of First Class (not being Chief Metropolitan Magistrate or Chief Judicial Magistrate)* with at least 3 years of experience, and
- *Two social workers* (at least one woman) actively involved in health, education, or welfare activities pertaining to children for at least 7 years or a practicing professional with a degree in child psychology, psychiatry, sociology, or law.

BOX 2: Child Welfare Committee (CWC).

CHILD WELFARE COMMITTEE
(One or more for every district)

Members:

- *Chairperson* and
- *Four other members* as the State Government may think fit to appoint (at least one woman and another, an expert on the matters concerning children).

To be appointed as a member of the Committee a person has to be actively involved in health, education, or welfare activities pertaining to children for at least 7 years or be a practicing professional with a degree in child psychology, psychiatry, or law or social work or sociology or human development.

The functions and responsibilities of the Committee:

- Taking notice of and receiving the children in need of care and protection
- Conducting inquiry on relevant issues under this Act
- Directing the conduction of social investigation and reviewing the report
- Directing the placement of a child in foster care
- Ensuring care, protection, appropriate rehabilitation, or restoration of children in need of care and protection based on the child's individual care plan
- Identifying registered institutions for placement of children requiring institutional support
- Conducting inspection visits of residential facilities for children in need of care and protection and recommending action for improvement
- Attempts to restore the abandoned or lost children to their families
- Declaration of an orphan abandoned and surrendered child as legally free for adoption after due inquiry
- Rehabilitation of sexually abused children under the protection of children from Sexual Offenses Act, 2012
- Coordinate with the police and other agencies involved in the care and protection of children
- Accessing appropriate legal services for children.

Tables 2 and 3 highlight the psychosocial and mental health assessments that are required to be done for children in need of care and protection and children in conflict with law.

Flowchart 5 depicts the process of JJA, 2015, in respect of a child in conflict with law apprehended by the police.

Psychosocial and Mental Health Assessment of Children in Conflict with the Law

When a heinous offense (minimum 7 years of imprisonment) is alleged to have been committed by a child who has completed or is above the age of 16 years, the JJB conducts a preliminary assessment. The preliminary assessment is performed by JJB to evaluate the child's mental and physical capacity to commit such an offense, ability to understand the consequences of the offense, and the circumstances in which he allegedly committed the offense. The JJB can seek assistance from assistance of psychologists or psycho-social workers or other experts who have experience of working with children in difficult circumstances. The assessment can be done in outpatient or inpatient setting as shown in **Flowchart 6**.

Under Section 15 of the Juvenile Justice (Care and Protection of Children) Act, 2015, a preliminary assessment is conducted for children aged 16–18 years accused of heinous offenses to determine whether they should be tried as adults. This assessment is carried out by the JJB with the assistance of experts, including psychiatrists, psychologists, and social workers. The evaluation

TABLE 2: Psychosocial and mental health assessment for children in need of care and protection.

Basic information	• Name, age, gender, date, and time of assessment • Circumstances leading to current institutionalization
Presenting problems	Clinical complaints
Family history	Current living arrangement, family relationships, child's attachment to parents, parenting practices, mental illness, and substance use in family members
Child's temperament	Sociability, emotionality, attention, activity level, adaptability, stubbornness, sensitivity to criticism, excessive shyness, aggressive tendency, etc.
Personal history	*Schooling history:* • Is the child attending school, if yes—current grade, if not—last grade, reasons for not attending school, academic performance, and history of truancy *Institutional history:* • Places lived in other places than family home (e.g., hostel, observation home, etc.), and duration of stay
Physical, emotional, and sexual abuse	*Example questions to ask:* • Has anyone physically hurt you? • Has anyone said something that made you feel sad/angry or humiliated? • Has anyone touched you inappropriately or shown you sexually explicit pictures/videos?
Work experiences	*Child labor experiences:* • Why had the child to work? • How did the child find work? • Place of work, working hours, and money earned
Mental health concerns	• *Evaluation for disorders and impact of childhood trauma* such as "emotional disorders, developmental disorders, behavioral disorders, stress and trauma-related disorders, and depression" • *Evaluation for substance use (current/past):* Substances used, first dose intake, usual dose intake, last dose intake, pattern of use, etc.
Brief mental status examination	General appearance, behavior, speech and language, thought process, orientation, cognition, etc.
Summary	• Main problems and concerns of the child, including protection and psychosocial issues • Current challenges and coping strategies
Document care plan	• List actions taken or planned by the assessment agency/case worker to assist the child • Emergency actions • Measures to address immediate concerns • Psychosocial interventions • Referrals to other agencies

focuses on three key aspects: (1) the mental and physical capacity of the child to commit the offense, (2) their ability to understand its consequences, and (3) the circumstances under which the offense was committed. The process involves interviews with the child, psychological assessments (if necessary), and a review of case history and social investigation reports. Based on the findings, if the child is deemed incapable of fully understanding the offense and its consequences, the case remains under the jurisdiction of the JJB. However, if the child is found capable of committing and understanding the offense, the case may be transferred to

TABLE 3: Psychosocial and mental health assessment for children in conflict with the law.

Basic information	Name, age, gender, date, and time of assessment, and circumstances leading to current institutionalization
Reason(s) for referral	Preliminary assessment and mental health evaluation
Family history (Circumstances)	• Current living arrangements, family relationships, child's attachment to parents, parenting practices, mental illness, and substance use in family members • Parents support and plan for child's safe development
Personal history (Circumstances)	• *Schooling history:* Is the child attending school, if yes—current grade, if not—last grade, reasons for not attending school, academic performance, behavioral history in school (suspensions, expulsions, etc.) • *Peer relationships*: Age of friends (mostly same, older, or younger), games/activities engaged in with friends, time spent with peers, extent of peer influence (e.g., on school attendance, breaking rules, substance use, actions about sexuality), and consequences of peer influence (trouble with school/parents/police, etc.) • *Institutional history:* Places lived in other places than family home (e.g. hostel, observation home, etc.), duration of stay
Trauma experiences (Circumstances)	*Loss, death, and grief:* Details of experience of loss of a loved one (separation or death), feelings of the child about it *Example questions to ask:* • Have you lost someone you were very close to? • When did it happen? • How do you feel about it? *Physical, emotional, and sexual abuse:* *Example questions to ask:* • Has anyone physically hurt you? • Has anyone said something that made you feel sad/angry or humiliated? • Has anyone touched you inappropriately or shown you sexually explicit pictures/videos?
Mental health concerns	• *Evaluation for disorders and impact of childhood trauma* such as "Emotional Disorders", developmental disorders, behavioral disorders, stress and trauma-related disorders, and depression • *Evaluation for substance use* concerns (current/past) • Substances used, first dose intake, usual dose intake, last dose intake, pattern of use, etc.
Awareness of consequences and Child's plan for his future	• *Social, interpersonal, and legal:* Can be verified using a similar story situation or narrative told in the third person (i.e., about someone else rather than directly about the child in question) • Child's understanding of why they have been brought for assessment • Child's understanding of the risk factors when explained to him and his plan for safe development
• Youth's strengths and deficits • Life skills needs and deficits	• *Emotional regulation* (understanding and managing emotions, e.g., anger) • *Empathy* (understanding other's emotional states and perspectives) • *Coping with stress* (identifying and preventing stressors and use of stress reduction techniques) • *Effective communication* (assertiveness in expression) • *Problem-solving and decision making* (defining the problems, choosing from possible solutions by weighing the pros and cons of each, and fair trial of the solution before choosing another solution) • *Healthy interpersonal relationships*

Contd...

Contd...

Brief mental status examination	General appearance and behavior, speech and language, thought process, orientation, cognition, etc.
Summary	Main concerns include vulnerability, pathology, and consequence. Interpretation of findings
Document care plan	• Measures to address immediate concerns • Psychosocial interventions • Referrals to other agencies

Flowchart 5: Juvenile Justice Act (JJA), 2015 highlights.

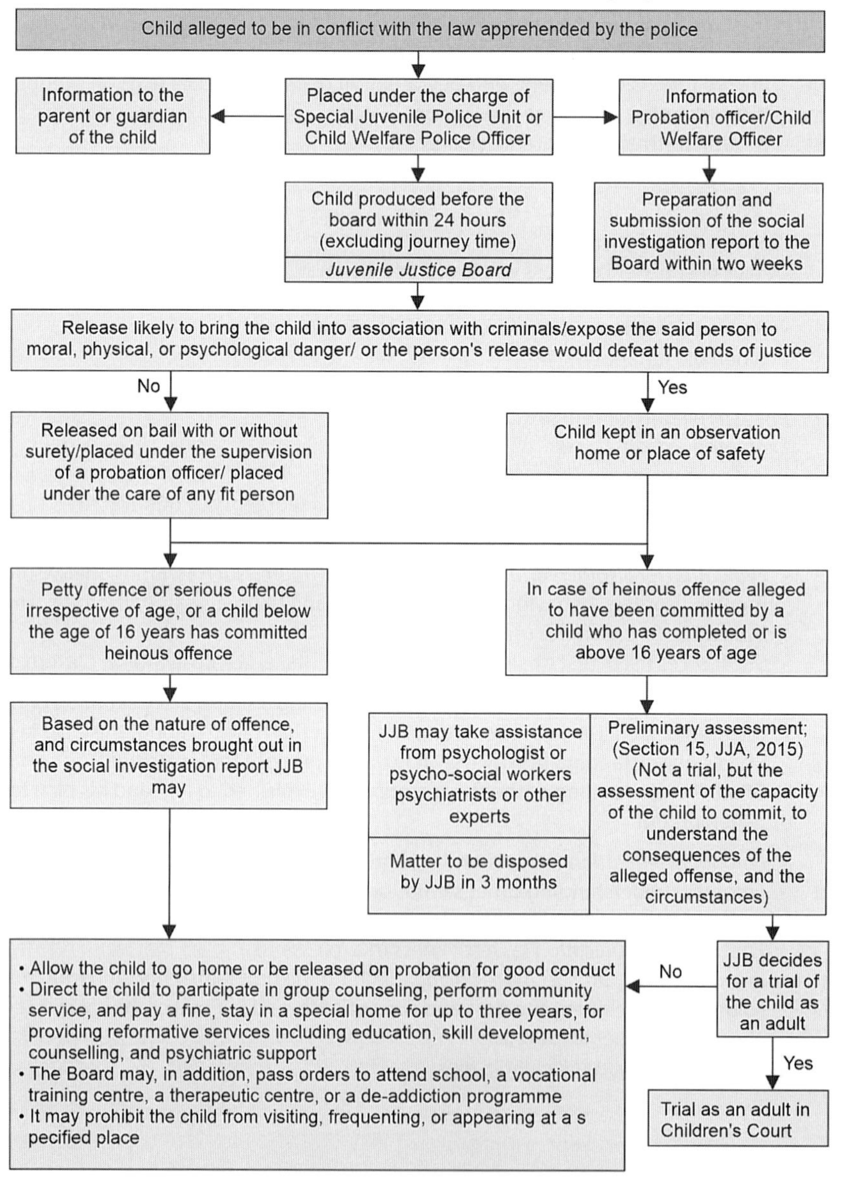

Flowchart 6: Assessment and reporting of the findings to the Juvenile Justice Board (JJB).

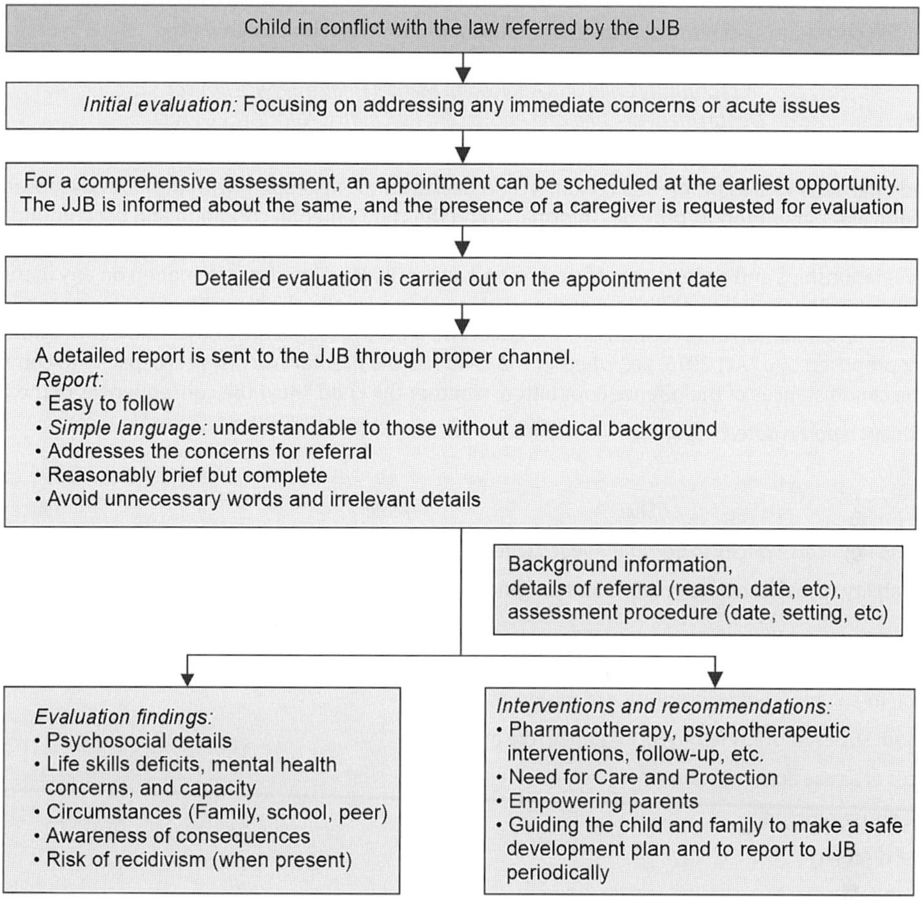

Child in conflict with the law referred by the JJB

↓

Initial evaluation: Focusing on addressing any immediate concerns or acute issues

↓

For a comprehensive assessment, an appointment can be scheduled at the earliest opportunity. The JJB is informed about the same, and the presence of a caregiver is requested for evaluation

↓

Detailed evaluation is carried out on the appointment date

↓

A detailed report is sent to the JJB through proper channel.
Report:
- Easy to follow
- *Simple language:* understandable to those without a medical background
- Addresses the concerns for referral
- Reasonably brief but complete
- Avoid unnecessary words and irrelevant details

Background information, details of referral (reason, date, etc), assessment procedure (date, setting, etc)

Evaluation findings:
- Psychosocial details
- Life skills deficits, mental health concerns, and capacity
- Circumstances (Family, school, peer)
- Awareness of consequences
- Risk of recidivism (when present)

Interventions and recommendations:
- Pharmacotherapy, psychotherapeutic interventions, follow-up, etc.
- Need for Care and Protection
- Empowering parents
- Guiding the child and family to make a safe development plan and to report to JJB periodically

the Children's Court for trial as an adult. The assessment must be conducted in a child-friendly manner, ensuring that the child receives legal aid, psychological support, and is not subjected to retraumatization **(Appendix 1)**.

CHILD CUSTODY EVALUATIONS

There are several laws governing custody and guardianship in India.

The Guardians and Wards (GAWA) Act, 1890

A secular law which provides for appointing a guardian for a minor. The guardian is charged with the custody of the ward.

The Hindu Marriage Act, 1955[7]

As per Section 26, the court may pass, revoke, suspend, or vary interim orders on child custody.

The Hindu Minority and Guardianship Act, 1956[8]

- Natural guardians of a Hindu minor:
  - In the case of a boy or an unmarried girl, the father, and after him, the mother
  - A minor who has not completed the age of 5 years shall 'ordinarily' be with the mother
- Natural guardianship of a minor adopted on:
  - Adoptive father and after him to the adoptive mother

APPENDIX 1: Preliminary assessment report proforma.

Psychosocial and Mental Health of Children in Conflict with the Law (Age 16–18 Years)
Preliminary Individual Assessment Report for Juvenile Justice Board[9,10]
Community Child and Adolescent Mental Health Service Project
Department of Child and Adolescent Psychiatry, NIMHANS-DWCD

As per the JJ Act 2015, the objective of the preliminary assessment of a child is to "evaluate the role of the child in the alleged offense as well as his mental condition and background". In keeping with this, the psychosocial and mental health assessment report provides information on the child's mental condition and background, namely the developmental level of the child, family history and relationships, school and education, involvement in child labor, peer relationships and experiences of trauma and abuse; it also provides information on any mental health disorders and developmental disabilities that the child may have. Finally, the report makes recommendations for treatment and rehabilitation interventions for the child. The report presents the above-said information using the framework proposed by JJ Act 2015, i.e., whether the child has the mental and physical capacity to commit the offense, the circumstances of the offense committed, whether the child knew the consequences of the offense.

This assessment report is dated:

Name of Child:

Age: *Sex:* *Male* *Place of origin:*

A. Mental and Physical Capacity to Commit Alleged Offense

The child's ability to make social decisions and judgments are compromised due to:

Life skills deficits (emotional dysregulation/difficulty coping with peer pressure/assertiveness and negotiation skills/problem-solving/conflict-resolution/decision-making)	
Neglect/poor supervision by family/poor family role models	
Experiences of abuse and trauma	
Substance abuse problems	
Intellectual disability	
Mental health disorder/developmental disability	
Any other (specify):	
No treatment/interventions provided so far to address the above issues	

*NA: Not applicable

B. Circumstances of Alleged Offense

Family history:

School history:

Child labor:

Peer relationships:

Contd...

Contd...

Abuse and trauma:

Mental health disorder/developmental disability:

C. Child's Knowledge of Consequences of Committing the Alleged Offense
Child's understanding of social/interpersonal and legal consequences of committing offense:

D. Other Observations and Issues

E. Recommendations

Islamic Law

- Custody vests with the mother until the son reaches the age of 7 years and the daughter reaches puberty. A mother cannot be deprived of this right unless she is disqualified and custody with her is found to be unfavorable to the child's welfare.

Parsi and Christian Law

The courts can issue interim orders for custody of the child.

The courts may refer the parents and child to mental health professionals for child custody evaluation and to help the court decide on the best interest of the child, type of custody, etc. The CCE involves the assessment of a child's social and developmental needs, the assessment of the parenting capacities of each parent, and the determination of the best fit between the child's needs and parental capacities to serve the child's best interest. Admission may be considered for 4–6 weeks for a multidisciplinary team evaluation. The duration of inpatient stay may be planned as follows: 2 weeks with each parent separately and 2 weeks with both parents together. A comprising if the child is found to have a mental illness during the evaluation, appropriate treatment should be initiated.

The purpose of the evaluation is not to confirm or deny the parties' allegations but to assist the court in making decisions regarding custody. The structure and approach to evaluation are depicted in **Flowchart 7** and **Table 4**.[11] **Table 5** highlights the areas which need to be assessed while interviewing a child.

Practical Tips to the Psychiatrists[12]

Psychiatrists play a critical role in evaluating children in conflict with the law or those requiring protection under the law. The assessment must be comprehensive, child-sensitive, and legally sound to aid the JJB, CWC, and other authorities in decision-making. Below are the key guidelines for psychiatrists conducting such assessments and submitting reports. Given the complexity of these cases involving children, it is always advisable to admit the child for a 360° assessment, ensuring a thorough evaluation of their mental health, family dynamics, environmental influences, crisis intervention, and rehabilitation needs. Always ensure the best interests of the child and follow a trauma-informed approach.

Flowchart 7: Structure of child custody evaluation.

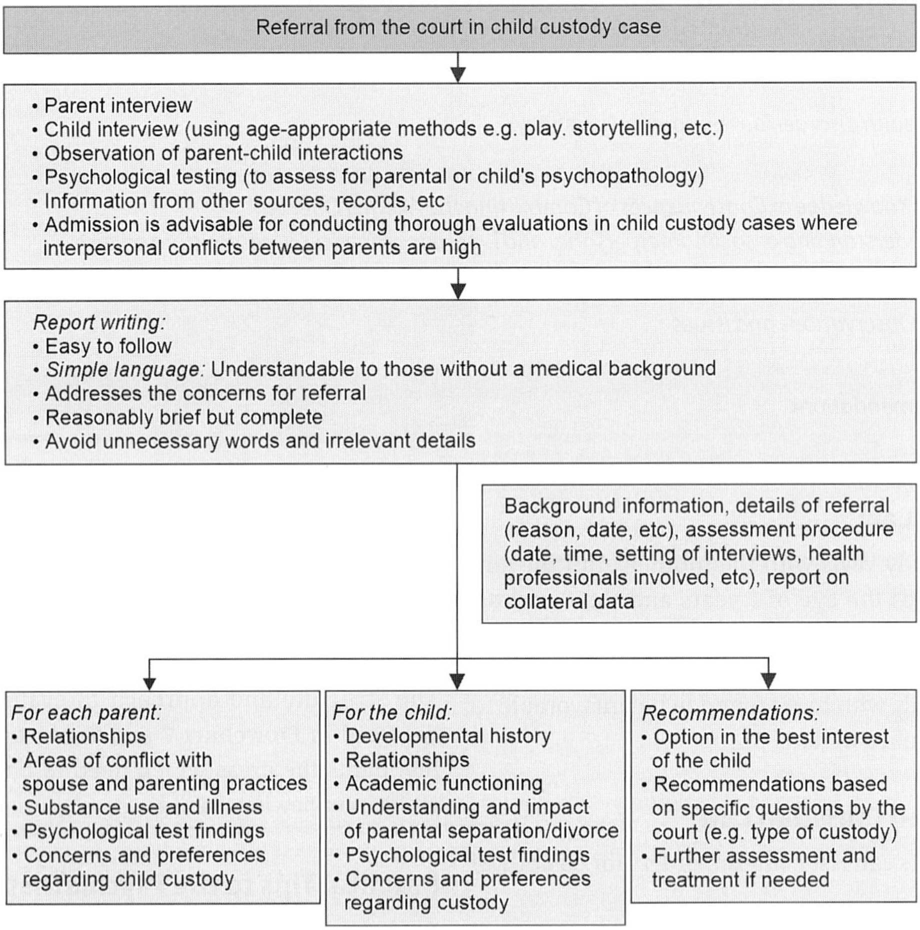

Referral from the court in child custody case

↓

- Parent interview
- Child interview (using age-appropriate methods e.g. play. storytelling, etc.)
- Observation of parent-child interactions
- Psychological testing (to assess for parental or child's psychopathology)
- Information from other sources, records, etc
- Admission is advisable for conducting thorough evaluations in child custody cases where interpersonal conflicts between parents are high

↓

Report writing:
- Easy to follow
- *Simple language:* Understandable to those without a medical background
- Addresses the concerns for referral
- Reasonably brief but complete
- Avoid unnecessary words and irrelevant details

Background information, details of referral (reason, date, etc), assessment procedure (date, time, setting of interviews, health professionals involved, etc), report on collateral data

↓

For each parent:
- Relationships
- Areas of conflict with spouse and parenting practices
- Substance use and illness
- Psychological test findings
- Concerns and preferences regarding child custody

For the child:
- Developmental history
- Relationships
- Academic functioning
- Understanding and impact of parental separation/divorce
- Psychological test findings
- Concerns and preferences regarding custody

Recommendations:
- Option in the best interest of the child
- Recommendations based on specific questions by the court (e.g. type of custody)
- Further assessment and treatment if needed

Maintain confidentiality unless disclosure is required for legal or safety reasons. Avoid leading questions and ensure noncoercive interactions. Assess in a neutral and unbiased manner without assuming guilt or victimhood. Provide psychological support to prevent distress or retraumatization.

For children accused of offenses, psychiatrists must conduct a preliminary assessment under Section 15 of the JJ Act, 2015, focusing on: (a) *Mental and Physical Capacity*: Evaluate cognitive abilities, impulse control, and emotional regulation, (b) *Understanding of Consequences:* Assess the child's comprehension of the offense and its impact, and (c) *Circumstances of the Offense:* Consider socio-environmental factors such as family, peer influence, substance use, or trauma history.

Children requiring protection (e.g., abandoned, abused, trafficked, or neglected children) must be assessed for: (a) *Physical Health:* Identify signs of abuse, malnutrition, neglect, or developmental delays, (b) *Trauma and Mental Health Issues:* Screen for post-traumatic stress disorder (PTSD), depression, anxiety, or behavioral disorders, and (c) *Family and Social*

TABLE 4: Information to be gathered from parent interviews.

Background details	• Name, age, and address
	• Personal history
	  – Education
	  – Occupation
	• Family history
	• Significant relationships other than family
	• Current living arrangement
	• Illness history (Medical or psychiatric, if yes—treatment history)
	• Substance use
	• Any other legal issues

Relationship with the spouse prior to separation/ divorce	• Beginning of relationship • Details of marriage • Relationships with in-laws • Decisions related to finances and childcare • Conflict resolution
History of current custody case	• Timeline of events • Reasons leading to separation or divorce • Other relevant details, e.g., about the legal process
Relationship with the spouse following separation/divorce	• Communication • Impact on childcare • Understanding of the child's needs • Understanding of the impact of disputes on child
Information regarding the child/children	• Name and age • Birth and developmental history • Temperament • *Schooling history:* Is the child attending school, if yes—current grade, if not—last grade, reasons for not attending school, academic performance, and behavioral history in school • Relationships • Illness history • Child's understanding of ongoing parental conflict
Desires regarding custody	Desires regarding custody

Environment: Assess whether returning to family is safe or if alternative care is needed.

A psychiatrist doing forensic assessments must submit a clear, objective, and legally sound report to the legal authorities. The report should outline clinical findings, including mental status, psychiatric diagnosis (if any), and a structured risk assessment covering self-harm, aggression, environmental risks, and likelihood of re-offending. Report must also include a logical explanation of findings in simple words, avoiding medical jargon to ensure clarity for legal authorities. Conclusions must be evidence-based, free from speculation or bias, relying on clinical examination, serial MSE, serial ward observations, and serial MMSE. The language of the report should remain neutral and factual, avoiding assumptions about guilt or victimhood.

Timely submission of the report is crucial to ensure that legal proceedings are not delayed. If psychiatrist require additional time for submitting comprehensive report, an interim

TABLE 5: Information to be gathered from child's interview.

Child's understanding of separation/divorce	• Is the child aware of the current situation? • If yes, who told the child about it? • What did each parent tell the child? • How does the child feel about each parent in the conflict? • Does the child feel responsible for the current situation? • Effect on relationships, academic performance, etc.
Child's perception of relationships	*Prior to the parental separation/divorce:* • *Attachment:* Parents and other family members • Friendships *Following the parental separation/divorce:* • Parents (Ask for any attempts by either parent to alienate the child from the other parent) • Friendships
Child's perception of impact of the parental separation/ divorce	Child's perspective of parental separation/divorce
Child's wishes about custody	• Whom does the child wish to stay with? Both parent/either parent? • What are the reasons for preferring one parent over the other? • How would the child feel if he/she had to live with the parent not preferred? • If the child were to live with either parent, how frequently would the child want to meet the other parent? • Three wishes
Assess for psychiatric symptoms/coping	Clinical symptoms and signs and coping

report should be submitted. This interim report should summarize initial observations, urgent concerns, and the expected timeline for the final report and at the same time ensuring the child receives necessary care and interventions without unnecessary delays. The final document must be well-structured, signed by the psychiatrist, and submitted confidentially to protect the child's privacy while guiding appropriate legal and rehabilitative actions.

SUMMARY AND CONCLUSION

To summarize, this chapter has provided basic information into various laws related to child mental healthcare and guidance for evaluating children and adolescents in clinical situations pertinent to these laws. Mental healthcare professionals need to familiarize themselves with these laws and evaluation procedures, given the frequency with which they may encounter such situations. Additionally, proper documentation, reporting, and collaboration with relevant agencies are essential to ensure comprehensive mental healthcare.

In conclusion, India has several key legislations work together to safeguard the rights and well-being of children and adolescents and individuals with mental or developmental disabilities. While the MHCA 2017 focuses on protecting the rights of persons with mental illness by ensuring access to affordable mental health services, promoting autonomy, and emphasizing least restrictive care, the RPWD 2016 expands the categories of disability and guarantees equality, nondiscrimination, and educational and employment opportunities. POCSO 2012 provides a robust, child friendly legal framework to prevent, report and prosecute sexual offenses against minors and JJA 2015 addresses both children in conflict with law and those in need of care and focusing on rehabilitation and social integration rather than punishment. Collectively, these laws uphold the dignity, safety, rights, and inclusion of vulnerable groups.

REFERENCES

1. Legislative Department, Ministry of Law and Justice, Government of India. (2025). The Mental Healthcare Act, 2017. [online] Available from https://lddashboard.legislative.gov.in/actsofparliamentfromtheyear/mental-healthcare-act-2017 [Last accessed 21 November, 2025].
2. Department of Empowerment of Persons with Disabilities (DEPwD), India. (2024). Latest Notified Guidelines for assessing the extent of specified disabilities dated 14.03.2024. [online] Available from https://depwd.gov.in/latest-notified-guidelines-for-assessing-the-extent-of-specified-disabilities-dated-14-03-2024/ [Last accessed 21 November, 2025].
3. Legislative Department, Ministry of Law and Justice, Government of India. (2012). The Gazette of India: Protection of Children from Sexual Offences Act 2012. [online] Available from https://ncpcr.gov.in/uploads/165648758662bbfea22021a_protection-of-children-from-sexual-offences-act-2012-english-hindi.pdf [Last accessed 21 November, 2025].
4. Ministry of Health and Family Welfare, Government of India. (2025). Guidelines and protocols medico legal care for survivors victims of sexual violence.[online] Available from https://mohfw.gov.in/?q=reports/guidelines-and-protocols-medico-legal-care-survivors-victims-sexual-violence [Last accessed 21 November, 2025].
5. APSAC Taskforce. (2023). Forensic Interviewing of Children. The American Professional Society on the Abuse of Children (APSAC); 2023. [online] Available from https://www.apsac.org/guidelines [Last accessed 21 November, 2025].
6. Legislative Department, Ministry of Law and Justice, Government of India. (2025). The Guardians and Wards Act, 1890. [online] Available from https://lddashboard.legislative.gov.in/actsofparliamentfromtheyear/guardians-and-wards-act-1890 [Last accessed 21 November, 2025].
7. Legislative Department, Ministry of Law and Justice, Government of India. (2025). The Hindu Marriage Act, 1955. [online] Available from https://lddashboard.legislative.gov.in/actsofparliamentfromtheyear/hindu-marriage-act-1955 [Last accessed 21 November, 2025].
8. Legislative Department, Ministry of Law and Justice, Government of India. (2025). The Hindu Minority and Guardianship Act, 1956. [online] Available from https://lddashboard.legislative.gov.in/actsofparliamentfromtheyear/hindu-minority-and-guardianship-act-1956 [Last accessed 21 November, 2025].
9. National Commission for Protection of Child Rights. The Juvenile Justice Care and Protection of Children Act 2015. [online] Available from https://ncpcr.gov.in/uploads/165648720662bbfd264b93a_the-juvenile-justice-care-and-protection-of-children-act-2015.pdf [Last accessed 21 November, 2025].
10. National Commission for Protection of Child Rights. (2023). Guidelines for Conducting Preliminary Assessment Under Section 15 of the Juvenile Justice (JJ) Act, 2015. [online] Available from https://ncpcr.gov.in/juvenile-justice-guidelines. [Last accessed 21 November, 2025].
11. Fuhrmann GSW, Zibbell RA, Fuhrmann GSW, Zibbell RA. Evaluation for Child Custody. Oxford: Oxford University Press; 2011.
12. Child Psychiatry Centre, Department of Child and Adolescent Psychiatry, NIMHANS. (2025). Reference for Preliminary Assessment Report Format. [online] Available from https://nimhanschildprotect.in/child-care-institutions/ [Last accessed 21 November, 2025].

Ethics in Child and Adolescent Psychiatry Practice

Shivanand Kattimani, Ragul Ganesh

INTRODUCTION

Ethics involves the moral principles that shape and guide an individual's attitude and behavior. Child and adolescent psychiatry (CAP) lies at the intersection of medicine, psychology, education, and law. Ethical practice in this field is uniquely complex due to the developmental immaturity of patients, the involvement of caregivers, and the often-ambiguous interface with institutions such as schools, child protection agencies, and the legal system. Practitioners are frequently challenged to make decisions that balance beneficence with respect for autonomy, confidentiality with duty to protect, and therapeutic care with legal mandates. Safeguarding the welfare of children is paramount not only in daily caregiving but also in research involving children. This importance is heightened, especially for children having developmental delays, orphans, fostered or adopted, migrants, refugees, victims of abuse, and in conflict with law, very young or having mental health difficulties. These conditions hinder effective communication of preferences, informed consent for treatment, and the seeking of assistance.

Ethical guidelines from various professional bodies [the American Psychiatric Association (APA), the Royal College of Psychiatrists (RCPsych), the American Medical Association (AMA), the World Psychiatric Association (WPA), and the Indian Psychiatric Society (IPS)] and Child and Adolescent Psychiatry organizations, including the American Academy of Child and Adolescent Psychiatry (AACAP), provide essential frameworks for ensuring ethical and high-quality care. These organizations help establish and maintain ethical standards in the field of psychiatry, particularly for the care of children and adolescents. The AACAP, while recognizing that a code of ethics cannot anticipate all circumstances, reiterates that it is a dynamic entity likely subject to revision and modification as future developments take place. It emphasizes its impartial use in all circumstances, and in case of ethical dilemmas to seek help from peers and appropriate professional resources.

ETHICAL PRINCIPLES IN CHILD AND ADOLESCENT PSYCHIATRY

The principles of beneficence and nonmaleficence in the medical profession, which emphasize "helping others and doing no harm," have been known from the era of Hippocrates. Thomas Beauchamp and James Childress laid the foundation for medical ethics, which has since been debated and expanded upon by subsequent scholars, further enriching the ethical framework in medicine.[1,2] Thus, principles of medical ethics such as autonomy, beneficence, nonmaleficence, and justice given by Beauchamp and Childress also apply in the practice of child and adolescent psychiatry. Although the core principles of bioethics apply, their interpretation must be developmentally and contextually informed.

The child and adolescent mental health professionals should be knowledgeable about the various developmental domains at various ages along with children's relationship with each and everyone in their immediate environment, including schools, social welfare agencies, etc.

Principles of Medical Ethics

Autonomy

Autonomy refers to the right of individuals to make informed decisions about their own lives. In medical practice, it pertains to understanding the choices given to them, the consequences that are likely to follow with each of the choices, and the decision to be conveyed to the treating doctor. Such informed decisions should be devoid of bias and done with maturity and clarity of mind so that persons in the patient's roles are responsible for their own decisions, irrespective of the consequences. In children, the capacity to make informed choices is evolving. Respect for autonomy is framed by age, cognitive ability, and emotional maturity. At the same time, development of trust between patient and the family is important for beneficial care to the child and respect for patient's privacy hold utmost importance for the establishment and maintenance of trust in therapeutic relationship.[3] Only if a minor perceives the physician to be trustworthy, he/she will reveal their feelings/thoughts to the physician providing care, with the assurance that the contents of the discussion will not be communicated to others without their permission.

Beneficence

Beneficence involves acting in the best interests of the patient. In case of children and adolescents, the major concern should be the welfare and optimal functioning and development of this group of individuals. The imperative to act in the child's best interest while minimizing harm guides most decisions. However, interpretations of "best interest" may differ between clinicians and caregivers. However, a child mental health professionals' judgements and actions should reflect "best interest of the child", overriding familial or societal pressures. Children's ability to understand about their "best interest" is hugely influenced by their cognitive maturity, and in such cases, caregivers or legal representatives' decision can be sought and a mutually informed decision can be made.

Nonmaleficence

Nonmaleficence means "do no harm", in case of children and adolescents, it means to avoid all actions that may be detrimental to the optimal development of the child or adolescent. It also calls for reduction in any harmful effects of the behaviors of significant others on children and adolescents at the individual, family, school, local community, or broader societal level. Children and adolescents grow in the warmth and gentle nurturance of the relationships of their families, making them emotionally vulnerable in their relationships with significant others. These vulnerabilities could lead to exploitation (emotional/physical) of children and adolescents without any complaints from their side. These vulnerabilities must be gauged by the child mental health professional and their ethical actions guided by this information. Emotional vulnerabilities of either the child/adolescent or their families should never be exploited for personal gains by the treating physician.

Justice

Justice in healthcare refers to fairness in the distribution of resources and treatment. In child and adolescent psychiatry, this principle underscores the need to ensure equitable access to mental health services, regardless of the patient's socioeconomic status, race, or geographical location. It is based on the belief that all lives are equal irrespective of age, gender, race, nationality, or socioeconomic status.

Mental healthcare professional should adhere to high ethical standards, which in addition to above mentioned principles also include:

- *Fidelity and truth telling:* Honesty is critical in building therapeutic relationships. This includes being transparent about diagnosis, treatment options, ensuring confidentiality while keeping in mind, the limits of confidentiality.
- *Integrity:* Upholding strong moral principles, acting consistently with values, and maintaining honesty, especially during difficult situations.
- *Informed consent:* Providing patients with comprehensive information about their conditions and treatment options to enable informed decision-making, respecting their autonomy.
- *Professionalism:* Maintaining high standards of competence, behavior, and integrity, adhering to ethical codes, and engaging in continuous improvement to provide optimal care.
- *Respect for persons and for emerging capacities:* It is important to recognize and treat every individual with dignity, compassion, and empathy, and respecting their rights and individuality. Also, adolescents especially must be included in decisions regarding their care, even if they cannot legally consent.
- *Veracity:* Being truthful and accurate with patients about their health status and treatment options to support informed consent.

Consent and Assent

In India, the legal age of maturity is 18 years. However, the Mental Healthcare Act (MHCA, 2017) introduces the concept of capacity-based decision making even for those under 18 years, in limited circumstances. Although guardians are vested by the responsibility for health and welfare of children and adolescents, their role and participation in deciding the kind of services and treatment they receive should be encouraged while keeping in mind their developmental age and stage.

For children below the age of consent, parents or legal guardians are the default decision makers. However, parental consent must be informed, voluntary, and documented. When both parents are involved, disagreements must be mediated with child welfare as the primary concern.[4]

Children over 7 years (or younger if developmentally capable) should be involved in decision making to the extent possible. Assent must be sought with developmentally appropriate explanations, and refusal should be respected in nonurgent situations.

Assent and consent during emergency situations are exceptional circumstances where lack of both assent and consent is considered secondary to the need for urgent medical care.

CASE VIGNETTE 1

Disagreement in Consent

A 12-year-old boy with ADHD was recommended medications for the same. The mother consented, but the father strongly objected. The clinical team held a joint meeting with both parents to mediate and emphasized that the child's functioning was being significantly impaired. After discussion, a trial was agreed upon with both parents informed of the expected benefits and side effects. At the same time, the boy was also engaged in the discussions and his views sought regarding initiation of medications. This opportunity also enabled the clinical team to include the boy in imparting information about expected benefits and possible side effects, thereby providing a window for development of mutual trust and confidence.

Confidentiality

It refers to protecting patient information and sharing it only with authorized individuals to maintain trust between patients and mental healthcare providers. Confidentiality is essential to therapeutic rapport, especially with adolescents. However, it is not "one-size-fits-all", and clinicians must explain limits of confidentiality upfront and apply discretions in disclosures to parents or institutions. They should be told about their confidentiality rights and limits of it in developmentally appropriate fashion in the first 1–2 sessions as and when the time and clinical situation allow. Additionally, any confidential information shared by family members about themselves or related others also should be upheld with the same integrity unless the information provided reveals concerning information posing a threat to the child/adolescent.

No information about the child/adolescent should be shared with any third party without the consent of the legal guardians, which in most cases are the parents of the child/adolescent.

Exceptions for upholding confidentiality include imminent risk of harm to self or others, suspected abuse [mandated under Protection of Children from Sexual Offences (POCSO) Act], and court orders. An effort should always be made to inform the child/adolescent and other related parties in advance whenever such a disclosure is necessary. In cases where the order for evaluation of a child/adolescent has come from administrative, legal, and educational purposes, the child/adolescent and others involved should be immediately informed of the nature and intent of assessment, its limitations and possible overriding of the right of confidentiality. In certain cases, where the adolescents are legally declared to be not under the control of their guardians (such situations being more common in western countries), the adolescent retains full confidentiality rights and this cannot be overruled by adult relatives.

Whenever information is required to be collected from multiple sources and informants, prior permission and clear understanding of the use of such information should be mutually decided between the physician, family members, and child/adolescent, unless there are immediate safety concerns.

CASE VIGNETTE 2

Confidentiality versus Safety

A 15-year-old girl disclosed suicidal thoughts while being treated for depressive episode but begged the therapist not to inform her parents. As risk assessment revealed a moderate to high risk of harm to self, the clinician informed the parents while offering ongoing support and explaining the rationale to the adolescent.

CASE VIGNETTE 3

A 16-year-old girl discloses self-harming behavior during therapy and also discloses occasional use of smoking tobacco in the past but requests that her parents not be informed. Physicians need to respect the minor's request for privacy, ensure confidentiality and at the same time consider the limits of confidentiality. In this scenario, the need to inform the parents is essential for ensuring the safety of the minor. The psychiatrist should discuss with the adolescent reasons behind their reservations for not disclosing the information to the parents. The adolescent should be helped to understand that involving the parents will mitigate the risk and will ease the treatment-seeking process. Parents can also act as gatekeepers to support them during times of crisis. The adolescent should feel confident in disclosing the information to parents and assure of their trust that the information will not be shared with others apart from parents. This preparation of the adolescent might require a few visits before the information can be shared and discussed with the family in presence/absence of the adolescent, as his/her wish may be.

Thus, by adhering to these ethical principles, mental healthcare professionals can navigate complex ethical dilemmas, provide high-quality care, and maintain the trust and respect of their patients and the broader community.

Relevance of Ethically Informed Approach in Mental Health Care

Psychiatrists need to be aware of the needs of their patients, which may be diverse in mental health care compared to other branches of health. Starting from screening, diagnosis, management and also in prevention measures for mental illness, ethical issues arise. Psychological and social impact is greater in persons seeking treatment in psychiatry. Even when persons are not medically sick, mental health issues and any attempt to address these shall affect them even when no patient-doctor relationship is formed. An ethical dilemma exists between a patient's autonomous choice for treatment and the responsibility of the doctor to act in the patient's best interests for the safety of the patient and others. The nature of ethical problems in psychiatry is multifaceted and complex. Consider a patient with a diagnosis of severe depression and with a suicidal attempt brought to the hospital by family members but refusing in-patient treatment. The issues here include the patient's right to choose their treatment and the psychiatrist's responsibility to act in the best interest of the patient's safety. In conventional sense, patient safety overrides his freedom to choose whether it is inpatient care or selection of treatment options. However, with implementation of Mental Healthcare Act (MHCA, 2017), individual rights are given more importance for adults in arriving at informed decision, in case of minors and for adults those who cannot make or convey informed decision this right is given to the nominated representative.

ETHICAL ISSUES IN CLINICAL PRACTICE

Ethical challenges in everyday clinical practice often arise around diagnosis, pharmacological treatment, psychotherapy boundaries, and handling emergencies.

Diagnosis and Labeling

Diagnostic labels can carry stigma and long-term implications, and thus caution is warranted in using these.[5] Identifying and diagnosing psychiatric disorders in children present significant challenges in clinical practice, with parental acceptance often being a major barrier to plan early intervention. A diagnosis can lead to stigma, shaping how children see themselves, and how others behave with them. It might influence their self-identity and affect their confidence and opportunities. Because children's brains and behaviors are still developing, what seems like a disorder could be a temporary phase. Many psychiatric symptoms overlap, and kids may struggle to express what they are feeling, leading to potential misdiagnosis. Cultural and environmental factors can also influence symptoms but are often overlooked. Once labeled, children may be steered toward medication-based treatments rather than considering modifying environmental or psychological factors.[6] A diagnosis can be necessary to access specialized services, but financial and social factors may create disparities in who gets diagnosed. While accurate diagnoses can lead to better support and understanding, they must be handled carefully, prioritizing the child's best interests and long-term well-being. Certain parents might have difficulty differentiating psychiatric disorders from social problems. Child psychiatrists are in a position to assess not only the child's behavior but also evaluate the environment in which these behaviors appear and decide on the need for a diagnosis. For example, chronic interparental discord can contribute to psychological distress in children, sometimes manifesting as dissociative disorders—often a maladaptive coping mechanism within dysfunctional family environments. Rather than viewing the child in isolation, a systemic perspective emphasizes the interconnected nature of family, recognizing and sharing with parties concerned that how parental functioning and child development continuously influence each other, goes a long way in the management of the child and family.

Psychopharmacology

In child and adolescent psychiatry, access to the best available evidence for treatment strategies is limited, and not all medications approved for adults receive the same approval for use in children.[7] Due to lack of a sound long-term database, long-term efficacy and side effects are always in question, many medications used in child psychiatry are off-label, and there is gross lack of information on the adverse effects of off-label use. Prescription writing and management is complex in children and adolescents in addition to the already existent challenges in decision making regarding diagnosis and management. In situations where a child/adolescent dissents but the caregiver consents to treatment, it may be beneficial and ethical to consider the health needs of the youngster and the psychological ramifications of treating the youngster against his/her wishes. Thus, it becomes important to explain the rationale, potential benefits and risks, and to actively involve caregivers in monitoring providing time and information for sufficient understanding of the case situation and explanation of professional opinion and various factors that guide the physicians' actions and recommendations for treatment.

Clear communication helps in building trust and ensures that the caregivers are well-informed, which is essential for effective collaboration and decision-making regarding the child's mental health care. The treatment and care of the child should also address their caregivers, parents, and other family members. Ethical problems related to treatment arise when the benefits of treatment for mental health problems in children are not clear. A careful assessment of risks and benefits is required in these cases and should be adequately explained to caregivers. Electroconvulsive therapy (ECT) is a recognized treatment for adults, and research and clinical practice have demonstrated that ECT is both effective and safe. However, concerns persist about the use of ECT in children and adolescents due to ethical issues surrounding use of ECT both for treatment and research in this age group.[8] These concerns necessitate careful consideration of the law of the land (MHCA, 2017 in case of India) and adherence to ethical standards to ensure the well-being of younger patients.

Psychotherapy and Boundaries

For psychotherapy to be effective for children and adolescents, establishing rapport and a safe environment with the child/adolescent and their parents/guardians remains the cornerstone. Clinicians must manage confidentiality, and it remains the most important point in developing and maintaining confidence of the child/adolescent regarding the safety of the therapeutic setting. Certain clear and generally agreed upon ethics-based rules apply to the practice of child and adolescent psychiatry, e.g., no sexual contact with the patient or family members (immediate or extended), while in therapy or even once the therapy has terminated, harsh/abusive treatment.

In the current world, the widespread use of electronic media for communication, such as email and social media, underscores the necessity for mental health professionals to be vigilant about the ethical challenges (e.g., privacy, safety, and efficacy) that may arise when interacting with child and adolescent patients and their families through these digital platforms. Ethical rules applying in these areas remain less clear than our basic, well-defined rules.

Another important area is respecting boundaries while dealing with children and adolescents. Boundary issues may seem to arise if, e.g., a preschooler wants to sit on the physicians' lap or hug him/her, offer invitations for home visits, etc. In situations like this, the child mental health professional should refrain from actions that confuse boundaries and blur the roles. Being asked personal questions is another challenge to be navigated with great expertise. Motivations behind asking these questions can be explored and an in-depth understanding of the adolescent can be attempted without providing any direct answer to such questions.

Adopting a demeanor of therapeutic neutrality (i.e., remaining neutral to the conflicts and desires of the child) guides the psychotherapeutic process. In this way, the physician will neither encourage nor discourage them but continue to remain invested and interested in understanding the motivation behind these desires.

It is important to be aware of physicians' own reactions and responses while working with children/adolescent. All emotional reactions may not be transference/countertransference but may be arising from the real-world issues in which the child is thriving.

Emergency Situations

In emergency situations, the child mental health professional may need to act without formal assent/parental consent. In addition to ethical principles, psychiatrists' actions during such situations may also be guided by the laws that apply in the area. For example, MHCA 2017 documents appropriate actions in emergency situations (physical restraint, hospitalization, and rapid tranquilization) while safeguarding the interests of the patient, family, and physician. Detailed justification and documentation of the situation and action taken is warranted, followed by debriefing to the family members.

Research

Biomedical and health research in psychiatry focuses on detecting, understanding causes, and developing strategies for promoting mental health, preventing and treating disorders, and rehabilitation.[9] Vulnerable populations, such as children and individuals with mental illnesses, require special protection in research due to their inability to make autonomous decisions and potential risk of coercion. Research involving these groups is justified only if it addresses their specific mental health priorities. Despite the challenges, pediatric research is crucial for ensuring safe and effective treatments for children, as relying on adult data can lead to adverse effects and less effective care. In countries like India, misconceptions about research emphasize the need for clear communication with participants and caregivers. Research proposals must demonstrate scientific rigor, balance potential benefits and harms, and involve experienced professionals, including child psychiatrists, to ensure ethical and effective study of children with mental illness in a supportive environment. The safety and well-being of the child should always remain the priority in research related to children/adolescents. All research protocols must be approved by the ethics committee of institutes prior to their implementation. It is the responsibility of the investigator to ensure informed decision making is encouraged and all potential risks and benefits of the research are clearly described to the guardians and to involved children/adolescents in a developmentally appropriate manner. Regardless of the risk, if a child refuses to assent/participate in research, it should be respected and undue attempts at coercion/manipulation should be avoided at all costs.

ETHICS AND LAW

Laws are characterized by consistency, universality, publication, acceptance, and enforceability, with violations of written rules resulting in specified punishment. Ethics, distinct from law, pertain to a code of behavior within specific groups, such as families, communities, or professional environments.

Child and adolescent psychiatrists should respect the child's right to privacy and maintain confidentiality, especially in cases involving legal matters.[10] The psychiatrist needs to be fully aware of the laws governing the medical and psychiatric practice including the Mental Healthcare Act.[11] Child and adolescent psychiatrists should also be aware of the laws regarding child abuse and neglect. Conflicts between the ethical principle of confidentiality and the duty of beneficence can arise, particularly when a child and adolescent psychiatrist learns about suspected child maltreatment. In such cases, psychiatrists must be mindful of relevant laws, including the POCSO Act, which mandates that "any person" who suspects or knows of a sexual offense against a child must report it.[12] Balancing these ethical and legal obligations is essential for the psychiatrist's practice. **Table 1** discusses the key differences between ethics and law. **Table 2** discusses the differences and similarities between ethics, moral values, societal values, and the law as applicable in practice of child and adolescent psychiatry. **Table 3** highlights specific ethical issues in special population groups within children and adolescents.

Competence in psychiatry involves evaluating an individual's functional ability to make informed decisions about their treatment. This competence can vary depending on the complexity of the decision at hand, with more complex decisions requiring higher levels of competence. Mental health professionals must assess whether a child possesses the necessary competence to make a specific decision. Competence involves understanding that there is a choice to be made, recognizing the consequences of different choices, and demonstrating the willingness, ability, and maturity to make an informed decision. Engaging young people ethically involves recognizing their

TABLE 1: Key differences between ethics and laws.

Sl no	*Domain*	*Ethics*	*Law*
1.	Source and authority	Derived from professional codes, ethical theories, and principles that guide conduct within the profession. Governed by professional organizations and ethical committees	Established by legislative bodies and enforced by the legal system. Governed by governmental authorities and courts
2.	Scope and flexibility	Provides a broad framework for decision-making, allowing for professional judgment and flexibility based on individual cases	Provide specific rules and regulations that must be followed, with less flexibility and room for interpretation
3.	Enforcement and consequences	Enforced by professional bodies through disciplinary actions, such as loss of licensure or professional disapproval	Enforced by the legal system through legal actions, penalties, fines, or imprisonment
4.	Focus and intent	Focuses on doing what is right and best for the patient, promoting well-being, and maintaining professional integrity	Focuses on ensuring compliance with established rules, protecting rights, and maintaining order and safety in society

TABLE 2: Difference and similarities between ethics, moral values, societal values, and law in child and adolescent psychiatry practice.

Sl no	*Domains*	*Ethics*	*Moral values*	*Social values*	*Laws*
1.	Concept	Guided by established principles and professional codes of conduct	Moral values are the personal beliefs held by individuals about what is right or wrong	Collective beliefs and norms held by a society or community about what is right and wrong, acceptable and unacceptable	Laws are formal rules and regulations enacted by legislative bodies and enforced by the legal system
2.	Key principles	Key ethical principles include respect for autonomy, beneficence, nonmaleficence, justice, confidentiality, and informed consent	These values are shaped by cultural, religious, and familial influences in the form of personal attitudes and can vary from person to person	These values are shaped by cultural, religious, and societal influences and can vary significantly between different groups	They provide a legal framework for ensuring the rights and responsibilities of individuals and organizations
3.	In relation to child/ adolescent	• *Autonomy:* Respecting the developing autonomy of children and adolescents by involving them in decision-making processes to an extent appropriate for their age and maturity • *Beneficence and non-maleficence:* Providing treatments that are in the best interest of the child or adolescent, and minimizing potential harm from interventions • *Confidentiality:* Ensuring that information shared by the child or adolescent is kept confidential, with clear communication about the limits of confidentiality	• *Respect for individual beliefs:* Understanding and respecting the personal values and beliefs of the child or adolescent, which may be influenced by their family, culture, and religion • *Personal integrity:* Encouraging honesty and integrity in interactions with the child or adolescent	• *Cultural norms:* Recognizing and respecting the cultural norms and social values that influence the behavior and attitudes of the child or adolescent • *Peer pressure:* Understanding the impact of peer pressure and social influences on the behavior and mental health of the child or adolescent	• *Consent laws:* Legal requirements for obtaining consent for treatment, including specific provisions for minors • *Confidentiality laws:* Legal standards for protecting patient information, with specific regulations for minors • *Mandatory reporting:* Laws requiring healthcare providers to report suspected cases of abuse or neglect to appropriate authorities

Contd...

Contd...

Sl no	*Domains*	*Ethics*	*Moral values*	*Social values*	*Laws*
4.	Regarding parent/caregiver	• *Informed consent:* Ensuring that parents or caregivers are fully informed about the diagnosis, treatment options, and potential risks and benefits, and obtaining their consent for treatment • *Respect for parental authority:* Balancing respect for parental authority with the need to act in the best interest of the child or adolescent • *Confidentiality:* Maintaining appropriate confidentiality, while also involving parents or caregivers in the treatment process as necessary	• *Parental values:* Acknowledging and respecting the moral values and beliefs of parents or caregivers, which may influence their decisions about their child's treatment • *Cultural sensitivity:* Being sensitive to cultural differences that may impact the family's approach to mental health and treatment	• *Family values:* Acknowledging and respecting the family values and social norms that influence the decisions and behavior of parents or caregivers • *Community expectations:* Understanding the expectations and norms of the community in which the family lives, and how these may impact the family's approach to mental health and treatment	• *Parental rights:* Legal rights of parents or guardians to make decisions on behalf of their minor children • *Custody and guardianship:* Laws governing custody and guardianship arrangements, which may impact decision-making in medical care • *Legal obligations:* Requirements for informing parents or caregivers about certain aspects of treatment and care
5.	Regarding friends	• *Confidentiality:* Protecting the privacy of the patient by not disclosing personal information to friends without appropriate consent • *Beneficence:* Encouraging supportive friendships that promote the well-being of the child or adolescent	• *Peer influence:* Recognizing the impact of peers on the moral development and behavior of the child or adolescent • *Supportive relationships:* Encouraging values of loyalty, honesty, and support in friendships	• *Social acceptance:* Recognizing the importance of social acceptance and the role of friendships in the social development of the child or adolescent • *Peer influence:* Understanding how social values and peer norms influence the behavior and mental health of the child or adolescent	*Privacy laws:* Legal requirements for maintaining the confidentiality of patient information, which extend to interactions with friends

Contd...

Contd...

Sl no	*Domains*	*Ethics*	*Moral values*	*Social values*	*Laws*
6.	Regarding teachers	• *Collaboration:* Working collaboratively with teachers to support the educational and mental health needs of the child or adolescent • *Confidentiality:* Sharing relevant information with teachers in a way that respects the confidentiality of the patient	• *Educational values:* Recognizing the moral values that teachers may hold regarding education, discipline, and student well-being • *Respect for authority:* Encouraging respect for teachers and their role in the child's or adolescent's development	• *Educational values:* Recognizing the societal values placed on education and the role of teachers in shaping the social and moral development of children and adolescents • *Disciplinary norms:* Understanding the social norms related to discipline and behavior in educational settings	• *Educational laws:* Regulations governing the sharing of information between healthcare providers and educational institutions • *Mandatory reporting:* Legal obligations for teachers to report suspected abuse or neglect, which may require coordination with healthcare providers
7.	In relation with other professionals	• *Professional boundaries:* Maintaining appropriate professional boundaries and collaborating with other healthcare providers to ensure comprehensive care • *Interdisciplinary collaboration:* Respecting the expertise of other professionals and working together to provide the best possible outcomes for the patient	• *Professional respect:* Upholding values of respect, honesty, and integrity in interactions with other professionals • *Shared goals:* Aligning moral values with the common goal of promoting the well-being of the child or adolescent	• *Professional norms:* Acknowledging the social values and norms that guide professional behavior and interactions in the healthcare setting • *Shared social goals:* Aligning the goals of various professionals with the broader social values related to child and adolescent well-being	• *Professional regulations:* Legal standards and regulations governing professional conduct and interactions between different healthcare providers • *Information sharing:* Laws that dictate how and when patient information can be shared between professionals and compliance with privacy regulations

Contd...

Contd...

Sl no	*Domains*	*Ethics*	*Moral values*	*Social values*	*Laws*
8.	Regarding legal authorities	• *Legal compliance:* Adhering to legal requirements and regulations in the practice of child and adolescent psychiatry • *Mandatory reporting:* Complying with mandatory reporting laws for cases of abuse, neglect, or harm, while balancing ethical obligations to the patient	• *Justice:* Upholding values of fairness and justice in interactions with legal authorities • *Advocacy:* Advocating for the rights and best interests of the child or adolescent within the legal system	• *Legal norms:* Understanding the social values that underpin legal norms and regulations, and how these influence the practice of child and adolescent psychiatry • *Public safety:* Recognizing the social values related to public safety and the protection of vulnerable populations, such as children and adolescents	• *Reporting requirements:* Legal mandates for reporting suspected abuse, neglect, or harm to appropriate authorities • *Court orders:* Legal orders that may affect the treatment and care of the child or adolescent, such as custody arrangements or mandated treatments • *Legal protections:* Laws that protect the rights of patients and ensure their safety and well-being within the healthcare system

TABLE 3: Specific ethics issues in special populations within the child and adolescent psychiatry practice.

Sl no	*Subpopulation*	*Specific issues related to ethics*			
		Autonomy	*Beneficence and nonmaleficence*	*Justice*	*Confidentiality*
1.	Adopted child	• Respect the child's right to know about their adoption at an age-appropriate level • Involve the child in discussions about their treatment and care	• Provide support for the unique psychological needs related to adoption • Avoid actions that might harm the child's sense of identity or security	Fair and equitable distribution of healthcare resources, treatments, and shortcomings	Maintain confidentiality regarding the child's adoption status unless disclosure is in the child's best interest and consent is obtained
2.	Victim of abuse	• Empower the child or adolescent by involving them in decision-making about their treatment • Respect their wishes regarding who is to be informed about their situation	• Provide trauma-informed care to minimize further psychological harm • Ensure safety and protection from further abuse	• Advocate for the child's rights and ensure they receive appropriate legal and social support • Treat offenders with a focus on rehabilitation and addressing underlying issues	Report abuse as mandated by law, while balancing the need to protect the child's privacy and confidentiality
3.	Drug abuse	Involve the adolescent in creating a treatment plan and respect their views on treatment options	• Provide evidence-based interventions that are most likely to benefit the adolescent • Avoid punitive approaches that may worsen their condition	See that treatment resources and accessibility are similar to that offered to any person	Maintain confidentiality but inform the adolescent of circumstances under which disclosure is necessary (e.g., risk of harm)
4.	Teenage pregnancy	Support the adolescent in making informed decisions about their pregnancy and future	• Provide comprehensive health care that addresses both physical and psychological needs • Offer nonjudgmental support and counseling	Ensure access to prenatal and postnatal care regardless of socioeconomic status	Report abuse as mandated by law, while balancing the need to protect the child's privacy and confidentiality
5.	Having genetically heritable disease	Involve the child or adolescent in discussions about their condition and potential implications	• Provide accurate information and supportive counseling to help them understand and manage their condition. • Avoid stigmatization and ensure their mental well-being is prioritized	Ensure access to care regardless of socioeconomic status or gender	Protect the privacy of genetic information and disclose it only with informed consent

Contd...

Contd...

Sl no	*Subpopulation*	*Specific issues related to ethics*			
		Autonomy	*Beneficence and nonmaleficence*	*Justice*	*Confidentiality*
6.	Having sexually transmitted disease (STD)	Encourage adolescents to take responsibility for their sexual health and involve them in decision-making about their treatment	• Provide appropriate medical treatment and education on preventing future infections • Avoid actions that may cause additional psychological harm	Ensure access to care regardless of socioeconomic status or gender, legal status, or nationality	Maintain confidentiality regarding STD diagnoses and treatment, while informing the adolescent about the limits of confidentiality (e.g., public health reporting requirements)
7.	Organ donor or recipient	Ensure that the child or adolescent fully understands the implications of organ donation or receipt and consents to it voluntarily	• Prioritize the health and well-being of both the donor and the recipient • Provide thorough medical and psychological evaluation and support	Ensure fair and equitable access to organ transplantation resources	Protect the privacy of both donors and recipients
8.	Euthanasia	• In jurisdictions where euthanasia is legal, respect the wishes of terminally ill adolescents who are deemed capable of making such decisions • Ensure that all decisions are made voluntarily and with full informed consent	• Prioritize palliative care and explore all options to alleviate suffering • Ensure that decisions are made with the primary goal of reducing suffering and improving quality of life	Ensure that the adolescent's rights and dignity are upheld throughout the process	Maintain confidentiality regarding discussions and decisions about euthanasia, respecting the adolescent's wishes and legal requirements
9.	Child labor	Support the child or adolescent in under-standing their rights and the implications of child labor	• Advocate for the child's removal from harmful labor conditions and provide necessary medical and psychological care • Work toward ensuring their access to education and a safe environment	Advocate for policies and practices that protect children from exploitation and ensure their rights are respected	Protect the privacy of the child or adolescent while ensuring that appropriate authorities are informed to take action

Contd...

Contd...

Sl no	Subpopulation	Specific issues related to ethics			
		Autonomy	**Beneficence and nonmaleficence**	**Justice**	**Confidentiality**
10.	Orphans	• *Age-appropriate involvement:* Involve orphans in decisions about their care to the extent appropriate for their age and maturity • *Empowerment:* Encourage orphans to express their preferences and concerns	• *Holistic care:* Address both the mental health and psychosocial needs of orphans • *Prevent harm:* Ensure that interventions do not cause additional trauma or distress	• *Equitable access:* Ensure that orphans have equal access to mental health services • *Advocacy:* Advocate for the rights and needs of orphans within the healthcare and social systems	*Privacy protection:* Protect the confidentiality of orphans, particularly in institutional settings
11.	Street children	• *Engagement:* Engage street children in their care decisions in a respectful and noncoercive manner • *Trustbuilding:* Establish trust to facilitate open communication	• *Comprehensive care:* Provide care that addresses immediate health needs and long-term psychosocial support • *Safety:* Ensure that interventions prioritize the safety and well-being of street children	• *Nondiscrimination:* Provide services without discrimination based on their street status • *Resource allocation:* Advocate for adequate resources to support the mental health needs of street children	*Secure communication:* Ensure confidentiality in interactions to protect the privacy and safety of street children
12.	Migrant population (moving out of their country for various reasons)	• *Cultural sensitivity:* Respect the cultural backgrounds and practices of migrant families in care decisions • *Informed consent:* Ensure that migrants fully understand treatment options and give informed consent	• *Culturally competent care:* Provide culturally appropriate and sensitive care to the specific needs of migrant children • *Minimize trauma:* Avoid interventions that may inadvertently retraumatize migrant children	• *Access to services:* Advocate for the removal of barriers to mental health services for migrant children • *Legal support:* Provide support in navigating legal systems to ensure migrant children receive necessary care	*Data protection:* Protect the personal information of migrant families, especially in cases involving immigration status

Contd...

Contd...

Sl no	*Subpopulation*	*Specific issues related to ethics*			
		Autonomy	***Beneficence and nonmaleficence***	***Justice***	***Confidentiality***
13.	Refugees (driven out of their home country due to persecution)	• *Empowerment:* Encourage refugees to participate actively in their treatment plans • *Cultural respect:* Respect cultural values and practices in treatment planning and delivery	• *Trauma-informed care:* Provide care that recognizes and addresses the impact of trauma and displacement • *Prevent retraumatization:* Ensure that care settings and interventions do not exacerbate trauma	• *Equal access:* Ensure refugees have equal access to mental health services, regardless of legal status • *Advocacy:* Advocate for policies that protect and support refugee children	*Privacy in services:* Maintain confidentiality to protect refugees from potential harm due to their legal or social status
14.	Children in conflict with the law	• *Involvement:* Involve children in conflict with the law in decisions about their mental health treatment • *Respectful interaction:* Treat them with respect and dignity throughout the treatment process	• *Rehabilitation focus:* Provide care aimed at rehabilitation and reintegration rather than punishment • *Prevent harm:* Ensure the environment and interventions do not cause additional psychological harm	• *Fair treatment:* Ensure that children in conflict with the law are treated fairly and justly within the legal and health-care systems • *Advocacy for rights:* Advocate for their rights to receive appropriate mental health care and support	*Protect privacy:* Maintain strict confidentiality to protect the child's legal and social standing

growing ability to make independent choices while also ensuring they receive the guidance and support necessary for their development. This balance between fostering autonomy and providing nurturance is crucial.

SUMMARY AND CONCLUSION

To summarize, ethics in child and adolescent psychiatry is a multifaceted and dynamic field, requiring practitioners to navigate complex principles. By adhering to core ethical principles, maintaining professional boundaries, and incorporating cultural and social considerations, psychiatrists can provide compassionate and effective care. Structured decision-making frameworks and case-based learning further enhance the ability to address ethical dilemmas thoughtfully and responsibly. Ultimately, the goal is to promote the mental health and well-being of children and adolescents while upholding the highest ethical standards in clinical practice and research.

In conclusion, the chapter discusses the ethical principles and challenges unique to the field of child and adolescent psychiatry. It emphasizes the importance of safeguarding the welfare of children, who are often vulnerable and lack autonomy, relying on parental guidance for care and decision-making. The principles of medical ethics, such as autonomy, beneficence, nonmaleficence, and justice, are also equally applicable to child psychiatric practice as is informed consent, age-appropriate communication. Sometimes ethical dilemmas are faced by psychiatrists, such as balancing a patient's autonomy choice with the responsibility to act in their best interest. There is need for high ethical standards in mental health care, regarding fidelity, integrity, confidentiality, informed consent, professionalism, and respect for persons. Ethical challenges in child and adolescent psychiatry, where decisions often impact family dynamics, and the child's developing autonomy should be carefully navigated.

REFERENCES

1. Beauchamp T, Childress J. Principles of Biomedical Ethics: Marking Its Fortieth Anniversary. Am J Bioeth. 2019;19(11):9-12.
2. Gillon R. Defending the four principles approach as a good basis for good medical practice and therefore for good medical ethics. J Med Ethics. 2015;41(1):111-6.
3. Goldsmith M, Roberts LW. Ethical Issues in Child and Adolescent Psychiatry. Focus J Life Long Learn Psychiatry. 2016;14(1):64-7.
4. Liverpool S, Pereira B, Hayes D, Wolpert M, Edbrooke-Childs J. A scoping review and assessment of essential elements of shared decision-making of parent-involved interventions in child and adolescent mental health. Eur Child Adolesc Psychiatry. 2021;30(9):1319-38.
5. Eriksen K, Kress VE. Beyond the DSM Story: Ethical Quandaries, Challenges, and Best Practices. SAGE; 2004.
6. Hinshaw SP. The stigmatization of mental illness in children and parents: developmental issues, family concerns, and research needs. J Child Psychol Psychiatry. 2005;46(7):714-34.
7. Cortese S, Adamo N, Giovane CD, Mohr-Jensen C, Hayes AJ, Carucci S, et al. Comparative efficacy and tolerability of medications for attention-deficit hyperactivity disorder in children, adolescents, and adults: a systematic review and network meta-analysis. Lancet Psychiatry. 2018;5(9):727-38.
8. Døssing E, Pagsberg AK. Electroconvulsive Therapy in Children and Adolescents: A Systematic Review of Current Literature and Guidelines. J ECT. 2021;37(3):158.
9. Carlson RV, Boyd KM, Webb DJ. The revision of the Declaration of Helsinki: past, present and future. Br J Clin Pharmacol. 2004;57(6):695-713.
10. Noiseux J, Rich H, Bouchard N, Noronha C, Carnevale FA. Children need privacy too: Respecting confidentiality in paediatric practice. Paediatr Child Health. 2019;24(1):e8-12.
11. Math SB, Basavaraju V, Harihara SN, Gowda GS, Manjunatha N, Kumar CN, et al. Mental Healthcare Act 2017 – Aspiration to action. Indian J Psychiatry. 2019;61(Suppl 4):S660-6.
12. Seth R, Srivastava RN. Child Sexual Abuse: Management and prevention, and protection of children from Sexual Offences (POCSO) Act. Indian Pediatr. 2017;54(11):949-53.

Children in Special Settings: Hospital Settings, Juvenile Home, Institutionalized Children (Special Problems and Special Considerations in Management)

Priti Arun, Shivangi Mehta, Ira Domun

INTRODUCTION

Almost 90% of children and adolescents are found to be living in low- and middle-income countries (LMICs)[1] with constrained mental health services. According to UNICEF, at least 50 million children in India are affected with mental health issues; 80–90% have not sought support.[1,2] The increasing burden of mental health problems among this population is a growing concern as most mental disorders have onset before the age of 25 years, more so within the period of adolescence. Hence, the affliction with a mental health disorder directly puts a brunt on the very foundation of life in aspects of personality, emotional stability, and academics, leading to its multidimensional effects throughout life. In India, children with mental health disorders are mostly undiagnosed and more often than not, their parents are hesitant to seek help or treatment from mental health professionals.

This chapter envisages children's specific issues in special settings such as hospital settings, institutions like observation homes, special homes for children in conflict with the law and places of safety for children in need of care and protection. It also includes some pertinent references to the institutions for children with special needs and those affected by HIV/AIDS. Further, the chapter highlights the legal policies, acts, and schemes implemented by the Government of India for the welfare and better development of these vulnerable children to safeguard their well-being. For most of the chapter, the word "children" has been used for both children and adolescents (and for both males and females).

CHILDREN IN HOSPITAL SETTINGS

Children and adolescents may need to visit a hospital for varied reasons. While most families prefer to take children to pediatric services for management of their illnesses/issues/problems, there are quite a few who would by themselves come to psychiatric services or have been referred by other health professionals, schools, or relatives for assessment and management of problems of different kinds (behavior problems, academic difficulties, developmental delays, psychiatric conditions, etc.). These evaluations are carried out initially in the outpatient services of the psychiatry department in a general hospital setting.

Outpatient Care

Available literature amply emphasizes on the fact that spaces used for assessment of children and adolescents should be child-friendly and equipped with activities and materials (such as toys, books, art supplies, etc.) that are enough for the duration of time the child/adolescent is required to be engaged. At the same time, it should be safe with durable furniture that minimizes potential injury. The waiting period before meeting the doctor is, on most occasions, long enough to make the child feel intimidated, irritable, and uncooperative for assessments. It is recommended to have physical spaces with walls painted with bright colors, having cartoon characters and other fables, simple toys and play material (blocks, art material, papers, and colored pens/pencils), blackboard/whiteboard with chalks/pens, etc., to keep them engaged while waiting. This kind of engaging and inviting environment may also aid in more compliance to come back, and in cases where repeat consultations are required. All health professionals attending to children/adolescents in these settings should be well-versed with these "how, why, and when" of these activities.[3]

Inpatient Care

The inpatient psychiatry services for children centers on the provision of a safe, structured, and supportive environment for the seriously ill children. Their needs and requirements are diverse and unique to their developmental age and stage and, therefore, the design, layout, and functionality of the inpatient services should meet the developmental needs of their age group. Also, active family involvement in daily care, treatment, and activities should be encouraged and implemented.

Children may have to receive inpatient care for different reasons, ranging from providing therapies for neurodevelopmental disorders and/or management of problem behaviors, eating disorders, psychosis, mood disorders, severe family relationship difficulties, risk of harm to self or to others, and many other psychiatric conditions. In addition to providing beds and space for patients and their accompanying family members, the services should also have large multipurpose group activity/therapy rooms, big enough interview rooms that can accommodate families, outdoor space for recreational activities, a playroom for play observation and play therapy, as and when needed. Safety and security should always be ensured.

Unlike adults, children and adolescents experience a range of emotions while getting admitted to psychiatry inpatient facilities, which can range from shame, embarrassment, stigma, and anger. Children often experience the absence of warmth and comfort of their homes, lack of structured routine (e.g., regular school routines), no friends, and free play time and area. They often experience social isolation, difficulties with relationships, and may be intimidated by authority and embarrassed by intimate examination.[4] Although younger children readily accept their parents' decisions and other authority figures, therefore, working with them becomes less difficult.

As opposed to adolescents who are in a developmental stage of wanting independence and privacy, which makes them experience specific challenges when hospitalization is required or advised. They experience a loss of control in almost all areas of their lives during hospitalization making them feel depressed, anxious, helpless, and with a feeling of loss of independence. They may feel helpless that they are not able to decide what time they get up, what time they eat/rest/study. Privacy is perceived to be lost at a time when self-consciousness is at its peak. As a result, they may either regress to a more dependent state of a young child or become defiant and noncompliant. They may not follow the rules of the ward, creating conflict and power struggles between them, their caregivers and the treating team. Adolescents from religious, ethnic, or cultural minority groups may face different and amplified challenges in addition to those mentioned above as they temporarily lose cultural supports. These issues become more challenging as young people are at an age when they become more aware of their personal and social differences and the resultant responses from others. Absence from schools (repeated absences in some cases due to repeated hospitalization) exposes them to discriminatory behavior (from school authorities and peers), leading to bullying, embarrassment, low self-esteem, anxiety, stigma, and may lay the ground for another major issue of school avoidance/school refusal. Such issues need to be tackled actively and are best done by promoting and maintaining active school liaison.

Parental reactions to children's illness and treatment should also be taken care of. Parents often feel guilty for their child's problems/illness and may respond in ways which are not helpful for their children, e.g., becoming overprotective. The financial status of the family should be kept in mind while making a postdischarge management plan, as children are dependent on families for follow-up. If families must come at frequent intervals and/or from far-off places, the cost of travel to hospitals poses additional stress to families, especially in financially compromised ones. Use of online modes for follow-up, coordination/liaison/back referral to nearby hospitals can be one of the solutions in such circumstances.

Besides, the family members have profound doubts and associated stigma attached to the seeking of mental healthcare facilities and labeling of mental illness for the child. This emphasizes on the need for providing information about the illness, management strategies, and all possible contributing factors (modifiable and nonmodifiable) for better planning of action and compliance on the part of the family.[5]

The laws related to treatment, admission of children, and adolescents are covered in another chapter of the book.

CASE VIGNETTE 1

Mr A, a 17-year-old male, presented with active suicidal ideation for 1 week. He was immediately admitted to the psychiatry ward. On further probing, he had been experiencing obscene mental imagery toward family members, which had caused significant distress and disturbed biological functions. A clinical diagnosis of moderate depression and comorbid obsessive compulsive disorder (OCD) was made. He was started on pharmacological and psychological therapy, to which he was responding well. However, there were concerns regarding his upcoming 12th-class board examinations. On improvement, he was sent for home paroles; however, the intrusive thoughts and images would hamper his study preparation at home. He was able to concentrate and prepare during his ward stay. Although a separate room was not available, a temporary provision of allowing him to study in the interview room at specified times of the day and at night under supervision of family members and nursing staff was made. His ward stay was extended, and he was given parole on the days of the examination to appear for his board examinations. He was discharged after the board examination, and he successfully passed his 12th examination.

Tip: This vignette exemplifies the adjustments made in management of the psychiatric condition, keeping in mind the special situation of the upcoming board examination, as not being able to give the examination would have posed additional challenges and stress for the patient and family.

In India, there are many barriers to implementation of quality services for children and adolescent mental health such as shortage of specialists, meager financial resources, stigma and cultural factors, for which intersectoral collaboration with various stakeholders (pediatricians, general psychiatrists, psychologists, educators, social workers, etc.) involved in the care of children and adolescents is required.[6]

CHILDREN IN INSTITUTIONS

India has the world's largest child population, constituting 40% of the nation's population.[7] Among these, children facing adversities grow up in institutions instead of their own homes among their families. The word "institution" is generally used for different kinds of residential facilities where many young boys and girls spend a significant duration of their lives. These facilities include, children's homes, care homes, juvenile detention facilities, orphanages, reform schools, institutes for those with physical and mental disabilities, etc. Those who have either lost a parent, cannot be supported by the family, had to be separated from the family because of abuse or ran away from home, have committed a crime, or were subject to trafficking or drug abuse are the ones who would be residing in institutions or shelter homes made for the purpose.[8]

In India, the state of Jammu and Kashmir alone is home to 31,710,000 orphan children. In India, 1.8 lakh children live in childcare facilities because their parents cannot provide for their basic needs, including clothing, food, and shelter.[7] According to the National Mental Health Survey 2016, the positive screener rate for intellectual disability (ID) was 0.6%[9] and was reported to be 2% as per a meta-analysis conducted in 2022.[10] Children with developmental disabilities, which include children with ID and autism spectrum disorder (ASD), also form a significant proportion of children residing in residential facilities as the families have either abandoned them or are not socioeconomically sound to provide care for them or the problem behaviors in these children are to an extent that keeping them in families becomes unmanageable.

Another group of children who reside in institutions are "children in conflict with law (CCL)", i.e., a child who is alleged or found to have committed an offense and has not completed 18 years of age on the date of commission of such offense and *"children in need of care and protection"*, i.e., a child who meets specific criteria, including being found without a home or means of subsistence, engaging in illegal labor, living on the streets or begging, residing with an abusive guardian, being at risk of drug abuse or trafficking, facing unconscionable exploitation, suffering from incurable diseases or disabilities, being a victim of armed conflict or natural disasters, or being at risk of early marriage.[11]

A Child Care Institution, as defined under the JJ-Act, 2015, means a "Children's Home, Open Shelter, Observation Home, Special Home, Place of Safety, Specialized Adoption Agency, and Fit Facility" recognized under the Act for providing care and protection to children who need such services. Children in conflict with the law are provided with residential care and protection here. Different kinds of residential facilities are defined and described in JJA, 2015, and described in another chapter on laws dealing with children and adolescents in this Section of the Book.

The objectives of residential care in an "Observation Home" as laid down in JJA, 2015, are:

- To ensure the safety, protection, and care of the alleged CCL during the period of inquiry.
- To support the child through the period of inquiry by ensuring that legal aid is accessible, ensure attendance at every hearing, and explain the process and progress of the case.
- To formulate an "Individual Care Plan" for each child based on background (familial situation, peer and neighborhood influences, and positive influences), needs and interests using appropriate methods—counseling sessions, interaction with the child's family, home visits, aptitude testing for education and vocational training, and consultation with physical and mental health professionals.

Table 1 enlists the different residential settings for children and adolescents.

TABLE 1: Different residential settings for children and adolescents.

	Observation home	*Special home*	*Place of safety*
Purpose	• For temporary reception, care and rehabilitation of any child alleged to be in conflict with law, during the pendency of any enquiry under this Act • For every child alleged to be in conflict with law who is not placed under the charge of parent or guardian	For rehabilitation of those children in conflict with law who are found to have committed an offense and who are placed thereby an order of the Juvenile Justice Board made under Section 18	To place a person above the age of 18 years or child in conflict with law, who is between the age of 16–18 years and is accused of or convicted for committing a heinous offense
Duration of care	Does not exceed 4 months	Does not exceed 3 years	During the process of inquiry or person convicted of committing an offense
Establishment	The State Government shall establish and maintain in every district or a group of districts, either by itself, or through voluntary or nongovernmental "observation homes"	The State Government shall establish and maintain in every district or a group of districts, either by itself, or through voluntary or nongovernmental, "Organizations Special Homes"	The State Government shall set up at least one place of safety in a State

Source: As under Section 41, JJ Act 2015.

The following are the objectives of care in "Special Home":

- Provide reformative services, including education, skill development, counseling, behavior modification therapy, and psychiatric support during stay in the "Special Home."
- Formulate, review, and implement an "Individual Care Plan" for each child based on understanding the child's background (familial situation, peer and neighborhood influences, and positive influences), needs and interests through appropriate use.
- Methods, including counseling sessions, interaction with the child's family, home visits, aptitude testing for education and vocational training, and consultation with physical and mental health professionals.
- Ensure that children accept responsibility, take accountability for the crime they were found to have committed, and begin a process of healing and transformation.
- Preparing the child for reintegration into the family and community with skills and a plan to ensure that they will not commit crime again.[12]

Effects of Institutional Care

Depending upon the age at which a child is institutionalized and the period of institutionalization, the impacts are varied. Ranging from insecure/disorganized attachment style to increased social desirability manifesting as increased sociality with overly friendly behavior, these children tend to have a close brush with substance abuse, crimes, and abuse of different types (emotional, physical, sexual, or a combination). This further leads to an array of emotional issues, such as fear of abandonment, loneliness, continuing abusive relationships, and risk of exploitation **(Fig. 1)**. Relationship disruption adversely affects the neuroendocrine system, and prolonged exposure to stress may cause brain

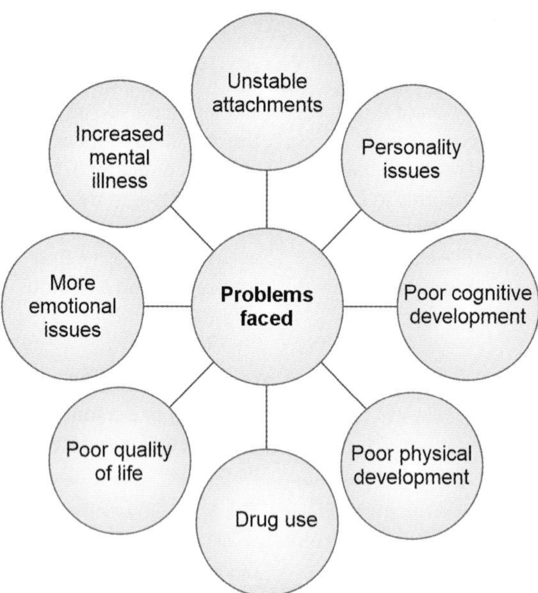

Fig. 1: Commonly faced issues by institutionalized children.
Source: Figure has been made by authors of the chapter, as per knowledge gained from cited sources.

damage that increases the risk of developing disorders in the future.[13]

Many studies report poor cognitive development, which tends to reverse if these children are adopted into families. The English Romanian Adoptees (ERA) Study team monitored 144 institutionalized children, most during their first month of life, and had impoverished early experiences with insufficient nutrition and little stimulation or interaction with caretakers. When psychological functioning was assessed at 6 years, only 25% of those who entered between the ages of 24 and 42 months had no impairment, compared to 70% of those who entered at <6 months. Poor quality institutional care that lasted longer than 6 months was highly associated with impaired cognitive performance and disinhibited indicators of attachment disorder.[14]

Similarly, children who are institutionalized for the first few years of their lives frequently have delayed physical development. Children who have been institutionalized or adopted and have experienced early institutionalization lag behind their peers who have grown up in families in terms of crucial physical development, including weight, height, and head circumference. Longer duration of institutional stays before adoption was strongly and linearly associated with a more delayed age-corrected growth in height in a meta-analysis of eight studies.[15]

Once adopted from orphanages and placed in families, a sizable body of research indicates that the deficiencies observed in institutionalized children might regress or continue to differing degrees in postinstitutionalized (PI) adoptees.[13,16]

In the context of housing and accommodation, the children, while growing, may experience changes in institutions depending on existing policies and foster care. These disruptions create a sense of instability and further impair the ability to weigh lifelong situations and obstacles to create a stable present and future, hence, a safe home.

Besides these, some more problems faced by institutionalized children include:

- *Education and accolades:* Lacking opportunities, stigma at the hands of society, and lack of motivation may contribute to children's inability to explore their academic potential. Further, due to a lack of close observation (primarily due to sparse staff availability), learning disabilities and neurodevelopmental disorders may go unseen and untreated in the children, hampering their academic success.
- *Health issues:* Overcrowding, poor hygiene, lack of nurturance, poor nutrition, scabies/fungal infections and other infectious illnesses are more commonly seen in institutionalized children.
- *Menstrual hygiene:* Using sanitary napkins or dirty clothes for prolonged periods may result in severe or fatal outcomes such as toxic shock syndrome, as these children lack proper

guidance, and poor-quality products make them more prone to infections.

- *Teenage pregnancy:* Female adolescents in institutional homes generally lack proper attachment skills, have a fear of abandonment, lack sex education, have exposure to the negative aspects of society and, hence, are more prone to this scarring experience, which in a way perpetuates and contributes to the vicious cycle of induction of children to institutions.
- *Drug use:* The institutionalized children are more predisposed to develop substance abuse and associated issues. In a Swedish study, 38% of children being studied had a history of being raised in foster care.[7]
- *Behavioral issues:* Behaviors such as conflict with authority, preoccupation with excessive fantasy, pathological lying, stealing, running away from home or school, learning difficulties, lack of impulse control (acting out, promiscuity, and sex crimes), and a fascination with fire or fire-lighting are commonly seen in children institutionalized both during and after institutionalization.
- *Conflict with law:* They are at a higher risk for criminal activities, which could be deduced from the circumstances mentioned above.
- *Quality of life (QoL):* Institutionalized children's quality of life is poorer than family-reared children. A Japanese study also found a significant difference in QoL between the two groups.[16,17]

What Needs to be Done?

The social pedagogy model places young people in residential care at the center of the services. It advocates for care workers to share the everyday lives of these young people. They also need to keep their educational aims at the center, and work alongside their family and community to achieve social integration.[18]

- *Adoption into family care:* To overcome the harmful effects of institutionalization, a safer environment with more love, affection, and social and cultural stimulation can be found in a home with a family. The benefits of integration into the family have been emphasized in **Flowchart 1** as well. This could be achieved via adoption or reintegration into biological families.
- *Building resilience to overcome child vulnerability:* Though resilience is attributed to possessing some strengths and protective factors,[19] the one defining element is the stable support system in the form of support from one stable and committed relationship with an adult—a parent, caregiver, or another adult.[20] The importance of resilience lies in the fact that resilient children beat the odds and manage to have excellent and robust well-being outcomes over the long term.
- *Reduce the carer-child ratio:* To increase the child's dependability and establish a stable relationship for them to learn about life goals, face challenges, and seek help and guidance, trained personnel should be caring for every child to the best of their ability.
- *Emphasize continuity of relationships:* The continuity of relationships, not just with the person providing care but with the peer group and kinship, goes a long way in children's emotional and social development.
- *Better staff training:* Given the poor conditions of children in institutions, not just in India but throughout the world, the staff employed at these institutions need to be better trained to handle the challenges presented to them, ensuring a smoother life journey for these children with adequate support.
- *Individualized care:* Every child is different, and not even siblings are the same; the needs, demands, and strategies that need to be implemented for the betterment of

Flowchart 1: A Model for improving children's care outcomes; a systemic cross-sectoral approach shall yield benefits across generations.

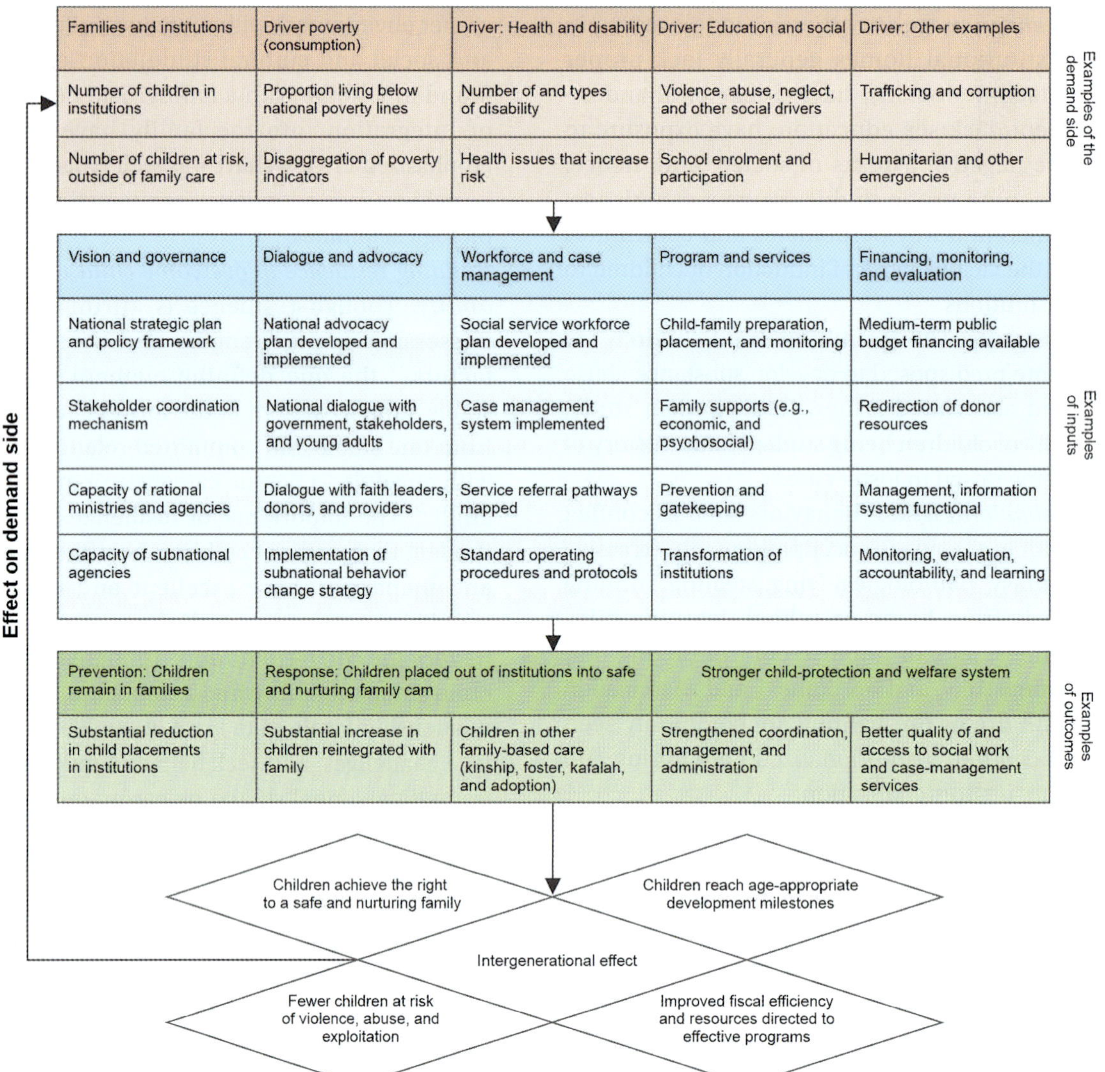

Source: Adapted from institutionalization and deinstitutionalization of children: A systematic and integrative review of evidence regarding effects on development.[18]

each institutionalized child need to be individualized.

- *Better funding for adequate provisions and opportunities:* Nothing comes free. So, to improve the status of these institutions and lower the strife of these children for basic amenities. These can be government-sanctioned or donations by citizens.

Flowchart 1 is a suggested care-model and explains (in orange) the various categories of children who may require instituionalization at different life stages, with respective drivers pushing the children into institutionalization. Followed by the resources (in blue) which can be developed and strengthened in order to improve the outcomes of institutionalized children from ground level to policy level. The possible outcomes (in green) include first and foremost if possible prevention of institutionalization; a favorable response of children being integrated into families/foster-care/etc.; and robust Child-protection and Welfare systems in place. If this stepwise model is followed positively, taking into consideration preventable errors, keeping in mind existing and upcoming welfare policies, we can influence the lives of children who are institutionalized or likely to be, in a beneficial manner.

Some Schemes by the Government of India

Mission Vatsalya[21]

The Ministry of Women and Child Development has implemented a centrally sponsored scheme, "Mission Vatsalya". "Mission Vatsalya" is a roadmap to achieve development and child protection priorities aligned with the Sustainable Development Goals (SDGs). The "Vatsalya" scheme replaced the Child Protection Services (CPS) in 2009–10. The mission aims to provide comprehensive care and protection to children. This includes children in need of care and protection (CNCP), children in conflict with the law (CCL), and children affected by HIV/AIDS. The scheme also aims to prevent child abuse and promote children's rights. It emphasizes child rights, advocacy, and awareness, strengthening the juvenile justice care and protection system with the motto "leave no child behind."

In the context of adoption:

i. The Child Adoption Resource Information and Guidance System (CARINGS), an online platform, has been developed to build bridges and create links through a robust web-based management system designed to bring transparency to the adoption system and curtail delays at various levels.
ii. Policy about adoption under the Juvenile Justice (Care and Protection of Children) Act, 2015 (as amended in 2021), the JJ Rules, 2022, and the Adoption Regulations, 2022, has been simplified with District Magistrate (DM) empowered to issue adoption orders instead of Court resulting in a reduction in pendency.
iii. *Enhanced accountability through child protection service:* The District Child Protection Unit (DCPU) has been assigned to conduct the Home Study Report of Prospective Adoptive Parents (PAPs), postadoption follow-ups, and scrutiny of the adoption applications for the perusal of the DMs concerned.
iv. Prospective Foster Parents have started registering in CARINGS in the new online module, which will promote noninstitutional care of older children. As soon as the competent authority makes a decision, institutionalized older children will be placed with a foster family after completing procedural requirements.

Noninstitutional care support: The guiding principles of the JJ Act provide for institutionalization as a measure of last resort and acknowledge that family-based care plays an essential role in the overall development of children. Children develop a sense of belonging and self-esteem, get religious and cultural identity, learn values, and grow up in a safe and secure environment under familial care.

The allocation of children to the State Government/UT Administrations for Non-institutional Care (i.e., Sponsorship, Foster Care, and Aftercare), including children who are orphans, children covered under the PM CARES for children scheme, children in conflict with law, child labor, child trafficking, child marriage, and Protection of Children from Sexual Offences (POCSO) victims under Mission Vatsalya Scheme for FY 2023–2024 has increased which reflects the commitment of government for extending family-based care to all children in difficult circumstances. 62,675 children were covered under noninstitutional care during FY 2022–2023, which increased from 29,331 children during FY 2021–2022, showing an increase of 113.6%.

Child helpline: As per Mission Vatsalya guidelines, the "Child Helpline" is run in coordination with State and District functionaries and integrated with the Emergency Response Support System 112 (ERSS-112) helpline of Ministry of Home Affairs. The Ministry also issued the Standard Operating Procedures (SoPs) of the Child Helpline on 31st March 2023. "Child Helpline Services" are now functional in all 36 States/UTs.

Scheme for Care and Support to Victims under Sections 4 and 6 of the Protection of Children from Sexual Offences Act, 2012[22]

The scheme provides integrated support and assistance to minor pregnant girl child victims under one roof. It facilitates immediate, emergency, and nonemergency access to services for long-term rehabilitation in terms of access to education, police assistance, medical (also comprising maternity, neonatal, and infant care), psychological, mental health counseling, legal support, noninstitutional care monthly support up to 18 years of age, and can be extended up to 23 years of age in exceptional circumstances by the concerned Child Welfare Committee, place of stay in CCI/Aftercare facilities and health insurance cover for the girl child victim and her newborn under one roof to enable access to justice and empowerment of such girl child victims.

CASE VIGNETTE 2

Ms D, a 9-year-old female, presented to Psychiatry OPD with episodes of screaming, fearfulness, and excessive clinginess to her mother for 2 months. These symptoms were precipitated by alleged sexual abuse by an adolescent boy. She was diagnosed with post-traumatic stress disorder (PTSD); additionally, she had an IQ of 77 (borderline intelligence).

The mother had lodged an FIR, despite resistance from her husband and family members; the alleged perpetrator was under custody; however, since he was an adolescent, he was likely to be released in a few months. The girl child had known this fact and revealed this during one-on-one therapy sessions, which would precipitate excessive anxiety in her. Besides this, the mother was also concerned that the locality was unsafe for her daughter, as several other males tried to break into the house after this news spread. The patient was responding well to a safe environment, therapy and medication; however, she would worsen even when sent on home parole.

Hence, after a discussion with family members, the treating team decided it would be best to send her to a care home where her family could meet her. She was sent to residential care facility for girls in the same city, where she comfortably attended classes and would meet her family members once fortnightly. Her medications and therapy were continued.

Tip: Vignette 2 highlights the integrated support and assistance facilities for the girl child victim of a sexual offense. Though it might seem that the girl was institutionalized, despite being the victim; the greater cause was addressed, since mother had concerns owing to the child's vulnerabilities, *home environment, unavailability of a 24*7 guardian to keep the child safe at home, and escort her to school, extracurricular activities, etc. These psycho-social issues were resolved with institutionalization. This case is an example that despite family care being the best option, in certain situations, institutionalization has to be opted for.*

PM CARES (Prime Minister's Citizen Assistance and Relief in Emergency Situation)[23]

It includes comprehensive support for children who have lost both their parents due to the coronavirus disease 2019 (COVID-19) pandemic through health insurance and education and to equip them for a self-sufficient existence with financial backing to reach 23 years of age. The PM CARES for Children scheme ensures, depending on the age of the child—support for boarding and lodging, assistance for preschool, school and higher education, health insurance, and financial support (monthly stipend from the age of 18 years and lump sum amount of ₹ 10 lakh on attaining 23 years of age).

Institutions for Differently-abled Children

Another important group of children and adolescents includes those with different abilities. One in every 10 children is born with or acquires a physical, mental, or sensory disability.[24] These translate into 40–90 million children, a substantial number.

Though the Indian healthcare system has taken some significant strides, the situation of differently-abled children remains deplorable, particularly in rural areas and among the lower socioeconomic population. They are subject to multiple deprivations and limited opportunities in several dimensions of their lives, like not being enrolled in schools, lower employment rates, limited awareness of entitlements and services available, and lack of social welfare support. Their families and caregivers also go through a lot of stress and challenges in having a person with a disability at home, which ultimately leads to grave discriminatory practices toward these children.[25] In the unfortunate event of being orphaned or abandoned by the family, these children land up in the institutions.

CASE VIGNETTE 3

Mr E, a 13-year-old boy belonging to LSES with Severe Intellectual disability, Autism and Metabolic syndrome, was brought by his mother (who herself had borderline intellectual capacity), frequenting the emergency department with acute aggression repeatedly. These episodes would usually be precipitated by psychosocial factors leading to a change in accommodation or sometimes due to a lack of sufficient funds to meet the basic needs of the child. Over years of multiple admissions, the child was enrolled in Daycare special needs school, i.e., GRIID (Government Rehabilitation Institute for Intellectual Disabilities), where he had shown improvement in behavioral issues and good participation. His care, however, took a toll on the widowed mother and 15-year-old sister, who were both diagnosed with dysthymia and were on regular medications and psychotherapy for the caregiver burden.

With every subsequent admission, it became increasingly evident that family members were not able to cater to the needs of this child, due to which child was worsening in terms of psychiatric symptoms, and their mental, as well as overall health was bearing the brunt. Hence, after much discussion with family members, it was finally decided to shift the patient to a long-term care facility, Pingalwada.

He is now doing well; his medications are being tapered slowly and steadily. However, family members are not allowed to meet him, for which his mother receives supportive psychotherapy, but his sister is able to do a job and focus on her career and growth.

Tip: Mr E exemplifies the efforts to rehabilitate a specially-abled adolescent in a special institution, where the typical modalities of rehabilitation did not seem to work for the adolescent and his family.

After offering the basic life necessities of food, clothing and shelter, the institutions try to give a structure to their life with the inculcation of social and cultural activities, regular health checkups by trained professionals, supervised medications for seizures, which are comorbid in about 70–80% of the children with disabilities predominantly intellectual disability and autism spectrum disorder.

The institutions aim for these children to have their own Aadhaar Cards and Bank Accounts for depositing and saving their disability pension which can subsequently cater to their needs as required by their own money so that they do not face financial constraints. All this meticulous planning and administration depends on the expertise and training of the service providers and their active involvement in the affairs. For places with staff with good values and humanitarian touch with the children, these children thrive despite their challenges (physical, emotional, and behavioral).

CASE VIGNETTE 4

Mr F was brought to an institution at the age of 6 years with his hearing and speech impairment comorbid with intellectual disability (mild). After initial hiccups, he developed a kinship with 2–3 boys—all mischievous and playing a lot. They were known to be full of energy and always in for the games. As they aged toward adolescence, Mr F started showing inappropriate sexual behavior; the other boys followed him and were then caught by the staff at the institution. Mr F was extra social and forthcoming to anyone visiting the institution. Everyone liked him to be a jolly and happy-go-lucky fellow who would fulfil his demands of chips, biscuits, ball, bat, and so on.

Gradually, it came to light that Mr F was the one leading others for this behavior. After a detailed evaluation with history from many people working in the institution over the years, he was diagnosed with ADHD and Conduct disorder and mild Intellectual Disability with Hearing and Speech impairment.

Despite medications (atomoxetine 40 mg and risperidone 4 mg), he was still getting rowdy and was always on the go. Although the medications decreased his sexual urges, for the rest of his behaviors he could now be involved in behavior therapy. He was doing well in 1:1 behavior therapy, followed his psychologist, and helped to manage some tasks with staff members at the institution but still could not be made to sit for >30 minutes at the special school where he was enrolled.

He was very fond of cricket and demanded a new bat almost every 4–5 days and 3–4 balls every day. His aggression increased on not getting these due to limited funds to the institute.

Gradually, it was decided by the treating team that his own disability pension could be used wisely to fulfil his demands of balls, bat, clothes, and shoes after the funds were exhausted.

Tip: Vignette 4 exemplifies the rehabilitation of a specially-abled adolescent with no family, yet having his own resources while living in a special institution.

CHILDREN IN NEED OF BOTH HIV PREVENTION AND CARE AND SUPPORT

In a country westernizing rapidly like India, another vital segment includes the vulnerability of a child living in a household with a chronically ill parent/caregiver in a high-risk setting due to HIV prevalence or proximity to high-risk behaviors. Due to poverty, family disintegration, household violence, disability, and social unrest, the number of these children is expected to increase in the future. These children are most vulnerable and are at increased risk of exposure to child labor, trafficking, prostitution, abduction, stigma, and discrimination. They are more susceptible than other children because they have already lost parental protection and care.

Why and how are these children vulnerable?

- Children of sex workers and other marginalized communities, such as rag pickers and street children, who are in exploitive situations and are especially vulnerable to HIV
- Girls who are increasingly at risk because of myths surrounding sexuality and STIs/HIV, such as the belief that if a man has sex with a virgin girl, he can be cured of STIs/HIV
- Media messages are mainly communicated through adult programs and literature like movies and magazines that glamorize alcohol, sex, and affluent lifestyles, tempting young people to succumb to potentially risky situations.
- Substance use among young people which makes them vulnerable to risky behavior and HIV
- Young boys and girls who are unaware of reproductive health issues and safe sex practices may experiment with unprotected sex and expose themselves to STIs/HIV
- Children who are caregivers of HIV-affected parents and thus have experienced trauma and the loss of childhood may also be infected by HIV.

Over the years, a better understanding of the HIV epidemic has emphasized the need to sensitize and educate service providers to respond urgently and more effectively to the needs of these vulnerable children infected and affected by HIV/AIDS. There is a need for life skills education that addresses both HIV prevention and care and support issues to prevent HIV infection, manage and cope with risky situations related to HIV, and help to cope with problems associated with HIV infection and care and support.

The "Life Skills Education" encourages children to acquire psychosocial skills, enabling them to acquire the following abilities:

- Understand sexual issues and sexuality to reduce their vulnerability to HIV
- Cope effectively with risky situations
- Practice safe sex behavior to reduce HIV risks
- Learn how to help and support other children

Children can acquire these skills only if they can learn and practice them in a supportive environment of peers and family. In this way, children can practice new, safe, and healthy behaviors, and build confidence in their day-to-day lives.[26-28]

SUMMARY AND CONCLUSION

To summarize, this chapter focuses on the difficulties faced by children and the healthcare system of India when dealing with children and adolescents in special settings. The special settings include Hospital Settings, institutions like observation homes, special homes for children in conflict with the law, places of safety for children in need of care and protection, institutions for especially abled children, and care for those affected by HIV/AIDS. Children in special settings require immense care, input, and facilitation from government and nongovernment organizations.

In conclusion, for vulnerable children and those in conflict with the law or need of care and protection, setting up and running the institutions is a step toward the care they need and the state's responsibility. It is of utmost importance to consolidate the functioning of these institutions with adequate amenities—both physical and emotional, staff training, employment of proper staff, funding, policies, and adoption into families—all these are the need of the hour. The MHCA 2017 has led to provision for separate wards for child and adolescent populations to decrease stigma and improve treatment seeking. Observation homes and special homes have replaced the remand home to decrease the stigma attached. The improvement in legislation is evident from the sequential amendments in child care laws like the Juvenile Justice Act and the POCSO, which have been landmark laws for the welfare of children in India.

REFERENCES

1. UNICEF. (2025). UNICEF report spotlights on the mental health impact of COVID-19 in children and young people. [online] Available from https://www.unicef.org/india/press-releases/unicef-report-spotlights-mental-health-impact-covid-19-children-and-young-people. [Last accessed November, 2025].
2. Ramaswamy S, Sagar JV, Seshadri S. A trans-disciplinary public health model for child and adolescent mental healthcare in low- and middle-income countries. Lancet Reg Health Southeast Asia. 2022;3:100024.
3. Srinath S, Jacob P, Sharma E, Gautam A. Clinical practice guidelines for assessment of children and adolescents. Indian J Psychiatry. 2019;61: 158-75.
4. Yates S, Payne M, Dyson S. Children and young people in hospitals: doing youth work in medical settings. J Youth Studies. 2009;12:77-92.
5. Kumar A. The Transformation of The Indian Healthcare System. Cureus. 2023;15:e39079.
6. Babatunde GB, van Rensburg AJ, Bhana A, Petersen I. Barriers and facilitators to child and adolescent mental health services in low-and-middle-income countries: a scoping review. Glob Soc Welf. 2021;8:29-46.
7. Rohta S. Institutional care for the vulnerable children in India: The perspective of institutional caregivers. Child Youth Serv Rev. 2021;121:105777.
8. Goldman PS, Bakermans-Kranenburg MJ, Bradford B, Christopoulos A, Ah Ken PL, Cuthbert C, et al. Institutionalisation and deinstitutionalisation of children 2: policy and practice recommendations for global, national, and local actors. Lancet Child Adolesc Health. 2020;4:606-33.
9. Ministry of Health and Family Welfare, Govt. of India. (2016). National Mental Health Survey, 2015-16. [online] Available from https://main.mohfw.gov.in/sites/default/files/National%20Mental%20Health%20Survey%2C%202015-16%20-%20Mental%20Health%20Systems_0.pdf. [Last accessed November, 2025].
10. Russell PSS, Nagaraj S, Vengadavaradan A, Russell S, Mammen PM, Shankar SR, et al. Prevalence of intellectual disability in India: A meta-analysis. World J Clin Pediatr. 2022;11: 206-14.
11. Ministry of Women and Child Development, Govt. of India. (2016). Juvenile Justice Act. [online] Available from https://www.childlineindia.org/pdf/j-j-act.PDF. [Last accessed November, 2025].
12. Vikaspedia. (2025). Objectives and approach of Child Care Institutions. [online] Available from https://vikaspedia.in/education/child-rights/

living-conditions-in-institutions-for-children-in-conflict-with-law/objectives-and-approach-of-child-care-institutions. [Last accessed November, 2025].

13. Rutter M, Bishop D, Pine D, Scott S, Stevenson JS, Taylor EA, et al. Rutter's Child and Adolescent Psychiatry, 5th Edition. United States: Wiley Blackwell; 2008: xv, 1230.
14. O'Connor TG, Rutter M. Attachment disorder behaviour following early severe deprivation: extension and longitudinal follow-up. English and Romanian Adoptees Study Team. J Am Acad Child Adolesc Psychiatry. 2000;39:703-12.
15. van IJzendoorn MH, Palacios J, Sonuga-Barke EJ, Gunnar MR, Vorria P, McCall RB, et al. Children in Institutional Care: Delayed Development and Resilience. Monogr Soc Res Child Dev. 2011;76:8-30.
16. Dozier M, Zeanah CH, Wallin AR, Shauffer C. Institutional Care for Young Children: Review of Literature and Policy Implications. Soc Issues Policy Rev. 2012;6:1-25.
17. Almas AN, Papp LJ, Woodbury MR, Nelson CA, Zeanah CH, Fox NA. The Impact of Caregiving Disruptions of Previously Institutionalized Children on Multiple Outcomes in Late Childhood. Child Dev. 2020;91:96-109.
18. van IJzendoorn MH, Bakermans-Kranenburg MJ, Duschinsky R, Fox NA, Goldman PS, Gunnar MR, et al. Institutionalisation and deinstitutionalisation of children 1: a systematic and integrative review of evidence regarding effects on development. Lancet Psychiatry. 2020;7:703-20.
19. Zolkoski SM, Bullock LM. Resilience in children and youth: A review. Children Youth Serv Rev. 2012;34:2295-303.
20. Centre on the Developing Child at Harvard University. (2015). In Brief: The Science of Resilience. [online] Available from http://www.developingchild.harvard.edu . [Last accessed November, 2025].
21. MissionVatsalya. [online] Available from https://wcd.nic.in/sites/default/files/GUIDELINES%20OF%20MISSION%20VATSALYA%20DATED%2005%20JULY%202022_1.pdf. [Last accessed November, 2025].
22. The Protection of Children from Sexual Offences. [online] Available from https://wcd.nic.in/sites/default/files/POCSO%20Act%2C%202012.pdf. [Last accessed November, 2025].
23. Ministry of Women and Child Development, Govt. of India. (2021). PM CARES (Prime Minister's Citizen Assistance and Relief in Emergency Situation Fund) for Children. [online] Available from https://pmcaresforchildren.in/. [Last accessed November, 2025].
24. National Legal Services Authority (Legal Services for Differently Abled Children) Scheme, 2021. https://patnahighcourt.gov.in/bslsa/pdf/ActsRules/131.pdf [Last accessed November, 2025].
25. Janardhana N, Muralidhar D, Naidu DM, Raghevendra G. Discrimination against differently abled children among rural communities in India: Need for action. J Nat Sci Biol Med. 2015;6:7-11.
26. World Health Organization. (2024). Global HIV Programme. [online] Available from www.who.int/teams/global-hiv-hepatitis-and-stis-programmes/hiv/treatment/treatment-and-care-in-children-and-adolescents. [Last accessed November, 2025].
27. USAID. (2012). India's HIV orphans and vulnerable children—generating evidence for policy practice. [online] Available from https://ovcsupport.org/wpcontent/uploads/Documents/Indias_HIV_Orphans_and_Vulnerable_Children_Generating_Evidence_for_Policy_and_Practice_1.pdf. [Last accessed November, 2025].
28. Department of Health and the Ministry of Justice, in consultation with the Welsh Assembly Government. (2017). Mental Health Act 2017. [online] Available from http://www.legislation.gov.uk/ukpga/2007/12/pdfs/ukpgaen_20070012_en.pdf . [Last accessed November, 2025].

Index

Page numbers followed by *b* refer to box, *f* refer to figure, *fc* refer to flowchart, and *t* refer to table.

A

D

E

N